HANDBOOK OF
CLINICAL ANESTHESIA

FIFTH EDITION

Paul G. Barash, MD

Professor, Department of Anesthesiology
Yale University School of Medicine
Attending Anesthesiologist
Yale–New Haven Hospital
New Haven, Connecticut

Bruce F. Cullen, MD

Professor, Department of Anesthesiology
University of Washington School of Medicine
Attending Anesthesiologist
Harborview Medical Center
Seattle, Washington

Robert K. Stoelting, MD

Emeritus Professor and Chair, Department of Anesthesia
Indiana University School of Medicine
Indianapolis, Indiana

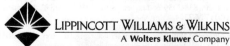

LIPPINCOTT WILLIAMS & WILKINS
A Wolters Kluwer Company

Philadelphia • Baltimore • New York • London
Buenos Aires • Hong Kong • Sydney • Tokyo

Acquisitions Editor: Brian Brown
Managing Editor: Franny Murphy
Developmental Editor: Grace R. Caputo, Dovetail Content Solutions
Marketing Manager: Angela Panetta
Production Editor: Dave Murphy
Designer: Doug Smock
Manufacturing Manager: Ben Rivera
Compositor: TechBooks
Printer/Binder: R.R. Donnelley, Crawfordsville

© 2006 by LIPPINCOTT WILLIAMS & WILKINS
530 Walnut Street
Philadelphia, PA 19106 USA
LWW.com

Library of Congress Cataloging-in-Publication Data
Handbook of clinical anesthesia / [edited by] Paul G. Barash, Bruce F. Cullen,
    Robert K. Stoelting—5th ed.
        p. ; cm.
    Includes bibliographical references and index.
    ISBN 0-7817-5793-2 (alk. paper)
    1. Anesthesiology—Handbooks, manuals, etc.   2. Anesthesia—Handbooks, manuals, etc.
I. Barash, Paul G.   II. Cullen, Bruce F.   III. Stoelting, Robert K.   IV. Clinical anesthesia.
    [DNLM: 1. Anesthesia—Handbooks.   2. Anesthetics—Handbooks.
    WO 231 H236 2006] RD82.2.H35 2006 617.9′6—dc22
                                                                    2005018775

Care has been taken to confirm the accuracy of the information presented and to
describe generally accepted practices. However, the authors, editors, and publisher are not
responsible for errors or omissions or for any consequences from application of the information in this book and make no warranty, expressed or implied, with respect to the currency,
completeness, or accuracy of the contents of the publication. Application of this information
in a particular situation remains the professional responsibility of the practitioner.

The authors, editors, and publisher have exerted every effort to ensure that drug
selection and dosages set forth in this text are in accordance with current recommendations
and practice at the time of publication. However, in view of ongoing research, changes in
government regulations, and the constant flow of information relating to drug therapy and
drug reactions, the reader is urged to check the package insert for each drug for any change
in indications and dosage and for added warnings and precautions. This is particularly
important when the recommended agent is a new or infrequently employed drug.

Some drugs and medical devices presented in this publication have Food and Drug
Administration (FDA) clearance for limited use in restricted research settings. It is the responsibility of health care providers to ascertain the FDA status of each drug or device planned
for use in their clinical practice.

To purchase additional copies of this book, call our customer service department
at (800) 638-3030 or fax orders to (301) 824-7390. International customers should call
(301) 714-2324.

Visit Lippincott Williams & Wilkins on the Internet: at LWW.com. Lippincott
Williams & Wilkins customer service representatives are available from 8:30 AM to 6 PM,
EST.

10 9 8 7 6 5 4 3

THIS EDITION OF CLINICAL ANESTHESIA IS
DEDICATED TO THE MEMORY AND SPIRIT OF
DANIEL BERNARD BARASH

Welcome to the fifth edition of the *Handbook of Clinical Anesthesia*. When first conceived, the *Handbook* was to be a bridge to the scope of knowledge required for superior clinical care. Although still the primary goal, the *Handbook* has become an integral part of the *Clinical Anesthesia* series, which now consists of the textbook *Clinical Anesthesia*, the *Handbook*, *Clinical Anesthesia for the PDA*, the *Review of Clinical Anesthesia* (edited by D. Silverman and N. Connelly), and *The Lippincott Interactive Anesthesia Library on CD-ROM*. The aim of the series is to facilitate rapid acquisition, comprehensive understanding and review of the scientific and clinical foundations of our specialty.

Because the *Handbook* parallels the parent textbook, *Clinical Anesthesia*, extensive changes in the fifth edition of the text mandated similar changes to this volume. Again, as with previous editions, information is transmitted in tables and graphics where possible to enhance rapid access to information. According to the American Board of Anesthesiology the immediate availability and appropriate integration of knowledge is a cornerstone of clinical management. "The ability to independently acquire and process information in a timely manner is central to assure individual responsibility for all aspects of anesthesiology care."

The *Handbook* still comprises two major sections. The first section, the text, takes the reader in a systematic fashion through the perioperative period, including preoperative evaluation, intraoperative management and anesthesia subspecialtics, as well as postoperative care. In this edition, to meet the realities of the world we live in, the Editors have added sections or chapters on: disaster preparedness and weapons of mass destruction, genomics, obesity (bariatric surgery) and new paradigms for perioperative patient management and cost containment.

The second section, the appendices, contains formulas, an ECG atlas; drug lists; the American Heart Association emergency resuscitation protocols for adult, pediatric, and neonatal patients. New to this section in the drug list appendix is the use of icons to alert the clinician to drugs that carry a 'black box' warning label from the Food and Drug Administration. Further, since many patients are treated with herbal compounds, a section on herbal medications has been added. In addition to the ASA Standards for Basic Anesthesia Monitoring and the ASA Difficult Airway

Algorithm, we have also supplied an appendix on other clinically relevant ASA Guidelines and Standards, which we are feel are part of the cornerstone of the safe practice of anesthesia.

We would like to acknowledge the contributors of the textbook *Clinical Anesthesia*. Although the *Handbook of Clinical Anesthesia* is the product of the Editors, its chapters were developed from the expert knowledge of the original contributors, reorganized and rewritten in a style necessary for a text of this scope. We would also like to thank our Administrative Assistants, Gail Norup, Ruby Wilson, and Deanna Walker, whose continued help has been a source of support. As always a special word of thanks is due to out colleagues at Lippincott William & Wilkins: Brian Brown, Senior Acquisitions Editor, David Murphy Senior Production Manager with the assistance of Grace Caputo, Project Director, Dovetail Content Solutions and Chris Miller, Project Manager, TechBooks. Their constructive comments during the process of writing and editing this book continue to demonstrate their commitment to medical education.

Paul G. Barash, MD
Bruce F. Cullen, MD
Robert K. Stoelting, MD

CONTRIBUTING AUTHORS

The authors would like to gratefully acknowledge the efforts of the contributors to the fifth edition of the textbook *Clinical Anesthesia*.

Stephen E. Abram, MD
J. Jeffrey Andrews, MD
Douglas R. Bacon, MD, MA
Robert L. Barkin, MBA, PharmD, FCP
Audrée A. Bendo, MD
Christopher M. Bernards, MD
Arnold J. Berry, MD, MPH
Frederic A. Berry, MD
David R. Bevan, MD
Barbara W. Brandom, MD
Ferne R. Bravermas, MD
Russell C. Brockwell, MD
Levon M. Capan, MD
Barbara A. Castro, MD
Frederick W. Cheney Jr., MD
Barbara A. Coda, MD
Edmond Cohen, MD
James E. Cottrell, MD
Joseph Cravero, MD
C. Michael Crowder, MD, PhD
Marie Csete, MD, PhD
Anthony J. Cunningham, MD
Jacek B. Cywinski, MD
Steven Deem, MD
Stephen F. Dierdorf, MD
François Donati, PhD, MD, FRCPC
John C. Drummond, MD, FRCPC
Thomas J. Ebert, MD, PhD
Jan Ehrenwerth, MD
John H. Eichhorn, MD
James B. Eisenkraft, MD
John E. Ellis, MD

Alex S. Evers, MD
Lynne R. Ferrari, MD
Jeffrey E. Fletcher, PhD
J. Sean Funston, MD
Steven I. Gayer, MD, MBA
Kathryn Glas, MD
Alexander W. Gotta, MD
John Hartung, PhD
Tara M. Hata, MD
Laurence M. Hausman, MD
Thomas K. Henthorn, MD
Simon C. Hillier, MB, ChB
Terese T. Horlocker, MD
Robert J. Hudson, MD, FRCPC
Anthony D. Ivankovitch, MD
Joel O. Johnson, MD, PhD
Raymond S. Joseph Jr., MD
Zeev N. Kain, MD, MBA
Ira S. Kass, MD
Jonathan D. Katz, MD
Brian S. Kaufman, MD
Charbel A. Kenaan, MD
Donald A. Kroll, MD, PhD
Carol Lake, MD, MBA, MPH
Noel W. Lawson, MD
Harish S. Lecamwasam
Wilton C. Levine, MD
Jerrold H. Levy, MD
Adam David Lichtman, MD
J. Lance Lichtor, MD
Spencer S. Liu, MD
Richard L. Lock, MD
David A. Lubarsky, MD, MBA
Timothy R. Lubenow, MD

Srinivas Mantha, MD
Joseph P. Mathew, MD
Michael S. Mazurek, MD
Kathryn E. McGoldrick, MD
Roger S. Mecca, MD
Sanford M. Miller, MD
Terri G. Monk, MD, MS
John R. Moyers, MD
Michael F. Mulroy, MD
Stanley Muravchick, MD, PhD
Glenn S. Murphy, MD
Michael J. Murray, MD, PhD
Steven M. Neustein, MD
Cathal Nolan, MB
Babatunde O. Ogunnaike, MD
Jerome F. O'Hara, Jr., MD
Charles W. Otto, MD, FCCM
Nathan Leon Pace, MD, MStat
Charise T. Petrovitch, MD
Mihai V. Podgoreanu, MD
Karen L. Posner, PhD
Donald S. Prough, MD
J. David Roccaforte, MD
Michael F. Roizen, MD
Gladys Romero, MD
Stanley H. Rosenbaum, MD
Henry Rosenberg, MD
Meg A. Rosenblatt, MD
William H. Rosenblatt, MD

Carl E. Rosow, MD, PhD
Nyamkhishig Sambuughin,
    PhD
Alan C. Santos, MD, MPH
Jeffrey J. Schwartz, MD
Margaret L. Schwarze, MD
Harry A. Seifert, MD, MSCE
Aarti Sharma, MD
Nikolaos Skubas, MD
Hugh M. Smith, MD, PhD
Karen J. Souter, MBBS,
    MSc, FRCA
M. Christine Stock, MD,
    FCCM, FACP
Christer H. Svensén, MD,
    PhD, DEAA, MBA
Stephen J. Thomas, MD
Miriam M. Treggiari, MD,
    MPH
Jeffery S. Vender, MD,
    FCCM, FCCP
J. Scott Walton, MD
Mark A. Warner, MD
Denise J. Wedel, MD
Paul F. White, PhD, MD,
    FANZCA
Charles W. Whitten, MD
Scott W. Wolf, MD
James R. Zaidan, MD, MBA

CONTENTS

SECTION I ■ INTRODUCTION TO ANESTHESIA PRACTICE

1 The History of Anesthesia   1

2 Practice and Operating Room Management   8

3 Experimental Design and Statistics   16

4 Occupational Health   22

5 Professional Liability, Quality Improvement, and Anesthetic Risk   32

SECTION II ■ BASIC PRINCIPLES OF ANESTHESIA PRACTICE

6 Cellular and Molecular Mechanisms of Anesthesia   40

7 Genomic Basis of Perioperative Medicine   49

8 Electrical and Fire Safety   61

9 Acid-Base, Fluids, and Electrolytes   74

10 Hemotherapy and Hemostasis   98

SECTION III ■ BASIC PRINCIPLES OF PHARMACOLOGY IN ANESTHESIA PRACTICE

11 Basic Principles of Clinical Pharmacology   120

12 Autonomic Nervous System: Physiology and Pharmacology   137

13 Nonopioid Intravenous Anesthesia   167

14 Opioids   186

15 Inhalation Anesthesia   208

16   Neuromuscular Blocking Agents   235

17   Local Anesthetics   255

SECTION IV ■ PREPARING FOR ANESTHESIA

18   Preoperative Evaluation and Management   272

19   Anesthesia for Patients with Rare
     and Coexisting Diseases   295

20   Malignant Hyperthermia and Other
     Pharmacogenetic Disorders   315

21   Delivery Systems for Inhaled Anesthetics   328

22   Airway Management   341

23   Patient Positioning   357

24   Monitoring the Anesthetized Patient   365

SECTION V ■ MANAGEMENT OF ANESTHESIA

25   Epidural and Spinal Anesthesia   390

26   Peripheral Nerve Blockade   417

27   Anesthesia for Neurosurgery   438

28   Respiratory Function in Anesthesia   464

29   Anesthesia for Thoracic Surgery   483

30   Cardiovascular Anatomy and Physiology   499

31   Anesthesia for Cardiac Surgery   518

32   Anesthesia for Vascular Surgery   543

33   Anesthesia and the Eye   572

34   Anesthesia for Otolaryngologic Surgery   583

35   The Renal System and Anesthesia
     for Urologic Surgery   596

36   Anesthesia and Obesity   619

37   Anesthesia and Gastrointestinal Disorders   629

38   Anesthesia for Minimally Invasive Procedures   637

39   Anesthesia and the Liver   644

40   Anesthesia for Orthopaedic Surgery   659

41   Anesthesia and the Endocrine System   677

42   Obstetric Anesthesia   694

43   Neonatal Anesthesia   711

44   Pediatric Anesthesia   726

45   Anesthesia for the Geriatric Patient   741

46   Anesthesia for Ambulatory Surgery   755

47   Monitored Anesthesia Care   767

48   Trauma and Burns   782

49   The Allergic Response   808

50   Drug Interactions   819

51   Anesthesia Provided at Alternative Sites   828

52   Office-Based Anesthesia   843

53   Anesthesia for Organ Transplantation   855

SECTION VI ■ POSTANESTHESIA AND CONSULTANT PRACTICE

54   Postoperative Recovery   870

55   Management of Acute Postoperative Pain   881

56   Chronic Pain Management   903

57   Anesthesia and Critical Care Medicine   918

58   Cardiopulmonary Resuscitation   943

59   Disaster Preparedness and Weapons of Mass Destruction   959

■ APPENDICES

A   Formulas   971

B   Electrocardiography Atlas   975

C American Heart Association (AHA) Resuscitation
   Protocols 1003

D American Society of Anesthesiologists Standards 1024

E The Airway Approach Algorithm and Difficult
   Airway Algorithm 1033

F Malignant Hyperthermia Protocol 1035

G Drug List 1037

H Herbal Medications 1110

Index 1119

CHAPTER 1 ■ THE HISTORY OF ANESTHESIA

Although most human civilizations evolved some method for diminishing patient discomfort, anesthesia, in its modern and effective meaning, is a comparatively recent discovery with traceable origins dating back 160 years (an epitaph on a monument to William T. G. Morton, one of the founders of anesthesia, reads "Before whom in all time Surgery was Agony") (Smith HM, Bacon DR: The history of anesthesia. In Barash PG, Cullen BF, Stoelting, RK [eds]: *Clinical Anesthesia*, pp 3–26. Philadelphia, Lippincott Williams & Wilkins, 2006).

I. ANESTHESIA BEFORE ETHER.
In addition to limitations in technical knowledge, cultural attitudes toward pain are often cited as reasons why humans endured centuries of surgery without effective anesthesia.

A. Early Analgesics and Soporifics (Table 1-1).

II. ALMOST DISCOVERY: HICKMAN, CLARKE, LONG, AND WELLS

A. William E. Clarke, a medical student, may have given the first ether anesthetic in Rochester, New York, in January 1842, for a dental extraction.

B. Crawford Williamson Long administered ether for surgical anesthesia to James M. Venable on March 30, 1842, in Jefferson, Georgia, for the removal of tumors on his neck. Long did not report his success until 1849 when ether anesthesia was already well known.

C. Horace Wells observed the "analgesic effects" of nitrous oxide when he attended a lecture-exhibition by an itinerant "scientist," Gardner Quincy Colton. A few weeks later, in January 1845, Wells attempted a public demonstration in Boston at the Harvard Medical School, but the experience was judged a failure.

D. W. T. G. Morton and October 16, 1846. The successful public demonstration of ether anesthesia by Morton in the Bullfinch Amphitheater of the Massachusetts

TABLE 1-1

EARLY ANALGESICS AND SOPORIFICS

Mandragora (soporific sponge)
Alcohol
Diethyl ether (known in the sixteenth century and perhaps as early as the eighth century)
Nitrous oxide (prepared by Joseph Priestly in 1773)

General Hospital is memorialized by the surgeon's statement to his audience at the end of the procedure, "Gentlemen, this is no humbug."

III. CHLOROFORM AND OBSTETRICS

A. James Young Simpson, a successful obstetrician of Edinburgh, Scotland, was among the first to use ether for the relief of pain in obstetrics. He became dissatisfied with ether and encouraged the use of chloroform.

B. Queen Victoria's endorsement of obstetric anesthesia resulted in acceptance of the use of anesthesia in labor.

C. John Snow took an interest in anesthetic practice soon after the news of ether anesthesia reached England in December 1846. Snow developed a mask that closely resembles a modern face mask and also introduced a chloroform inhaler.

IV. THE SECOND GENERATION OF INHALED

ANESTHETICS. Throughout the second half of the nineteenth century, the pattern of fortuitous discovery that brought nitrous oxide, diethyl ether, and chloroform forward between 1844 and 1847 continued (ethyl chloride, ethylene, cyclopropane, divinyl ether).

A. All potent anesthetics of this period were explosive save for chloroform whose hepatic and cardiac toxicity limited use in America.

B. Charles Suckling, a British chemist created halothane in 1953 and it was introduced into clinical practice in 1956 by Michael Johnstone.

C. Enflurane and its isomer isoflurane were the result of the search for fluoriniated liquid anesthetics of greater stability (synthesized by Ross Terrell in 1963 and 1965 but not introduced into clinical practice until the 1970s). Isoflurane was nearly abandoned because of difficulties in its purification.

D. Desflurane was released in 1992 and sevoflurane (halogenated only with fluorine) was released in 1994. Sevoflurane is more potent than desflurane and is minimally irritating to the airways, making it a useful agent for inhaled inductions, especially in pediatric patients.

V. REGIONAL ANESTHESIA

A. Carl Koller introduced cocaine as a topical anesthetic for ophthalmic surgery with a report to the Congress of German Ophthalmologists in Heidelberg on September 15, 1884.

B. American surgeons, including William Halsted and Richard Hall, described use of cocaine for topical anesthesia in multiple sites as well as subcutaneous injection to produce nerve blocks (brachial plexus).

C. The term "spinal anesthesia" was coined in 1885 by a neurologist, Leonard Corning, although it is likely he actually performed an epidural injection.

    1. The technique of lumbar puncture was described by Heinrich Quincke of Kiel, Germany.

    2. Procaine was introduced as an alternative to the more toxic cocaine.

    3. In 1944, Edward Tuohy of the Mayo Clinic introduced the Tuohy needle to facilitate the use of continuous spinal techniques.

D. In 1949, Martinez Curbelo of Havana, Cuba, used Tuohy's needle and a ureteral catheter to perform the first **continuous epidural anesthetic.**

E. In 1902, Harvey Cushing coined the phrase "regional anesthesia" for his technique of blocking either the brachial plexus or sciatic plexus under direct vision during general anesthesia to decrease anesthetic requirements and provide postoperative pain.

F. John J. Bonica's many contributions to anesthesiology during his periods of military, civilian, and university service at the University of Washington included development of a multidisciplinary pain clinic and publication of the text *The Management of Pain.*

VI. ANESTHESIA MACHINES AND MECHANICAL VENTILATION

A. **Early Anesthesia Delivery Systems.** John Snow created ether inhalers and Joseph Clover, another British physician, was the first to administer chloroform in known concentrations through the "Clover bag."

B. Critical to increasing patient safety was the development of a machine capable of delivering calibrated amounts of gas and volatile anesthetics (also carbon dioxide absorbance, vaporizers, ventilators).

VII. CONTROL OF THE AIRWAY

A. Joseph Clover was the first to urge the now universal practice of thrusting the patient's jaw forward to overcome obstruction of the upper airway by the tongue. Clover was also the first to perform cricothyrotomy for emergency treatment of upper airway obstruction following induction of anesthesia.

B. **Tracheal Intubation in Anesthesia**
   1. The development of techniques and instruments for tracheal intubation ranks among the major advances in the history of anesthesiology.
   2. The first use of elective oral tracheal intubation (placed by palpation) for an anesthetic was described in 1878 by a Scottish surgeon, William Macewan, for a patient with an oral tumor.
   3. Albert Kirstein in Berlin devised the first direct-vision laryngoscope in 1895.
   4. Robert Miller of San Antonio introduced a slender straight laryngoscope blade (passes under the epiglottis) in 1941 and Robert Macintosh of Oxford University introduced a curved largyngoscope blade (passed anterior of the epiglottis) in 1943.
   5. Arthur Guedel began a series of experiments in 1926 designed to develop a cuffed tracheal tube.
   6. Frank Robershaw of Manchester, England, introduced a double-lumen endobronchial tube in 1953.
   7. A. I. J. Brain described the laryngeal mask airway in 1983.

VIII. PATIENT MONITORING

A. Two American surgeons, George W. Crile and Harvey Cushing, advocated systemic blood pressure monitoring during anesthesia. In 1902, Cushing applied the Riva Rocci cuff for blood pressure measurements to be recorded on an anesthesia record.

B. The discovery and widespread use of electrocardiography, pulse oximetry, blood gas analysis, capnography, and neuromuscular blockade monitoring have reduced patient morbidity and mortality and revolutionized anesthesia practice.

   1. Severinghaus states, "Pulse oximetry is arguably the most important technological advance ever made in monitoring the well-being and safety of patients during anesthesia, recovery, and critical care."

   2. Breath to breath continuous monitoring and waveform display of carbon dioxide (infrared absorption) concentrations in the respired gases confirms endotracheal intubation (rules out accidental esophageal intubation).

IX. INTRAVENOUS MEDICATIONS IN ANESTHESIA

A. Thiopental was synthesized in 1932 and first administered to a patient at the University of Wisconsin in March 1934. The successful introduction of thiopental into clinical practice was a result of the work of John S. Lundy at the Mayo Clinic, who began an active assessment of thiopental during June 1934.

B. **Ketamine** was synthesized in 1962 and introduced into clinical practice in 1970. Its analgesic properties are increasingly utilized.

C. **Propofol** was tested clinically in 1977 and its antiemetic effects have made it an agent of choice in total intravenous anesthesia cases.

D. **Opioids**

   1. Fentanyl was synthesized in 1960 and was followed by sufentanil and alfentanil.

   2. Remifentanil, an ultra-short-acting opioid, was introduced in 1996 (rapid onset and rapid metabolism by nonspecific tissue esterases make this drug useful during continuous intravenous infusion when precise pain control and predictable offset are preferable).

E. **Antiemetics** have evolved relatively recently and have been driven by incentives to limit hospitalization expenses and to improve patient satisfaction.

1. Droperidol, released in the early 1960s, became widely used until recent concerns regarding prolongation of the QT interval on the electrocardiogram.
2. Corticosteroids were first recognized to have antiemetic effects by oncologists treating intracranial edema from tumors.
3. Ondansetron was the first serotonin 5HT3 antagonist introduced for antiemetic effects.

X. MUSCLE RELAXANTS

A. Curare was used by Arthur Lawen of Leipzig to produce surgical relaxation in an anesthetized patient, but his report was not widely appreciated (not surprising because tracheal intubation and controlled ventilation of the lungs were not known techniques at this time).
B. On January 23, 1942, Harrold Griffith and his resident, Enid Johnson, anesthetized and intubated the trachea of a patient before injecting curare early in the course of an appendectomy. Their report of the successful use of curare in 25 patients launched a revolution in anesthetic care.
C. In 1906, Hunt and Taveaux prepared succinylcholine and studied its cardiac effects in curarized rabbits. As a result, the paralyzing effects of succinylcholine were not recognized. Subsequently, succinylcholine was introduced as a muscle relaxant in 1949.

XI. HEMODYNAMIC CONTROL

A. Unrestrained venesection killed U.S. president George Washington when in 1799 he was drained of nine pints of blood in 24 hours following a throat infection.
B. In 1900, Karl Landsteiner and Samuel Shattock independently helped lay the scientific basis of all subsequent transfusions by recognizing that blood computability was based upon different blood groups.

XII. ANESTHESIA ORGANIZATION AND EDUCATION

A. Anesthesiology evolved slowly as a medical specialty in the United States and ether remained the dominant anesthetic.

1. During the late nineteenth century, small communities were often served by a single physician who assigned a nurse to "drop" ether under his direction.
2. In larger towns, doctors practiced independently and did not welcome the role of being placed in what they perceived to be the subordinate role of anesthetist, while their competitors enhanced their surgical reputation and collected the larger surgical fee.

B. Organized Anesthesiology

   1. The Long Island Society of Anesthetists, founded in 1905, was America's first specialty anesthesia society, with annual dues of $1.00. In 1911, the Long Island Society became the New York Society of Anesthetists and the annual fee increased to $3.00.
   2. Francis Hoffer McMechan was a practicing anesthesiologist in Cincinnati until 1915 when crippling rheumatoid arthritis ended his operating room career. McMechan was the editor of the first journal devoted to anesthesia, *Current Researches in Anesthesia and Analgesia*.

CHAPTER 2 ■ PRACTICE AND OPERATING ROOM MANAGEMENT

Practice and operating room management issues are assuming increasing importance in the daily activities of anesthesiologists (Lock RL, Eichhorn JH: Practice and operating room management. In Barash PG, Cullen BF, Stoelting RK [eds]: *Clinical Anesthesia*, pp 27–62. Philadelphia, Lippincott Williams & Wilkins, 2006).

I. ADMINISTRATIVE COMPONENTS OF ALL ANESTHESIOLOGY PRACTICES

A. Operational and Information Resources
1. The American Society of Anesthesiologists (ASA) provides extensive resource materials to its members regarding practice management (Table 2-1).
2. These documents are updated regularly by the ASA through its committees and House of Delegates.

B. Internet
1. A modern anesthesiology practice must use the information resources (journals, textbooks, electronic bulletin boards) provided by the Internet.
2. The Web site for the American Society of Anesthesiologists is **asahq.org**.

C. The Credentialing Process and Clinical Privileges
1. The system of credentialing a health care professional and granting clinical privileges is motivated by the assumption that appropriate education, training, and experience, along with the absence of an excessive number of adverse patient outcomes, increase the likelihood that the health care professional will deliver high-quality care.
2. Models for credentialing anesthesiologists are offered by the ASA.
3. The **National Practitioner Data Bank** is a central repository of licensing and credentials information about physicians. The data bank is maintained by the federal government, and adverse events involving a physician (substance abuse, malpractice litigation,

TABLE 2-1
PRACTICE MANAGEMENT MATERIALS PROVIDED BY THE
AMERICAN SOCIETY OF ANESTHESIOLOGISTS

The Organization of an Anesthesia Department
Guidelines for Delineation of Clinical Privileges in
  Anesthesiology
Guidelines for a Minimally Acceptable Program of Any
  Continuing Education Requirement
Guidelines for the Ethical Practice of Anesthesiology
Ethical Guidelines for the Anesthesia Care of Patients with
  Do-Not-Resuscitate Orders or Other Directives that Limit
  Treatment
Guidelines for Patient Care in Anesthesiology
Guidelines for Expert Witness Qualifications and Testimony
Guidelines for Delegation of Technical Anesthesia Functions for
  Nonphysician Personnel
The Anesthesia Care Team
Statement on Conflict of Interest
Statement on Economic Credentialing
Statement on Member's Right to Practice
Statement on Routine Preoperative Laboratory and Diagnostic
  Screening

revocation or limitation of the physician's license)
must be reported to it via the appropriate state board
of medical registration.
4. An important issue in granting clinical privileges,
especially in procedure-oriented specialties such as
anesthesiology, is whether it is reasonable to grant
"blanket" privileges (the right to do everything
traditionally associated with the specialty).
5. Initial board certification after the year 2000 by the
American Board of Anesthesiology will be time limited
and subject to periodic testing and recertification. This
requirement will encourage an ongoing process of
continued medical education (CME).
D. Medical Staff Participation and Relationships
1. Medical staff activities are increasingly important in
achieving a favorable accreditation status from the
Joint Commission on the Accreditation of Healthcare
Organizations (JCAHO).
2. Anesthesiologists should be active participants in
medical staff activities (Table 2-2).
E. Establishing Standards of Practice and Understanding the
"Standard of Care"

TABLE 2-2
EXAMPLES OF THE ANESTHESIOLOGIST AS A PARTICIPANT IN MEDICAL STAFF ACTIVITIES

Credentialing
Peer review
Transfusion review
Operating room management
Medical direction of same-day surgery units
Medical direction of postanesthesia care units
Medical direction of intensive care units
Medical direction of pain management services and clinics

1. American anesthesiology is one of the leaders in establishing practice standards that are intended to maximize the quality of patient care and help guide anesthesiologists to make difficult decisions, including those about the risk-benefit and cost-benefit aspects of specific practices (Table 2-3).
2. The standard of care is the conduct of and the skill of a prudent practitioner that can be expected at all times by a reasonable patient.
   a. Failure to meet the standard of care is considered malpractice.
   b. Courts have traditionally relied on medical experts to give opinions as to what is the standard of care and whether or not it has been met in an individual case.
3. Anesthesiology has been very active in publishing standards of care (see Table 2-3).
   a. A practice guideline has some of the same elements as a standard of practice but is intended more to guide judgment, largely through algorithms.
   b. Practice guidelines serve as potential vehicles for helping to eliminate unnecessary procedures and to limit costs.
   c. Guidelines do not define the standard of care, although adherence to the outlined principles should provide the anesthesiologist with a reasonably defensible position.
4. JCAHO standards focus on credentialing and privileges, verification that anesthesia services are of uniform quality, continuing education, and documentation of preoperative and postoperative evaluations.

TABLE 2-3

MATERIALS PROVIDED BY THE AMERICAN SOCIETY OF ANESTHESIOLOGISTS DESIGNED TO ESTABLISH PRACTICE STANDARDS

Standards (Minimum Requirements for Sound Practice)
Basic Standards for Preanesthesia Care
Standards for Basic Anesthesia Monitoring
Standards for Postanesthesia Care

Guidelines (Recommendations for Patient Management)
Guidelines for Ambulatory Surgical Facilities
Guidelines for Critical Care in Anesthesiology
Guidelines for Nonoperating Room Anesthetizing Locations
Guidelines for Regional Anesthesia in Obstetrics

Practice Guidelines
Practice Guidelines for Acute Pain Management in the
  Perioperative Setting
Practice Guidelines for Management of the Difficult Airway
Practice Guidelines for Pulmonary Artery Catheterization
Practice Guidelines for Difficult Airway

Practice Parameters
Pain Management
Transesophageal Echocardiography
Sedation by Nonanesthesia Personnel
Preoperative Fasting
Avoidance of Peripheral Neuropathies
Fast-Track Management of Coronary Artery Bypass Graft
  Patients

     5. Another type of regulatory agency is the peer review
organization (PRO), whose objectives include issues
related to hospital admissions and quality of care.
- F. Policy and Procedure
  1. An important organizational aspect of an anesthesia
     department is a policy and procedure manual.
  2. This manual includes specific protocols for areas
     mentioned in the JCAHO standards, including
     pre-anesthetic evaluation, safety of the patient during
     anesthesia, recording of all pertinent events during
     anesthesia, and release of the patient from the
     postanesthesia care unit.
- G. Meetings and Case Discussion
  1. There must be regularly scheduled departmental
     meetings.

2. JCAHO requires that there be at least monthly meetings at which risk management and quality improvement activities are documented and reported.

H. **Malpractice Insurance**
   1. **Occurrence** means that if the insurance policy was in force at the time of the occurrence of an incident resulting in a claim, the physician will be covered.
   2. **Claims made** provides coverage only for claims that are filed when the policy was in force ("tail coverage" is needed if this policy is not renewed annually).
   3. A new approach in medical risk management and insurance is advocating immediate full disclosure to the victim or survivors (shift the culture of blame with punishment to a just culture with restitution).

II. PRACTICE ESSENTIALS

A. **The "job market" for anesthesiologists** is being influenced by the number of residents being trained, geographic maldistribution of anesthesiologists, and marketplace forces as reflected by managed care organizations and the real and potential impact on numbers of surgical procedures. By 2001 it was perceived that there was a shortage of anesthesia providers.

B. **Types of practice** include academic practice, private practice, and salaried employees in private practice.

C. **Billing and collecting** may be based on calculations according to units and time, a single predetermined fee independent of time, or fees bundled with all physicians involved in the surgical procedure.
   1. Billing for specific procedures becomes irrelevant in systems with prospective "capitated" payments for large numbers of patients (a fixed amount per enrolled member per month [PMPM]).
   2. The federal government has issued a new regulation allowing individual states to "opt out" of the requirement that a nurse anesthetist be supervised by a physician to meet Medicare billing requirements.

D. **Antitrust Considerations**
   1. The law is concerned solely with the preservation of competition within a defined marketplace and the rights of the consumer.
   2. The market is not threatened by the exclusion of one physician from the medical staff of a hospital.

E. **Exclusive service contracts** state that anesthesiologists seeking to practice must be members of the group holding the exclusive contract.
   1. In some instances, members of the group may be terminated without due process by the medical staff.
   2. Economic credentialing (opposed by the ASA) is defined as the use of economic criteria unrelated to quality of care or professional competency for granting or renewing hospital privileges.
F. **Hospital Subsidies.** Modern economic realities may necessitate anesthesiology practice groups to recognize that patient care revenue, after overhead is paid, does not provide sufficient compensation to attract and retain the number and quality of staff necessary. A direct cash subsidy from the hospital may be negotiated to augment practice revenue in order to maintain benefits while increasing the pay of staff members to a market-competitive level.

III. MANAGED CARE AND NEW PRACTICE ARRANGEMENTS

A. Managed care systems for health care delivery exist as a mechanism to control and then reduce health care costs by having independent reviewers and decision makers who are not physicians rendering the care limit the health care services being delivered to large groups of patients.
B. A public backlash against the limitations on medical care services led to decreased expansion of managed care and to some easing of the restrictions on services in many plans.
C. **Value-based anesthesia practice** is an attempt to balance the relationship of cost of care and patient outcomes. Because data available for statistical analysis of costs and outcomes is difficult to generate, the widespread applicability of this approach in everyday anesthesia practice remains to be developed.

IV. HIPAA. Implementation of the privacy rule of the Health Insurance Portability and Accountability Act (HIPAA) creates significant changes in how medical records and patient information are handled. Under HIPAA, patients' names may not be used on an OR board if there is any chance that

anyone not directly involved in their care could see them.

V. EXPANSION INTO PERIOPERATIVE MEDICINE, HOSPITAL CARE, AND HYPERBARIC MEDICINE

A. Formalized **preoperative screening clinics** operated and staffed by anesthesiologists could replace the historical practice of sending patients to primary care physicians or consultants for "preoperative clearance."

B. Anesthesiologists can become the coordinators of postoperative care, especially in the realm of providing comprehensive pain management.

VI. OPERATING ROOM MANAGEMENT

A. Current emphasis on cost containment and efficiency requires anesthesiologists to take an active role in eliminating dysfunctional aspects of OR practice (first-case morning start times).
   1. It is the anesthesiologist with the insight, overview, and unique perspective who is best qualified to provide leadership in an OR.
   2. An important aspect of OR organization is materials management.

B. **Scheduling Cases**
   1. Anesthesiologists need to participate in scheduling of cases as the number of anesthesia professionals is dependent on daily caseload, including "off-site" diagnostic areas.
   2. The majority of operating rooms utilize either block scheduling (preassigned guaranteed OR time with an agreed cut-off time), open scheduling (first come, first served), or a combination.
   3. **Computerization** will likely benefit every operating room.

C. **Pre-op Clinic.** An anesthesia preoperative evaluation clinic (APEC) usually results in more efficient running of the operating room and avoidance of unanticipated cancellations or delays.

D. **Anesthesiology Personnel Issues.** In light of the current and future shortage of anesthesia professionals, managing and maintaining a stable supply promises to dominate the OR landscape for years.

E. **Cost and Quality Issues**

1. Health care accounts for approximately 14% of the Gross Domestic Product and anesthesia (directly and indirectly) represents 3 to 5% of total health care costs.
2. Anesthesia drug expenses represent a small portion of the total perioperative costs but the great number of doses administered contributes substantially to the aggregate total cost to the institution.
   a. Reducing fresh gas flow from 5 L/min to 2 L/min wherever possible would save approximately $100 million annually in the United States.
   b. More expensive techniques and drugs may reduce indirect costs (propofol infusion is more expensive but may decrease PACU time and reduce nausea and vomiting)
   c. For long surgical procedures, newer and more expensive drugs may offer limited benefits over older and less expensive longer acting alternatives.
   d. It is estimated that the 10 highest expenditure drugs account for more than 80% of the anesthetic drug costs at some institutions.

CHAPTER 3 ■ EXPERIMENTAL DESIGN AND STATISTICS

The practitioner of scientific medicine must be able to read the language of science to independently assess and interpret the scientific literature and the increasing emphasis on statistical methods (Pace NL: Experimental design and statistics. In Barash PG, Cullen BF, Stoelting RK [eds]: *Clinical Anesthesia*, pp 63–75. Philadelphia, Lippincott Williams & Wilkins, 2006).

I. **DESIGN OF RESEARCH STUDIES.** The **case report** engenders interest and the desire to experiment but is not sufficient evidence to advance scientific medicine.

   A. **Sampling**
      1. A **sample** is a subset of a **target population** that is intended to allow the researcher to generalize the results of the small sample to the entire population.
      2. The best hope for a representative sample of the population would be realized if every subject in the population had the same chance of being in the experiment (**random sampling**). However, most clinical anesthesia studies are limited to using those patients who are available (**convenience sampling**).

   B. **Control groups** may be self-control or parallel control groups versus historical control groups (studies using historical controls are more likely than those using self-controls or parallel controls to show a benefit from a new therapy).

   C. **Random allocation of treatment groups** is helpful to avoid research bias in entering patients into specific study groups (random allocation is most commonly accomplished by computer-generated random numbers).

   D. **Blinding** refers to masking from the view of both the patient and experimenter the experimental group to which the subject has been assigned.
      1. A single-blind study is when the patient is unaware of the treatment given (patient expectations from a treatment could influence results).

      2. A double-blind study is when the subject and the data collector are ignorant of the treatment group (best way to test a new therapy).

  E. Types of Research Design
      1. Longitudinal studies evaluate changes over time using research subjects chosen **prospectively** (cohort) or **retrospectively** (case control). Retrospective studies are a primary tool of epidemiology.
      2. Cross-sectional studies evaluate changes at a certain point in time.

  F. Hypothesis Formulation
      1. The researcher starts the work with some intuitive feel for the phenomenon to be studied (biologic hypothesis).
      2. The biologic hypothesis becomes a statistical hypothesis during research planning.

  G. Logic of Proof
      1. If sample values are sufficiently unlikely to have occurred by chance (alpha [p] <0.05), the **null hypothesis** (assumes there is no difference) is rejected.
      2. Because statistics deal with probabilities and not certainties, there is a chance that decisions made concerning the null hypothesis are erroneous.
        a. Type I (alpha) error is wrongly rejecting the null hypothesis (false positive). The smaller the chosen alpha, the smaller the risk of a type I error.
        b. Type II (beta) error is failing to reject the null hypothesis (false-negative). Variability in the population increases the chance of type II error. Increasing the number of subjects (very important in research design for controlled clinical trials), raising the alpha value, and dealing with large differences between two conditions decrease the chances of a type II error.

II. STATISTICAL TESTING

  A. Statistics is a method for working with sets of numbers (X and Y) and determining if the values are different. Statistical methods are necessary because there are sources of variation in any data set, including random biologic variation and measurement error. These errors make it difficult to avoid bias and to be precise.

TABLE 3-1
DATA TYPES

Data types	Definition	Examples
Interval		
Discrete	Data measured with an integer-only scale	Age Parity
Continuous	Data measured with a constant-scale interval	Blood pressure Temperature
Categorical		
Dichotomous	Binary data	Mortality Gender
Nominal	Qualitative data that cannot be ordered or ranked	Eye color Drug category
Ordinal	Data ordered, ranked, or measured without a constant-scale interval	ASA physical status Pain score

- B. **Data Structure.** Properly assigning a variable to the correct data type is essential for choosing the correct statistical technique (Table 3-1).
- C. **Descriptive statistics** are intended to describe the sample of numbers obtained and to characterize the population from which the sample was obtained. The two summary statistics most frequently used are the **central location** and **variability** (Table 3-2).
- D. **Inferential Statistics**
  1. The testing of hypotheses or significance testing is the main focus of inferential statistics (Table 3-3).
  2. General guidelines relate the variable type and the experimental design to the choice of statistical test (Table 3-4).
     - a. The **Student's *t* test** is used to compare the values of the means of two populations. The **paired *t* test** is used when each subject serves as his or her own control (before and after measurements in the same patient decrease variability and increase statistical power). An **unpaired *t* test** is used when measurements are taken on two groups of subjects.
     - b. The most versatile approach for handling comparisons of means among more than two groups is called **analysis of variance** (ANOVA).

TABLE 3-2
DESCRIPTIVE STATISTICS

Central Location for Interval Variables
Arithmetic mean (average of the numbers in the data set)
Median (middle-most number or number that divides the
    samples into two equal parts; not affected by very high or
    low numbers)
Mode (number in a sample that appears most frequently)

Spread or Variability
Standard deviation (SD; approximates the spread of the sample
    data; 1 SD encompasses roughly 68% of the sample and
    population members, whereas 3 SDs encompass 99%)

Confidence Intervals
Standard error of the mean (approximates the precision with
    which the population center is known)

---

    c. For parametric statistics (*t* tests and ANOVA), it is
    assumed that the populations follow the normal
    distribution.
    d. Robustness and non-parmetric tests can be used
    when there is concern that the populations do not
    follow a normal distribution.

TABLE 3-3
**INFORMATION NECESSARY TO ACCEPT OR REJECT THE
NULL HYPOTHESIS**

Confirm that experimental data conform to the assumptions of
    the intended statistical test
Choose a significance level (alpha)
Calculate the test statistic
Determine the degree(s) of freedom
Find the critical value for the chosen alpha and the degree(s) of
    freedom from the appropriate theoretical probability
    distribution
If the test statistic exceeds the critical value, reject the null
    hypothesis
If the test statistic does not exceed the critical value, do not
    reject the null hypothesis

TABLE 3-4
WHEN TO USE WHAT

Variable type tests	One-Sample	Two-Sample tests	Multiple-Sample tests
Dichotomous or nominal	Binomial distribution	Chi-square test	Chi-square test
Ordinal	Chi-square test	Chi-square test, nonparametric tests	Chi-square test, nonparametric tests
Continuous or discrete	z or t distribution	Unpaired t test, paired t test, nonparametric tests	Analysis of variance, nonparametric analysis of variance

E. **Interpretation of Results**
   1. Scientific studies do not end with the statistical test (statistical significance does not always equate with biologic relevance).
   2. Even small, clinically unimportant differences between groups can be detected if the sample size is sufficiently large. If the sample size is small, there is a greater chance that confounding variables may explain any difference.
   3. If the experimental groups in a properly designed study are given three or more doses of a drug, the reader should expect to observe a steadily increasing or decreasing dose-response relationship.
   4. In comparing alternative therapies, the confidence that a claim for a superior therapy is true depends on study design.
      a. The strength of the evidence concerning efficacy is least for an anecdotal case report; next in importance is a retrospective study, then a prospective series of patients compared with historical controls, and finally a randomized, controlled clinical trial.
      b. The greatest strength for a therapeutic claim is a series of randomized, controlled clinical trials confirming the same hypothesis.

III. READING JOURNAL ARTICLES

A. The clinician with limited time should select journal articles to read that are relevant (determined by the specifics of one's anesthetic practice) and credible (function of the merits of the research methods).
B. Although the statistical knowledge of most physicians is limited, these skills of critical appraisal of the literature can be learned and can greatly increase the efficiency and benefit of journal reading.
C. **Systematic review** is a new type of research method in which a focused question drives the research. To answer the question, data are obtained from randomized clinical trials already in the medical literature rather than from direct experimentation.
   1. The American Society of Anesthesiologists (ASA) has developed a process for the creation of practice parameters that include a variant form of systematic reviews.

CHAPTER 4 ■ OCCUPATIONAL HEALTH

Anesthesia personnel spend long hours in an environment (the operating room) filled with many potential hazards (exposure to vapors from chemicals, ionizing radiation, and infectious agents and psychological stress engendered by the high-stakes nature of the practice) (Berry AJ, Katz JD: Occupational health. In Barash PG, Cullen BF, Stoelting RK [eds]: *Clinical Anesthesia*, pp 76–98. Philadelphia, Lippincott Williams & Wilkins, 2006).

I. PHYSICAL HAZARDS

A. Anesthetic Gases

1. Reports on the effects of chronic environmental exposure to anesthetics have included epidemiologic surveys, in vitro studies, cellular research, and studies in laboratory animals and humans. Areas addressed include fertility and spontaneous abortion, incidence of congenital malformations, mortality rate, incidence of cancer, hematopoietic diseases, liver disease, neurologic disease, and psychomotor and behavioral changes produced by exposure to anesthetics.

2. **Anesthetic Levels in the Operating Room.** Appropriate scavenging and adequate air exchange in the operating room significantly lowers levels of waste anesthetic gases.

3. **Epidemiologic studies** are difficult to interpret and results often do not withstand scientific scrutiny.

4. **Reproductive outcomes studies** suggest there is a slight increase in the risk of spontaneous abortion and congenital abnormalities in offspring for female physicians working in the operating room. The routine use of scavenging has been implemented since the time of most of these studies and there was no risk of spontaneous abortion in studies of personnel who worked in scavenged environments.

    a. Retrospective surveys of large numbers of women who worked during pregnancy indicate that negative reproductive outcomes may be related to job-related conditions (increased work hours, hours worked while standing, occupational fatigue associated with preterm birth) other than exposure to trace anesthetic gases.

   b. Routine use of scavenging techniques has generally lowered environmental anesthetic levels in the operating room and may make it difficult to prove any adverse effects using epidemiologic data.

5. **Neoplasms and Other Nonreproductive Diseases.** Overall, there appears to be some evidence that the operating room environment produces a slight increase in the rate of spontaneous abortion and cancer in female anesthesiologists and nurses. Mortality risks from cancer and heart disease for anesthesiologists do not differ from those for other medical specialists.

6. **Laboratory Studies**
   a. **Cellular effects.** Nitrous oxide administered in clinically useful concentrations affects hematopoietic and neural cells by irreversibly oxidizing the cobalt atom of vitamin B12 from an active to inactive state. This inhibits methionine synthetase and prevents the conversion of methyltetrahydrofolate to tetrahydorfolate, which is required for DNA synthesis, assembly of myelin sheath, and methyl substitutions in neurotransmitters. Inhibition of methionine synthetase in individuals exposed to high concentrations of nitrous oxide may result in anemia and polyneuropathy, but chronic exposure to trace levels does not appear to produce these effects.
   b. Anesthetics are not mutagenic (carcinogenic) using the Ames bacterial assay. Analyses of sister chromatid exchanges or formation of micronucleated lymphocytes to assess for genotoxicity in association with anesthetic exposure have been negative.
   c. Anesthetists working where waste gas scavenging is not used have increased fractions of micronucleated lymphocytes compared to those practicing in a scavenged operating room (significant unclear).

7. **Reproductive Outcome.** Data from animals fail to confirm alterations in female or male fertility or reproduction with exposure to subanesthetic

TABLE 4-1
EXAMPLES OF RECOMMENDED THRESHOLD LIMITS FOR
OCCUPATIONAL EXPOSURE TO ANESTHETIC AGENTS[a]

Country	Nitrous Oxide	Enflurane	Isoflurane
United States (NIOSH)	25	2	2
United States (ACGIH)	50	75	not determined
Great Britain	100	50	50
Norway	100	2	2
Sweden	100	10	10

[a]Time-weighted average in parts per million (ppm).
NIOSH, National Institute of Occupational Safety and Health; ACGIH,
American Conference on Governmental Industrial Hygienists.

    concentrations of currently used inhaled drugs (other
possible factors must also be considered, including
stress, alterations in work schedule, and fatigue).

8. **Effects of Trace Anesthetic Levels on Psychomotor
   Skills.** Studies to clarify whether low concentrations of
   anesthetics alter psychomotor skills are inconclusive.
9. **Recommendations of the National Institute for
   Occupational Safety and Health (NIOSH)** (Table 4-1).
   Despite the use of scavenging devices, there is a need
   for continued monitoring of anesthetic levels in the
   operating room and routine attention to equipment
   maintenance (Table 4-2).
10. **Anesthetic Levels in the Postanesthesia Care Unit**
    a. As patients awaken from general anesthesia, waste
       anesthetic gases are released into the environment
       of the postanesthesia care unit (PACU) (especially if
       patient's tracheas are still intubated when they
       arrive in the PACU).
    b. NIOSH threshold limits for anesthetic gases can be
       obtained in the PACU by ensuring adequate room
       ventilation and fresh gas exchange and by
       discontinuing the anesthetic gases in sufficient time
       prior to leaving the operating room.
B. **Chemicals**
   1. **Methylmethacrylate** concentrations in the operating
      room (allowable exposure 100 ppm) may be
      decreased by scavenging devices.
   2. **Allergic reactions** have been attributed to exposure of
      anesthesiologists to vapors of methylmethacrylate and
      inhaled anesthetics.

TABLE 4-2

SOURCES OF OPERATING ROOM CONTAMINATION

Anesthetic Techniques
Failure to turn off gas flow control valves at end of an anesthetic
Turning gas flow on before placing mask on patient
Poorly fitting masks (especially with induction of anesthesia)
Flushing the circuit
Filling of anesthesia vaporizers
Uncuffed or leaking tracheal tubes (pediatrics) or poor-fitting
    laryngeal mask airways
Pediatric circuits (Jackson-Rees version of Mapleson D system)
Sidestream sampling carbon dioxide and anesthetic gas analyzers

Anesthesia Machine Delivery System and Scavenging System
Open/closed system
Occlusion/malfunction of hospital disposal system
Maladjustment of hospital disposal system vacuum
Leaks
High-pressure hoses or connectors
Nitrous oxide tank mounting
O rings
CO_2 absorbent canisters
Low-pressure circuit

Other Sources
Cryosurgery units
Cardiopulmonary bypass circuits

3. **Latex sensitivity** has become a common source of
   allergic reactions among operating room personnel
   (12.5 to 15.8% of anesthesiologists are sensitive to
   latex). Irritant or contact dermatitis from wearing
   latex-containing gloves accounts for about 80% of
   reactions to latex (Table 4-3). Use of powderless
   gloves will limit exposure to ambient latex antigens.
C. **Radiation** exposure (fluoroscopic guidance procedures) is
   a function of total exposure intensity and time, distance
   from the source of radiation, and use of shielding.
   1. Pregnant workers should limit the dose to <500 mrem
      during the gestation period.
   2. Radiation exposure should be monitored with film
      badges in all anesthesia personnel at risk.
D. **Noise** pollution may approach unacceptable levels in the
   operating room (75 to 90 decibels [db] is produced by
   ventilators, suction equipment, music, and conversation;

TABLE 4-3
TYPES OF REACTIONS TO LATEX GLOVES

Reaction	Signs/Symptoms	Cause	Management
Irritant contact dermatitis	Scaling, drying, cracking of skin	Direct skin irritation by gloves, powder, soaps	Identify reaction, avoid irritant, possible use of glove liner, use of alternative product
Type IV delayed hypersensitivity	Itching, blistering, crusting (delayed 6 to 72 hours)	Chemical additives used in manufacturing (such as accelerators)	Identify offending chemical, or alternative without chemical additive, possible use of glove liner
Type I immediate hypersensitivity		Proteins found in latex	Identify reaction, avoid latex-containing products, use of nonlatex or powder-free, low-protein gloves by co-workers
Localized contact urticaria	Itching, hives in area of contact with latex (immediate)		Antihistamines, topical/systemic steroids
Generalized reaction	Runny nose, swollen eyes, generalized rash or hives, bronchospasm, anaphylaxis		Anaphylaxis protocol

safe noise exposure level for 8 hours is considered to be 90 db).

E. **Human factors** that exist in the operating room (configuration and placement of equipment [ergonomics], constant vigilance [mental fatigue], interpersonal relationships, and communication) remain the greatest potential source contributing to patient morbidity and mortality. Production pressure is an organizational concern that has the potential to create an environment in which issues of productivity supersede those of safety.

F. **Work hours and night call** can contribute to fatigue and impaired performance of complex cognitive tasks such as monitoring and vigilance. Demands associated with night call have been identified as the most stressful aspect of anesthesia practice.

1. Sleep deprivation and circadian disruption have deleterious effects on cognition, performance, mood, and health (acute sleep deprivation resembles alcohol intoxication).

2. Residents in the sleep-deprived condition demonstrated progressive impairment of alertness and had longer response latency to vigilance probes utilizing the anesthesia simulator but there were no significant differences in the clinical management of the simulated patients between the rested and sleep-deprived groups.

3. Subsequent to a period of sleep deprivation, performance does not return to normal levels until 24 hours of rest and recovery has occurred.

4. The Accreditation Council for Graduate Medical Education and its Residency Review Committees have set universal standards that limit resident duty hours to 80 hours per week and no more than 30 hours at any one time.

5. Naps prior to the start of call as well as the use of caffeine improve alertness during long shifts.

II. INFECTION HAZARDS

A. Anesthesia personnel are at risk for acquiring infections from both patients and other personnel (Table 4-4). Viral infections are the greatest threat to health care workers and are spread most often by the respiratory route. Transmission of blood-borne pathogens (hepatitis virus and human immunodeficiency virus [HIV]) can be prevented by mechanical barriers or vaccination (hepatitis B). Hand washing between patients, appropriate use of gloves, and use of needleless or protected needle safety devices are the best protections for health care workers from the risks of contracting infections from patients.

B. **OSHA Standards, Universal Precautions, and Isolation Precautions**

1. Universal precautions for preventing transmission of blood-borne infections should be used for all patient contacts (Table 4-5).

2. General infection-control practice recommends use of gloves when a health care worker comes in contact

TABLE 4-4
SOURCES OF INFECTION FROM PATIENTS

Respiratory Viruses
Influenza A or B (vaccination, amantadine)
Respiratory syncytial virus

Herpes Viruses
Varicella-zoster virus (chicken pox or shingles; susceptible hospital
   personnel with exposure to the virus should not have direct
   patient contact from the 10th to 21st day after exposure)
Herpes simplex (spread by direct contact with body fluids, as
   during tracheal intubation)
Herpetic whitlow (consider limiting direct patient care because this
   virus can infect susceptible individuals; acyclovir may shorten
   course of primary cutaneous infection)
Cytomegalovirus (source usually an infected infant or
   immunosuppressed patient)
Rubella (vaccination recommended for susceptible health care
   personnel)
Measles (vaccination recommended for susceptible health care
   personnel)
Severe Acute Respiratory Syndrome (SARS) (emerging respiratory
   tract infection caused by coronavirus, high fever followed by
   headache and occasionally pneumonia and acute respiratory
   distress syndrome; prevent spread by isolation of infected
   patients)

Viral Hepatitis
Hepatitis A
Hepatitis B (significant risk for nonimmunized health care
   personnel who have contact with blood and possibility of
   needlesticks; vaccination is recommended for susceptible health
   care personnel)
Hepatitis C (high rate of chronic hepatitis often progressing to
   cirrhosis, risk after infected needle stick is 2 to 4%)

Human Immunodeficiency Virus-1
Rate of seroconversion in health care workers sustaining a
   percutaneous exposure (needlestick injury) is about 0.3% with
   conversion usually occurring within 6 to 12 weeks after
   exposure; estimated risk of patient-transmitted infection to the
   anesthesiologist is between 0.001% and 0.129%; utilize
   universal precautions in managing known and high-risk patients
   (see Table 4-5)

Creutzfeldt-Jakob Disease
Tuberculosis (increased incidence in immigrants from countries
   with a high incidence of this disease and in alcoholics, homeless
   persons, immunosuppressed patients, and intravenous drug
   users)

TABLE 4-5

UNIVERSAL PRECAUTIONS

1. All needles, blades, and sharp instruments should be handled so as to prevent accidental injuries, and all should be considered potentially infected. Disposable sharp items should be placed in puncture-resistant containers located as close as is practical to the area in which they are used. Needles should not be recapped, bent, broken, or removed from disposable syringes prior to placing them in appropriate disposable containers.
2. Gloves should be worn when touching mucous membranes or open skin of all patients. When the possibility exists of exposure to blood, body fluid, or items soiled with these, gloves should be used. With some procedures such as endoscopy, during which aerosolization or splashes of blood or secretions are likely to occur, wearing of masks, eye coverings, and gowns is indicated. Gloves and body coverings should be removed and disposed of properly after patient contact.
3. Frequent hand washing, especially between patient contacts and after removal of gloves, should be encouraged. If hands are accidentally contaminated with blood or other body fluids, they should be washed as soon as possible.
4. Ventilation devices for resuscitation should be available at appropriate locations to prevent the need for emergency mouth-to-mouth resuscitation.
5. Health care workers who have exudative lesions or weeping dermatitis should not participate in direct patient-care activities until the condition resolves.

with patient mucous membranes or oral fluids, such as during tracheal intubation and pharyngeal suctioning.
C. **Viruses in Laser Plumes**
  1. Viable viruses have been found in plumes produced by laser vaporization of tissues that contain viruses.
  2. To protect operating room personnel from exposure to the viral and chemical contents of the laser plume, it is recommended that the tubing from a smoke evacuator be held within 2.5 cm of the tissue being vaporized.

III. EMOTIONAL CONSIDERATIONS

A. **Stress** from working in the operating room (similar to that experienced by air traffic controllers) may reflect an excessive workload, the necessity for making many difficult decisions, night duty, fatigue, increasing reliance on technology, interpersonal tensions, and concerns about liability and night call.

B. Substance Use, Abuse, and Dependence

1. Substance abuse (particularly use of potent, short-acting opioids) is often considered an occupational hazard for anesthesiologists.

2. Causative factors of substance abuse specific to the specialty of anesthesiology include job stress, lack of external recognition, availability of addictive drugs (resulting in a need to audit distribution of drugs within the operating room), and a susceptible premorbid personality.

3. Potential consequences of substance abuse are multiple. When the anesthesiologist's professional conduct is impaired to the extent that it is apparent to his or her colleagues, the disease is approaching its end stage (death) (Table 4-6).

4. Disciplinary action taken against a physician impaired by substance abuse must be reported to the National Practitioner Data Bank. Health care professionals suffer from chemical dependency (including alcohol abuse) at a rate roughly equivalent to that of the general population (8 to 12%).

5. Controversy remains about the ultimate career path of the anesthesiologist in recovery from chemical dependency. Because of contradictory data, no universal recommendation can be made about reentry into the practice of anesthesiology after treatment. The American Board of Anesthesiology has established a policy for candidates with a history of alcoholism or illegal use of drugs.

IV. THE AGING ANESTHESIOLOGIST

A. In contrast to other industries, little research has been directed toward challenges faced by older anesthesiologists (commercial pilots are required to take regular medical examinations).

B. An area of particular difficulty for anesthesiologists is maintaining the stamina required for long work shifts and night call.

TABLE 4-6

SIGNS OF SUBSTANCE ABUSE AND ADDICTION

Social (Outside the Hospital)
Withdrawal from leisure activities, friends, family
Uncharacteristic or inappropriate behavior in social settings
Impulsive behavior (overspending, gambling)
Domestic turmoil (separation from spouse, child abuse, sexual
    problems)
Change in behavior of spouse or children
Legal problems (arrested for driving while intoxicated)

Health
Deterioration in personal hygiene
Accidents
Numerous health complaints (frequent need for medical attention
    for unrelated illnesses)

Professional (In the Hospital)
Sign out ever-increasing quantities of opioids
Charting becomes sloppy and unreadable
Unusual changes in behavior (wide mood swings)
Prefer to work alone, decline relief, frequently relieve others,
    volunteer for additional cases and call, stay in hospital even
    when not on duty
Frequent requests for bathroom relief
Difficult to find between cases
Insist on personally administering opioids in the PACU
Wear long-sleeved gowns (hide needle marks) and combat
    subjective feeling of cold

V. MORTALITY AMONG ANESTHESIOLOGISTS

   A. It is debatable whether or not anesthesiologists are
      subject to premature death compared to other physicians.
      Data from the American Medical Association concluded
      there was no difference in age-specific mortality among
      anesthesiologists and internists.
   B. **Suicide** is an occupational hazard for anesthesiologists,
      perhaps reflecting the high degree of stress associated with
      the care of anesthetized patients. A malpractice lawsuit
      or suspension of privileges may result in suicidal ideation.

CHAPTER 5 ■ PROFESSIONAL LIABILITY, QUALITY IMPROVEMENT, AND ANESTHETIC RISK

In anesthesia, as in other areas of life, everything does not always go as planned (Posner KL, Cheney FW, Kroll DA: Professional liability, quality improvement, and anesthetic risk. In Barash PG, Cullen BF, Stoelting RK [eds]: *Clinical Anesthesia*, pp 99–108. Philadelphia, Lippincott Williams & Wilkins, 2006). Undesirable outcomes may occur regardless of the quality of care provided. An anesthesia risk management program can work in conjunction with a program for quality improvement to minimize the liability risks of practice while ensuring the highest quality of care for patients.

I. PROFESSIONAL LIABILITY

A. Tort System
1. A tort may be loosely defined as a civil wrongdoing. Negligence is one type of tort. **Malpractice** refers to any professional misconduct, but its use in legal terms typically refers to professional negligence.
2. To be successful in a malpractice suit, the patient-plaintiff must prove four elements of negligence (Table 5-1).
3. Although the burden of proof of causation ordinarily falls on the patient-plaintiff, it may, under special circumstances, be shifted to the physician-defendant under the doctrine of *res ipsa loquitur* ("the thing speaks for itself") (Table 5-2).
4. **Damages** in a malpractice suit are characterized as **general damages** (pain and suffering as a direct result of the injury), **special damages** (medical expenses, lost income), and **punitive damages** (rarely invoked in malpractice suits). Determining the dollar amount of damages is the responsibility of the jury.

B. Standard of Care
1. Because medical malpractice usually involves issues beyond the comprehension of lay jurors and judges,

TABLE 5-1
ELEMENTS REQUIRED TO PROVE MALPRACTICE

Duty (established when patient seen preoperatively, expected by patient that anesthesiologist will adhere to the standard of care)

Breach of duty (determined often by expert witnesses)

Causation (judge and juries determine if the breach of duty was the proximate cause of the injury)

Damages (breach of standard of care was the cause of damage)

the court establishes the standard of care in a particular case by the testimony of **expert witnesses**.
2. Expert witnesses differ from factual witnesses mainly in that they may give opinions.
3. The trial court judge has sole discretion in determining whether a witness may be qualified as an expert.

C. **Causes of Suits**
1. The leading causes of injuries for which suits are filed against anesthesiologists are death, nerve damage (spinal cord injury, peripheral nerve injury), and brain damage. The causes of death and brain damage most often reflect airway management problems. Nerve damage, especially to the ulnar nerve, often occurs despite apparently adequate positioning. Chronic pain management is an increasing source of malpractice claims against anesthesiologists.
2. The anesthesiologist is more likely to be the target of a lawsuit if an untoward outcome of a procedure occurs because the physician-patient relationship is often incomplete (the patient rarely chooses the anesthesiologist, the preoperative visit is brief, and a different anesthesiologist may administer the anesthesia).

D. **What to Do If Sued** (Table 5-3)

TABLE 5-2
ELEMENTS NECESSARY TO PROVE *RES IPSA LOQUITUR*

The injury would not typically occur in the absence of negligence.

The injury was caused by something under the exclusive control of the anesthesiologist.

The injury must not be attributable to any contribution on the part of the patient.

The evidence for the explanation of events is more accessible to the anesthesiologist than to the patient.

TABLE 5-3
STEPS TO TAKE WHEN NAMED IN A LAWSUIT

Do not discuss the case with others.
Never alter any records.
Gather all pertinent records.
Make notes relating to your recall of events.
Work closely with your attorney.

II. RISK MANAGEMENT AND QUALITY IMPROVEMENT

A. Aspects of risk management most directly relevant to the liability exposure of the anesthesiologist include prevention of patient injury, adherence to standards of care, documentation, and patient relations.

B. Important factors in the prevention of patient injury are vigilance, up-to-date knowledge, adequate monitoring (American Society of Anesthesiologists [ASA] Standards for Basic Anesthetic Monitoring; see Appendix D), equipment checklists, and equipment maintenance with documentation of service performed. The ASA Web site may be reviewed for any changes in ASA Standards of Practice as well as a review of ASA Guidelines.

C. If a critical incident occurs during the conduct of an anesthetic, it is helpful to write a note in the patient's medical record describing the event, drugs used, time sequence, and who was present.

D. Whenever an anesthetic complication becomes apparent postoperatively, appropriate consultation should be obtained and the department or institutional risk management group should be notified. If the complication is likely to lead to prolonged hospitalization or permanent injury, the liability insurance carrier should be notified.

E. **Jehovah's Witnesses**
   1. Patients have well-established rights, and among these is the right to refuse specific treatment because of religious beliefs.
   2. As a general rule, physicians are not obligated to treat all patients who seek treatment in elective situations. Emergency medical care imposes greater constraints on the treating physician, because there is no opportunity to provide continuity of care in a

TABLE 5-4
SOURCES OF INPUT FOR THE NATIONAL PRACTITIONER DATA BANK

Medical malpractice payments (any payment made on behalf of a physician in response to a written complaint or claim)
License actions by medical boards
Professional review or clinical privilege actions taken by hospitals and other health care entities (professional societies)
Actions taken by the Drug Enforcement Agency
Medicare/Medicaid exclusions

life-threatening situation without the initial physician's continued involvement.

3. Exceptions to patients' rights include parturients and adults who are the sole support of minor children. In these instances, it may be necessary to seek a court order to proceed with a refused medical therapy such as a blood transfusion.

F. **National Practitioner Data Bank** (Table 5-4)

III. QUALITY IMPROVEMENT IN ANESTHESIA PRACTICE

A. It is generally accepted that attention to quality will improve patient safety and satisfaction with anesthesia care.

B. Quality improvement programs are generally guided by requirements of the Joint Commission on Accreditation of Healthcare Organizations (JCAHO).

C. **Structure, Process, and Outcome: The Building Blocks of Quality**

1. Although quality of care is difficult to define, it is generally accepted that it is composed of three components: structure (setting in which care is provided), process of care (pre-anesthetic evaluation plus continual attendance and monitoring during anesthesia), and outcome.

2. A quality improvement program focuses on measuring and improving these basic components of care.

3. Continuous quality improvement (CQI) focuses on system errors (controllable and solvable) as opposed to random errors (difficult to prevent).

   a. A CQI program may focus on undesirable outcomes as a way to identify opportunities for improvement in the structure and process of care (peer review is critical to this process).

   b. An extension of CQI is total quality management (TQM), which extends beyond patient care to include all aspects of the patient care delivery system.

D. **Difficulty of Outcome Measurement in Anesthesia**

   1. Improvement in quality of care is often measured by a decrease in the rate of adverse outcomes.

   2. Adverse outcomes are rare in anesthesia, making measurement of improvement difficult. To complement outcome measurements, anesthesia CQI programs can focus on critical incidents (events that cause or have the potential to cause patient injury if not noticed or corrected in a timely manner [ventilator disconnect]), sentinel events (isolated events that may indicate a systems problem [syringe swap with subsequent analysis of confusing labeling]), and human errors (inevitable yet potentially preventable by appropriate system safeguards).

E. **JCAHO Requirement for Quality Improvement**

   1. Anesthesia care is an important function of patient care that has been identified by the JCAHO. It is important that policies and procedures for administration of anesthesia be consistent in all locations within the hospital. Specific JCAHO standards address pre-anesthetic assessment and planning, informed consent, intraoperative monitoring, and postanesthesia recovery.

   2. In 2004, JCAHO adopted patient safety goals for accredited organizations (Table 5-5).

   3. JCAHO requires all sentinel events to undergo Root Cause Analysis.

TABLE 5-5

JCAHO PATIENT SAFETY GOALS FOR ACCREDITED ORGANIZATIONS

Improved accuracy of patient identification
Improved effectiveness of communication among caregivers
Elimination of wrong site/wrong procedure surgery
Improved safety of infusion pumps
Improved effectiveness of clinical alarm systems

   F. **Measuring Quality: Approaches to Data Collection**
1. Methods for collection of CQI data in anesthesia include retrospective records review and self-reporting by the care providers that track critical incidents and sentinel events.
2. Standardization of definitions (hypotension, blood loss) is important.

   G. **Peer review** is an integral part of quality improvement programs and refers to the review of cases by members of one's specialty. This is commonly integrated into a quality improvement program in the context of the mortality and morbidity conference.

IV. MORTALITY AND MAJOR MORBIDITY RELATED TO ANESTHESIA (Tables 5-6 and 5-7)

TABLE 5-6

RECENT ESTIMATES OF ANESTHESIA-RELATED DEATH

Time period	Country	Data sources/methods	Anesthesia-related death
1989–1999	United States	Cardiac arrests within 24 hours of surgery (72,959 anesthetics) in a teaching hospital	0.55/10,000 anesthetics
1992–1994	United States	Suburban teaching hospital anesthetics and 115 deaths) (37,924 anesthetics)	0.79/10,000 anesthetics
1995–1999	United States	Urban teaching hospital (146,548 anesthetics and 232 deaths)	0.75/10,000 anesthetics
1995–1997	Holland	All deaths within 24 hours or patients who remained comatose 24 hours postoperatively (869,483 anesthetics and 811 deaths)	1.4/10,000 anesthetics
1990–1995	Western Australia	Deaths within 48 hours or deaths in which anesthesia was considered a contributing factor	1/40,000 anesthetics
1994–1996	Australia	Deaths reported to the committee (8,500,000 anesthetics)	0.16/10,000 anesthetics
1992–2002	Japan	Deaths because of life-threatening events in the operating room (3,855,384 anesthetics) in training hospitals	0.1/10,000 anesthetics
1994–1998	Japan	Questionnaires to training hospitals (2,363,038 anesthetics)	0.21/10,000 anesthetics
1989–1995	France	ASA 1–4 patients undergoing anesthesia (101,769 anesthetics and 24 cardiac arrests within 12 hours postanesthesia)	0.6/10,000 anesthetics
1994–1997	United States	Pediatric patients from 63 hospitals (1,089,200 anesthetics)	0.36/10,000 anesthetics

TABLE 5-7
RATES OF SELECTED ANESTHESIA COMPLICATIONS

Complication	Time period	Country	Specific complication	Results
Nerve injury	1995	United States	Ulnar neuropathy following noncardiac surgery	0.5%
	1995–1997	United States	Persistent ulnar neuropathy following patients diagnostic or noncardiac procedures with anesthesia	1/2729
	1980–1981	United States	Ulnar neuropathy after general anesthesia	0.26%
	1957–1991	United States	Lower extremity motor neuropathy following surgery in lithotomy position	1/3608
Awareness and recall	1997–1998	Sweden	Awareness and recall associated with general anesthesia procedures	18/11,785
	1990	Great Britain	Awareness with recall in adults following surgery	0.2%
	1994–1995	Finland	Awareness in patients >12 years old having general anesthesia	0.4%
Eye injuries and visual changes	1999	United States	New onset blurred vision lasting >3 days	4.2%
	1986–1998	United States	New onset visual loss or visual changes lasting >30 days after noncardiac surgery	1,125,234
Dental injury	1988–1992	United States	Eye injury after nonocular surgery	0.056%
	1987–1997	United States	Dental injuries within 7 days of anesthesia patients that required intervention	1/4537

CHAPTER 6 ■ CELLULAR AND MOLECULAR MECHANISMS OF ANESTHESIA

Despite the importance of general anesthesia and more than 100 years of active research, the molecular mechanisms responsible for anesthetic action remain one of the unsolved mysteries of pharmacology (Evers AS, Crowder CM: Cellular and molecular mechanisms of anesthesia. In Barash PG, Cullen BF, Stoelting RK [eds]: *Clinical Anesthesia*, pp 111–132. Philadelphia, Lippincott Williams & Wilkins, 2006). Molecular and genetic tools are becoming available that should allow for major insights into anesthetic mechanisms in the next decade. A wide variety of structurally unrelated compounds (steroids to elemental xenon) are capable of producing anesthesia suggesting that multiple molecular mechanisms may be operative.

I. WHAT IS ANESTHESIA?

A. The components of the anesthetic state include unconsciousness, amnesia, analgesia, immobility, and attenuation of autonomic nervous system responses to noxious stimulation.

B. Anesthesia is always defined by drug-induced changes in behavior or perception. As such, anesthesia can only be defined and measured in the intact organism.

II. HOW IS ANESTHESIA MEASURED?

A. To study the pharmacology of anesthetic action, a quantitative measurement of anesthetic potency is essential. This is provided in the concept of minimum alveolar concentration (MAC).

   1. MAC is defined as the alveolar partial pressure (PA) of a gas (end-tidal concentration) at which 50% of humans will not move in response to a surgical skin incision (in animals, in response to a noxious stimulus such as a tail clamp).

      a. MAC is the standard for determining the potency of volatile anesthetics.

   b. MAC is reproducible and constant over a wide range of species.
   c. The quantal nature of MAC (either anesthetized or not anesthetized with no partially anesthetized data point possible) makes it difficult to compare MAC measurements with concentration-response curves obtained in vitro.
2. A MAC equivalent for intravenous anesthetics is the plasma concentration of the drug required to prevent movement in response to a noxious stimulus in 50% of subjects.
3. The PA is an accurate reflection of the anesthetic concentration in the plasma and brain tissue at 37°C.

III. WHERE IN THE CENTRAL NERVOUS SYSTEM DO ANESTHETICS WORK?

A. Plausible sites of action of general anesthetics include the spinal cord, brainstem, and cerebral cortex. Peripheral sensory receptors are not important sites of anesthetic action.
B. Spinal Cord
   1. The spinal cord is probably the site at which anesthetics act to inhibit purposeful responses to noxious stimulation (end-point for determination of MAC).
   2. Anesthetic actions at the spinal cord cannot explain either amnesia or unconsciousness.
C. Reticular Activating System
   1. It has long been speculated that the reticular activating system, a diffuse collection of brainstem neurons, is involved in the effects of general anesthetics on consciousness.
   2. A role for the brainstem in anesthetic action is supported by changes in somatosensory evoked potentials (increased latency and decreased amplitude indicating that anesthetics inhibit information transfer through the brainstem).
   3. Within the reticular formation is a set of pontine noradrenergic neurons (locus coeruleus) that innervates a number of targets in the basal forebrain and cortex. It is likely that the tuberomammillary nucleus and its associated pathway are sites of sedative action of anesthetics (propofol, barbiturates) that act on γ-aminobutyric acid (GABA) receptors.

D. **Cerebral Cortex.** Anesthetics alter cortical electrical activity as evidenced by the consistent changes in surface electroencephalogram patterns recorded during anesthesia. Inhalation anesthetics may depress the excitability of thalamic neurons, thus blocking thalamocortical communication and inducing loss of consciousness.
E. There is no basis for identifying a single anatomic site responsible for anesthesia.

IV. HOW DO ANESTHETICS INTERFERE WITH THE ELECTROPHYSIOLOGIC FUNCTION OF THE NERVOUS SYSTEM?

A. There are multiple mechanisms by which anesthetics could inhibit vital central nervous system (CNS) functions.
   1. **Pattern Generators.** Evidence that clinical concentrations of anesthetics have effects on pattern-generating neuronal circuits in the CNS is provided by the observation that most anesthetics exert profound effects on frequency and pattern of breathing (respiratory pattern generators in the brainstem).
   2. **Neuronal Excitability.** Evidence indicates that anesthetics can hyperpolarize (create a more negative resting membrane potential) spinal motor neurons and cortical neurons.
   3. **Synaptic function** is widely considered to be the most likely subcellular site of general anesthetic action. Neurotransmission across both excitatory and inhibitory synapses is markedly altered by general anesthetics.
      a. Enhancement of inhibitory transmission is observed with propofol, etomidate, and inhalational anesthetics.
      b. Clinical concentrations of general anesthetics can depress inhibitory postsynaptic potentials in the hippocampus and spinal cord.
      c. **Presynaptic effects.** Neurotransmitter release from glutamatergic synapses is inhibited by clinical concentrations of volatile anesthetics.
      d. **Postsynaptic effects.** A wide variety of anesthetics (barbiturates, etomidate, propofol, volatile

anesthetics) affect synaptic function by enhancing the postsynaptic response to GABA.

B. **Anesthetic Actions on Ion Channels.** Ion channels are one likely target of anesthetic action. Ion channels can be described according to the stimuli to which they respond by opening or closing (mechanism of gating).

 1. **Anesthetic Effects on Voltage-Dependent Ion Channels**
    a. The notion that voltage-dependent sodium channels are insensitive to anesthetics may not be correct.
    b. **Voltage-dependent calcium channels** serve to couple electrical activity to specific cellular functions, usually by opening to allow calcium to enter the cell and by activating calcium-dependent secretion of neurotransmitters into the synaptic cleft. Anesthetics inhibit these channels at concentrations estimated to be two to five times that necessary to produce anesthesia (this insensitivity makes these channels unlikely major targets of anesthetic action).
    c. **Potassium channels** include voltage-gated second-messenger and ligand-activated inward-rectifying channels. High concentrations of volatile and intravenous anesthetics are required to affect the function of voltage-gated potassium channels. Rectifying potassium channels are relatively insensitive to sevoflurane and barbiturates.

 2. **Anesthetic Effects on Ligand-Gated Channels.** Selective effects of anesthetics on these channels could influence excitatory and inhibitory neurotransmission in the CNS.
    a. **Glutamate-activated ion channels** include N-methyl-D-aspartate (NMDA) receptors to which ketamine (not other anesthetics) selectively binds, suggesting that this receptor may be the principal molecular target for the anesthetic actions of this drug.
    b. **GABA-activated ion channels** mediate the postsynaptic response to GABA (the most important inhibitory neurotransmitter in the CNS) by selectively allowing chloride ions to enter and

thereby hyperpolarize neurons. $GABA_A$ receptors are probable molecular targets for anesthetics. Barbiturates, benzodiazepines, etomidate, propofol, and volatile anesthetics all modulate $GABA_A$ receptor function.

C. **Anesthetic Effects on Second Messenger–Activated Ion Channels**
   1. A variety of substances, referred to as chemical second messengers (cyclic nucleotides, calcium ions, hydrogen ions, inositol phosphates, adenosine triphosphate), are known to modulate the function of ion channels.
   2. Calcium-dependent potassium channels are inhibited by clinical concentrations of anesthetics that may contribute to excitatory effects of low concentrations of anesthetics and to the convulsant properties of some anesthetic agents.

V. WHAT IS THE CHEMICAL NATURE OF ANESTHETIC TARGET SITES?

A. **The Meyer-Overton Rule**
   1. Although there is a consensus that anesthetics act by affecting the function of ion channels, considerable controversy remains as to the molecular interactions underlying these functional effects.
   2. Because a wide variety of structurally unrelated compounds obey the Meyer-Overton rule (potency of anesthetic gases is correlated with their solubility in olive oil), it has been reasoned that all anesthetics are likely to act at the same molecular site (unitary theory of anesthesia).
   3. The anesthetic site is likely to be amphipathic, having both polar and nonpolar characteristics.
   4. **Exceptions to the Meyer-Overton Rule**
      a. Halogenated compounds exist (fluorothyl) that are structurally similar to the inhaled anesthetics but are convulsants rather than anesthetics.
      b. In the series of *n*-alkanols, anesthetic potency increases from methanol dodecanol, and all longer alkanols lack anesthetic properties (cutoff effect).
      c. Compounds that deviate from the Meyer-Overton rule suggest that anesthetic target sites are also defined by other properties, including size and shape.

      d. The fact that enantiomers of anesthetics differ in their potency as anesthetics argues against the Meyer-Overton rule and favors a protein-binding site.

   5. Pressure Reversal. Evidence indicates that pressure reverses anesthesia by producing excitation that physiologically counteracts depression rather than by acting as an anesthetic antagonist at the anesthetic site of action.

B. Lipid Versus Protein Targets. There are several possible molecular targets that anesthetics might interact with to produce their effects on the function of ion channels and other proteins. Anesthetics might dissolve in the lipid bilayer, causing physiochemical changes in the membrane structure that alter the ability of membrane proteins to undergo conformational changes important for their function. Alternatively, anesthetics could bind directly to proteins (either ion channels or modulatory proteins) so as to interfere with binding of a neurotransmitter or the ability of the protein to undergo conformational changes important for its function.

   1. Lipid Theories of Anesthesia

      a. The lipid theory of anesthesia postulates that anesthetics dissolve in lipid bilayers of biologic membranes and produce anesthesia when they reach a critical concentration in the membrane (membrane–gas solubility coefficients of anesthetic gases in pure lipids correlate with anesthetic potency).

      b. Membrane perturbation. More sophisticated versions of the lipid theory require that anesthetic molecules cause perturbation in the properties of the membrane.

      c. Membrane expansion. Clinical concentrations of anesthetics dissolved in membranes do increase membrane volume (critical volume hypothesis), but the small magnitude of this effect, coupled with its inability to explain the cutoff effect, make it unlikely that membrane expansion is the explanation for general anesthesia.

      d. Membrane disordering. Anesthetics can disorder the packing of phospholipids in biologic membranes (increase membrane fluidity). These changes produced by anesthetics can be mimicked by changes in temperature of $<1°C$, making it unlikely that this is the explanation for general anesthesia.

2. **Protein Theories of Anesthesia**
   a. The Meyer-Overton rule may also be explained by the interaction of anesthetics with hydrophobic sites on protein. Direct interactions of anesthetic molecules with proteins would also provide explanations for exceptions from this rule, because any protein-binding site is likely to be defined by properties such as size and shape in addition to its solvent properties.
   b. **Evidence for anesthetic binding to proteins.** A variety of physical techniques (x-ray diffraction, nuclear magnetic resonance spectroscopy) have confirmed that anesthetic molecules can bind in the hydrophobic core of proteins and the size of the binding site can account for the cutoff effect.
   c. **Direct evidence for anesthetic binding to proteins** is stereoselectivity.
3. Current evidence strongly supports proteins rather than lipids as the molecular targets for anesthetic action.

VI. HOW ARE THE EFFECTS OF ANESTHETICS ON MOLECULAR TARGETS LINKED TO ANESTHESIA IN THE INTACT ORGANISM?

A. It is likely that anesthetics affect the function of a number of ion channels and signaling proteins, probably via direct anesthetic–protein interactions. A number of approaches have been used to try to link anesthetic effects observed at a molecular level to anesthesia in intact animals.

B. **Pharmacological Approaches**
1. α-2 agonists decrease halothane MAC but also have their own inherent CNS depressant effects.
2. Development of a specific antagonist for anesthetics would provide a useful tool for linking anesthetic effects at the molecular level to anesthesia in the intact organism.
3. Evidence is consistent with the conclusion that volatile anesthetics affect the function of a large number of important neuronal proteins and no one

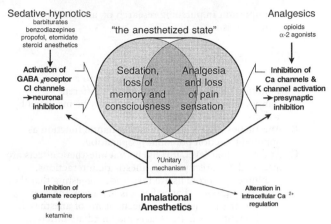

FIGURE 6-1. Multiple sites of action model for the mechanism of anesthesia. The model proposes that presynaptic inhibition (calcium channel inhibition and potassium channel activation) are responsible for analgesic effects, whereas postsynaptic GABA$_A$ receptor activation is responsible for sedation and amnesia. The overlapping circles indicate that these two different mechanisms of action are not mutually exclusive; some anesthetic drugs exert predominant effects on calcium and potassium channels and some exert predominant effects on GABA$_A$ receptors, whereas volatile anesthetics influence both. Inhibition of glutamate receptor function is an alternative pathway by which ketamine and perhaps the volatile anesthetics produce anesthesia.

    target is likely to mediate all of the effects of these drugs.

  C. Genetic Approaches. Genetic techniques that alter structure of the putative anesthetic targets may result in changes in sensitivity to anesthetics (known to exist between individuals and animal species).

    1. Inhibition of excitatory neurotransmitter release may be important in anesthetic action.

    2. Experiments involving GABA$_A$ receptors and model anesthetic binding proteins have demonstrated that single amino acid changes can drastically alter anesthetic potency or affinity.

    3. The GABA α-1 subunit mediates the sedative and amnestic actions of benzodiazepines.

    4. The demonstration that the general anesthetic actions of propofol and etomidate can be blocked by a single mutation in a subunit of GABA$_A$ receptors is

important in pursuing research on anesthetic
mechanisms.

VII. CONCLUSIONS

A. Anesthetic actions cannot be localized to a specific
anatomic site in the CNS, but in fact different
components of the anesthetic state may be mediated by
actions at disparate sites.
B. Anesthetics preferentially affect synaptic function as
opposed to action potential propagation.
C. At a molecular level, it is likely that anesthetic effects are
mediated by direct protein–anesthetic interactions.
   1. Numerous proteins are involved, suggesting that the
   unitary theory of anesthesia is incorrect and that
   there are at least several mechanisms of anesthesia.
   2. Different anesthetic targets may mediate different
   components of the anesthetic state (Fig. 6-1).

CHAPTER 7 ■ GENOMIC BASIS OF PERIOPERATIVE MEDICINE

I. **GENETIC BASIS OF DISEASE.** Human biological diversity involves interindividual variability in morphology, behavior, physiology, development, susceptibility to disease, and response to stressful stimuli and drug therapy (*phenotypes*) (Podgoreanu MV, Mathew JP: Genomic basis of perioperative medicine. In Barash PG, Cullen BF, Stoelting RK [eds]: *Clinical Anesthesia*, pp 133–148. Philadelphia, Lippincott Williams and Wilkins, 2006). This phenotypic variation is determined, at least in part, by differences in the specific genetic makeup (*genotype*) of an individual. Completion of the Human Genome Project provides the discipline of genomics with basic resources to study the functions and interactions of all genes in a systematic fashion, including their interaction with environmental factors, and to translate the findings into clinical and societal benefits. To integrate this new generation of genetic results into clinical practice, perioperative physicians need to understand the patterns of human genome variation, the methods of population-based genetic investigation, and the principles of gene and protein expression analysis.

A. **Overview of Human Genetic Variation.** Although the human DNA sequence is 99.9% identical between individuals, the variations may greatly affect a person's disease risk. Rare genetic variants (*mutations*) are responsible for monogenic disorders (hypertrophic cardiomyopathy, long-QT syndrome, sickle cell anemia). Most of the genetic diversity in the population is attributable to more widespread DNA sequence variations (*polymorphisms*), which can be either nucleotide base substitutions (*single nucleotide polymorphisms*, SNPs), short sequence repeats (*microsatellites*), or insertion/deletion of one or more nucleotides (*indels*), and may or may not be associated with a specific phenotype (Fig. 7-1). Complex phenotypes can be viewed as the integrated effect of many susceptibility genes and many environmental exposures

(Fig. 7-2). The proportion of phenotypic variance that is the result of genetic factors is referred to as *heritability*.
B. **Genetic Analysis of Complex Disease.** Most ongoing research on complex disorders focuses on identifying genetic polymorphisms that enhance susceptibility to given conditions. Both the candidate gene and genome scan approaches can be implemented using one of two fundamental methods of identifying polymorphisms

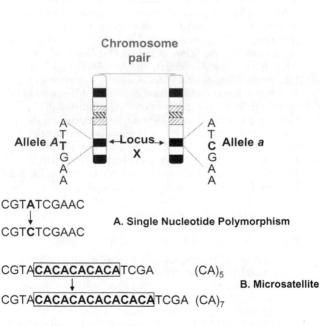

FIGURE 7-1. Categories of genetic polymorphisms. **A.** *Single nucleotide polymorphism (SNP)* can be silent or have functional consequences ranging from changes in amino acid sequence to premature termination of protein synthesis. **B.** *Microsatellite polymorphism* with varying number of dinucleotide (CA) repeats. **C.** *Insertion/deletion polymorphism. Locus*—the location of a gene/genetic marker in the genome; *alleles*—alternative forms of a gene/genetic marker; *genotype*—the observed alleles for an individual at a genetic locus; *heterozygous*—two different alleles are present at a locus; *homozygous*—two identical alleles are present at a locus.

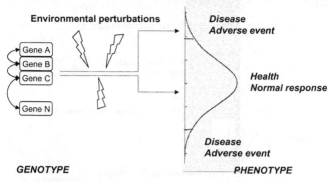

FIGURE 7-2. Common diseases (coronary artery disease, hypertension, diabetes, cancer) and individual responses to various perturbations (drug administration, hemodynamic challenge, surgical stress, trauma) are complex, involving multiple gene–gene interactions (*polygenic*) and gene-environment interactions (*multifactorial*) to produce a final clinical outcome, or *phenotype.*

affecting common diseases: linkage analysis or association studies in human populations.

1. **Linkage analysis** is used to identify the chromosomal location of gene variants related to a given disease. This approach has been used successfully to map hundreds of genes for rare, monogenic disorders.

2. **Genetic association studies** examine the frequency of specific genetic polymorphisms in a population-based sample of unrelated diseased individuals and appropriately matched unaffected controls. Accumulating evidence suggests that specific genotypes are associated with a variety of organ-specific perioperative adverse outcomes, including neurocognitive dysfunction, renal compromise, vein graft restenosis, postoperative thrombosis, vascular reactivity, and death.

C. **Large-Scale Gene and Protein Expression Profiling.** Genomic approaches are anchored in the concept of transcription of messenger RNA (mRNA) from a DNA template, followed by translation of RNA into protein (Fig. 7-3). While the human genome contains only about 30,000 genes, it is believed that there are approximately 200,000 distinct proteins in humans. Preconditioning can

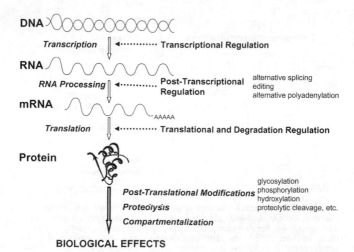

DNA

Transcription   ◄·········· **Transcriptional Regulation**

RNA

RNA Processing   ◄·········· **Post-Transcriptional Regulation**   alternative splicing / editing / alternative polyadenylation

mRNA

Translation   ◄·········· **Translational and Degradation Regulation**

Protein

Post-Translational Modifications   glycosylation / phosphorylation / hydroxylation / proteolytic cleavage, etc.
Proteolysis
Compartmentalization

BIOLOGICAL EFFECTS

FIGURE 7-3. Central dogma of molecular biology. Protein expression involves two main processes, RNA synthesis (*transcription*) and protein synthesis (*translation*), with many intermediate regulatory steps.

be induced by various triggers including intermittent ischemia, osmotic or redox stress, heat shock, toxins, and interestingly, inhaled anesthetics. *Proteomics* is the study of the sequence, modification, and function of all proteins in a biological system at a given time. Integrated genomic and proteomic data analysis may be applied in perioperative medicine to elucidate individual responses to surgical injury and provide useful prognostic information.

II. GENOMICS AND PERIOPERATIVE PROFILING.

Perioperative complications are significant, costly, variably reported, and often imprecisely detected. There is a critical need for accurate, comprehensive perioperative outcome databases. There is striking variability in patient responses to surgical procedures, anesthetic agents, hemodynamic challenge, and the pharmacopoeia used in the perioperative period. It is becoming increasingly recognized that specific genotypes may also predict adverse perioperative outcomes in otherwise healthy individuals. Such adverse outcomes will develop only in patients whose combined burden of genetic and environmental risk factors exceeds a certain threshold, which may vary with age.

A. **Genetic Susceptibility to Adverse Perioperative Cardiovascular Outcomes.** It is commonly accepted that patients who have underlying cardiovascular disease are at risk for adverse cardiac events after surgery, but identifying patients at the highest risk of perioperative myocardial infarction remains difficult. There is a proven role for genetic influences in the incidence and progression of coronary artery disease (CAD). On a genetic level, functional allelic variations likely modulate, each with a small overall contribution and relative risk, individual susceptibility to develop such adverse myocardial events, and the manifestation, severity, and prognosis of the disease process. Evidence has linked various genotypes to mechanistic pathways known to be involved in triggering or modulating the severity of perioperative myocardial injury, including thrombosis, inflammatory response, or vascular reactivity. The acute phase response or stress response to surgery is characterized by an increase in fibrinogen concentration, platelet adhesiveness, and plasminogen activator inhibitor-1 (PAI-1) production. One of the most common inherited prothrombotic risk factors is a point mutation in coagulation factor V resulting in resistance to activated protein C. Genetic variants modulating the magnitude of the postoperative inflammatory response have been identified. Variability in the β-2-adrenergic receptor gene has been associated with increased mean arterial blood pressure to the stress stimuli of tracheal intubation.

B. **Genetic Variability and Perioperative Event-Free Survival.** Increasing evidence suggests that the ACE gene indel polymorphism may influence post-CABG complications. A functionally important amino acid alteration in the β-3 integrin chain of the glycoprotein IIb/IIIa platelet receptor (PlA2 polymorphism) is associated with an increased risk (odds ratio of 4:7) for major adverse cardiac events (may be related to a genetically modulated prothrombotic tendency).

C. **Genetic Susceptibility to Adverse Perioperative Neurologic Outcomes.** Despite advances in surgical and anesthetic techniques, significant neurologic morbidity continues to occur following cardiac surgery (remains poorly explained by procedural risk factors, suggesting that environmental and genetic factors may interact to determine disease onset, progression, and recovery). The pathophysiology of perioperative neurological injury is thought to involve complex interactions between primary pathways associated with atherosclerosis and thrombosis, and secondary response pathways like inflammation, vascular reactivity, and direct cellular injury. Many functional genetic variants have been reported in each of these mechanistic pathways involved in modulating the magnitude and the response to neurological injury, which may have implications in chronic as well as acute perioperative neurocognitive outcomes. There may be a role for platelet activation in the pathophysiology of adverse neurological sequelae. Genetic variants in surface platelet membrane glycoproteins, important mediators of platelet adhesion and platelet–platelet interactions, have been shown to increase the susceptibility to prothrombotic events.

D. **Genetic Susceptibility to Adverse Perioperative Renal Outcomes.** Acute renal dysfunction is a common, serious complication of cardiac surgery. Inheritance of certain genetic polymorphisms is associated with acute renal injury following CABG surgery.

E. **Genetic Variants and Risk for Prolonged Postoperative Mechanical Ventilation.** Prolonged mechanical ventilation (inability to extubat patient by 24 hours postoperatively) is a significant complication following cardiac surgery, and genetic variants in the renin–angiotensin pathway and in proinflammatory cytokine genes have been associated with respiratory complications post cardiopulmonary bypass. A next crucial step in understanding the complexity of adverse perioperative outcomes is to assess the contribution of variations in many genes simultaneously and their interaction with traditional risk factors to the longitudinal prediction of outcomes in individual patients.

III. PHARMACOGENOMICS AND ANESTHESIA.
Pharmacogenomics is used to describe how inherited variations in genes modulating drug actions are related to interindividual variability in drug response. Such variability in drug action may be pharmacokinetic or pharmacodynamic (Fig. 7-4).

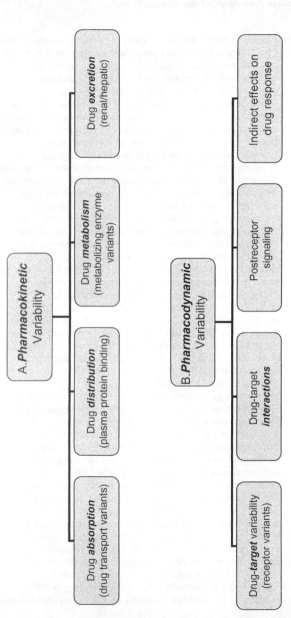

FIGURE 7-4. Pharmacogenomic determinants of individual drug responses operate by pharmacokinetic and pharmacodynamic mechanisms.

A. **Pseudocholinesterase Deficiency**. Characterization of the genetic basis for plasma pseudocholinesterase deficiency in 1956 was of fundamental importance to anesthesia and the further development and understanding of genetically determined differences in drug response. More than 20 variants have since been identified in the butyrylcholinesterase gene, and pharmacogenetic testing is currently not recommended in the population at large, but only as an explanation for an adverse event.

B. **Genetics of Malignant Hyperthermia**. Malignant hyperthermia (MH) is a rare autosomal dominant genetic disease of skeletal muscle calcium metabolism, triggered by administration of general anesthesia with volatile anesthetic agents or succinylcholine in susceptible individuals. It is becoming increasingly apparent that MH susceptibility results from a complex interaction between multiple genes and the environment (such as environmental toxins). Because of the polygenic determinism and variable penetrance, direct DNA testing in the general population for susceptibility to MH is currently not recommended whereas testing in individuals from families with affected individuals has the potential to greatly reduce mortality and morbidity.

C. **Genetic Variability and Response to Anesthetic Agents**. Anesthetic potency as defined by the minimum alveolar concentration (MAC) of an inhaled anesthetic varies approximately 10% among individuals. This observed variability may be explained by interindividual differences in multiple genes that underlie responsiveness to anesthetics, by environmental or physiological factors (brain temperature, age), or by measurement errors. Evidence of a genetic basis for increased anesthetic requirements is suggested by the observation that desflurane requirements are increased in subjects with red hair versus dark hair. Genetic approaches have been used in mammalian models to provide mechanistic insight into the molecular basis of anesthetic action in humans utilizing animal models (transgenic, knockout, and knock in animals). Inhaled anesthetics appear to mediate their effects by acting on several receptor targets. Unlikely receptors for MAC include the $GABA_A$ (despite their compelling role in IV anesthetic-induced immobility), 5-HT3, AMPA, kainate, acetylcholine and α–2 adrenergic receptors, and potassium channels. Glycine, NMDA receptors, and sodium channels remain likely candidates.

D. **Genetic Variability and Response to Pain.** Similar to the observed variability in anesthetic potency, the response to painful stimuli and analgesic manipulations varies among individuals. The sources of variability in the report and experience of pain and analgesia are multifactorial, including factors extrinsic to the organism (cultural factors, or circadian rhythms) and intrinsic factors (age, gender, hormonal status, or genetic makeup). Furthermore, pain behavior in response to noxious stimuli and its modulation by the central nervous system in response to drug administration or environmental stimuli may be strongly influenced by genetic factors. In addition to genetic control of peripheral nociceptive pathways, considerable evidence exists for genetic variability in the descending central pain modulatory pathways, potentially explaining the interindividual variability in analgesic responsiveness.

E. **Genetic Variability in Response to Other Drugs Used Perioperatively** (Table 7-1). There are more than 30 families of drug-metabolizing enzymes in humans, most with genetic polymorphisms shown to influence enzymatic activity. Of special importance to anesthesiologists is the *CYP2D6*, which is involved in the metabolism of several drugs including analgesics (codeine, dextromethorphan), cardiac antidysrhythmics (flecainide, propafenone, quinidine), and diltiazem. Genetic variation in drug targets (receptors) can have profound effects on drug efficacy. Carriers of certain susceptibility alleles have no manifest QT-interval prolongation or family history of sudden death until a QT-prolonging drug challenge is superimposed. Predisposition to QT-interval prolongation (considered a surrogate for risk of life-threatening ventricular arrhythmias) has been responsible for more drug withdrawals from the market than any other category of adverse event.

IV. GENOMICS AND CRITICAL CARE

A. **Genetic Variability in Response to Injury.** Systemic injury (including trauma and surgical stress), shock, or infection trigger physiological responses of fever, tachycardia, tachypnea, and leukocytosis that collectively define the systemic inflammatory response syndrome. The large interindividual variability in the magnitude of response

TABLE 7-1

EXAMPLES OF GENETIC POLYMORPHISMS INVOLVED IN VARIABLE RESPONSES TO DRUGS USED IN THE PERIOPERATIVE PERIOD

Drug class	Gene name (gene symbol)	Effect of polymorphism
Pharmacokinetic variability		
β-blockers	Cytochrome P450 2D6 (CYP2D6)	Enhanced drug effect
Codeine, dextromethorphan	CYP2D6	Decreased drug effect
Ca-channel blockers	Cytochrome P450 3A4 (CYP3A4)	Uncertain
Alfentanil	CYP3A4	Enhanced drug response
Angiotensin-II receptor type 1 blockers	Cytochrome P450 2C9 (CYP2C9)	Enhanced blood pressure response
Warfarin	CYP2C9	Enhanced anticoagulant effect, risk of bleeding
Phenytoin	CYP2C9	Enhanced drug effect
ACE-inhibitors	Angiotensin-I converting enzyme (ACE)	Blood pressure response
Procainamide	N-acetyltransferase 2 (NAT2)	Enhanced drug effect
Succinylcholine	Butyrylcholinesterase (BCHE)	Enhanced drug effect
Digoxin	P-glycoprotein (ABCB1, MDR1)	Increased bioavailability
Pharmacodynamic variability		
β-blockers	β–1 and β–2 adrenergic receptors (ADRB1, ADRB2)	Blood pressure and heart rate response, airway responsiveness to β-2 agonists
QT-prolonging drugs (antiarrhythmics, cisapride)	Sodium and potassium ion channels (SCN5A, KCNH2, KCNE2, KCNQ1)	Long QT syndrome, risk of *torsade de pointes* Long QT syndrome, risk of *torsade de pointes*
Aspirin, glycoprotein IIb/IIIa inhibitors	Glycoprotein IIIa subunit of platelet glycoprotein IIb/IIIa (ITGB3)	Variability in antiplatelet effects
Phenylephrine	Endothelial nitric oxide synthase (NOS3)	Blood pressure response

to injury, including activation of inflammatory and coagulation cascades, apoptosis, and fibrosis, suggests the involvement of genetic regulatory factors.

B. **Functional Genomics of Injury.** The standard "single-gene" paradigm is insufficient to adequately describe the tissue response to severe systemic stimuli. Instead, organ injury might better be defined by patterns of altered gene and protein expression.

V. FUTURE DIRECTIONS

A. **Integration of "omic" Information: System Biology Approaches.** The Human Genome Project provides the sequence of nucleotides, localization of genes, and amino acid sequences in encoded proteins. Proteomics complements genome-based approaches by enabling the identification and characterization of differential protein expression, turnover and localization, post-translational modifications, and interaction with other biological molecules.

B. **Targeted Drug Development.** Genomic and proteomic approaches are rapidly becoming platforms for all aspects of drug discovery and development. The human genome contains about 30,000 genes encoding for approximately 200,000 proteins, which represent potential drug targets.

C. **Ethical Considerations.** There is a risk for discrimination against individuals who are genetically predisposed for a medical disorder. Another ethical concern is the transferability of genetic tests across ethnic groups, particularly in the prediction of adverse drug responses as it is known that most polymorphisms associated with variability in drug response show significant differences in allele frequencies among populations and racial groups.

VI. **CONCLUSIONS.** The Human Genome Project has revolutionized all aspects of medicine, allowing us to assess the impact of genetic variability on disease taxonomy, characterization, and outcome, and individual responses to various drugs and injuries. Information gleaned through genomic approaches is already unraveling long-standing mysteries behind general anesthetic action and adverse responses to drugs used perioperatively. For the anesthesiologist, this may soon translate into prospective risk assessment incorporating genetic profiling of markers important in thrombotic, inflammatory, vascular, and neurologic responses to perioperative stress, with implications ranging from individualized additional preoperative testing and physiological optimization to choice of perioperative monitoring strategies and critical care resource utilization. Furthermore, genetic profiling of drug-metabolizing enzymes, carrier proteins, and receptors, using currently available high-throughput molecular technologies, will enable personalized choice of drugs and dosage regimens tailored to suit a patient's pharmacogenetic profile.

CHAPTER 8 ■ ELECTRICAL AND FIRE SAFETY

The myriad electronic devices in the modern operating room greatly improve patient care and safety but also subject the patient and operating room personnel to increased risks (Ehrenwerth J, Seifert HA: Electrical and fire safety. In Barash PG, Cullen BF, Stoelting RK [eds]: *Clinical Anesthesia*, pp 149–174. Philadelphia, Lippincott Williams & Wilkins, 2006).

I. PRINCIPLES OF ELECTRICITY

A. A basic principle of electricity is known as Ohm's law and is represented by the equation $E = I \times R$ (electromotive force in volts = current in amperes times resistance in ohms).
  1. Ohm's law forms the basis for the physiologic equation in which the blood pressure is equal to the cardiac output times the systemic vascular resistance (BP = CO × SVR).
  2. Electrical power is measured as watts (voltage × amperage).
B. The amount of electrical work done (watt-second or joule) is a common designation for electrical energy expended (energy produced by a defibrillator is measured in joules).

II. DIRECT AND ALTERNATING CURRENTS

A. Flow of electrons (current) through a conductor is characterized as direct current (electron flow is always in the same direction) or alternating current (electron flow reverses direction at a regular interval).
B. **Impedance** is the sum of forces that oppose electron movement in an alternating current circuit.
C. **Capacitance** is the ability of a capacitor (two parallel conductors separated by an insulator) to store charge.
  1. In a direct current circuit, the charged capacitor plates (battery) do not result in current flow unless a resistance is connected between the two plates and the capacitor is discharged.

2. Stray capacitance is capacitance that is not designed into the system but is incidental to the construction of the equipment (all alternating current operating equipment produces stray capacitance even though not turned on).

III. ELECTRICAL SHOCK HAZARDS

A. Alternating and Direct Currents

1. Whenever an individual contacts an external source of electricity, an electrical shock is possible (requires approximately three times as much direct current as alternating current to cause ventricular fibrillation).
2. A short-circuit occurs when there is zero impedance with a high current flow.

B. Source of Shocks

1. Electrical accidents or shocks occur when a person becomes part of or completes an electrical circuit (Fig. 8-1).
2. Damage from electrical current is a result of disruption of normal electrical function of cells

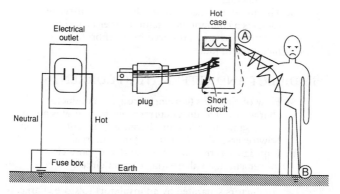

FIGURE 8-1. When a faulty piece of equipment without an equipment ground wire is plugged into an electrical outlet not containing a ground wire, the instrument case becomes energized ("hot"). If an individual touches the case (**A**), he or she will receive a shock (*dashed line* depicts path of electrical current) because he or she is standing on earth (**B**) and completes the circuit.

(skeletal muscle contracture, ventricular fibrillation) or dissipation of electrical energy (burn).

3. The severity of an electrical shock is determined by the amount of current and the duration of current flow.

   a. Macroshock describes large amounts of current flow that can cause harm or death.

   b. Microshock describes small amounts of current flow and applies only to the electrically susceptible patient (external conduit that is in direct contact with the heart [pacing wire, saline-filled central venous pressure catheter]) in whom even minute amounts of current (1 mA, which is the threshold of perception) may cause ventricular fibrillation.

4. Very high-frequency current (see Section IV) does not excite contractile tissue and does not cause cardiac dysrhythmias.

C. Grounding

   1. To fully understand electrical shock hazards and their prevention, one must have a thorough knowledge of the concepts of grounding. In electrical terminology, grounding is applied to electrical power and equipment.

   2. **Electrical Power: Grounded**

      a. Electrical utilities universally provide power to homes that are grounded (by convention, the earth ground potential is zero).

      b. Electrical shock is an inherent danger of grounded power systems (an individual standing on ground or in contact with an object that is referenced to ground needs only one additional contact point to complete the circuit).

      c. Modern wiring systems have added a third wire (low-resistance pathway through which the current can flow to ground) to decrease the severity of a potential electrical shock (Fig. 8-2).

   3. **Electrical Power: Ungrounded**

      a. The numerous electronic devices, along with power cords and puddles of saline-filled solutions on the floor, tend to make the operating room an electrically hazardous environment for both patients and personnel.

      b. In an attempt to decrease the risk of electrical shock, the power supplied to most operating

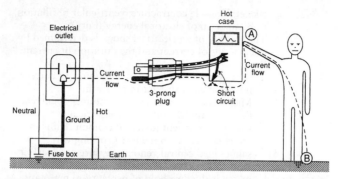

FIGURE 8-2. When a faulty piece of equipment containing an equipment ground wire is properly connected to an electrical outlet with grounding protection, the electrical current (*dashed line*) will preferentially flow down the low-resistance ground wire. An individual touching the instrument case (**A**) and standing on the earth (**B**) will still complete the circuit; however, only a small part of the current will flow through the individual.

                rooms is ungrounded (current isolated from ground).

    c. Supplying ungrounded power to the operating room requires the use of an isolation transformer (Fig. 8-3).

    d. The isolated power system provides protection from macroshock (Fig. 8-4).

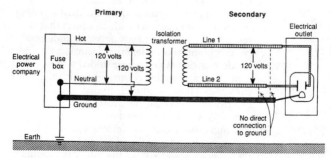

FIGURE 8-3. In the operating room, the isolation transformer converts the grounded power on the primary side to an ungrounded power system on the secondary side of the transformer. There is no direct connection from the power on the secondary side to ground. The equipment ground wire, however, is still present.

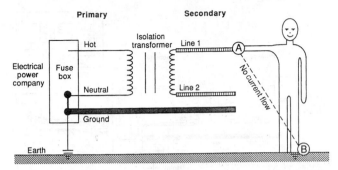

FIGURE 8-4. A safety feature of the isolated power system is illustrated. An individual contacting one side of the isolated power system (**A**) and standing on the ground (**B**) will not receive a shock. In this instance, the individual is not contacting the circuit at two points and thus is not completing the circuit.

    e. A faulty piece of equipment plugged into an isolated power system does not present a shock hazard.

D. The Line Isolation Monitor

    1. The line isolation monitor is a device that continuously monitors the integrity of the isolated power system (measures the impedance to ground on each side of the isolated power system).

    2. If a faulty piece of equipment is connected to the isolated power system, this will, in effect, change the system to a conventional grounded system; yet the faulty piece of equipment will continue to function normally.

        a. The meter of the line isolation monitor indicates the amount of leakage in the system resulting from any device plugged into the isolated power system.

        b. Visual and audible alarms are triggered if the isolation from ground has been degraded beyond a predetermined limit (Fig. 8-5).

    3. If the line isolation monitor alarm is triggered, the first step is to determine if it is a true fault.

        a. If the gauge reads between 2 and 5 mA, there probably is too much electrical equipment plugged into the circuit (all alternating current-operated devices have some capacitance and associated leakage current).

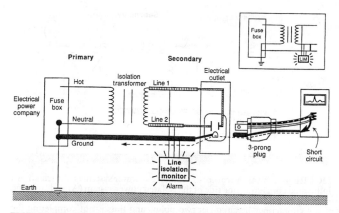

FIGURE 8-5. When a faulty piece of equipment is plugged into the isolated power system, it decreases the impedance from line 1 or line 2 to ground. This is detected by the line isolation monitor, which sounds an alarm. The faulty piece of equipment does not present a shock hazard but converts the isolated power system into a grounded power system.

    b. If the gauge is reading >5 mA, it is likely that a faulty piece of equipment is present in the operating room. This equipment may be identified by unplugging each piece of equipment until the alarm is silenced.

    c. If the faulty piece of equipment is not essential, it should be removed from the operating room for repair. If it is a vital piece of life-support equipment, it can be safely used but no other piece of electrical equipment should be connected during the remainder of the case, or until the faulty piece of equipment can be removed.

  4. The line isolation monitor is not designed to provide protection from microshock.

E. Ground Fault Circuit Interrupter

  1. The ground fault circuit interrupter (circuit breaker) is used to prevent individuals from receiving an electrical shock in a grounded power system (monitors both sides of the circuit for equality of current flow, and if a difference is detected, the power is immediately interrupted).

  2. The disadvantage of using a ground fault circuit interrupter in the operating room is that it interrupts the power without warning. A defective piece of equipment can no longer be used, which might be a problem if it were necessary for life support.

F. Microshock

1. In the electrically susceptible patient (one who has a direct external connection to the heart such as a CVP catheter or transvenous pacing wires), ventricular fibrillation can be produced by a current that is below the threshold of human perception (1 mA).

2. The stray capacitance that is part of any alternating current-powered electrical instrument may result in significant amounts of charge buildup on the case of the instrument.

   a. An individual who simultaneously touches the case of this instrument and the electrically susceptible patient may unknowingly cause a discharge to the patient that results in ventricular fibrillation.

   b. An intact equipment ground wire provides a low-resistance pathway for leakage current and constitutes the major source of protection against microshock in the electrically susceptible patient.

   c. The anesthesiologist should never simultaneously touch an electrical device and a saline-filled central venous pressure catheter or external pacing wires (wear rubber gloves).

3. Modern patient monitors are designed to electrically isolate all direct patient connections from the power supply of the monitor by placing a very high impedance between the patient and the device (limits the amount of internal leakage through the patient connection to <0.01 mA).

G. The objective of electrical safety is to make it difficult for electrical current to pass through people (patient and anesthesiologist should be isolated from ground as much as possible).

1. The isolation transformer is used to convert grounded power to ungrounded power. The line isolation monitor warns that isolation of the power from ground has been lost in the event that a defective piece of equipment has been plugged into one of the isolated circuit outlets.

2. All equipment that is plugged into the isolated power system has an equipment ground wire that provides an alternative low-resistance pathway enabling

potentially dangerous currents (macroshock) to flow to the ground. The ground wire also dissipates leakage currents and protects against microshock in the electrically susceptible patient.

3. All electrical equipment must undergo routine maintenance, service, and inspection to ensure that it conforms to designated electrical safety standards. Records of the routine maintenance service must be kept.

4. Electrical power cords should be located overhead (subject to crush if left on floor) or placed in areas of low traffic.

5. Multiple-plug extension boxes should not be left on the floor where they can come in contact with electrolyte solutions.

IV. ELECTROSURGERY

A. The electrosurgical unit (ESU), invented by Professor William T. Bovie, operates by generating high-frequency currents (radiofrequency range). Heat is generated whenever a current passes through a resistance. By concentrating the energy at the tip of the "Bovie pencil," the surgeon can accomplish either therapeutic cutting or coagulation.

1. High-frequency currents have a low tissue penetration and do not excite contractile cells (direct contact with the heart does not cause ventricular fibrillation).

2. High-frequency electrical energy generated by the ESU interferes with signals from physiologic monitors.

B. The ESU cannot be safely operated unless the energy is properly routed from the unit through the patient and back to the unit via a large surface area dispersive electrode (often erroneously referred to as the "ground plate") (Fig. 8-6).

1. Because the area of the return plate is large, the current density is low and no harmful heat or tissue destruction occurs.

2. If the return plate is improperly applied to the patient or if the cord connecting the return plate to the ESU is broken, the high-frequency electrical current will seek an alternate return path (leads for the ECG, temperature probe), perhaps resulting in a

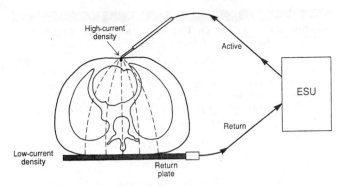

FIGURE 8-6. A properly applied ESU return plate. The current density at the return plate is low, resulting in no danger to the patient.

serious burn to the patient at this return site (high-current density generates heat) (Fig. 8-7).

3. In most modern ESUs, the power supply is isolated from ground to protect the patient from burns by eliminating alternate return pathways. The isolated ESU does not protect the patient from burns if the return electrode does not make proper contact with the patient.

4. The most important factor in preventing patient burns from the ESU is proper application of the return plate (Table 8-1).

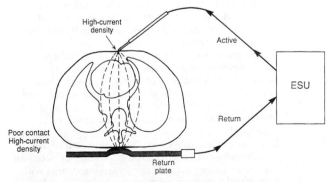

FIGURE 8-7. An improperly applied ESU return plate. Poor contact with the return plate results in a high-current density (heat) and a possible burn to the patient.

TABLE 8-1

PROPER APPLICATION OF THE ELECTROSURGICAL UNIT DISPERSIVE RETURN PLATE

Appropriate amount of electrolyte gel
Intact return wire
Ensure that electrolyte gel has not dried on plate from a prior use
Place as close as possible to operative site
Place below thorax if patient has an artificial cardiac pacemaker

   5. The need for higher than normal settings should
      initiate an inspection of the return plate and
      cable.
C. A bipolar ESU is when the current passes only between
   the two blades of a pair of forceps.
   1. Because the active and return electrodes are the two
      blades of the forceps, it is not necessary to attach
      another dispersive electrode to the patient.
   2. The bipolar ESU generates less power than the
      unipolar ESU and is mainly used for ophthalmic and
      neurologic surgery.
D. The use of a unipolar ESU (also electroconvulsive
   therapy) may cause electrical interference, which could
   be interpreted by an automatic implantable
   cardioverter-defibrillator (AICD) as a ventricular
   tachydysrhythmia, resulting in delivery of a
   defibrillation pulse to the patient.
E. In the presence of an oxygen-enriched environment, a
   spark from the ESU can serve as the ignition source for
   fuels (plastics such as anesthesia face masks, tracheal
   tubes), causing fires with associated injuries to patients
   and operating room personnel.
   1. The risk of surgical fires should be considered
      whenever the ESU is used in close proximity to
      oxygen-enriched environments (an airway, head and
      neck surgery using monitored anesthesia care and
      delivery of supplemental oxygen [oxygen is heavier
      than air and tends to accumulate in folds of
      drapes]).
   2. Tenting of the drapes to allow dispersion of any
      accumulated oxygen and/or its dilution by room air
      or use of a circle anesthesia breathing system with
      minimal to no leak of gases around the anesthesia
      mask will decrease the risk of ignition from a spark
      generated by an ESU.

V. **CONDUCTIVE FLOORING** is not necessary in anesthetizing areas where flammable anesthetics are not used.

VI. ENVIRONMENTAL HAZARDS

A. Potential hazards in the operating room include electrical shock to the patient and operating room personnel and the presence of cables and power cords to electrical equipment and monitoring devices (ceiling mounts).
B. Modern monitoring devices include an isolated patient input from the power supply of the device.
C. All health care facilities are required to have a source of emergency power (electrical generators, battery-operated light sources including laryngoscope).

VII. ELECTROMAGNETIC INTERFERENCE (EMI)

A. Wireless communication devices (cellular telephones, cordless telephones, walkie-talkies) emit EMI.
B. There is concern that EMI could interfere with implanted pacemakers or various types of monitoring devices in critical care areas.
   1. Cellular telephones should be kept at least 6 inches from a pacemaker.
   2. Cellular telephones do not seem to interfere with automatic implantable cardioverter-defibrillators (AICDs).

VIII. CONSTRUCTION OF NEW OPERATING ROOMS

A. The National Fire Protection Association (NFPA) standards for health care facilities no longer require isolated power systems or line isolation monitors in areas designated for use of only nonflammable anesthetics.
B. The decision to install isolated power is determined by two factors: Is the operating room a wet location (presence of blood, fluid, saline solutions) and if so, is an interruptible power supply acceptable?
   1. When power interruption is acceptable, a ground fault circuit interrupter is permitted as a protective means.

2. When power interruption would be unacceptable, an isolated power system and a line isolation monitor are preferred.

IX. FIRE SAFETY

A. Fires in the operating room are just as much a danger today as they were 100 years ago when patients were anesthetized with flammable anesthetic agents (Table 8-2).
B. Dangers of fires are burns to patients and operating room personnel and release of toxic compounds (carbon monoxide, ammonia, hydrogen chloride, cyanide) when plastics burn.
   1. The endotracheal tube may act as a blowtorch type of flame, resulting in severe injury to the trachea and lungs (laser-resistant endotracheal tubes).
   2. Leakage of gases around an uncuffed tube in the presence of the ESU can ignite flammable endotracheal tubes (minimize risk by keeping the inspired oxygen concentration as low as possible).

TABLE 8-2
ELEMENTS NECESSARY FOR A FIRE TO START (FIRE TRIAD)

Heat (Ignition Source)
Electrical surgical unit
Lasers
Electrical tools
Fiberoptic light cords

Fuel
Prep agents (alcohol)
Paper drapes
Hair
Alimentary gases
Ointments
Anesthesia equipment (breathing circuit hoses, masks, endotracheal tubes, laryngeal mask airways, volatile anesthetics, carbon dioxide absorbents)

Oxidizer
Air
Oxygen
Nitrous oxide

      3. In critically ill patients requiring high concentrations of oxygen during a surgical tracheostomy, it may be prudent not to use the ESU.

      4. Diffusion of nitrous oxide into the abdomen may create a fire hazard during laparoscopic surgery (carbon dioxide will not support combustion).

C. Fires on the patient are most likely during surgery in and around the head and neck where the patient is receiving monitored anesthesia care and supplemental oxygen (facemask or nasal cannulae).

      1. Oxygen should be treated as a drug and administered to provide optimum benefits (titrated to desired level).

      2. Tenting the drapes and using an adhesive sticky drape that seals the operative site from the oxygen flow will reduce the risk of a fire.

      3. Pooling of prep solutions may result in alcohol vapors that are flammable.

D. Desiccated carbon dioxide absorbents in the presence of volatile anesthetics (especially sevoflurane) may result in an exothermic reaction (fires may occur involving the breathing circuit).

E. If a fire occurs, the first step is to interrupt the fire triad by removing one component (best accomplished by removing the oxidizer).

      1. Disconnecting a burning endotracheal tube from the anesthetic circuit will usually result in the fire going out (not recommended to remove a burning endotracheal tube as may cause even greater harm to the patient).

      2. When the endotracheal tube fire is extinguished, it is safe to remove the tracheal tube and inspect the patient's airway by bronchoscopy followed by reintubation.

      3. If the fire is on the patient, extinguishing it with a basin of saline is a rapid and effective intervention.

         a. Paper drapes are impervious to water and throwing water or saline on them is likely to be ineffective.

         b. After removing the burning drapes from the patient the flame is extinguished with a fire extinguisher.

F. Prep solutions with alcohol should be dry before surgery begins.

CHAPTER 9 ■ ACID-BASE, FLUIDS, AND ELECTROLYTES

As a consequence of underlying diseases and therapeutic manipulations, surgical patients may develop potentially harmful disorders of acid-base equilibrium, intravascular and extravascular volume, and serum electrolytes (Prough DS, Wolf SW, Funston JS, Svensén CH: Acid-base, fluids and electrolytes. In Barash PG, Cullen BF, Stoelting RK [eds]: *Clinical Anesthesia*, pp 175–207. Philadelphia, Lippincott Williams & Wilkins, 2006). Precise perioperative management of acid-base status, fluids, and electrolytes may limit perioperative morbidity and mortality.

I. OVERVIEW OF ACID-BASE EQUILIBRIUM

   A. The conventional approach to describing acid-base equilibrium is the Henderson-Hasselbalch equation (Fig. 9-1).
   B. Because the concentration of bicarbonate is largely regulated by the kidneys, whereas carbon dioxide is controlled by the lungs, the emphasis on acid-base interpretation has been to examine disorders in terms of metabolic disturbances (bicarbonate primarily increased or decreased) and respiratory disturbances ($PaCO_2$ primarily increased or decreased) (Fig. 9-2).
   C. The negative logarithm of the hydrogen ion concentration is described as the pH.
      1. A pH of 7.4 corresponds to a hydrogen ion concentration of 40 nmol/L.
      2. From a pH of 7.2 to 7.5, the curve of hydrogen ion concentration is relatively linear, and for each change of 0.01 pH unit from 7.4, the hydrogen ion concentration can be estimated to increase (pH values >7.4) or decrease (pH values >7.4) by 1 nmol/L.

$$pH = 6.1 + \log [HCO_3]/0.03 \times PaCO_2$$

FIGURE 9-1. Henderson-Hasselbalch equation.

P_{CO_2} (lungs)

$\uparrow$

$$CO_2 + H_2O = H_2CO_3 = H^+ + HCO_3^-$$

$\downarrow$

Kidney

FIGURE 9-2. Acid-base balance reflects the retention or elimination of carbon dioxide or bicarbonate ions by the lungs or kidneys, respectively.

II. METABOLIC ALKALOSIS (pH >7.45 AND BICARBONATE >27 mEq/L)

A. Metabolic alkalosis is the commonest acid-base abnormality in critically ill patients (Table 9-1).

B. Metabolic alkalosis exerts multiple physiologic effects (Table 9-2).

C. Recognition of hyperbicarbonatremia in the preoperative serum electrolyte concentration justifies arterial blood gas analysis and should alert the anesthesiologist to the possibility that the patient is hypovolemic or hypokalemic.

D. Acute or chronic increases and decreases in $PaCO_2$ produce predictable effects on arterial pH and the serum bicarbonate concentration (Table 9-3).

E. Treatment of metabolic alkalosis (Table 9-4).

III. METABOLIC ACIDOSIS (pH <7.35 AND BICARBONATE <21 mEq/L)

A. Two types of metabolic acidosis occur based on whether the calculated anion gap is normal or

TABLE 9-1
CAUSES OF METABOLIC ALKALOSIS

Generating Factors
Nasogastric suction
Chronic diuretic administration
Excessive bicarbonate loads
Posthypercapnic state (abrupt correction of chronic hypercapnia)

Maintenance Factors (Continued Stimulus for Renal Resorption of Bicarbonate)
Decreased effective arterial volume
Hypokalemia
Renal failure

TABLE 9-2
PHYSIOLOGIC EFFECTS PRODUCED BY METABOLIC ALKALOSIS

Hypokalemia (potentiates effects of digoxin; evokes ventricular cardiac dysrhythmias)

Decreased serum ionized calcium concentration

Compensatory hypoventilation (may be exaggerated in patients with chronic obstructive pulmonary disease or those who have received opioids; compensatory hypoventilation rarely results in a $PaCO_2$ >55 mm Hg)

Arterial hypoxemia (reflects effect of compensatory hypoventilation)

Increased bronchial tone (may contribute to atelectasis)

Leftward shift of oxyhemoglobin dissociation curve (oxygen less available to tissues)

Decreased cardiac output

Cardiovascular depression and cardiac dysrhythmias (result of inadvertent iatrogenic respiratory alkalosis added to pre-existing metabolic alkalosis during anesthetic management)

increased (Table 9-5). The commonly measured cation (sodium) usually exceeds by 9 to 13 mEq/L the total concentration of anions (chloride, bicarbonate).

B. Metabolic acidosis exerts multiple physiologic effects (Table 9-6).

TABLE 9-3
EFFECTS OF ACUTE AND CHRONIC CHANGES IN $PaCO_2$ ON ARTERIAL pH AND SERUM BICARBONATE CONCENTRATION

Decreased $PaCO_2$

pH increases 0.1 unit and serum bicarbonate decreases 2 mEq/L for each acute 10 mm Hg decrease in $PaCO_2$.

pH will nearly normalize if hypocarbia is sustained.

Serum bicarbonate will decrease 5–6 mEq/L for each chronic 10 mm Hg decrease in $PaCO_2$.[a]

Increased $PaCO_2$

pH decreases 0.05 unit and serum bicarbonate increases 1 mEq/L for each acute 10 mm Hg increase in $PaCO_2$.

pH will return toward normal if hypercarbia is sustained.

Serum bicarbonate will increase 4 mEq/L for each chronic 10 mm Hg increase in $PaCO_2$.

[a]Hospitalized patients rarely develop chronic compensation for hypocarbia because of stimuli that enhance distal tubular resorption of sodium.

TABLE 9-4
TREATMENT OF METABOLIC ALKALOSIS

Etiologic Therapy
Expansion of intravascular fluid volume (intraoperative fluid
   management with 0.9% saline (lactated Ringer's solution
   provides additional substrate for generation of bicarbonate)
Administration of potassium
Avoid iatrogenic hyperventilation of the patient's lungs

Nonetiologic Therapy
Acetazolamide (causes renal bicarbonate wasting)
Hydrogen (ammonium chloride, arginine hydrochloride,
   hydrochloric acid [must be injected into a central vein])

TABLE 9-5
CLASSIFICATION OF METABOLIC ACIDOSIS

Normal Anion Gap
Renal tubular acidosis
Diarrhea
Carbonic anhydrase administration
Early renal failure
Saline administration

High Anion Gap (>13 mEq/L)
Uremia
Excess production of lactic acid or keto acids
Increased retention of waste products (sulfate, phosphate)
Ingestion of excess amounts of aspirin
Ingestion of ethylene glycol or methanol

TABLE 9-6
PHYSIOLOGIC EFFECTS PRODUCED BY METABOLIC
ACIDOSIS

Decreased myocardial contractility
Increased pulmonary vascular resistance
Decreased systemic vascular resistance
Impaired response of the cardiovascular system to endogenous and
   exogenous catecholamines
Compensatory hyperventilation

TABLE 9-7

ANESTHETIC IMPLICATIONS OF METABOLIC ACIDOSIS

Monitor arterial blood gases and pH
Possible exaggerated hypotensive responses to drugs and positive-pressure ventilation of the patient's lungs (reflects hypovolemia)
Consider monitoring with an intra-arterial catheter and pulmonary artery catheter
Maintain previous degree of compensatory hyperventilation

    C. Anesthetic implications of metabolic acidosis are proportional to the severity of the underlying process (Table 9-7).
    D. Treatment of metabolic acidosis (Table 9-8).

IV. RESPIRATORY ALKALOSIS (pH >7.45 AND $PaCO_2$ <35 mm Hg)

    A. The development of spontaneous respiratory alkalosis in a previously normocarbic patient requires prompt evaluation (Table 9-9).
    B. Respiratory alkalosis exerts multiple physiologic effects (Table 9-10).
    C. Treatment of respiratory alkalosis is recognition and treatment of the underlying problem.
        1. Correction of hypoxemia or hypoperfusion-induced lactic acidosis should result in resolution of the associated increases in respiratory drive.
        2. Preoperative recognition of chronic hyperventilation necessitates maintenance intraoperatively of a similar $PaCO_2$.

TABLE 9-8

TREATMENT OF METABOLIC ACIDOSIS

Reverse primary pathophysiologic process (hypoperfusion, arterial hypoxemia)
Sodium bicarbonate (measure arterial blood gases and pH about 5 minutes after intravenous administration; unlikely to be efficacious in treatment of lactic acidosis)
Preload may require assessment via echocardiography
Maintain compensatory hyperventilation

TABLE 9-9

CAUSES OF RESPIRATORY ALKALOSIS

Hyperventilation syndrome (diagnosis of exclusion, most often
  encountered in emergency department)
Iatrogenic hyperventilation
Pain
Anxiety
Arterial hypoxemia
Central nervous system disease
Systemic sepsis

V. RESPIRATORY ACIDOSIS (pH <7.35 AND PaCO$_2$ >45 mm Hg)

A. Respiratory acidosis may be acute (absence of renal
  bicarbonate retention) or chronic (renal retention of
  bicarbonate returns the pH to near normal).

B. Respiratory acidosis occurs because of a decrease in
  minute ventilation and/or an increase in carbon dioxide
  production (Table 9-11).

C. Anesthetic Implications
  1. Patients with chronic hypercarbia because of
    intrinsic pulmonary disease require careful
    preoperative evaluation (arterial blood gas and pH
    determinations), anesthetic management (direct
    arterial blood pressure monitoring and frequent
    arterial blood gas measurements), and postoperative
    care (pain control, often with neuraxial opioids, and
    mechanical support of ventilation).
  2. Administration of opioids and sedatives, even in low
    doses, may cause hazardous depression of
    ventilation.

TABLE 9-10

PHYSIOLOGIC EFFECTS PRODUCED BY RESPIRATORY ALKALOSIS

Hypokalemia (potentiates toxicity of digoxin)
Hypocalcemia
Cardiac dysrhythmias
Bronchoconstriction
Hypotension
Decreased cerebral blood flow (returns to normal over 8–24 hr
  corresponding to the return of cerebrospinal fluid pH to normal)

TABLE 9-11
CAUSES OF RESPIRATORY ACIDOSIS

Decreased Alveolar Ventilation
Central nervous system depression (opioids, general anesthetics)
Peripheral skeletal muscle weakness (neuromuscular blockers, myasthenia gravis)
Chronic obstructive pulmonary disease
Acute respiratory failure

Increased Carbon Dioxide Production
Hypermetabolic states
Sepsis
Fever
Multiple trauma
Malignant hyperthermia
Hyperalimentation

    3. Intraoperatively, a patient with chronic hypercapnia should be ventilated to maintain a normal pH (an abrupt increase in alveolar ventilation may produce profound alkalemia because renal excretion of bicarbonate is slow).

  D. Treatment of acute respiratory acidosis is elimination of the causative factor (opioids, muscle relaxants) and mechanical support of ventilation as needed. Chronic respiratory acidosis is rarely managed with mechanical ventilation but rather with efforts to improve pulmonary function so as to permit more effective elimination of carbon dioxide.

  E. In patients requiring mechanical ventilation for respiratory failure, ventilation with a lung-protective strategy may result in hypercapnia, which in turn has been managed with alkalinization.

VI. PRACTICAL APPROACH TO ACID-BASE INTERPRETATION

  A. Rapid interpretation of a patient's acid-base status involves integration of data provided by arterial blood gas, pH, and electrolyte measurements, and history.

  B. After obtaining these data, a stepwise approach facilitates interpretation (Table 9-12).

    1. The pH status usually indicates the primary process (acidosis or alkalosis).

    2. If the $PaCO_2$ and the pH change reciprocally but the magnitude of the pH and bicarbonate changes is not

TABLE 9-12

SEQUENTIAL APPROACH TO ACID-BASE INTERPRETATION

Is the pH life threatening, requiring immediate intervention?
Does the pH reflect a primary acidosis or alkalosis?
Could the arterial blood gas and pH readings represent an acute
   change in $PaCO_2$?
If there is not evidence of an acute change in $PaCO_2$, is there
   evidence of a chronic respiratory disturbance or of an acute
   metabolic disturbance?
Are appropriate compensatory changes present?
Is an anion gap present?
Do the clinical data fit the acid-base picture?

consistent with a simple acute respiratory
disturbance, a chronic respiratory or metabolic
problem (>24 hours) should be considered (pH
becomes nearly normal as the body compensates).
3. If neither an acute nor chronic respiratory change
   could have resulted in the arterial blood gas
   measurements, then a metabolic disturbance must
   be present.
4. Compensation in response to metabolic disturbances
   is prompt via changes in $PaCO_2$ whereas renal
   compensation for respiratory disturbances is slower.
5. Failure to consider the presence or absence of an
   increased anion gap results in an erroneous
   diagnosis and failure to initiate appropriate
   treatment. Correct assessment of the anion gap
   requires correction for hypoalbuminemia.

VII. FLUID MANAGEMENT—PHYSIOLOGY

A. Body Fluid Compartments
1. Accurate replacement of fluid deficits necessitates an
   understanding of the distribution spaces of water,
   sodium, and colloid.
2. Total body water approximates 60% of total body
   weight (42 liters in a 70-kg adult).
   a. Total body water consists of intracellular fluid
      (28 liters) and extracellular fluid (14 liters).
   b. Plasma volume is about 3 liters, whereas red
      blood cell volume is about 2 liters.
3. Sodium is present principally in the extracellular
   fluid (140 mEq/L), whereas potassium is present
   principally in the intracellular fluid (150 mEq/L).

4. Albumin is the most important oncotically active constituent of extracellular fluid (4 g/dL).
B. **Regulation of extracellular fluid volume** is influenced by aldosterone (enhances sodium resorption), antidiuretic hormone (enhances water resorption), and atrial natriuretic peptide (enhances sodium and water excretion).

VIII. FLUID REPLACEMENT THERAPY

A. **Maintenance Requirements for Water, Sodium, and Potassium**
   1. In healthy adults sufficient water is required to balance gastrointestinal losses (100 to 200 mL/day), insensible losses (500 to 1,000 mL/day representing respiratory and cutaneous losses), and urinary losses (1,000 mL/day)
   2. Water maintenance requirements are often calculated on the basis of body weight. For a 70-kg adult, daily water maintenance requirements are about 2,500 mL (Table 9-13).
   3. Renal sodium conservation is highly efficient, such that the average daily maintenance requirement in an adult is about 75 mEq.
   4. The average daily maintenance requirement of potassium is about 40 mEq. Physiologic diuresis induces an obligate potassium loss of at least 10 mEq for every 1,000 mL of urine.
   5. Electrolytes such as chloride, calcium, and magnesium do not require short-term replacement, although they must be supplied during chronic intravenous fluid maintenance.
B. **Dextrose**
   1. Addition of glucose to maintenance fluid solutions is indicated only in those patients considered to be at

TABLE 9-13
MAINTENANCE WATER REQUIREMENTS

	mL/kg/hr	mL/kg/day
1–10 kg	4	100
11–20 kg	2	50
>20 kg	1	20

risk for the development of hypoglycemia (infants, patients on insulin therapy). Otherwise, the normal hyperglycemic response to surgical stress is sufficient to prevent hypoglycemia.

   a. Iatrogenic hyperglycemia can limit the effectiveness of fluid resuscitation by inducing an osmotic diuresis.
   b. In critically ill patients tight control of plasma glucose concentrations (80 to 110 mg/dL) may reduce morbidity and mortality.
C. **Surgical Fluid Requirements**
   1. **Water and Electrolyte Composition of Fluid Losses**
      a. Surgical patients require replacement of plasma volume and extracellular fluid secondary to hemorrhage and tissue manipulation (third-space loss).
      b. Lactated Ringer's solution is often selected for replacement of third-space losses as well as for gastrointestinal secretions.
   2. **Fluid Shifts During Surgery**
      a. In addition to maintenance fluids and replacement of estimated blood loss, a guideline for third-space loss is 4 mL/kg/hr for operations involving minimal tissue trauma, 6 mL/kg/hr for those involving moderate trauma, and 8 mL/kg/hr for those involving extreme tissue trauma.
      b. Perioperative fluid management may influence postoperative morbidity (thirst, dizziness, nausea) and this influence may by specific to the types of surgery and types of fluid used. Postoperative complications may be less in fluid-restricted patients.
   3. **Mobilization of Expanded Interstitial Fluid.** The reverse of third-space translocation of fluid (mobilization and return of accumulated fluid to the extracellular fluid volume and plasma— "deresuscitation") occurs about 72 hours postoperatively. Hypervolemia and/or pulmonary edema may occur at this time in patients with compromised renal and/or cardiac function.

IX. COLLOIDS, CRYSTALLOID, AND HYPERTONIC SOLUTIONS

A. **Physiology and Pharmacology**
   1. Intravenous fluids vary in oncotic pressure, osmolarity, and tonicity.

TABLE 9-14
POSSIBLE ADVANTAGES AND DISADVANTAGES OF COLLOID VERSUS CRYSTALLOID INTRAVENOUS FLUIDS

	Advantages	Disadvantages
Colloid	Smaller volume infused	Greater cost
	Prolonged increase in plasma volume	Coagulopathy (dextran >hetastarch)
	Greater peripheral edema	Pulmonary edema (capillary leak states)
	Less cerebral edema	Decreased glomerular filtration rate
		Osmotic diuresis (low molecular weight dextran)
Crystalloid	Lower cost	Transient hemodynamic
	Greater urinary flow	Peripheral edema (protein dilution)
	Replaces interstitial fluid	Pulmonary edema (protein dilution plus high pulmonary artery occlusion pressure

    2. When the capillary membrane is intact, fluids containing colloid, such as albumin or hydroxyethyl starch, preferentially expand plasma volume rather than intracellular fluid volume.

  B. Clinical Implications of Choices Between Alternative Fluids

    1. Despite relative advantages and disadvantages, there is no evidence to support the superiority of either colloid-containing or crystalloid-containing solutions (Table 9-14).

    2. Despite a commonly held opinion, the risk of pulmonary edema seems to be independent of the selection of a crystalloid- or colloid-containing solution.

    3. Colloid-induced expansion of the plasma volume redistributes slowly, such that diuretic therapy is often required if pulmonary edema develops.

    4. There appears to be no important clinical difference in pulmonary function after administration of crystalloid or colloid solutions in the absence of hypervolemia.

TABLE 9-15

CONDITIONS ASSOCIATED WITH DEFICITS IN BLOOD
VOLUME AND EXTRACELLULAR FLUID VOLUME

Trauma	Pancreatitis
Burns	Bowel obstruction
Sepsis	Chronic systemic hypertension
Chronic diuretic use	Prolonged gastrointestinal losses

C. **Implications of Crystalloid and Colloid Infusions on
   Intracranial Pressure.** Despite a commonly believed
   clinical notion, the risk of increased intracranial
   pressure seems to be independent of the selection of a
   crystalloid- or colloid-containing solution.
D. **Clinical Implications of Hypertonic Fluid
   Administration.** The theoretical advantages of
   hypertonic/hyperoncotic fluids seem most likely to be
   effective in the treatment of hypovolemic patients who
   have decreased intracranial compliance.

X. FLUID STATUS: ASSESSMENT AND MONITORING

A. The preoperative clinical assessment of blood volume
   and extracellular fluid volume begins with the
   recognition of conditions in which deficits are likely to
   occur (Table 9-15).
B. Physical signs of hypovolemia are insensitive and
   nonspecific (Table 9-16).
   1. A normal blood pressure reading may represent
      relative hypotension in an elderly or chronically
      hypertensive patient. Conversely, substantial
      hypovolemia may occur despite an apparently
      normal blood pressure and heart rate.

TABLE 9-16

SIGNS AND SYMPTOMS OF HYPOVOLEMIA

Oliguria (rule out renal failure, stress-induced endocrine response)
Hypotension in supine position (implies blood volume deficit
  >30%)
Positive tilt test (increase in heart rate >20 beats/min and decrease
  in systolic blood pressure >20 mm Hg when patient assumes the
  standing position)

TABLE 9-17

LABORATORY EVIDENCE OF HYPOVOLEMIA

Hemoconcentration (hematocrit is a poor indicator of blood
  volume)
Azotemia (may be influenced by events unrelated to blood volume)
Low urine sodium concentration (<20 mEq for every 1000 mL of
  urine)
Metabolic alkalosis
Metabolic acidosis (reflects organ hypoperfusion)

    2. Elderly patients may demonstrate orthostatic
       hypotension despite a normal blood volume.
    3. Young, healthy subjects can tolerate an acute blood
       loss equivalent to 20% of their blood volume while
       exhibiting only postural tachycardia and variable
       postural hypotension.
    4. Orthostatic changes in central venous pressure,
       coupled with assessment of the response to fluid
       infusion, may represent a useful test of the adequacy
       of blood volume.

C. **Laboratory Evidence of Hypovolemia** (Table 9-17)
    1. Hematocrit is a poor indicator of blood volume
       because it is influenced by the time elapsed since
       hemorrhage and the volume of asanguineous fluid
       replacement.
      a. Hematocrit is virtually unchanged by acute
         hemorrhage; later, hemodilution occurs as fluids
         are administered or as fluid shifts from the
         interstitial to the intravascular space.
      b. If the intravascular fluid volume has been
         restored, hematocrit measurement will reflect red
         blood cell mass more accurately and can be used
         to guide transfusion.
    2. Blood urea nitrogen and serum creatinine levels may
       be increased if hypovolemia is sufficiently prolonged
       (both measurements may also be influenced by
       events unrelated to blood volume). Although
       hypovolemia does not cause metabolic alkalosis,
       extracellular fluid volume depletion is a potent
       stimulus for the maintenance of metabolic alkalosis.

D. **Intraoperative Clinical Assessment**
    1. Visual estimation is the simplest technique for
       quantifying intraoperative blood loss, as seen on
       operative sponges and drapes.

TABLE 9-18

CLINICAL INDICATORS OF THE ADEQUACY OF INTRAOPERATIVE BLOOD VOLUME REPLACEMENT

Heart rate (tachycardia is insensitive and nonspecific)
Blood pressure
Central venous pressure
Urinary output
Arterial oxygenation and pH

2. Adequacy of intraoperative blood volume replacement cannot be ascertained by any single modality (Table 9-18).
3. Preservation of the blood pressure, accompanied by a central venous pressure of 6 to 12 mm Hg in the presence of a volatile anesthetic, suggests an adequate blood volume.
   a. During profound hypovolemia, indirect measurement of blood pressure may significantly underestimate true blood pressure, emphasizing the potential value of direct blood pressure measurements in selected patients.
   b. An additional advantage of direct arterial pressure monitoring may be recognition of increased systolic blood pressure variation accompanying positive pressure ventilation in the presence of hypovolemia.
4. Urinary output usually decreases precipitously (<0.5 mL/kg/hr) in the presence of moderate to severe hypovolemia.

E. Oxygen Delivery as a Goal of Management
   1. No intraoperative monitor is sufficiently sensitive or specific to detect hypoperfusion in all patients.
   2. In high-risk surgical patients, systemic oxygen delivery ≥ 600 mL/m2/min (equivalent to a cardiac index of 3 L/m2/min, and hemoglobin concentration equivalent to 14 g/dL) may result in improved outcome.

XI. ELECTROLYTES

A. **Physiologic Role of Electrolytes** (Table 9-19)
B. **Sodium**
   1. Disorders of sodium concentration (hyponatremia, hypernatremia) usually result from relative excesses

TABLE 9-19

PHYSIOLOGIC ROLE OF ELECTROLYTES

Sodium	Osmolarity
	Extracellular fluid volume
	Action potential
Potassium	Transmembrane potential
	Action potential
Calcium	Excitation-contraction
	Neurotransmission
	Enzyme function
	Cardiac pacemaker activity
	Cardiac action potential
	Bone structure
Phosphorus	Stores energy (adenosine triphosphate)
	Component of second messengers (cyclic adenosine monophosphate)
	Component of cell membranes (phospholipids)
Magnesium	Enzyme cofactor (sodium-potassium pump)
	Controls potassium movement into cells
	Membrane excitability
	Bone structure

or deficits of water. Regulation of the quantity and concentration of electrolytes is accomplished primarily by the endocrine and renal systems.

2. **Hyponatremia** (<130 mEq/L) is the most common electrolyte disturbance in hospitalized patients (most often postoperative or acute intracranial disease) and is most often a result of excess total body water.
   a. Signs and symptoms of hyponatremia depend on the rate at which the plasma sodium concentration decreases and the severity of the decrease (Table 9-20).
   b. Many patients develop hyponatremia as a result of the syndrome of inappropriate antidiuretic hormone secretion (SIADH). The cornerstone of SIADH management is free water restriction and elimination of precipitating causes (Table 9-21).
   c. Inappropriately rapid correction of hyponatremia (>12 mEq/L in 24 hours or 25 mEq/L in 48 hours) may result in neurologic sequelae (central pontine myelinolysis or the osmotic demyelination syndrome).
   d. Hypertonic saline (1 to 2 mL/kg/hr) is indicated in patients with severe hyponatremia (<120 mEq/L)

TABLE 9-20
SIGNS AND SYMPTOMS OF HYPONATREMIA

Neurologic
Altered consciousness (sedation to coma)
Seizures
Cerebral edema

Gastrointestinal
Loss of appetite
Nausea and vomiting

Muscular
Cramps
Weakness

who have developed seizures. Intravenous administration of furosemide may be useful by increasing free water clearance. Once the plasma sodium concentration exceeds 120 to 125 mEq/L, water restriction alone is usually sufficient.

3. **Hypernatremia** (>150 mEq/L) is usually the result of decreased total body water.

   a. Signs and symptoms of hypernatremia most likely reflect the effect of dehydration on neurons and the presence of hypoperfusion caused by hypovolemia (Table 9-22). When hypernatremia develops abruptly, the associated sudden brain shrinkage may stretch and disrupt cerebral vessels, leading to subdural hematoma, subarachnoid hemorrhage, and venous thrombosis.

   b. Postoperative neurosurgical patients who have undergone pituitary surgery are at particular risk of developing transient or prolonged diabetes insipidus, leading to hypernatremia.

TABLE 9-21
PRECIPITATING CAUSES OF INAPPROPRIATE ANTIDIURETIC HORMONE SECRETION

Hypovolemia
Pulmonary disease
Central nervous system trauma
Endocrine dysfunction
Drugs that mimic antidiuretic hormone

TABLE 9-22

SIGNS AND SYMPTOMS OF HYPERNATREMIA

Neurologic
Thirst
Weakness
Hyperreflexia
Seizures
Intracranial hemorrhage

Cardiovascular
Hypovolemia

Renal
Polyuria or oliguria
Renal insufficiency

    c. **Treatment** of hypernatremia is influenced by the clinical assessment of extracellular fluid volume (Table 9-23).
  C. Potassium
    1. **Hypokalemia** (<3.0 mEq/L) may result from acute redistribution of potassium from the extracellular to the intracellular fluid (total body potassium concentration is normal) or from chronic depletion of total body potassium. With chronic potassium loss, the ratio of intracellular to extracellular

TABLE 9-23

TREATMENT OF HYPERNATREMIA

Sodium Depletion (Hypovolemia)
Hypovolemia correction (0.9% saline)
Hypernatremia correction (hypotonic fluids)

Sodium Overload (Hypervolemia)
Enhance sodium removal (loop diuretics, dialysis)
Replace water deficit (hypotonic fluids)

Normal Total Body Sodium (Euvolemia)
Replace water deficit (hypotonic fluids)
Control diabetes insipidus (DDAVP, vasopressin, chlorpropamide)
Control nephrogenic diabetes insipidus (restrict sodium and water intake, thiazide diuretics)

TABLE 9-24

SIGNS AND SYMPTOMS OF HYPOKALEMIA

Cardiovascular
Cardiac dysrhythmias (premature ventricular contractions)
ECG changes (widened QRS segment, ST segment depression,
    first-degree atrioventricular heart block)
Potentiates digitalis toxicity
Postural hypotension

Neuromuscular
Skeletal muscle weakness (hypoventilation)
Hyporeflexia
Confusion

Renal
Polyuria
Concentrating defect

Metabolic
Glucose intolerance
Potentiation of hypercalcemia and hypomagnesemia

potassium remains relatively constant, whereas acute redistribution of potassium substantially changes the resting potential difference across cell membranes.

a. Plasma potassium concentration poorly reflects total body potassium and hypokalemia may occur with high, normal, or low total body potassium. The plasma potassium concentration (98% of potassium is intracellular) correlates poorly with total body potassium stores. Total body potassium approximates 50 to 55 mEq/kg. As a guideline, a chronic decrease in serum potassium of 1 mEq/L corresponds to a total body deficit of about 200 to 300 mEq.

b. Signs and symptoms of hypokalemia reflect the diffuse effects of potassium on cell membranes and excitable tissues (Table 9-24).

c. Cardiac rhythm disturbances are among the most dangerous complications of hypokalemia. Although no clear threshold has been defined for a level of hypokalemia below which safe conduct of anesthesia is compromised, serum potassium concentrations <3.5 mEq/L may be associated with an increased incidence of perioperative

TABLE 9-25

TREATMENT OF HYPOKALEMIA

Correct Precipitating Factors
Alkalosis
Hypomagnesemia
Drugs

Mild Hypokalemia (>2.0 mEq/L)
Infuse potassium chloride up to 10 mEq/hr iv

Severe Hypokalemia (<2.0 mEq/L, ECG changes, intense skeletal muscle weakness)
Infuse potassium chloride up to 40 mEq/hr iv
Continuously monitor the ECG

     dysrhythmias (atrial fibrillation/flutter in cardiac surgical patients).

d. Potassium depletion may induce defects in renal concentrating ability, resulting in polyuria.

e. Hypokalemia causes skeletal muscle weakness and, when severe, may even cause paralysis.

f. Treatment of hypokalemia consists of potassium repletion, correction of alkalosis, and discontinuation of offending drugs (diuretics, aminoglycosides) (Table 9-25). Hypokalemia secondary only to acute redistribution may not require treatment. Oral potassium chloride (chloride deficiency may limit the ability of the kidneys to conserve potassium) is preferable to intravenous replacement if total body potassium stores are decreased. Intravenous potassium replacement at a rate of >20 mEq/hr should be continuously monitored with the electrocardiogram (ECG).

2. **Hyperkalemia** (>5 mEq/L) is most often because of renal insufficiency or drugs that limit potassium excretion (nonsteroidal anti-inflammatory drugs, angiotensin-converting enzyme inhibitors, cyclosporine, potassium-sparing diuretics). The electrocardiogram is an insensitive and nonspecific method of detecting hyperkalemia.

a. Signs and symptoms of hyperkalemia primarily involve the central nervous and cardiovascular systems (Table 9-26).

TABLE 9-26
SIGNS AND SYMPTOMS OF HYPERKALEMIA

Cardiovascular
Cardiac dysrhythmias (heart block)
ECG changes (widened QRS segment, tall peaked T waves, atrial
asystole, prolongation of P-R interval)

Neuromuscular
Skeletal muscle weakness
Paresthesias
Confusion

    b. Treatment of hyperkalemia is designed to
    eliminate the cause, to reverse membrane
    hyperexcitability, and to remove potassium from
    the body (Table 9-27).
D. Calcium
  1. Hypocalcemia (ionized calcium <4.0 mg/dL) occurs
  as a result of parathyroid hormone deficiency
  (surgical parathyroid gland damage or removal,
  burns, sepsis) or because of calcium chelation or
  precipitation (hyperphosphatemia, as from cell lysis
  secondary to chemotherapy).
    a. The hallmark of hypocalcemia is increased
    neuronal membrane irritability and tetany
    (Table 9-28).

TABLE 9-27
TREATMENT OF SEVERE HYPERKALEMIA[a]

Reverse Membrane Effects
Calcium (10% calcium chloride iv over 10 min)

Transfer Potassium into Cells
Glucose (D10W) and regular insulin (5–10 U regular insulin for
every 25–50 g glucose)
Sodium bicarbonate (50 to 100 mEq over 5 to 10 minutes)
B-2 agonists

Remove Potassium from Body
Diuretics (proximal or loop)
Potassium-exchange resins
Hemodialysis (removes 25–50 mEq/hr)

[a] >7 mEq/L, ECG changes.

TABLE 9-28

SIGNS AND SYMPTOMS OF HYPOCALCEMIA

Cardiovascular
Cardiac dysrhythmias
ECG changes (prolongation of the Q-T interval, T-wave inversion)
Hypotension
Congestive heart failure

Neuromuscular
Skeletal muscle spasm
Tetany
Skeletal muscle weakness
Seizures

Pulmonary
Laryngospasm
Bronchospasm
Hypoventilation

Psychiatric
Anxiety
Dementia
Depression

---

      b. Decreased total serum calcium concentration occurs in as many as 80% of critically ill and postsurgical patients, but few patients develop ionized hypocalcemia (multiple trauma, following cardiopulmonary bypass, massive transfusion [citrate]).

      c. Treatment of hypocalcemia (Table 9-29).

  2. Hypercalcemia (ionized calcium >5.2 mg/dL) occurs when calcium enters the extracellular fluid more rapidly than the kidneys can excrete the excess.

TABLE 9-29

TREATMENT OF HYPOCALCEMIA

Administer calcium
10 mL of 10% calcium gluconate iv over 10 min, followed by a
   continuous infusion 500–1,000 mg of calcium orally every 6 hr
Administer vitamin D
Monitor electrocardiogram

TABLE 9-30

SIGNS AND SYMPTOMS OF HYPERCALCEMIA

Cardiovascular
Hypertension
Heart block
Digitalis sensitivity

Neuromuscular
Skeletal muscle weakness
Hyporeflexia
Sedation to coma

Renal
Nephrolithiasis
Polyuria (renal tubular concentration defect)
Azotemia

Gastrointestinal
Peptic ulcer disease
Pancreatitis
Anorexia

Clinically, hypercalcemia most commonly results from an excess of bone resorption over bone formation, usually secondary to malignant disease, hyperparathyroidism, or immobilization.
  a. Signs and symptoms (Table 9-30).
  b. Treatment of hypercalcemia in the perioperative period includes saline infusion and administration of furosemide to enhance calcium excretion (urine output should be maintained at 200 to 300 mL/hr).
E. **Phosphate** provides the primary energy bond in ATP and creatinine phosphate.
  1. **Hypophosphatemia** (<2.5 mg/dL) is associated with neurologic manifestations, hematologic abnormalities, and immune dysfunction (susceptible to sepsis). Hyperventilation decreases serum phosphate concentrations.
  2. **Hyperphosphatemia** (>5.0 mg/d:) is corrected by eliminating the cause (renal failure) and correcting associated hypocalcemia.
F. **Magnesium** is principally intracellular and is necessary for enzymatic reactions.

TABLE 9-31
SIGNS AND SYMPTOMS OF HYPOMAGNESEMIA

Cardiovascular
Coronary vasospasm
Cardiac dysrhythmias (especially after myocardial infarction or
  following cardiopulmonary bypass)
Refractory ventricular fibrillation
Congestive heart failure

Neuromuscular
Neuronal irritability (tetany)
Skeletal muscle weakness
Sedation
Seizures

Miscellaneous
Dysphagia
Anorexia
Nausea
Hypokalemia (magnesium-induced potassium wasting)
Hypocalcemia (magnesium-induced suppression of parathyroid
  hormone secretion)

1. **Hypomagnesemia** (<1.8 mg/dL) is common in
   critically ill patients, most likely reflecting
   nasogastric suctioning and inability of the renal
   tubules to conserve magnesium. Hypomagnesemia
   can aggravate digoxin toxicity and congestive heart
   failure.
   a. Signs and symptoms (Table 9-31).
   b. Treatment of hypomagnesemia (Table 9-32).
      During magnesium repletion, the patellar reflexes

TABLE 9-32
TREATMENT OF HYPOMAGNESEMIA

Administer magnesium[a]
Intravenous magnesium 8–16 mEq over 1 hr followed by
  2–4 mEq/hr
Intramuscular magnesium 10 mEq every 4–6 hrs

[a]MgSO4 1 g = 8 mEq; MgCl2 1 g = 10 mEq.

TABLE 9-33

SIGNS AND SYMPTOMS OF HYPERMAGNESEMIA

	Plasma Magnesium Concentration (mg/dL)
Normal	1.8–2.5
Therapeutic range (pre-eclampsia)	5–8
Hypotension	3–5
Deep tendon hyporeflexia	5
Somnolence	7–12
Deep tendon areflexia	7–12
Hypoventilation	>12
Heart block	>12
Cardiac arrest	>12

should be monitored frequently and magnesium withheld if they become suppressed. During intravenous infusion of magnesium, it is important to continuously monitor the ECG to detect cardiotoxicity.

2. **Hypermagnesemia** (>2.5 mg/dL) is usually iatrogenic (treatment of pregnancy-induced hypertension or premature labor).
   a. Signs and symptoms (Table 9-33).
   b. Hypermagnesemia antagonizes the release and effect of acetylcholine at the neuromuscular junction, manifesting as potentiation of the action of nondepolarizing muscle relaxants.
   c. Treatment of neuromuscular and cardiac toxicity produced by hypermagnesemia can be promptly but transiently antagonized by calcium, 5 to 10 mEq intravenously (iv). Urinary excretion of magnesium can be increased by expanding the extracellular fluid volume and inducing diuresis with a combination of furosemide and saline. In emergency situations and in patients with renal failure, magnesium may be removed by dialysis.

CHAPTER 10 ■ HEMOTHERAPY AND HEMOSTASIS

The administration of blood products should be undertaken only with a complete understanding of those hazards and of the potential benefits (Drummond JC, Petrovich CT: Hemotherapy and hemostasis. In Barash PG, Cullen BF, Stoelting RK [eds]: *Clinical Anesthesia*, pp 208–244. Philadelphia, Lippincott Williams & Wilkins, 2006).

I. RISKS OF BLOOD PRODUCT ADMINISTRATION

A. **Infectious Risks Associated with Blood Product Administration** (Table 10-1)
   1. The rate of viral infectivity has decreased dramatically in the last two decades (Table 10-2).
   2. Universal nucleic acid testing (NAT) for HIV and the hepatitis C virus (HCV) has reduced the frequency of transmission of those agents to very low levels.

B. **Noninfectious Risks Associated with Blood Product Administration** (Table 10-3)
   1. **Immunologically mediated transfusion reactions** can occur as a result of the presence of antibodies that are either constitutive (anti-A, anti-B) or that have been formed as a result of prior exposure to donor red blood cells (RBCs), white blood cells, platelets, and/or proteins.
      a. **Acute hemolytic transfusion reactions (AHTR)** against foreign RBCs often manifests as hemolysis of the donor RBCs leading to acute renal failure, disseminated intravascular coagulation, and death. Hypotension and hemoglobinuria and diffuse bleeding may be the only clues that a hemolytic transfusion reaction has occurred during anesthesia. If a reaction is suspected, the transfusion should be stopped and the identity of the patient and the labeling of the blood rechecked. Management has three main objectives—maintenance of systemic blood

TABLE 10-1
INFECTIOUS RISKS ASSOCIATED WITH BLOOD PRODUCT ADMINISTRATION

Hepatitis A, B, C, D, and E
Human T-cell lymphotropic viruses (HTLV-1, HTLV-2)
Human immunodeficiency viruses 1 and 2
Cytomegalovirus
West Nile virus
Epstein-Barr virus
Prions (Creutzfeldt Jacob and variant Creutzfeldt Jacob)
Contaminating bacteria
Parasites (malaria)

TABLE 10-2
ESTIMATES OF THE RATE (PER DONOR EXPOSURE) OF TRANSFUSION-TRANSMITTED DISEASE

Hepatitis B (HBV)	1 / 350,000
Hepatitis C (HCV)	1 / 2,000,000
Human immunodeficiency virus (HIV)	1 / 2,000,000
Human T-cell lymphotrophic virus (HTLV)	1 / 2,900,000

TABLE 10-3
THE NONINFECTIOUS ADVERSE REACTIONS ASSOCIATED WITH BLOOD PRODUCT ADMINISTRATION AND THEIR APPROXIMATE INCIDENCES

Adverse reaction	Incidence
Acute hemolytic transfusion reactions	1 / 25,000–50,000
Delayed hemolytic transfusion reactions	1 / 2500
Minor allergic reactions	1 / 200–250
Anaphylactic/toid reactions	1/25,000–50,000
Febrile reactions	1 / 200
Transfusion-related acute lung injury (TRALI)	1 / 5000
Graft-versus-host disease	Rare
Immunomodulation	(?) 1 / 1

pressure, preservation of renal function, and the prevention of DIC.

b. **Reactions to donor proteins** (minor allergic reactions) cause urticarial reactions in 0.5% of all transfusions. Mild symptoms can be treated with diphenhydramine. Infrequently a more severe form of allergic reaction involving anaphylaxis will occur in which the patient experiences dyspnea, bronchospasm, hypotension, laryngeal edema, chest pain, and shock (occurs when patients with hereditary IgA deficiency who have been sensitized by previous transfusions or pregnancy are exposed to blood with "foreign" IgA protein).

c. **White cell–related transfusion reactions** (febrile reactions) may occur as a result of antibody attack on donor leukocytes. The febrile response occurs in about 1% of all red blood cell transfusions. Typically, the patient experiences a temperature increase of more than 1 degree centigrade within 4 hours of a blood transfusion and defervesces within 48 hours.

2. **Transfusion-related acute lung injury (TRALI)** is a noncardiogenic form of pulmonary edema associated with blood product administration. Beginning within 6 hours after transfusion, and often more rapidly, the patient develops dyspnea, chills, fever, and noncardiogenic pulmonary edema. Chest x-ray reveals bilateral infiltrates. Diuretics are not indicated as the pulmonary edema is noncardiogenic.

3. **Graft-versus-host disease (GVHD)** occurs when viable donor lymphocytes are transfused into immuno-compromised patients. The donor lymphocytes may become engrafted, proliferate, and establish an immune response against the recipient. GVHD typically progresses rapidly to pancytopenia and the fatality rate is very high. GVHD has been reported only after the transfusion of cellular blood components. It has not occurred following transfusion of FFP, cryoprecipitate, or frozen red cells. Irradiation remains the only effective means for preventing GVHD.

4. **Immunomodulation.** Alteration of immune function has been associated with allogenic transfusion. Transfused white cells are thought to be the

TABLE 10-4
CONSEQUENCES OF MASSIVE BLOOD TRANSFUSIONS

Hypothermia (slows coagulation and causes sequestration of platelets)
Volume overload
Dilutional coagulopathy (manifests as deficiencies of platelets and clotting factors)
Decreases in 2,3-diphosphoglycerate (2,3-DPG) (left shifting of the oxyhemoglobin dissociation curve)
Acid-base changes
Hyperkalemia
Citrate intoxication
Microaggregate delivery

mediators of the immunity attenuating effects. These observations have led to the development and application of techniques for leukocyte depletion (leukoreduction) of donor blood products.

C. **Other Noninfectious Risks Associated with Transfusion**
   1. Massive transfusion of large volumes of stored blood can have several consequences (Table 10-4).

II. BLOOD PRODUCTS AND TRANSFUSION THRESHOLDS

A. **Red Blood Cells**
   1. The contemporary transfusion trigger for general medical-surgical patients is a Hct of 21% and a Hb of 7.0 g/dL (Table 10-5).
   2. The Practice Guidelines for Blood Component Therapy developed by the American Society of Anesthesiologists (ASA) state that "red blood cell transfusion is rarely indicated when the hemoglobin concentration is greater than 10 g/dL and is almost always indicated when it is less than 6 g/dL."
   3. Ultimately the decision to transfuse red blood cells should be made based on the clinical judgment that the oxygen carrying capacity of the blood must be increased.
   4. **Compensatory Mechanisms During Anemia** (Table 10-6)
   5. **Isovolemic Anemia Versus Acute Blood Loss**
      a. With acute blood loss, hypovolemia induces stimulation of the adrenergic nervous system,

TABLE 10-5

CONDITIONS THAT MAY DECREASE TOLERANCE FOR ANEMIA AND INFLUENCE THE RBC TRANSFUSION THRESHOLD

Increased oxygen demand
  Hyperthermia
  Hyperthyroidism
  Sepsis
  Pregnancy
Limited ability to increase cardiac output
  Coronary artery disease
  Myocardial dysfunction (infarction, cardiomyopathy)
  β-adrenergic blockade
  Inability to redistribute cardiac output
Low SVR states
  Sepsis
  Postcardiopulmonary bypass
  Occlusive vascular disease (cerebral, coronary)
Left shift of the Oxyhemoglobin dissociation curve
  Alkalosis
  Hypothermia
Abnormal hemoglobins
  Presence of recently transfused Hb (decreased 2,3-DPG)
  HbS (sickle cell disease)
Acute anemia (limited 2,3-DPG compensation)
Impaired oxygenation
  Pulmonary disease
  High altitude
Ongoing or imminent blood loss
  Traumatic/surgical bleeding
  Placenta previa or accreta, abruption, uterine atony
  Clinical coagulopathy

TABLE 10-6

COMPENSATORY MECHANISMS THAT MAINTAIN OXYGEN DELIVERY DURING ISOVOLEMIC HEMODILUTION

Increased cardiac output
Redistribution of cardiac output
Increased oxygen extraction
Changes in oxygen–hemoglobin affinity

TABLE 10-7

INDICATIONS (EXPRESSED AS CURRENT PATIENT PLATELET COUNT) FOR THE ADMINISTRATION OF PLATELETS

Nonbleeding patients without other abnormalities of hemostasis	10,000/mm^3
Lumbar puncture, epidural anesthesia, central line placement, endoscopy with biopsy, liver biopsy or laparotomy in patients without other abnormalities of hemostasis	50,000/mm^3
Intended procedures in which closed cavity bleeding might be especially hazardous (neurosurgery)	100,000/mm^3
To maintain platelets during ongoing bleeding and transfusion	50,000/mm^3
To maintain platelets during DIC with ongoing bleeding	50,000/mm^3

leading to vasoconstriction and tachycardia. Increased cardiac output does not contribute.

    b. In chronically anemic patients, cardiac output increases as the hemoglobin decreases to approximately 7 to 8 g/dL.

B. **Platelets** (Table 10-7). One platelet unit will typically increase platelet count by 5 to 10,000/mm^3. However, the increase must be verified by platelet count, especially in patients who may have been alloimmunized by frequent platelet administration.

C. **Fresh Frozen Plasma** (Table 10-8)

D. **Cryoprecipitate** contains Factor VIII, the von Willebrand factor (vWF), fibrinogen, fibronectin, and Factor XIII (Table 10-9).

TABLE 10-8

INDICATIONS FOR THE ADMINISTRATION OF FRESH FROZEN PLASMA

Correction of single coagulation factor deficiencies for which specific concentrates are not available (principally Factor V)

Correction of multiple coagulation factor deficiencies (DIC, with evidence of microvascular bleeding and PT and/or aPTT >1.5 times normal)

Urgent reversal of warfarin therapy (prothrombin complex concentrate [II, VII, IX, X] is an alternative)

Correction of microvascular bleeding during massive transfusion (>1 blood volume) when PT/aPTT cannot be obtained in a timely manner

TABLE 10-9
INDICATIONS FOR THE ADMINISTRATION OF CRYOPRECIPITATE

Prophylaxis before surgery or treatment of bleeding in patients with congenital dysfibrinogenemias

Microvascular bleeding when there is a disproportionate decrease in fibrinogen (DIC and massive transfusion) with fibrinogen <80–100 mg/dL (FFP is the first-line component for the factor depletion associated with massive transfusion)

Prophylaxis before surgery or treatment of bleeding in Hemophilia A and vWD if concentrates are unavailable or ineffective

Bleeding as a result of uremia that is unresponsive to DDAVP

III. BLOOD CONSERVATION STRATEGIES
(Table 10-10)

IV. THE JEHOVAH'S WITNESS will accept neither administration of homologous blood products nor the readministration of autologous products that have left the circulation (significant personal discretion and many will accept procedures that maintain extracorporeal blood in continuity with the circulation).

V. COLLECTION AND PREPARATION OF BLOOD PRODUCTS FOR TRANSFUSION

   A. **RBCs** for transfusion are first collected in bags containing citrate-phosphate-dextrose-adenine (CPDA) or CPD solution. The citrate chelates the calcium present in blood and prevents coagulation.

TABLE 10-10
BLOOD CONSERVATION TECHNIQUES

Preoperative autologous donation (hip replacement, scoliosis surgery)

Acute normovolemic hemodilution

Intraoperative blood salvage (cell savers, risk of air embolism)

Postoperative blood salvage

Pharmacologic agents

   Erythropoietin

   Blood substitutes (hemoglobin and nonhemoglobin-based oxygen carrying solutions)

   DDAVP

   Antifibrinolytics

TABLE 10-11

MAJOR RBC SURFACE ANTIGEN INCIDENCE (%) IN THE U.S. POPULATION

Group	Whites	Blacks
O	45	49
A	40	27
B	11	20
AB	4	4
Rh (D)	85	92

   1. Packed RBCs are prepared by centrifugation (hematocrit of about 70 to 75%, contains 50 to 70 mL of residual plasma in a total volume of 250 to 275 mL and has a shelf life of 35 days). The administration of one unit of packed RBCs will increase the Hb and Hct of a 70 kg adult by approximately 1 g/dL and 3% respectively.

B. **Compatibility testing** involves three separate procedures.

   1. ABO, Rhesus Typing (Table 10-11)

   2. **The antibody screen** (indirect Coomb's test) is performed to identify recipient antibodies against RBC antigens. The likelihood that the antibody screen will miss a potentially dangerous antibody has been estimated to be no more than 1 in 10,000.

   3. **The Crossmatch** (donor RBCs are mixed with recipient serum) requires about 45 minutes to complete and is carried out in three phases: (1) the immediate phase, (2) incubation phase, and (3) antiglobulin phase.

     a. The immediate phase requires only 1 to 5 minutes and detects ABO incompatibilities. Determining the ABO blood group type and Rh status alone yields the probability that the transfusion will be compatible in 99.8% of instances.

     b. The second phase, the incubation phase, requires 30 to 45 minutes and detects antibodies primarily in the Rh system.

     c. The third phase (antiglobulin phase crossmatch or the indirect antiglobulin test) is performed only on blood yielding a positive antibody screen and requires 60 to 90 minutes.

C. **Type and screen orders** are used preoperatively for surgical cases in which it is unlikely that the blood will

TABLE 10-12

PREFERRED ORDER FOR SELECTING BLOOD IN THE ABSENCE OF COMPATABILITY TESTING

Type-specific, partially crossmatched blood
Uncrossmatched blood (urgent situations when need blood before compatibility testing can be completed)
  Group O RBCs until there is time to complete ABO and Rh testing
  Rh-negative blood is preferable if the patient's Rh type is unknown or if the patient is a woman of child-bearing age
  Nongroup O patients who have received group O red cells approximating one patient blood volume (10–12 units) during the period of acute blood loss should not be switched back to their own ABO group unless testing has been performed to confirm that significant titers of Anti-A or Anti-B antibodies are not present

actually be transfused. The ABO and Rh status of the patient is determined and the antibody screen is performed. If the antibody screen is negative, type-specific uncrossmatched blood will result in a hemolytic reaction in less than 1/50,000 units.

D. **Emergency Transfusions** (Table 10-12)
E. **Platelets**
   1. One unit of platelets will increase the platelet count of a 70-kg recipient by 5 to 10,000/mm^3.
   2. Platelets bear both ABO and human leukocyte (HLA) antigens. ABO compatibility is ideal (but not required) because incompatibility shortens the life span of the platelet. Platelets do not carry the Rh antigen.
   3. Platelets should be administered through a 170-micron filter.
F. **Fresh frozen plasma (FFP).** Plasma is separated from the RBC component of whole blood by centrifugation. To preserve the two labile clotting factors (V and VIII), it is frozen promptly and thawed only immediately prior to administration. FFP must be ABO compatible.
G. **Solvent Detergent Plasma**
   1. One of the principle hazards of FFP administration has been virus transmission.
   2. Three procedures, pasteurization, photochemical treatment, and solvent detergent (SD) treatment, have been used to inactivate viruses.

H. **Cryoprecipitate** is the precipitate that remains when FFP is thawed slowly. It is a concentrated source of factor VIII, factor XIII, vWF, and fibrinogen.
   1. One unit of cryoprecipitate contains sufficient fibrinogen to increase fibrinogen levels 5 to 7 mg/dL (bags contain 10 or 20 units).
   2. ABO compatibility is not essential because of the limited antibody content of the associated plasma vehicle (10 to 20 mL).
   3. Viruses can be transmitted with cryoprecipitate.

VI. THE HEMOSTATIC MECHANISM

A. Normal "hemostasis" involves a series of physiologic checks and balances that assure that blood remains in an invariably liquid state as it circulates throughout the body but, once the vascular network is violated, transforms rapidly to a solid state (coagulation). Coagulation must inevitably be complemented by processes for eliminating clot that is no longer needed for hemostasis (fibrinolysis).

B. **The Nomenclature of Coagulation** (Table 10-13)

C. **The Coagulation Mechanism**
   1. The classical, dual cascade (intrinsic and extrinsic pathway) model of coagulation is now recognized to be an inadequate representation of in vivo coagulation (leaves it unclear why either type of hemophiliac could not simply clot via the unaffected pathway).
   2. Activation of the coagulation process begins when a breach in the vascular endothelium exposes blood to the membrane bound protein, tissue factor (TF).
   3. The prothrombinase complex catalyzes the conversion of prothrombin to thrombin. It is this initial formation of thrombin in small amounts that advances the coagulation process to the more efficient "amplification" phase that follows.
   4. **Amplification** of coagulation includes activation of adjacent platelets and Factors V, VIII, and IX. The net result of this amplification stage is the availability of activated platelets and activated factors V, VIII, and IX.
   5. **Propagation** is characterized by an explosive generation of thrombin.

TABLE 10-13
FACTOR NOMENCLATURE AND HALF-LIVES

Factor	Synonyms	In vivo half-life (hours)
I	Fibrinogen	100–150
II	Prothrombin	50–80
III	Tissue thromboplastin, tissue factor	
IV	Calcium ion	
V	Proaccelerin, labile factor	24
VII	Serum prothrombin conversion 6 accelerator (SPCA), stable factor	
VIII	Antihemophilic factor (AHF)	12
vWF	von Willebrand factor	24
IX	Christmas factor	24
X	Stuart Prower factor, Stuart factor, Autoprothrombin	25–60
XI	Plasma thromboplastin antecedent (PTA)	0–80
XII	Hageman factor	50–70
XIII	Fibrin stabilizing factor (FSF)	150
Prekallikrein	Fletcher factor	35
HMW kininogen	Fitzgerald, Flaujeac, or Williams factor; contact activation cofactor	150

6. **Additional Principles of Coagulation** (Table 10-14)
D. **Fibrinolysis** leads to the dissolution of fibrin clots and recanalizes vessels that have been occluded by thrombosis.
  1. **The Formation of Plasmin**
     a. Fibrinolysis involves primarily the production of plasmin, an active fibrinolytic enzyme.
     b. Plasmin is formed by the conversion of plasminogen to plasmin. Plasminogen circulates and when it comes into contact with fibrin binds to it. Once bound to the fibrin surface, plasminogen is converted to plasmin by tissue plasminogen activator (t-PA).

TABLE 10-14

CHARACTERISTICS OF COAGULATION

Most clotting factors circulate in an inactive form.

Most clotting factors are synthesized by the liver.

Factor VIII is a large two-molecule complex (vWF and coagulant factor VIII).

Absence of vWF causes two hemostatic abnormalities.
  Defect in primary hemostasis because of a failure of platelet adhesion to the sites of vascular injury.
  Clinical hemophilia A because of an absence of circulating factor VIII:C.

Synthesis of the vWF occurs in endothelial cells and megakaryocytes 4.

Clotting factors II, VII, IX, and X require vitamin K for completion of their synthesis in the liver
  Warfarin administration displaces vitamin K and the vitamin K–dependent factors are not carboxylated.
  Factor VII has the shortest half-life and is the first clotting factor to disappear from the circulation when a patient is placed on warfarin or begins to develop vitamin K deficiency

Factors V and VIII (labile factors) have short storage half-lives (massive transfusion with stored blood leads to a dilutional coagulopathy because of diminished activity of factors V and VI)

   c. When plasmin is released into the bloodstream it is immediately neutralized by α-2 antiplasmin.

2. **Tissue plasminogen activator** is produced by vascular endothelial cells. If a clot begins to form on the normal endothelial surface, several mechanisms, including the elaboration of t-PA from endothelial cells, will rapidly inhibit clot formation or lead to its dissolution.

3. **Fibrin degradation products** (FDPs) are removed from the blood by the liver, kidney, and reticuloendothelial system. If the FDPs are produced at a rate that exceeds their normal clearance, they will accumulate. In high concentrations, FDPs impair platelet function, inhibit thrombin, and prevent the cross-linking of fibrin strands.

4. **Excess circulating plasmin** leads to a bleeding tendency. In pathologic conditions in which the fibrinolytic system produces large quantities of plasmin (primary fibrinolysis or secondary fibrinolysis [DIC]), the antiplasmin capacity may be

TABLE 10-15
MECHANISMS THAT REGULATE AND CONTROL COAGULATION

Endothelial inhibition (intact endothelium has properties that limit platelet aggregation and coagulation and induce fibrinolysis should a clot form)

Thromboxane-prostcyclin balance

Nitric Oxide and ADPase (effects of prostacyclin are potentiated by nitric oxide [formerly called endothelium-dependent relaxing factor])

Inhibition of coagulation
  Clotting factors circulate in an inactive form
  Normal blood flow dilutes activated clotting factors
  Liver removes activated clotting factors
  Need for a phospholipid surface localizes clot formation

Native (endogenous) anticoagulant mechanisms
  Thrombin, thrombomodulin, and protein C and protein S
  Thrombin and Antithrombin III (ATIII)

In the absence of heparin, ATIII has a relatively low affinity for thrombin
  When heparin is bound to ATIII, the efficiency of binding of ATIII to thrombin and the other factors increases dramatically
  Congenital ATIII deficiency can lead to thrombotic events
  Acquired deficiencies of ATIII (liver disease, prolonged heparin administration, nephrotic syndrome, DIC, sepsis, pre-eclampsia, fatty liver of pregnancy, following surgery)
  Tissue factor pathway inhibitor (TFPI)

Heparin sulfate (coats endothelial surface)

exceeded and plasmin may circulate. Excess plasmin can lead to a coagulopathy.
  E. **Control of Coagulation—The Checks and Balances** (Table 10-15)

VII. LABORATORY EVALUATION OF THE HEMOSTATIC MECHANISM

  A. **Laboratory Evaluation of Primary Hemostasis**
    1. **Platelet count** (does not reflect platelet activity) is the first test ordered in the evaluation of primary hemostasis (normal platelet counts range between 50,000 and 440,000/mm^3 and counts below 150,000/mm^3 are defined as thrombocytopenia). Spontaneous bleeding is unlikely in patients with

platelet counts >10 to 20,000/mm^3. With counts from 40 to 70,000/mm^3, bleeding induced by surgery may be severe.

2. **Bleeding time** is an accepted clinical test of platelet function. Both poor platelet function and thrombocytopenia can prolong the bleeding time (normal range is 2 to 9 minutes). Despite the fact that bleeding time reliably becomes progressively prolonged as platelet count falls below 80,000/mm^3, there are no convincing data to confirm that bleeding time is a reliable predictor of the bleeding that will occur in association with surgical procedures.

B. **Laboratory Evaluation of Coagulation**
   1. **Evolution of the Prothrombin Time (PT) and the Partial Thromboplastin Time (PTT).** In 1936, when Quick introduced the PT to clinical medicine, sufficient "thromboplastin" was used to yield a clotting time of approximately 12 seconds. Under these circumstances, even patients lacking factors VIII or IX showed normal clotting times. However, when "dilute" thromboplastin (or a "partial" thromboplastin) was used in lieu of the "12-second reagent," hemophiliacs showed much longer clotting times than did healthy controls. The two different pathways could be tested individually simply by varying the amount and type of thromboplastin added to blood.
   2. **Prothrombin time (PT)** evaluates the coagulation sequence initiated by tissue factor (TF) and leading to the formation of fibrin without the participation of factors VIII or IX (classical extrinsic pathway).
      a. The normal PT is 10 to 12 seconds (prolonged if deficiencies, abnormalities, or inhibitors of factors VII, X, V, II, or I are present).
      b. When prothrombin levels are only 10% of normal, the increase in the PT may be only 2 seconds. PT will not be prolonged until the fibrinogen level is below 100 mg/dL.
      c. A prolonged PT is most likely to represent a deficiency or abnormality of factor VII. Because factor VII has the shortest half-life of the clotting factors synthesized in the liver, factor VII is the

clotting factor that first becomes deficient with liver disease, vitamin K deficiency or warfarin therapy.

   d. **International Normalized Ratio.** A difficulty with the PT test is that many different thromboplastin reagents are used. This results in wide variation in normal values, which makes comparison of PT results between laboratories difficult. The International Normalized Ratio was introduced to circumvent this difficulty.

3. **Partial thromboplastin time** (PTT) assesses the function of the classical intrinsic (time to fibrin strand formation) and final common pathways. It entails the addition of a "partial thromboplastin" and calcium to citrated plasma.

   a. Normal aPTT values are between 25 and 35 seconds.

   b. The aPTT is most sensitive to deficiencies of factors VIII and IX, but, as is the case with the PT, levels of these factors must be reduced to approximately 30% of normal values before the test is prolonged. Heparin prolongs the aPTT but with high levels will also prolong PT. As with the PT, the level of fibrinogen must also be reduced to 100 mg/dL before the aPTT is prolonged.

4. **Activated clotting time** (ACT) is similar to the aPTT in that it tests the ability of blood to clot in a test tube and is dependent on factors that are all "intrinsic" to blood (the classical intrinsic pathway of coagulation).

   a. The automated ACT is widely used to monitor heparin therapy in the operating room. Normal values are in the range of 90 to 120 seconds.

   b. The ACT is far less sensitive than the aPTT to factor deficiencies in the classical intrinsic coagulation pathway.

5. **Thrombin time** (TT) is a measure of the ability of thrombin to convert fibrinogen to fibrin.

   a. The TT is prolonged when there is an inadequate amount of fibrinogen (<100 mg/dL) or when the fibrinogen molecules that are present are abnormal (dysfibrinogenemia as in advanced liver disease).

   b. The normal TT is <30 seconds.

6. **Reptilase Time**
   a. When the TT is prolonged, the reptilase time can be used to differentiate between the effects of heparin and FDPs. A prolonged TT and a normal reptilase time suggests the presence of heparin. Prolongation of both TT and reptilase time will occur in the presence of FDPs, or when fibrinogen level is low.
   b. The normal reptilase time is 14 to 21 seconds.
7. **Fibrinogen Level**
   a. Normal values are between 160 and 350 mg/dL (below 100 mg/dL may be inadequate to produce a clot).
   b. Fibrinogen is rapidly depleted during DIC.
   c. A marked increase in fibrinogen may occur in response to stress including surgery and trauma (hypercoagulable state).
C. **Laboratory Evaluation of Fibrinolysis**
   1. **Fibrin Degradation Products (FDP) and D-Dimer**
      a. FDPs will be increased in any state of accelerated fibrinolysis (advanced liver disease, cardiopulmonary bypass, administration of exogenous thrombolytics [streptokinase], DIC).
      b. D-dimer is specific to conditions in which extensive lysis of the cross-linked fibrin of mature thrombus is occurring, in particular DIC but also deep venous thrombosis and pulmonary embolism.
D. **The thromboelastogram** provides a measure of the mechanical properties of evolving clot as a function of time. A principal advantage of this test is that the steps it measures require the integrated action of all the elements of the hemostatic process: platelet aggregation, coagulation, and fibrinolysis.
E. **Interpretation of Tests of the Hemostatic Mechanism** (Table 10-16)
   1. The most commonly ordered coagulation tests are the platelet count, PT, aPTT, and occasionally BT. Coagulation defects that appear most often are revealed as abnormal values of PT and/or aPTT.
   2. When a greater disruption of the hemostatic mechanism is suspected, further tests, including fibrinogen, TT, and assays for FDPs and the D-dimer, may be ordered.

TABLE 10-16

INTERPRETATION OF COAGULATION TESTS

Platelet count	Bleeding time	aPT	PT	TT	Fibrinogen	FDPs	Possible causes	Example
D	N or D	N	N	N	N	N	Decreased production, sequestration Increased consumption Immune destruction	Radiation, chemotherapy, splenomegaly Tissue damage
N	I	N	N	N	N	N	Platelet dysfunction	Drugs (ASA, NSAIDs), uremia, mild von Willebrand's disease
N	I	I	N	N	N	N	Severe vWF deficiency	von Willebrand's disease
N	N	I	N	N	N	N	Factor deficiency Factor inhibition Antiphospholipid antibody	Hemophilia A or B Low-dose heparin Lupus anticoagulant
N	N	N	I	N	N	N	Factor VII deficiency	Early liver disease Early vitamin K deficiency Early warfarin therapy

					Mechanism	Condition
N	I	I	N	N	Multiple factor deficiencies	Late vitamin K deficiency
N	I	I	N	N		Late warfarin therapy[a]
N	N	I	I	N		Heparin therapy
D	I	I	I	N	Dilution of factors and platelets	Massive transfusion
D	I	I	I	I	Hypercoagulable state with or without decreased production of clotting factors	DIC[b]
D	I	I	I	N		Advanced liver disease

I, increased; D, decreased; N, normal; aPTT, activated plasma partial thromboplastin time; PT, prothrombin time; TT, thrombin time; FDPs, fibrin degradation products; vWF, von Willebrand factor; NSAIDs, nonsteroidal anti-inflammatory drugs; DIC, disseminated intravascular coagulation.

[a] Bleeding time may also be prolonged in association with a marked aPTT increase.

[b] DIC may be distinguished by the presence of D-dimers.

TABLE 10-17
COMMON COAGULATION PROFILES
Platelet count decreased (normal aPTT and PT)
Decreased platelet production
Consumption of platelets
Sequestration of platelets
Prolonged BT (normal platelet count, aPTT, PT)
Antiplatelet drug ingestion (NSAIDs, ASA)
Uremia
vWD
Heparin
Prolonged PT (normal platelet count and aPTT)
Vitamin K deficiency
Warfarin administration
Early liver dysfunction
Factor VII deficiency
Acquired coagulation factor inhibitors
Prolonged PT, aPTT, and TT (normal platelet count)
Heparin
Dysfibrinogenemia

    F. Common Coagulation Profiles (Table 10-17). The interpretation of coagulation tests may be made difficult by the fact that patients who develop a bleeding diathesis in the perioperative period may have more than one bleeding disorder (DIC and coagulopathy as a result of massive transfusion) and may also have a surgical cause for bleeding.

VIII. DISORDERS OF HEMOSTASIS: DIAGNOSIS AND TREATMENT (Table 10-18)

    A. The preoperative history is invaluable in the identification of disorders of hemostasis.
        1. Abnormalities of primary hemostasis, usually caused by reduced platelet number or function, will be revealed by evidence of "superficial" (skin and mucosal) bleeding including easy bruising, petechiae, prolonged bleeding from minor skin lacerations, recurrent epistaxis, and menorrhagia.
        2. Coagulation abnormalities are associated with "deep" bleeding events including hemarthroses or hematomas after blunt trauma.
    B. Hereditary Disorders of Hemostasis (Table 10-19)

TABLE 10-18

CLASSIFICATION AND TREATMENT OF DISORDERS OF HEMOSTASIS

Classification
Abnormal bleeding
Abnormal clotting
Involve platelets
Involve clotting factors
Presence of absence of inhibitors (FDPs)
Hereditary
Acquired

Treatment
Hemostatic agents (platelets and/or clotting factors)
Pharmacologic agents (desmopressin, antiplatelet drugs, vitamin K, warfarin, heparin, aprotinin, antifibrinolytic agents, protamine, fibrinolytics)

    C. Acquired Disorders of Hemostasis (Table 10-20)
       1. It is helpful to classify bleeding disorders according to which of the three hemostatic processes are involved: primary hemostasis (platelet disorders), coagulation (clotting factor disorders), fibrinolysis (production of inhibitors such as FDPs), or some combination of the three.

TABLE 10-19

HEREDITARY DISORDERS OF HEMOSTASIS

von Willebrand's Disease (vWD)
  Most common hereditary bleeding disorder (approximately 1% of the general population though it is overtly symptomatic in only about 10% of those afflicted)
  Result of abnormal synthesis of the von Willebrand factor (vWF), which is important for binding of platelets to sites of vascular injury and for coagulation
  Diagnosis based on history (abnormal bleeding from mucosal surfaces)
  Platelet count, the aPTT and the PT, may be normal
  Treatment is DDAVP and factor concentrate
Hemophilia A (deficient or functionally defective factor VIII:C)
Hemophilia B (Christmas disease) (deficiency or abnormality of factors IX)
Hemophilia C (deficiency or abnormality of factor XI)

TABLE 10-20

ACQUIRED DISORDERS OF HEMOSTASIS

Acquired Disorders of Platelets
Thrombocytopenia
Uremia
Drugs (inhibit platelet aggregation)
   Cyclo-oxygenase inhibitors (aspirin is the prototype)
   Cox-2 inhibitors reduce prostacyclin generation by vascular
      endothelial cells and tilt the natural balance toward platelet
      aggregation (increased rate of myocardial ischemic events)
   Dipyridamole
   ADP receptor antagonists (ticlopidine, clopidogrel)
   Glycoprotein IIb/IIIa receptor antagonists (management of acute
      coronary syndromes)
   Herbal medications (ginkgo, ginseng, garlic, ginger) and
      vitamins (vitamin E)
Myeloproliferative and myelodysplastic syndromes
**Acquired Disorders of Clotting Factors (including anticoagulant
   therapy)**
   Vitamin K deficiency (prolongation of the PT)
   Warfarin therapy (competes with vitamin K for the
      carboxylation binding sites, administered for prevention of
      deep venous thrombosis and pulmonary embolism and to
      patients with atrial fibrillation and patients with prosthetic
      heart valves)
Heparin Therapy (inhibits coagulation principally through its
   interaction with one of the body's natural anticoagulant
   proteins, anti-thrombin III)
Low molecular weight heparin (LMWH)
   Heparin induced thrombocytopenia/thrombosis (relatively
      uncommon with LMWH)
   Heparin in cardiopulmonary bypass (protamine is titrated
      against ACT for heparin reversal)
   Inhibitors of Xa (fondaparinux, idraparinux)
**Acquired Combined Disorders of Platelets and Clotting Factors
   with Increased Fibrinolysis**
   Liver disease
Disseminated Intravascular Coagulation (DIC)
   Diagnosis (increased PT aPTT, thrombocytopenia, decreased
      fibrinogen level, presence of FDPs and D-dimer)
   Treatment should focus on management of the underlying
      condition (septicemia, evacuation of the uterus, correction of
      hypovolemia, acidosis and hypoxemia)

2. It is useful to use the results of coagulation tests to determine whether the clinical problem involves primary hemostasis (decreased platelet count, increased bleeding time), coagulation (prolonged PT and aPTT, decreased factor levels), fibrinolysis (increased FDPs, increased D-dimer), or some combination of the three.

D. **Heparin in Cardiopulmonary Bypass.** A common practice is to maintain ACT 400 to 500 seconds for the duration of bypass.

E. **Direct thrombin inhibitors** are utilized during cardiopulmonary bypass when heparin is contraindicated. With the exception of bivalirudin, there is no antidote.

CHAPTER 11 ■ BASIC PRINCIPLES OF CLINICAL PHARMACOLOGY

Comprehensive knowledge of clinical pharmacology is a prerequisite to the practice of anesthesiology (Hudson RJ, Henthorn TK: Basic principles of clinical pharmacology. In Barash PG, Cullen BF, Stoelting RK [eds]: *Clinical Anesthesia*, pp 247–274. Philadelphia, Lippincott Williams & Wilkins, 2006).

I. TRANSFER OF DRUGS ACROSS MEMBRANES

A. Biologic membranes consist of a lipid bilayer with a nonpolar core and polar elements on their surfaces. Proteins are embedded in the lipid bilayer. The nonpolar core hinders passage of water-soluble molecules, so that only lipid-soluble molecules easily traverse cell membranes.
   1. Absorption, distribution, metabolism, and excretion of drugs require their transfer across cell membranes.
   2. Most drugs traverse cell membranes to reach their sites of action.
B. Transport Processes
   1. **Passive diffusion** occurs when a concentration gradient exists across a cell membrane (the rate of passive transfer is directly proportional to the concentration gradient and lipid solubility of the drug).
   2. **Active transport** of drugs through cell membranes (hepatocytes, renal tubular cells) is an energy-requiring process (pumping against concentration gradients) that is both specific and saturable.
C. **Effects of Molecular Properties**
   1. Most drugs are too large to pass through cellular membrane channels and must traverse the lipid component of cell membranes.
   2. Almost all drugs are either weak acids or weak bases and are present in both ionized and nonionized forms at physiologic pH. The nonionized form is more lipid soluble and able to traverse cell membranes easily.
   3. **Ion trapping.** If there is a pH gradient across a cell membrane, the drug will be trapped on the side that

TABLE 11-1
ROUTES OF ADMINISTRATION

Oral Administration
Absorption from the gastrointestinal tract highly variable
Must traverse the liver before entering the systemic circulation
(hepatic first-pass effect is reason oral dose must be smaller than
intravenous dose for some drugs; metabolism of some drugs by
the gastrointestinal mucosa also contributes to the first-pass
effect)

Sublingual Administration
Drugs pass directly into the systemic circulation
Limited absorption area (only highly lipid-soluble drugs
efficacious by this route)

Transcutaneous Administration
Limited to lipid-soluble drugs (fentanyl)
Delayed onset

Intramuscular and Subcutaneous Injection
Sustained effect

Intrathecal, Epidural, and Perineural Injection

Inhalational Administration

Intravenous Injection
Rapid achievement of therapeutic concentrations

has the higher ionized fraction because only the
nonionized drug is diffusible.

II. DRUG ABSORPTION

  A. Except after intravenous injection, all drugs must
     dissolve in water to reach the circulation.
  B. **Route of Administration** (Table 11-1)
  C. **Bioavailability** is defined as the fraction of the total
     dose that reaches the systemic circulation (decreased by
     incomplete absorption, first-pass hepatic effect, and
     pulmonary uptake).

III. DRUG DISTRIBUTION

  A. Highly perfused organs (brain, heart, kidneys, lungs,
     liver) receive most of the initially injected drug.

Delivery to skeletal muscles, skin, and fat is slower, and equilibration may take several hours to achieve.

1. Capillary membranes are freely permeable in most tissues (except in the brain), so drugs pass quickly into the extracellular space. Subsequent distribution varies according to the physicochemical properties of the drug.
   a. Distribution of water-soluble drugs such as neuromuscular blockers is essentially limited to extracellular fluid.
   b. Lipid-soluble drugs such as propofol easily cross cell membranes and are therefore distributed much more extensively.
2. Drugs accumulate in tissues because of binding to tissue components, pH gradients, or uptake of lipophilic drugs into fat.
3. Binding of drugs to plasma proteins influences distribution to other tissues (only free unbound drug can cross capillary membranes).

B. **Redistribution**
1. Following initial distribution of a lipid-soluble drug (thiopental, fentanyl, propofol) to highly perfused tissues (brain), the plasma concentration decreases as other tissues take up drug, creating a concentration gradient from the brain to the blood (drug diffuses back into blood for redistribution to tissues that are still taking up drug).
2. Recovery from an induction dose of thiopental is predominantly dependent on redistribution. If repeated injections are given, the concentration of thiopental increases in peripheral tissues (limits redistribution), and termination of drug action becomes increasingly dependent on the much slower process of drug elimination.

C. **Placental Transfer**
1. Most lipid-soluble drugs with low molecular weights cross the placenta by simple diffusion, whereas water-soluble drugs (neuromuscular blockers) do not cross the placenta to a significant extent.
2. Fetal pH is slightly lower than maternal pH; this causes the ionized fraction of weak bases (opioids, local anesthetics) to be higher in the fetus (ion trapping).

IV. DRUG ELIMINATION

A. **Elimination** occurs either by excretion of unchanged drug (kidneys excrete water-soluble drugs such as neuromuscular blockers) or by metabolism (the liver converts drug to a water-soluble metabolite that is likely to undergo renal excretion). Pulmonary excretion is the major route of elimination for inhaled gases.

   1. The volume of blood that is cleared of drug by the kidneys is analogous to creatinine clearance.
   2. Many drugs are cleared by more than one route such that total drug clearance is equal to the sum of the clearances of all the elimination pathways.

B. **Hepatic Drug Clearance**

   1. Drug clearance by the liver is dependent on hepatic blood flow, the intrinsic ability of the liver to irreversibly eliminate the drug from the blood (extraction ratio), and the extent of drug binding to plasma protein.

      a. Hepatic clearance of drugs with extraction ratios <0.3 is independent of changes in hepatic blood flow but very sensitive to the liver's ability to metabolize the drug (this is influenced by disease, inhibition or induction of drug-metabolizing enzymes, and interindividual differences). Drugs with low hepatic extraction ratios have capacity-limited clearance (Figs. 11-1 and 11-2).

      b. Hepatic clearance of drugs with hepatic extraction ratios >0.7 is dependent on changes in hepatic blood flow but insensitive to liver enzyme activity. Drugs with high hepatic extraction ratios have flow-limited clearance (Figs. 11-1 and 11-2).

      c. Drugs can be classified as having high, intermediate, or low hepatic extraction ratios (Table 11-2).

   2. **Physiologic, Pathologic, and Pharmacologic Alterations in Hepatic Drug Clearance**

      a. Congestive heart failure decreases drug clearance by decreasing both intrinsic clearance and hepatic blood flow (lidocaine clearance is decreased and risk of systemic toxicity is increased).

      b. Cirrhosis of the liver decreases clearance of drugs with high hepatic extraction ratios (decreased hepatic blood flow) and low hepatic extraction ratios (decreased hepatic enzyme activity) (see Table 11-2).

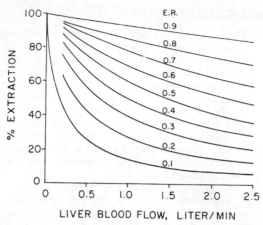

FIGURE 11-1. The effect of changes in hepatic blood flow on extraction of drugs with different extraction ratios (ER).

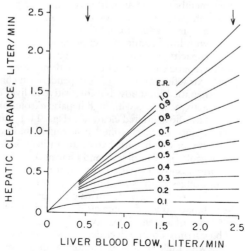

FIGURE 11-2. The effect of changes in hepatic blood flow on hepatic clearance of drugs with different extraction ratios (ER).

TABLE 11-2
CLASSIFICATION OF DRUGS ACCORDING TO HEPATIC EXTRACTION RATIOS

Low	Intermediate	High
Diazepam	Alfentanil	Alprenolol
Lorazepam	Midazolam	Bupivacaine
Methadone	Methohexital	Diltiazem
Phenytoin	Vecuronium	Fentanyl
Rocuronium		Ketamine
Theophylline		Lidocaine
Thiopental		Meperidine
		Metoprolol
		Morphine
		Naloxone
		Nifedipine
		Propofol
		Propranolol
		Sufentanil
		Verapamil

    c. It is logical to assume that clearance of drugs with high hepatic extraction ratios will be decreased during anesthesia (hypotension, effects of volatile anesthetics) and surgery (intra-abdominal surgery).

C. **Renal Drug Clearance**
    1. Although the kidneys can metabolize drugs, their major function in drug elimination is to excrete drugs and metabolites produced elsewhere (primarily the liver) into the urine. Renal clearance of drugs is determined by the net effect of glomerular filtration rate, tubular secretion, and tubular resorption.
        a. Glomerular filtration rate (about 20% of the plasma flow) cannot eliminate drugs efficiently (even if no drug is bound to proteins only about 20% can be removed by this mechanism).
        b. If a drug is neither secreted nor reabsorbed by the renal tubules, renal drug clearance will be equal to glomerular clearance.
        c. Clearance of drugs filtered by glomeruli or secreted by the proximal renal tubules may be decreased by subsequent resorption from renal tubules. Highly lipid-soluble

TABLE 11-3
DRUGS WITH SIGNIFICANT DEPENDENCE ON RENAL EXCRETION

Aminoglycosides	Pancuronium
Atenolol	Penicillins
Cephalosporins	Pipecuronium
Digoxin	Procaineamide
Doxacurium	Pyridostigmine
Edrophonium	Rocuronium
Nadolol	Quinolones
Neostigmine	

drugs (e.g., thiopental) are almost completely reabsorbed and have virtually no renal clearance.
2. **Physiologic, Pathologic, and Pharmacologic Alterations in Renal Drug Clearance**
    a. Renal drug clearance is proportional to creatinine clearance, even for drugs eliminated primarily by tubular secretion.
    b. Doses of drugs dependent on renal excretion must be decreased in the presence of renal failure or low cardiac output states (Table 11-3).

V. DRUG METABOLISM

A. Metabolism of drugs to more water-soluble compounds (this occurs principally in the liver but is also possible in the kidneys, lungs, and gastrointestinal tract) facilitates the ultimate excretion of metabolites into the bile and urine.
  1. Metabolites are usually less active pharmacologically than the parent drug (the exception may be metabolites of some of the benzodiazepines).
  2. Drug metabolism is more important in terminating the effects of drugs that are not extensively redistributed or when large or repeated doses are administered.
B. **Biotransformation Reactions**
  1. **Phase I reactions** either hydrolyze, oxidize, or reduce the parent compound.
    a. **The Cytochromes P450 (CYA)** are enzymes that catalyze most biotransformations.
    b. CYP is a superfamily of related enzymes. CYP families that share $\geq 40\%$ sequence identity are denoted by an Arabic numeral (CYP2).

TABLE 11-4

SUBSTRATES OF CYP3A4 ENCOUNTERED IN ANESTHESIOLOGY

Acetaminophen	Lidocaine
Alfentanil	Methadone
Alprazolam	Midazolam
Bupivacaine	Nicardipine
Cisapride	Nifedipine
Codeine	Omeprazole
Cortisol	Pantoprazole
Diazepam	Ropivacaine
Digitoxin	Statins
Diltiazem	Sufentanil
Felodpine	Verapamil
Fentanyl	Warfarin
Granisetron	

Subfamilies that share ≥55% identity are designated sequentially using a letter (CYP3A). Individual members of a family are assigned a second numeral (CYP3A4).

c. CYP isoenzymes from families 1, 2, and 3 effect 70 to 80% of all phase I metabolism of clinically used drugs.

d. CYP3A4 is the single most important enzyme accounting for 40 to 45% of all CYP-mediated metabolism (Tables 11-4 and 11-5).

TABLE 11-5

SUBSTRATES IN THE CYP2 FAMILY ENCOUNTERED IN ANESTHESIOLOGY

CYP2D6	Captopril
	Codeine
	Hydrocodone
	Metoprolol
	Ondansetron
	Propranolol
	Timolol
CYP2C9	Diclofenac
	Ibuprofen
	Indomethacin
CYP2C19	Diazepam
	Omeprazole
	Propranolol
	Warfarin

TABLE 11-6
FACTORS AFFECTING BIOTRANSFORMATION

Genetics (plasma cholinesterase)
Age (fetus and neonates have decreased capacity)
Enzyme induction
Liver disease
Renal disease
Anesthesia
Surgery

   2. **Phase II reactions** are characterized by conjugation
      with endogenous substrates such as glucuronic acid,
      acetate, and amino acids.
      a. Men have greater capacity for most phase II
         reactions.
      b. Smoking increases the metabolism of many drugs
         secondary to enzyme induction by polycyclic
         hydrocarbons in tobacco smoke.
      c. Renal failure decreases CYP activity not only in
         the kidneys but also the intestine and liver
         (primarily as a result of down-regulation of CYP
         gene expression).
   C. **Factors Affecting Biotransformation** (Table 11-6)

VI. BINDING OF DRUGS TO PLASMA PROTEINS

   A. The protein-bound fraction of a drug functions as a
      dynamic reservoir that buffers acute changes in the free
      drug concentration.
   B. **Binding proteins** include albumin (the most important
      drug-binding protein) and α-1 acid glycoprotein (its
      concentration increases in many acute and chronic
      illnesses [Table 11-7]).

TABLE 11-7
DRUGS THAT BIND TO α-1 ACID GLYCOPROTEIN

Alfentanil	Methadone
Alprenolol	Propranolol
Bupivacaine	Quinidine
Disopyramide	Ropivacaine
Fentanyl	Sufentanil
Lidocaine	Verapamil
Meperidine	

TABLE 11-8

FACTORS AND CONDITIONS AFFECTING DRUG BINDING TO PROTEINS

Lipid solubility
Acid-base disturbances
Accumulation of endogenous compounds
Pregnancy
Neonates
Age and gender
Liver disease
Renal disease
Inflammatory diseases
Cancer
Acute myocardial infarction
Catabolic states

    C. Factors and Conditions Affecting Drug Binding
    (Table 11-8)

VII. PHARMACOKINETIC PRINCIPLES

    A. The concentration of drug at its site or sites of action is a fundamental determinant of its pharmacologic effects.
      1. The concentration at the active site is a function of the concentration of drug in the blood.
      2. The change in drug concentration over time in the blood, at the site of action, and on other tissues is a result of complex interactions of various biologic factors with the physicochemical characteristics of the drug.
    B. Pharmacokinetic Concepts
      1. Rate Constants and Half-Lifes
        a. The disposition of most drugs follows **first-order** kinetics in which a constant fraction of the drug is removed during a finite period of time. This fraction is equivalent to the rate constant of the process.
        b. Rather than using rate constants, the rapidity of pharmacokinetic processes is often described by half-lifes (time necessary for the concentration to change by a factor of 2). Five half-lifes are considered sufficient time to completely remove a drug from the circulation.

2. **Volumes of Distribution**
   a. The volume of distribution (dose of drug injected/plasma concentration of drug) is an "apparent" volume that is necessary to explain the concentration of drug in a hypothetical compartment. If a drug is extensively distributed (lipid soluble), then the plasma concentration will be low and the volume of distribution large.
   b. Because the volume of distribution is a mathematical approximation, it cannot be correlated with the anatomic and physiologic factors that influence drug distribution.
   c. A large volume of distribution reflects extensive tissue uptake of a drug so that only a small fraction of the total amount of drug remains in the blood and accessible to clearance mechanisms (the larger the volume of distribution, the longer the elimination half-life).
   d. Calculation of volume of distribution immediately after intravenous injection of the drug is described as volume of distribution initial (Vdi) in contrast to calculation after equilibrium is achieved between tissues, which is described as volume of distribution at steady state (Vdss).
   e. Decreased protein binding results in an increased volume of distribution.
3. **Total drug clearance** is that portion of the volume of distribution from which drug is completely removed in a given time interval (analogous to creatinine clearance).

C. **Compartmental Pharmacokinetic Models**
   1. **One-Compartment Model.** Although for most drugs the one-compartment model is an oversimplification, it does illustrate the basic relationships between clearance, volume of distribution, and elimination half-life.
   2. **Two-Compartment Model** (Fig. 11-3)
      a. Immediately after intravenous injection into the central compartment, the beginning of drug transfer to the peripheral compartment (rate constant determines rapidity of transfer) occurs. As drug builds up in the peripheral compartment, some amount passes back to the central compartment. Drug is irreversibly cleared from the plasma only via the central compartment.

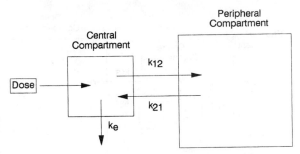

FIGURE 11-3. A two-compartment pharmacokinetic model.

    b. There are two discrete phases in the decline of the plasma concentration (Fig. 11-4). The initial rapid decrease ("distribution phase") is largely because of passage of drug from the plasma (central compartment) into tissues (peripheral compartment). The distribution phase is followed by a slower decline in the plasma concentration ("elimination phase") because of drug elimination from the central compartment.

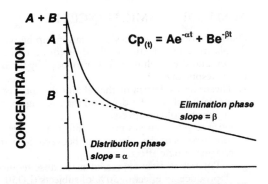

FIGURE 11-4. A schematic graph of the plasma concentration, on a logarithmic scale, versus time for a drug with a distribution phase preceding the elimination phase (two-compartment or biexponential kinetics).

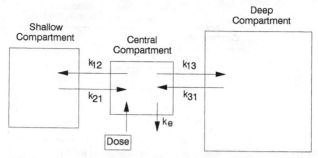

FIGURE 11-5. A three-compartment pharmacokinetic model.

   3. **The three-compartment model** distinguishes
      between rapidly equilibrating ("shallow") peripheral
      compartments and more slowly equilibrating
      ("deep") peripheral compartments (Fig. 11-5).
      Distribution of drugs between compartments
      (intercompartmental clearance) occurs.
      a. Most pharmacokinetic models are developed
         using population modeling in which
         pharmacokinetic parameters are estimated using
         all the concentration versus time data from the
         entire group of subjects in a single stage.

VIII. PHARMACODYNAMIC PRINCIPLES

   A. Pharmacodynamics defines the relationship between
      the plasma concentration of the drug (or at its site of
      action) and the resultant effects produced by the drug.
   B. **Dose-Response Curves**
      1. These curves determine the relationship between
         increasing doses of a drug and the ensuing changes
         in pharmacologic effects.
      2. Dose-response curves provide information regarding
         four aspects of the relationship between dose and
         pharmacologic effect.
         a. **Potency** is often expressed as the dose required to
            produce an effect in 50% of subjects (ED50).
         b. **Slope** of the dose-response curve indicates the
            rate of increase in effect as the dose is increased.
         c. **Efficacy** is the maximum effect produced by the
            drug.

      d. Variability in potency, slope, and efficacy is present when multiple subjects are used to generate dose-response curves.

C. Concentration-Response Relationships

  1. When a drug is infused at a constant rate intravenously, the plasma concentration initially increases rapidly and approaches a steady-state level after about five elimination half-lifes. The corresponding pharmacologic effect initially increases slowly, then more rapidly, and eventually reaches a steady state. When the drug is discontinued, the plasma concentration decreases promptly but the pharmacologic effect persists. There is always a lag time between changes in plasma concentration of a drug and its pharmacologic effect.

  2. At steady state, the plasma concentration of drug is in equilibrium with the concentrations throughout the body and is directly proportional to the steady-state concentration at the site of action. The **CPss50** is the steady-state plasma concentration producing 50% of the maximal response (determined from the concentration-response curve).

D. Dose-Receptor Interactions

  1. The biochemical and physiologic effects of many drugs, neurotransmitters, and hormones result from the binding of these compounds to receptors, which initiates changes in cellular function.

  2. At the neuromuscular junction, only 20 to 25% of the postjunctional nicotinic cholinoceptors need to bind acetylcholine to produce skeletal muscle contraction (75 to 80% of receptors are classified as "spare receptors"). Because most receptors must be occupied by an antagonist before transmission is affected, the existence of spare receptors accounts for the "margin of safety" of neuromuscular transmission.

  3. Binding of drugs to receptors changes cellular function by alterations in receptor-linked membrane ion channels (ionophores) or changes in guanine nucleotide binding proteins (**G** proteins) (Table 11-9).

  4. Receptors are not static entities, but rather dynamic cellular components that adapt to their environment (sequestration, down-regulation, up-regulation).

E. Agonists, Partial Agonists, and Antagonists (Table 11-10)

TABLE 11-9
DRUG-RECEPTOR INTERACTIONS

Receptor–Ionophore Complex
Acetylcholine (causes channels to open, leading to an influx of sodium and skeletal muscle contraction)
γ-aminobutyric acid (causes channels to open, leading to influx of chloride and hyperpolarization of cell membrane)
Benzodiazepines (same as γ-aminobutyric acid)
Intravenous anesthetics (same as γ-aminobutyric acid)

Guanine Nucleotide-Binding Proteins (G Proteins)
β-adrenoceptors (activate G proteins, which leads to a change in intracellular concentrations of second messengers [calcium, cyclic adenosine monophosphate])

IX. DRUG INTERACTIONS (Table 11-11)

X. CLINICAL APPLICATION OF PHARMACO-KINETICS AND PHARMACODYNAMICS TO ADMINISTRATION OF INTRAVENOUS AGENTS. Exquisite control of anesthetic blood (and effect site) concentrations is possible with inhaled anesthetics but to achieve similar degrees of control of intravenously administered anesthetics requires infusion

TABLE 11-10
AGONISTS, PARTIAL AGONISTS, AND ANTAGONISTS

Agonists
Drugs that bind to receptors and produce an effect
Differences in potency reflect differences in affinity for receptor

Partial Agonists
Drugs that cannot produce a maximal effect even at high concentrations

Antagonists
Drugs that bind to receptors but do not produce an effect
Competitive antagonists bind reversibly to receptors, and their blocking effect can be overcome with high concentrations of agonists (anticholinesterase drugs that increase the concentration of acetylcholine to overcome the effects of nondepolarizing muscle relaxants)
Noncompetitive antagonists bind irreversibly to receptors

TABLE 11-11
DRUG INTERACTIONS

Anticholinesterase drugs combined with anticholinergic drugs
Mixing acidic drugs (thiopental) with basic drugs (opioids, muscle
   relaxants) results in a precipitate
Absorption of drugs onto plastic in delivery systems or
   cardiopulmonary bypass circuits (nitroglycerin, fentanyl)
Vasoconstrictors added to solutions containing local anesthetics
Drugs that alter absorption of other drugs (ranitidine,
   metoclopramide)
Competition for common protein binding sites
Drugs that alter enzyme activity necessary for clearance of
   concomitantly administered drugs
Opioids and opioid antagonists
Synergistic effect of opioids and benzodiazepines
Synergistic effect of volatile anesthetics and muscle relaxants

devices and software to manage pharmacokinetic
principles.

A. **Infusion Pumps** (Table 11-12)
B. **Pharmacokinetic and Pharmacodynamic Principles of
   Drug Infusions.** Optimal dosing requires use of
   multicompartmental pharmacokinetic models utilizing
   computer simulation.
C. **Rise to Steady-State Concentration.** The drug
   concentration versus time profile for the rise to steady
   state is the mirror image of its elimination profile.
D. **Target-Controlled Infusions (TCI)**
   1. To accomplish TCI, mathematical calculations of
      the pharmacokinetic events that convert a dose into
      a plasma or effect site concentrations are interfaced
      between the anesthesiologist and infusion pump by
      means of a computer.
   2. TCI principles have been applied to intravenous
      anesthesia, postoperative analgesia, and
      patient-controlled sedation.

TABLE 11-12

DESIRABLE FEATURES FOR INTRAVENOUS INFUSION PUMPS

Low acquisition and operating costs
Accuracy over a wide range of flow rates to allow use with
    multiple drug formulations in adult and pediatric patients
Small size and battery backup for transportation of patients
Controls that allow rapid changes in drug delivery rate
Pause function without alarm
Programmability
    Drug identification
    Ability to enter patient characteristics
    Computer interface for data acquisition and control
    Target-controlled infusion capability
Displays
    All programmed parameters
    Current infusion rate and cumulative dose
    Visible in low ambient light
Safety features
    Drug identification
    Audio and visual alarms (empty drug reservoir, air in line,
        occlusion, impending battery failure)

CHAPTER 12 ■ AUTONOMIC NERVOUS SYSTEM: PHYSIOLOGY AND PHARMACOLOGY

Anesthesiology is the practice of autonomic nervous system (ANS) medicine (Lawson NW, Johnson JO: Autonomic nervous system: Physiology and pharmacology. In Barash PG, Cullen BF, Stoelting RK [eds]: *Clinical Anesthesia*, pp 275–333. Philadelphia, Lippincott Williams & Wilkins, 2006). Data recorded on the anesthesia record often reflect ANS function and homeostasis. Drugs used during anesthesia as well as painful stimulation and disease states frequently produce ANS-related side effects.

I. **FUNCTIONAL ANATOMY.** The ANS is divided into the sympathetic nervous system (SNS, adrenergic system) and the parasympathetic nervous system (PNS, cholinergic system) (Fig. 12-1). The SNS and PNS produce complementary effects on the activity of various organ systems (Table 12-1).

   A. **Central Autonomic Organization**
   1. The principal site of ANS integration is the hypothalamus (blood pressure control, temperature regulation, stress responses).
   2. Vital centers for hemodynamic and ventilatory control are located in the medulla oblongata and pons.
   3. ANS hyperreflexia is an example of spinal cord mediation of ANS reflexes without integration of function from higher inhibitory centers.

   B. **Peripheral Autonomic Nervous System Organization** (Fig. 12-2)
   1. The cell body of the preganglionic neuron originates in the central nervous system (CNS) and synapses in an autonomic ganglion (adrenal medulla is an exception). Preganglionic fibers are myelinated (rapid conducting).
   2. Postganglionic neurons arise from the autonomic ganglia and are distributed to effector organs.

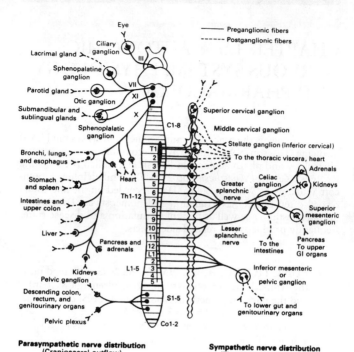

FIGURE 12-1. Schematic distribution of the craniosacral (parasympathetic) and thoracolumbar (sympathetic) nervous systems. Parasympathetic preganglioinic fibers pass directly to the organ that is innervated (discrete and limited effects). Activation of the sympathetic fibers produces a more diffuse physiologic response.

Postganglionic fibers are unmyelinated (slow conducting).

  a. The 22 pairs of SNS (paravertebral) ganglia are located nearer to the spinal cord than to the innervated organ.
  b. The PNS ganglia are located in or near the innervated organ.
3. Activation of the SNS produces a diffuse physiologic response (mass reflex), whereas activation of the PNS produces more discrete responses. For example, vagal stimulation may produce bradycardia with no effect on intestinal motility.

TABLE 12-1

HOMEOSTATIC BALANCE BETWEEN DIVISIONS OF THE AUTONOMIC NERVOUS SYSTEM

Heart	Sympathetic nervous system	Parasympathetic nervous system
Sinoatrial node	Tachycardia	Bradycardia
Atrioventricular node	Increased conduction	Decreased conduction
His-Purkinje system	Increased automaticity and conduction velocity	Minimal effect
Myocardium	Increased contractility, conduction velocity, automaticity	Minimal decrease in contractility
Coronary vessels	Constriction (alpha1) and dilation (beta1)	
Blood vessels		
Skin and mucosa	Constriction	Dilation
Skeletal muscle	Constriction (α1) > dilation (β-2) Dilation (β)	Dilation
Pulmonary	Constriction	Dilation
Bronchial smooth muscle	Relaxation	Contraction
Gastrointestinal tract		
Gallbladder	Relaxation	Contraction
Gut motility and secretions	Decreased	Increased
Bladder		
Detrusor	Relaxation	Contraction
Trigone	Contraction	Relaxation
Glands (nasal, lacrimal, salivary, pancreatic)	Vasoconstriction and reduced secretion	Stimulation of secretions
Sweat glands	Diaphoresis (cholinergic)	No effect
Apocrine glands	Thick and odiferous secretions	No effect
Eye		
Pupil	Mydriasis	Miosis
Ciliary	Relaxation for far vision	Contraction for near vision

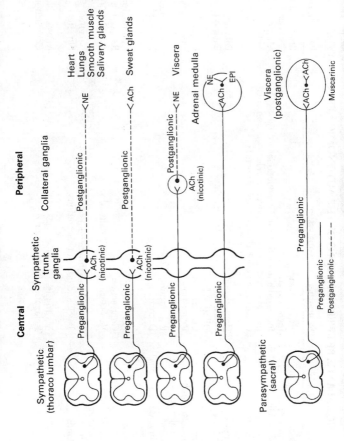

FIGURE 12-2. Schematic diagram of the efferent autonomic nervous system.

C. **Autonomic Innervation**
   1. **Heart.** SNS and PNS innervation of the heart (via the stellate ganglion) influences heart rate (chronotropism), strength of contraction (inotropism), and coronary blood flow.
      a. The PNS cardiac vagal fibers are distributed mainly to the sinoatrial and atrioventricular nodes, such that the main effect of cardiac vagal stimulation is chronotropic (strong vagal stimulation can arrest sinoatrial node firing and block impulse conduction to the ventricles).
      b. The SNS has the same supraventricular distribution as the PNS but with stronger distribution to the ventricles (normal SNS tone maintains contractility about 20% above that in the absence of SNS stimulation).
   2. **Peripheral Circulation.** The SNS is the most important regulator of the peripheral circulation. Basal ANS tone maintains arteriolar diameter at about 50% of maximum, thus permitting the potential for further vasoconstriction or vasodilation. By functioning as a reservoir for about 80% of the blood volume, small changes in venous capacitance produced by SNS-mediated venoconstriction produce large changes in venous return.

II. AUTONOMIC NERVOUS SYSTEM—NEUROTRANSMISSION

A. Transmission of impulses across the nerve terminal junctional sites (synaptic cleft) of the peripheral ANS occurs through the mediation of liberated chemicals (neurotransmitters). These neurotransmitters interact with a receptor on the end organ to evoke a biologic response.
B. **Parasympathetic Nervous System Neurotransmission**
   1. **Acetylcholine (ACh)** is the neurotransmitter at preganglionic nerve endings of the SNS and PNS and at postganglionic nerve endings of the PNS.
   2. The ability of a receptor to modulate the function of an effector organ is dependent on rapid recovery to its baseline state after stimulation. ACh removal occurs by rapid hydrolysis by acetylcholinesterase (true cholinesterase) (Fig. 12-3).

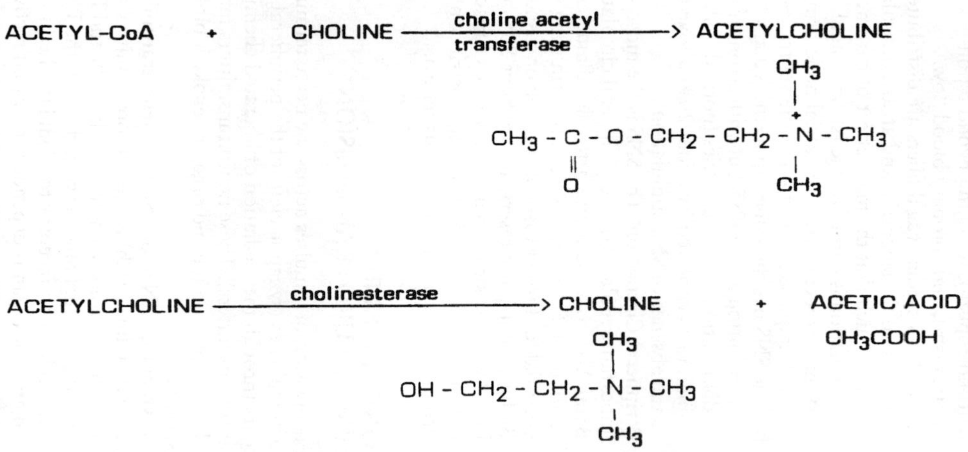

ACETYL-CoA + CHOLINE $\xrightarrow{\text{choline acetyl transferase}}$ ACETYLCHOLINE

$$CH_3 - C - O - CH_2 - CH_2 - \overset{\overset{\displaystyle CH_3}{|}}{\underset{\underset{\displaystyle CH_3}{|}}{N}} - CH_3$$
$$\underset{\displaystyle O}{\overset{\displaystyle \|}{}}$$

ACETYLCHOLINE $\xrightarrow{\text{cholinesterase}}$ CHOLINE + ACETIC ACID

$$OH - CH_2 - CH_2 - \overset{\overset{\displaystyle CH_3}{|}}{\underset{\underset{\displaystyle CH_3}{|}}{N}} - CH_3 \qquad CH_3COOH$$

FIGURE 12-3. Synthesis and metabolism of acetylcholine.

Pseudocholinesterase (plasma cholinesterase) is not physiologically significant in the termination (hydrolysis) of ACh action.

C. **Sympathetic Nervous System Neurotransmission**
1. Norepinephrine is the neurotransmitter at postganglionic nerve endings of the SNS (except in the sweat glands, where ACh is the neurotransmitter).
   a. Adenosine triphosphate (ATP) is released with norepinephrine and thus functions as a coneurotransmitter.
   b. Epinephrine is the principal hormone released by chromaffin cells (which function as postganglionic SNS neurons) into the circulation to function as a neurotransmitter hormone.
2. **Catecholamines: The First Messenger**
   a. Endogenous catecholamines are dopamine (neurotransmitter in the CNS), norepinephrine, and epinephrine. A catecholamine (including synthetic catecholamines) is any compound with a catechol nucleus (benzene ring with two adjacent hydroxyl groups) and an amine-containing side chain (Fig. 12-4).
   b. The effects of endogenous or synthetic catecholamines on adrenergic receptors can be indirect (little intrinsic activity but stimulate release of stored neurotransmitter) and direct.
3. **Inactivation** of catecholamines is by reuptake back into presynaptic nerve terminals, by extraneuronal uptake, diffusion, and metabolism (Fig. 12-5).

III. RECEPTORS

A. Receptors appear to be protein macromolecules on cell membranes, which when activated by an agonist (ACh or norepinephrine) lead to a response by an effector cell. An antagonist is a substance that attaches to the receptor (prevents access of an agonist) but does not elicit a response by the effector cell.
B. **Cholinergic receptors** are subdivided into muscarinic (postganglionic nerve endings) and nicotinic (autonomic ganglia, neuromuscular junction) receptors. ACh is the neurotransmitter at cholinergic receptors. Atropine is a specific antagonist at muscarinic receptors.

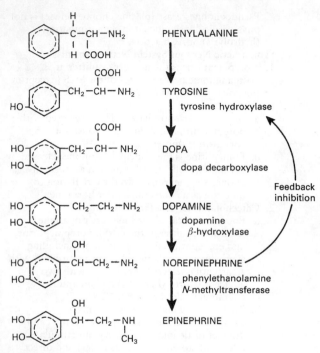

FIGURE 12-4. Synthesis of catecholamines.

C. **Adrenergic receptors** are subdivided into α, β, and *dopaminergic*, with subtypes for each category (Table 12-2).
   1. **α-Receptors in the Cardiovascular System**
      a. **Coronary arteries.** Postsynaptic α-2 receptors predominate in the large epicardial conductance vessels (they contribute about 5% to total coronary artery resistance, which is why phenylephrine has little influence on resistance to blood flow in coronary arteries), while postsynaptic α-2 receptors predominate in small coronary artery resistance vessels. Density of α-2 receptors in coronary arteries increases in response to myocardial ischemia.

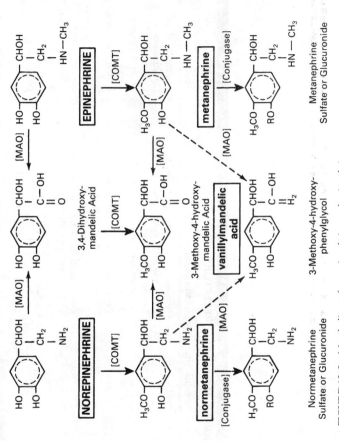

FIGURE 12-5. Metabolism of norepinephrine and epinephrine.

145

TABLE 12-2

CLASSIFICATION OF ADRENERGIC RECEPTORS

Receptor	Synaptic site	Anatomic site	Action
α-1	Postsynaptic	Peripheral vascular smooth muscle	Constriction
		Renal vascular smooth muscle	Constriction
		Epicardial coronary arteries	Constriction
		Myocardium	Positive inotropy
		Renal tubules	Antidiuresis
α-2	Presynaptic	Peripheral vascular smooth muscle	Inhibit norepinephrine release
		Central nervous system	Sedation
			Decreased mean alveolar concentration
	Postsynaptic	Endocardial coronary arteries	Constriction
		Central nervous system	Inhibition of insulin release
			Analgesia
			Natriuresis
			Diuresis

Receptor	Synaptic location	Tissue	Effect
β-1	Postsynaptic	Myocardium	Positive inotropy
			Positive chronotropy
		Coronary arteries	Dilation
		Kidneys	Renin release
β-2	Presynaptic	Myocardium	Accelerates norepinephrine release
	Postsynaptic	Peripheral vascular smooth muscle	Dilation
		Myocardium	Positive inotropy
			Positive chronotropy
		Bronchial smooth muscle	Dilation
		Renal vessels	Dilation
Dopamine$_1$	Postsynaptic	Blood vessels (renal, mesentery, coronary)	Dilation
		Renal tubules	Natriuresis
			Diuresis
		Juxtaglomerular cells	Renin release
Dopamine$_2$	Presynaptic	Postganglionic sympathetic nerves	Inhibits norepinephrine release
	Postsynaptic	Renal and mesenteric vessels	?Constriction

b. **Myocardium.** Postsynaptic α-1 receptors exert a positive inotropic effect (phenylephrine increases myocardial contractility) and contribute to the development of cardiac dysrhythmias (α-1 antagonists such as prazosin and phentolamine exert an antidysrhythmic effect).

c. **Peripheral Vessels.** Presynaptic α-2 vascular receptors mediate vasodilation, whereas postsynaptic α-1 and α-2 vascular receptors mediate vasoconstriction. Postsynaptic α-2 vascular receptors predominate on the venous side of the circulation (an α-1 agonist such as methoxamine produces minimal venoconstriction). Actions attributed to postsynaptic α-2 receptors include arterial and venous vasoconstriction, platelet aggregation, inhibition of insulin release, inhibition of bowel motility, and inhibition of antidiuretic hormone release.

2. **α-Receptors in the Kidneys.** The α-1 receptors dominate in the renal vasculature (vasoconstriction modulates renal blood flow), whereas α-2 receptors predominate in the renal tubules, especially the loops of Henle (which stimulate water and sodium excretion).

3. **β-Receptors in the Cardiovascular System**

a. **Myocardium.** Postsynaptic β-1 receptors and presynaptic β-2 receptors probably play similar roles in the regulation of heart rate and myocardial contractility. Increased circulating catecholamine levels associated with congestive heart failure result in down-regulation of β-1 receptors with relative sparing of β-2 and α-1 receptors (β-2 and α-1 receptors increasingly mediate the inotropic response to catecholamines during cardiac failure).

b. **Peripheral Vessels.** Postsynaptic vascular β receptors are predominantly β-2.

4. **β-Receptors in the Kidneys.** β-1 receptors are more prominent than β-2 receptors in the kidneys, and their activation results in renin release.

D. **Adrenergic Receptor Numbers or Sensitivity**

1. Receptors are dynamically regulated by a variety of conditions (ambient concentrations of catecholamines and drugs and genetic factors),

resulting in altered responses to catecholamines and ANS stimulation.

2. Alteration in the number or density of receptors is referred to as up-regulation or down-regulation. Chronic treatment with clonidine or propranolol results in up-regulation and a withdrawal syndrome if the drug is acutely discontinued.

IV. AUTONOMIC NERVOUS SYSTEM REFLEXES

A. **Arterial baroreceptors,** located in the carotid sinus and aortic arch, react to alterations in stretch caused by changes in blood pressure (Fig. 12-6).

1. Volatile anesthetics (halothane > isoflurane) interfere with baroreceptor function; thus, anesthetic-induced decreases in blood pressure may not evoke changes in heart rate.

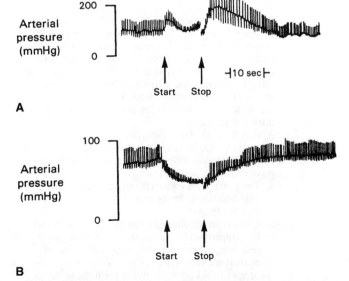

FIGURE 12-6. Blood pressure and heart rate response to a Valsalva maneuver (A, normal; B, abnormal in a patient with cervical quadriplegia).

2. Compliance of stretch receptors and their sensitivity may be altered by carotid sinus atherosclerosis (carotid artery disease may be a source of hypertension rather than a result).

B. **Venous baroreceptors,** located in the right atrium and great veins, produce an increased heart rate when the right atrium is stretched by increased filling pressures (Bainbridge reflex). Slowing of the heart rate during spinal anesthesia may reflect activation of venous baroreceptors as a result of decreased venous return.

V. CLINICAL AUTONOMIC NERVOUS SYSTEM PHARMACOLOGY

A. Drugs that modify ANS activity can be classified by their site of action and the mechanism of action or pathology (antihypertensives) for which they are administered.

B. **Cholinergic Drugs**

1. **Anticholinesterases** (neostigmine, pyridostigmine, edrophonium) inhibit activity of acetylcholinesterase, which normally destroys ACh by hydrolysis. As a result of this inhibition, ACh accumulates at muscarinic and nicotinic receptors. Simultaneous administration of an anticholinergic drug protects patients against undesired muscarinic effects (bradycardia, salivation, bronchospasm, intestinal hypermotility) without preventing nicotinic effects of ACh (reversal of nondepolarizing muscle relaxants).

2. **Anticholinergic drugs** (atropine, scopolamine, glycopyrrolate) interfere with the muscarinic actions of ACh by competitive inhibition of cholinergic postganglionic nerves.

   a. There are marked variations in sensitivity to anticholinergic drugs at different muscarinic sites (see Table 18-6).

   b. **Central anticholinergic syndrome** is characterized by symptoms that range from sedation to delirium, presumably reflecting inhibition of muscarinic receptors in the CNS by anticholinergics (unlikely with glycopyrrolate, which cannot easily cross the blood-brain barrier). Treatment is with physostigmine. Its tertiary amine structure allows it to cross the blood-brain barrier rapidly, whereas other anticholinesterases are quaternary ammonium compounds that lack the lipid solubility necessary to gain prompt entrance into the CNS.

C. **Hemodynamics**
1. Adrenergic agonists include drugs characterized as vasopressors (sympathomimetics) and inotropes (catecholamines). Most adrenergic agonists activate both α and β receptors, with the predominant dose-related pharmacologic effect being the expression of this mixed receptor activation (Table 12-3).
2. Hemodynamic effects evoked by adrenergic agonists include changes in heart rate (chronotropism), cardiac contractility (inotropism), conduction velocity of the cardiac impulse (dromotropism), cardiac rhythm, and systemic vascular resistance. Effects of these drugs on capacitance veins (venous return) may be as important as inotropic actions and more important than arteriolar effects (Table 12-4).
3. **Low-output syndrome** is present when there are abnormalities of the heart, blood volume, or blood flow distribution (when present for more than 1 hour usually reflects all three components).
   a. Septic shock is the most common distributive abnormality and volume repletion is an important initial consideration.
   b. Treatment of cardiogenic shock requires multiple autonomic interventions.
4. **Adverse Effects.** Side effects of α agonists most often reflect excessive α- or β-receptor activity.

D. **Adrenergic Agonists**
1. **Methoxamine** is a pure arterial vasoconstrictor that increases systemic vascular resistance and decreases cardiac output, even though blood pressure is increased. Few clinical indications remain for use of this drug, although a single intravenous dose may terminate paroxysmal atrial tachycardia reflexly through baroreceptor stimulation.
2. **Phenylephrine** is considered a pure α agonist, but unlike methoxamine, this drug produces greater venoconstriction than arterial constriction. As a result, venous return and blood pressure are increased.

TABLE 12-3
DOSES AND PRINCIPAL SITES OF ACTION OF ADRENERGIC AGONISTS

Agent	Bolus (iv)	Continuous infusion	α-1	α-2	β1	β-2	DA-1	DA-2
Methoxamine	5–10 mg		+++++	?	0	0	0	
Phenylephrine	50–100 μg	0.15 μ/kg/min (10 mg in 250 mL, 40 μg/ml)	+++++	?	+/-	0	0	
Norepinephrine		0.1 μg/kg/min (4 mg in 250 mL, 16 μg/mL)	++++++	++++++	+++	0	0	
Epinephrine	2–8 μg[a], 0.3–0.5 mg[b]	0.015 μg/kg/min (1 mg in 250 mL, 4 μg/mL)	+++++	+++	+++++	++	0	
Ephedrine	5–10 mg		++	?	+++	++	0	
Dopamine		2–10 μg/kg/min (200 mg in 250 mL, 800 μg/mL)	+ to ++++	?	+++	++	+++	?
Dobutamine		2–10 μg/kg/min (250 mg in 250 mL, 1 mg/mL)	+/-	?	++++	++	0	
Isoproterenol		1–5 μg/min (1 mg in 250 mL 4 μg/mL)	0	0	++++++	++++++	0	

DA, dopamine.

[a]Dose to treat hypotension.

[b]Dose to treat cardiac arrest.

TABLE 12-4
HEMODYNAMIC EFFECTS OF ADRENERGIC AGONISTS

Agent	Heart rate	Cardiac output	Systemic vascular resistance	Venous return	Renal blood flow
Methoxamine	Decreased	Decreased	Increased	No change	Decreased
Phenylephrine	Decreased	Decreased	Increased	Increased	Decreased
Norepinephrine	Decreased	Decreased	Increased	Increased	Decreased
Epinephrine	Increased	Increased	Increased	Increased	Decreased
Ephedrine	Increased	Increased	Increased	Increased	Unpredictable
Dopamine	No change	Increased	Decreased to no change	Increased	Increased
Dobutamine	Increased	Increased	Decreased to no change	Unpredictable	Increased to no change
Isoproterenol	Increased	Increased	Decreased	Decreased	Increased to no change

      a. Side effects. Excessive vasoconstriction produced by phenylephrine can elicit baroreceptor-mediated bradycardia with associated decreases in cardiac output. Increased systemic vascular resistance may further contribute to decreases in cardiac output and increases in myocardial oxygen requirements.

      b. Clinical uses. Phenylephrine is administered as a single dose (50 to 100 mg iv) to treat anesthetic-induced decreases in blood pressure, hypotension during cardiopulmonary bypass, and as a continuous infusion to maintain perfusion pressure during cerebral and peripheral vascular procedures. Use of phenylephrine to maintain perfusion pressures during cerebral and peripheral vascular procedures must be done cautiously, because it can evoke myocardial ischemia in susceptible patients.

3. Norepinephrine and methoxamine produce similar dose-related hemodynamic effects characterized by greater α than β effects.

      a. Vasoconstriction increases systemic blood pressure but may also decrease tissue blood flow (especially renal blood flow) and increase myocardial oxygen requirements.

      b. Continuous infusion of norepinephrine (must be via a centrally placed intravenous catheter) to maintain systolic blood pressure above 90 mm Hg requires invasive monitoring and attention to fluid management.

      c. In clinical conditions characterized by a low perfusion pressure and high flow (vasodilation) and maldistribution of flow, norepinephrine has been shown to improve renal and splanchnic blood flow by increasing perfusion pressure provided the patient has been volume resuscitated.

4. Epinephrine. The α effects of epinephrine predominate in renal and cutaneous vasculature to decrease blood flow, whereas β effects increase blood flow to skeletal muscles.

      a. Side effects. Cardiac dysrhythmias are a hazard of excess β stimulation.

      b. Clinical uses. Epinephrine is administered to (1) treat asthma (0.3 to 0.5 mg subcutaneously), (2) treat cardiac arrest or life-threatening allergic reactions (0.3 to 0.5 mg iv), (3) produce hemostasis (1:200,000 or 5 μg/mL injected subcutaneously or submucosally), (4) prolong regional anesthesia (0.2 mg added to local anesthetic solutions for spinal block or as a 1:200,000 concentration for epidural block), or (5) provide a bloodless arthroscopic field by large volume infusions of dilute epinephrine-containing solutions (1:200,000) (unpredictable absorption of epinephrine especially in denuded cancellous bone may result in overdose and acute heart failure, pulmonary edema, cardiac dysrhythmias, and cardiac arrest in otherwise healthy patients).

5. **Ephedrine** produces cardiovascular effects that resemble those produced by epinephrine; however, its potency is greatly decreased, although its duration of action is about 10 times longer than that of epinephrine. Venoconstriction is greater than arterial constriction; thus, venous return and cardiac output are improved. A β effect increases heart rate and further facilitates cardiac output. The α and β effects of ephedrine result in a modest and predictable increase in blood pressure.

    a. **Side effects.** Tachycardia and cardiac dysrhythmias are possible but less likely to occur than after administration of epinephrine.

    b. **Clinical uses.** Ephedrine is the most commonly used vasopressor (5 to 10 mg iv) to treat decreases in blood pressure produced by anesthesia (especially regional blocks) and is considered the drug of choice in obstetrics because uterine blood flow directly parallels ephedrine-induced increases in blood pressure. It is appropriate to administer ephedrine as a temporizing measure to restore perfusion pressure while the underlying cause of hypotension is corrected. Even relatively low doses of dopamine can cause renal artery vasoconstriction when added into the preexisting high levels of endogenous catecholamines commonly seen in acutely injured patients.

6. **Isoproterenol** is a nonspecific β agonist that lacks α-agonist effects. Cardiac output is increased by virtue of increases in heart rate as well as increased myocardial contractility, whereas decreases in

systemic vascular resistance contribute to decreased afterload.

   a. **Side effects.** Myocardial ischemia may be evoked in vulnerable patients (increased myocardial oxygen requirements because of tachycardia and increased myocardial contractility paralleled by decreased coronary oxygen delivery because of decreased diastolic blood pressure). Increases in cardiac output may be diverted to nonvital tissues such as skeletal muscles.

   b. **Clinical uses.** Isoproterenol is most often administered as a continuous intravenous infusion for the treatment of congestive heart failure associated with bradycardia, asthma, or pulmonary hypertension. This catecholamine acts as a chemical cardiac pacemaker in the presence of complete heart block.

7. **Dobutamine** is a synthetic catecholamine derived from isoproterenol that acts directly on β-1 receptors and does not cause norepinephrine release or stimulation of dopamine receptors. Weak α-1 agonist effects of dobutamine may be unmasked by β blockade. Dobutamine produces a positive inotropic effect with minimal effects on heart rate and systemic vascular resistance (an advantage over isoproterenol).

   a. **Side effects.** Increases in automaticity of the sinoatrial node and increases in conduction of cardiac impulses through the atrioventricular node and ventricles occur, emphasizing the need for caution in administering this drug to patients with atrial fibrillation or other tachydysrhythmias. Dobutamine may increase heart rate more than epinephrine for a given increase in cardiac output.

   b. **Clinical uses.** Dobutamine is most often administered (2 to 30 μg/kg/min iv) for its inotropic effects in patients with poor myocardial contractility, such as after cardiopulmonary bypass.

8. **Dopamine** is an agonist at dopaminergic (0.5 to 2 μg/kg/min iv [renal dose of dopamine but maybe more imagined than real]), β (2 to 10 μg/kg/min iv), and α (>10 μg/kg/min iv) receptors. Infusion rates >10 μg/kg/min iv may produce sufficient

vasoconstriction to offset desirable dopaminergic (increases renal blood flow) and β-(increased cardiac output) receptor stimulation. Despite the apparent dose-response dependency of dopamine, a wide variability of individual responses has been observed.

a. **Side effects.** Tachycardia and cardiac dysrhythmias occur infrequently. Extravasation of dopamine can produce gangrene. Pulmonary artery pressure may be increased, detracting from the use of dopamine in patients with right-sided heart failure. Insulin secretion is inhibited, explaining the common occurrence of hyperglycemia during infusion of dopamine.

b. **Clinical uses.** Dopamine is most often administered as a continuous intravenous infusion (2 to 10 μg/kg/min) for its inotropic and diuretic effects in patients with poor myocardial contractility, such as following cardiopulmonary bypass.

9. **Combination therapy** is most often with dopamine and dobutamine in an attempt to maximize positive inotropic effect with less vasoconstriction.

E. **Clonidine** is a centrally acting selective partial α-2 agonist. It is an antihypertensive drug by virtue of its ability to decrease central sympathetic outflow.

1. **Side Effects.** Sedation, bradycardia, and dry mouth from sympatholytics are common. Abrupt discontinuation of clonidine, as before surgery, may result in rebound hypertension, especially if the daily dose is >1.2 mg. This hypertension may be confused with a response to emergence from anesthesia, but it is typically delayed for about 18 hours. Transdermal administration of clonidine is an alternative to the oral route, because an intravenous preparation is not available. Life-threatening hypertension after withdrawal may be treated with nitroprusside.

2. **Clinical Uses.** In addition to its antihypertensive effect, clonidine administered preoperatively (5 μg/kg orally) attenuates SNS reflex responses such as those associated with direct laryngoscopy or surgical stimulation and greatly decreases anesthetic requirements (40% or more) for volatile drugs or opioids. When placed in the subarachnoid or epidural space, this drug produces analgesia that may be accompanied by sedation and bradycardia but not depression of ventilation.

F. **Dexmedetomidine** is a more selective α-2 agonist than clonidine. A stereoselective ability to interact with receptors resulting in decreased anesthetic requirements is evidence for an "anesthetic receptor."
   1. This drug produces excellent sedation (no depression of ventilation but upper airway obstruction may occur), produces analgesia, reduces blood pressure and heart rate (promotes hemodynamic stability) and greatly decreases plasma catecholamines.
   2. The loading infusion of 1 μg/kg is administered over 10 minutes in a monitored setting.

VI. NONADRENERGIC SYMPATHOMIMETIC AGENTS

A. **Vasopressin** and its congener, desmopressin, are exogenous preparations of the endogenous antidiuretic hormone (ADH).
   1. Clinical uses of vasopressin have included treatment of diabetes and as an adjunct to treatment of gastrointestinal bleeding and esophageal varices.
   2. New clinical indications for vasopressin include support of patients with septic shock, and cardiac arrest (40 IU in 40 mL intravenously) secondary to ventricular fibrillation or pulseless ventricular tachycardia.
B. **Adenosine** is an endogenous by-product of adenosine triphosphate, which when administered intravenously has negative chronotropic effects on the sinoatrial node as well as negative dromotropic effects on the atrioventricular node. The principal clinical use of adenosine is termination of paroxysmal supraventricular tachycardia (6 mg iv [100 to 150 μg/kg iv for pediatric patients]).
C. **Amrinone** is a phosphodiesterase inhibitor that is administered intravenously (loading dose followed by a continuous infusion) and increases cardiac output by positive inotropic effects as well as vasodilation with resulting decreases in systemic vascular resistance.
D. **Milrinone** is a more potent phosphodiesterase inhibitor that lacks effects on platelets and may be useful for short-term intravenous therapy of congestive heart failure.
E. **Digoxin** is administered principally to treat congestive heart failure and control supraventricular

tachydysrhythmias such as atrial fibrillation. A therapeutic effect occurs within 10 minutes (0.25 to 1.0 mg iv for adults). Signs of digitalis toxicity (cardiac dysrhythmias, gastrointestinal disturbances) must be inquired about when evaluating patients preoperatively. Digitalis toxicity is enhanced by hypokalemia or injection of calcium. Iatrogenic hyperventilation of the lungs with associated hypokalemia should be avoided during anesthesia. Most recommend continuation of digitalis therapy in the perioperative period, especially when the drug is being administered for heart rate control. Prophylactic preoperative administration of digitalis preparations is controversial but may be of unique value in elderly patients undergoing thoracic surgery.

VII. ADRENERGIC ANTAGONISTS-SYMPATHOLYTICS

A. α *Antagonists* produce orthostatic hypotension, tachycardia, and miosis.
   1. **Phentolamine** is a nonselective and competitive antagonist at α-1 and α-2 receptors; it is typically administered (2 to 5 mg iv) until adequate control of blood pressure is achieved. Tachycardia reflects continued presynaptic release of norepinephrine owing to α-2 receptor blockade.
   2. **Prazosin** is a selective postsynaptic α-1 antagonist that leaves intact the negative feedback mechanism for norepinephrine release that is mediated by presynaptic α-2 activity. This drug is useful in the preoperative preparation of patients with pheochromocytoma.
B. β *Antagonists* are distinguished by differing pharmacokinetic and pharmacodynamic characteristics (Table 12-5).
   1. **Side effects** of β antagonists include heart block, worsening of congestive heart failure, bronchospasm, vasoconstriction (of coronary arteries), and inhibition of insulin release. Excessive SNS activity (hypertension, angina) may accompany abrupt withdrawal of β antagonists, presumably reflecting prior up-regulation of β receptors caused by chronic suppression of agonist activity.

TABLE 12-5
PHARMACOKINETICS OF β ANTAGONISTS

Agent	Relative B-1 selectivity	Membrane stabilizing activity	Intrinsic sympathomimetic activity	Elimination half-time (hr)	Lipid solubility	Route of elimination
Propranolol	0	+	0	3–4	+++	Hepatic
Nadolol	0	0	0	14–24	0	Renal
Timolol	0	0	0	4–5	+	Hepatic Renal
Pindolol	0	+	++	3–4	+	Hepatic Renal
Esmolol	++	0	0	0.16	?	Plasma esterase
Acebutol	+	+	+	3–4	0	Hepatic
Atenolol	++	0	0	6–9	0	Renal
Metoprolol	++	0	0	3–4	+	Hepatic

2. **β-1 selectivity (cardioselective)** implies greater safety in treatment of patients with obstructive pulmonary disease, diabetes mellitus, or peripheral vascular disease because β-2 agonist effects (bronchodilation, vasodilation) presumably are maintained. The clinical significance of membrane-stabilizing activity (a local anesthetic effect on myocardial cells at high doses) or intrinsic sympathomimetic activity (partial β agonist activity at low doses) is not documented. Because of their selectivity, the use of β-blockers has extended to include treatment of congestive heart failure.

3. **Propranolol** is a nonselective β antagonist that may be administered in single intravenous doses of 0.1 to 0.5 mg (maximum dose about 2 mg) to slow heart rate during anesthesia. Additive negative inotropic or chronotropic effects with inhaled or injected anesthetics are likely to occur but have not been a significant clinical problem.

4. **Timolol** is administered as a topical preparation for the treatment of glaucoma. There may be sufficient systemic absorption to cause bradycardia and hypotension that are resistant to reversal with atropine.

5. **Esmolol** is a cardioselective β-1 antagonist administered as a single intravenous bolus (0.5 mg/kg) or as a continuous intravenous infusion (50 to 200 μg/kg/min) to produce rapid and short duration decreases in heart rate and blood pressure. A unique feature is rapid hydrolysis by plasma esterases, allowing precise control of drug effect during continuous intravenous infusion.

6. **Mixed Antagonists. Labetalol** produces selective α-1 and nonselective β antagonist effects. Administered as a single dose (0.05 to 0.15 mg/kg iv over 2 minutes), this drug is useful in controlling hypertension and tachycardia in response to painful stimulation during general anesthesia. Although the magnitude is less than with β antagonists, worsening of congestive heart failure or appearance of bronchospasm may follow administration of labetalol.

VIII. CALCIUM ENTRY BLOCKERS interact with cell membranes to interfere with movement of calcium into cells through ion-specific channels (known as slow

TABLE 12-6

COMPARATIVE EFFECTS OF CALCIUM ENTRY BLOCKERS

	Verapamil	Nifedipine	Diltiazem
Dose			
Intravenous (μg/kg)	75–150	5–15	75–150
Oral (mg every 8 hr)	80–160	10–20	60–90
Negative inotropic	+	0	0/+
Negative chronotropic	+	0	0/+
Negative dromotropic	+ + + +	0	+ + +
Coronary artery vasodilation	+ +	+ + + +	+ + +
Systemic vasodilation	+ +	+ + + +	+ +
Bronchodilation	0/+	0/+	
Elimination half-time (hr)	2–7	4–5	4
Route of elimination	Renal	Renal	Hepatic

channels because their transition among the resting, activated, and inactivated states is delayed compared with fast sodium channels).

A. Calcium entry blockers are a heterogeneous group of drugs with dissimilar structures and different electrophysiologic and pharmacologic properties. These drugs are most useful for the treatment of supraventricular tachydysrhythmias and coronary artery vasospasm (Table 12-6).

B. **Verapamil** is the drug of choice for termination of supraventricular dysrhythmias, and it is also effective in slowing the heart rate in patients with atrial fibrillation and atrial flutter. There is a dose-dependent increase in the P-R interval on the electrocardiogram and a delay in conduction of cardiac impulses through the atrioventricular node.

　　1. Caution must be exercised when treating patients with Wolff-Parkinson-White syndrome because verapamil may increase conduction velocity in the accessory tract.

　　2. Unlike β antagonists, verapamil does not increase airway resistance in patients with obstructive pulmonary disease.

C. **Nifedipine** is more effective than nitroglycerin for treatment of angina pectoris because of coronary artery vasospasm.

1. Vasodilation results in compensatory tachycardia, and cardiac output may increase as a result of afterload reduction.
2. Administration of nifedipine is useful during anesthesia when there is evidence of myocardial ischemia associated with hypertension.

D. **Diltiazem** is an effective coronary artery vasodilatory but a poor peripheral vasodilator; it may produce bradycardia.

E. **Nicardipine** produces vasodilation of coronary arterioles without altering activity of the sinus node or conduction of cardiac impulses through the atrioventricular node.

F. **Nimodipine** is a highly lipophilic drug that produces somewhat selective vasodilation of cerebral arteries, resulting as a favorable effect on the severity of neurologic deficits caused by cerebral vasospasm following subarachnoid hemorrhage.

G. **Calcium entry blockers** may exhibit additive myocardial depressant effects with volatile anesthetics, which may also interfere with inward calcium movement. Opioids do not seem to alter the response to calcium entry blockers. Calcium entry blockers seem to augment the effects of both depolarizing and nondepolarizing muscle relaxants in a manner similar to that of "mycin" antibiotics.

IX. CONVERTING ENZYME INHIBITORS

A. Inhibitors of angiotensin-converting enzyme (captopril, enalapril, lisinopril) prevent the conversion of angiotensin I to angiotensin II. These drugs are effective in the treatment of congestive heart failure and essential hypertension as well as renovascular and malignant hypertension.

B. Side effects are minor, with the principal cardiovascular effect being systemic vascular resistance.

X. VASODILATORS

A. Vasodilators decrease blood pressure by dose-related direct effects on vascular smooth muscle independent of α or β receptors (Table 12-7). These drugs may evoke baroreceptor-mediated increases in heart rate. Combination with α antagonist may be necessary to

TABLE 12-7
DOSES AND SITES OF ACTION OF VASODILATORS

Agent	Bolus (adult, iv)	Continuous infusion (adult, iv)	Site of action	Onset	Duration
Hydralazine	5–10 mg		Arterial	15–20 min	4–6 hrs
Nitroprusside	50–100 μg	0.25–5 μg/kg/min (50 mg in 250 mL, 200 μg/mL)	Arterial and venous	1–2 min	2–5 min
Nitroglycerin		0.25–3 μg/kg/min (50 mg in 250 mL, 200 μg/mL)	Venous and arterial	2–5 min	3–5 min
Diazoxide	300 mg		Arterial	3–5 min	5–12 hrs

offset this reflex tachycardia (maintain heart rate <100 beats/min).

B. **Hydralazine** (5 to 10 mg iv every 10 to 20 minutes) is useful to control perioperative hypertension.

C. **Nitroprusside** is administered as a continuous infusion (0.25 to 0.5 μg/kg/min iv) using an infusion pump and continuous monitoring of blood pressure. The dose is increased slowly as needed to control hypertension or to produce controlled hypotension. Rarely is more than 3 to 5 μg/kg/min of nitroprusside required in an anesthetized patient. Acute hypertensive responses can be treated with single intravenous doses of 50 to 100 μg.

   1. The hypotensive effect of nitroprusside reflects direct relaxation of arterial and venous smooth muscle, causing decreases in preload and afterload. Hypotensive effects of nitroprusside are potentiated by volatile anesthetics and blood loss.

   2. **Side Effects.** The ferrous iron of nitroprusside reacts with sulfhydryl groups in red blood cells and releases cyanide, which is reduced to thiocyanate in the liver. High doses of nitroprusside (>10 μg/kg/min iv) may result in cyanide toxicity. There is no evidence that renal or hepatic diseases increase the likelihood of cyanide toxicity.

      a. **Diagnosis.** Tachyphylaxis, increased venous oxygen tension, and metabolic acidosis signal the development of cyanide toxicity (cyanide binds to cytochrome oxidase causing cellular hypoxia) and the need to discontinue the infusion of nitroprusside immediately.

      b. **Treatment** of cyanide toxicity is with sodium thiosulfate (150 mg/kg iv in 50 mL of water) administered over 15 minutes to speed the conversion of cyanide to thiocyanate.

D. **Nitroglycerin** is administered as a continuous infusion (0.25 to 3.0 μg/kg/min iv) to treat myocardial ischemia. Its predominant action is on venules, causing increased venous capacitance and decreased venous return.

   1. Control of hypertension with nitroglycerin is less reliable than with nitroprusside, emphasizing the minimal effect of this drug on arterial smooth muscle.

   2. Unlike nitroprusside, nitroglycerin poses no risk of cyanide toxicity. For this reason, nitroglycerin may

be chosen over nitroprusside to control hypertension associated with pregnancy-induced hypertension.

E. **Diazoxide** is administered as a single dose (3 to 5 mg/kg iv every 5 min) to treat hypertensive emergencies. This drug has a greater effect on resistance than capacitance vessels, thus decreasing afterload with little or no effect on preload. Ability to titrate blood pressure to a given level, as with nitroprusside, is not possible with diazoxide.

CHAPTER 13 ■ NONOPIOID INTRAVENOUS ANESTHESIA

The concept of intravenous anesthesia has evolved from primarily induction of anesthesia to that of total intravenous anesthesia (White PF, Romero G: Nonopioid intravenous anesthesia. In Barash PG, Cullen BF, Stoelting RK [eds]: *Clinical Anesthesia*, pp 334–352. Philadelphia, Lippincott Williams & Wilkins, 2006). This change has been spurred by the development of rapid, short-acting intravenous hypnotic, analgesic, and muscle relaxant drugs, as well as reliable, easier-to-use infusion equipment (Table 13-1 and Fig. 13-1). Because the desired pharmacologic properties are not equally important in every clinical situation, the anesthesiologist must make the choice that best fits the needs of the individual patient and the operative procedure.

I. GENERAL PHARMACOLOGY OF INTRAVENOUS ANESTHETICS

A. Mechanism of Action

1. A widely accepted theory is that intravenous hypnotics (benzodiazepines, barbiturates, propofol, etomidate, ketamine) exert their primary effects through an interaction with the inhibitory neurotransmitter, γ-aminobutyric acid (GABA) (Fig. 13-2).

2. Activation of the GABA-receptor complex increases transmembrane chloride conductance (results in hyperpolarization and functional inhibition of the postsynaptic neuron).

3. Benzodiazepines increase the efficiency of the coupling between GABA and its receptor (ceiling effect).

4. Barbiturates and propofol appear to decrease the dissociation of GABA from its receptor.

5. Ketamine's central nervous system (CNS) effects appear to be primarily related to its antagonistic activity at the N-methyl-D-aspartate (NMDA) receptor. In addition, ketamine inhibits neuronal sodium channels (modest local anesthetic activity) and calcium channels (cerebral vasodilation).

6. Dexmedetomidine is a centrally active α-2 adrenergic agonist that produces potent sedative and

TABLE 13-1

DESIRABLE CHARACTERISTICS OF AN INTRAVENOUS ANESTHETIC

Stable in solution
Absence of pain on injection (venoirritation) or tissue damage from extravasation
Low potential to release histamine
Rapid onset
Prompt metabolism to inactive metabolites
Efficient clearance/redistribution mechanisms
Benign cardiovascular and/or ventilatory effects
Decrease in cerebral blood flow and metabolism
Prompt and complete return of consciousness
Absence of adverse postoperative effects (nausea, vomiting, delirium, headache)

   analgesic-sparing properties and reduces sympathetic outflow from the central nervous system

B. **Pharmacokinetics and Metabolism**

1. The rapid onset of the CNS effect of most intravenous anesthetics can be explained by their high lipid solubility and relatively high cerebral blood flow.

2. The pharmacokinetics of intravenous hypnotics are characterized by rapid distribution and subsequent redistribution into several hypothetical compartments, followed by elimination (Table 13-2).

   a. The primary mechanism for terminating the CNS effects of drugs used for the intravenous induction of anesthesia is redistribution from a central highly perfused compartment (brain) to larger and well-perfused peripheral compartments (muscle, fat).

   b. Most intravenous anesthetic agents are eliminated via hepatic metabolism (some metabolites are active) followed by renal excretion of more water-soluble metabolites.

   c. For most drugs, the hepatic enzyme systems are not saturated at clinically relevant drug concentrations, and the rate of drug elimination will decrease as an exponential function of the drug's plasma concentration (first-order kinetics).

   d. High steady-state plasma concentrations are achieved with prolonged infusions, hepatic enzyme

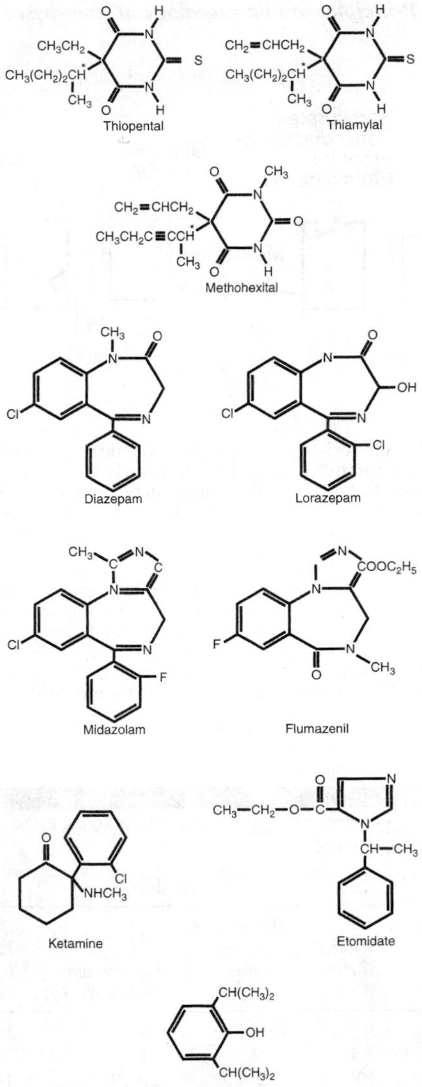

FIGURE 13-1. Chemical structures of nonopioid intravenous anesthetics.

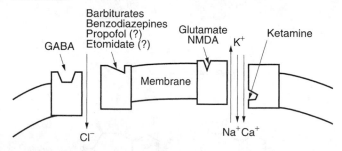

Extracellular

Intracellular

FIGURE 13-2. A model depicting the postsynaptic receptor sites for the inhibitory neurotransmitter γ-aminobutyric acid (GABA) and the excitatory neurotransmitter glutamate in the central nervous system. When GABA occupies the receptor, it allows inward flux of chloride ions resulting in hyperpolarization of the cell membrane and subsequent resistance of the neurons to stimulation by excitatory neurotransmitters. Barbiturates, benzodiazepines, and possibly propofol and etomidate decrease neuronal excitability by enhancing the effect of GABA at this receptor complex. When glutamate occupies the binding site of N-methyl-D-aspartate (NMDA) subtype of the glutamate receptor, the channel opens and allows sodium, potassium, and calcium ions to enter or leave the cell. Flux of these ions leads to depolarization of the postsynaptic neuron and initiation of an action potential. Ketamine blocks these open channels, thus inhibiting the excitatory response to glutamate.

TABLE 13-2

PHARMACOKINETIC VALUES FOR INTRAVENOUS ANESTHETIC DRUGS

Drugs	Protein binding (%)	Volume at steady state (L/kg)	Clearance (mL/kg/min)	Elimination half-time (h)
Thiopental	85	2.5	3.4	11
Methohexital	85	2.2	11	4
Propofol	98	2–10	20–30	14–23
Midazolam	94	1.1–1.7	6.4–11	1.7–2.6
Diazepam	98	0.7–1.7	0.2–0.5	20–50
Lorazepam	98	0.8–1.3	0.8–1.8	11–22
Etomidate	75	2.5–4.5	18–25	2.9–5.3
Ketamine	12	2.5–3.5	12–17	2–4

The "Distribution" spanning header covers: Protein binding (%), Volume at steady state (L/kg), and Clearance (mL/kg/min).

systems can become saturated, and the elimination rate becomes independent of the drug concentration (zero-order kinetics).

    e. Perfusion-limited clearance describes hepatic clearance of drugs (etomidate, propofol, ketamine, methohexital, midazolam) in which extraction is largely dependent on delivery to the liver (hepatic blood flow decreases with upper abdominal surgery, increasing age).

3. The **elimination half-time** $(T1/2\beta)$ is the time required for the plasma concentration to decrease 50%.

    a. Wide variations in $T1/2\beta$ reflect differences in volume of distribution (Vd) and/or clearance.

    b. Careful titration of an anesthetic drug to achieve the desired clinical effect is necessary to avoid drug accumulation and the resultant prolonged CNS effects after the infusion has been discontinued.

4. Context-sensitive half-time is the time necessary for the plasma concentration to decrease 50% in relation to the duration of the infusion (important for determining recovery after varying length infusions of sedative–hypnotic drugs).

5. Many factors contribute to interpatient variability in the pharmacokinetics of intravenous sedative–hypnotic drugs (Table 13-3).

C. Pharmacodynamic Effects

1. The principal pharmacologic effect of intravenous anesthetics is to produce dose-dependent CNS depression (dose-response curves) manifesting as sedation and hypnosis (Fig. 13-3).

2. When steady-state plasma concentrations are achieved, it can be presumed that the plasma

---

TABLE 13-3

FACTORS THAT CONTRIBUTE TO INTERPATIENT VARIABILITY IN PHARMACOKINETICS

Degree of protein binding
Efficiency of renal and hepatic clearance mechanisms
Aging (lean body mass decreases)
Preexisting diseases (hepatic, renal, cardiac)
Drug interactions
Body temperature

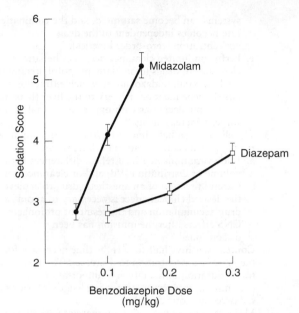

FIGURE 13-3. Dose-response relationships for sedation with midazolam and diazepam. The level of sedation was rated as 2 (awake and alert) to 6 (asleep).

concentration is in equilibrium with the effect-site (receptor) concentration.

a. **Efficacy** of an intravenous anesthetic relates to the maximum effect that can be achieved with respect to some measure to CNS function (benzodiazepines less efficacious than barbiturates in depressing electrical activity in the brain).

b. **Potency** relates to the quantity of drug necessary to obtain the maximum CNS effect.

3. Most sedative–hypnotic drugs (exception is ketamine) cause a proportional reduction in cerebral metabolism ($CMRO_2$) and cerebral blood flow (CBF) resulting in a decrease in intracranial pressure (ICP).

a. On the electroencephalogram (EEG), it is likely that sedative doses will produce activation of high-frequency activity, whereas anesthetic doses produce a burst-suppression pattern.

    b. Most sedative–hypnotic drugs can cause occasional EEG seizure-like activity (differentiate between the epileptogenic activity [methohexital] and myoclonic-like phenomena [etomidate]) despite also acting as anticonvulsants. Myoclonic activity is considered to be the result of an imbalance between excitatory and inhibitory subcortical centers owing to unequal degrees of suppression of these centers by the hypnotic drug.

  4. Most sedative–hypnotics (exception is ketamine) lower intraocular pressure in parallel with effects on ICP and blood pressure.

  5. With the exception of ketamine (and to a lesser extent etomidate), intravenous anesthetics produce dose-dependent depression of ventilation (transient apnea followed by decreased tidal volume).

  6. Many different factors contribute to the hemodynamic changes associated with intravenous induction of anesthesia (Table 13-4).

  7. Most intravenous sedative–hypnotic drugs lack intrinsic analgesic activity (exception is ketamine, which has pronounced analgesic-like activity).

D. Hypersensitivity (Allergic) Reactions

  1. Allergic reactions to intravenous anesthetics and/or their solubilizing agents, although rare, can be life threatening.

  2. With the exception of etomidate, all intravenous induction drugs have been alleged to cause some histamine release.

  3. Although propofol does not normally trigger histamine release, life-threatening allergic reactions have been reported, especially in patients with a

TABLE 13-4

FACTORS THAT CONTRIBUTE TO HEMODYNAMIC EFFECT OF INTRAVENOUS INDUCTION

Drugs
Blood volume
Sympathetic nervous system tone
Speed of injection
Cardiovascular drugs
Preanesthetic medication
Direct effects on cardiac contractility and/or peripheral vasculature

history of allergy to other drugs (most often muscle relaxants).

4. Barbiturates may precipitate episodes of acute intermittent porphyria in vulnerable patients (benzodiazepines, ketamine, etomidate, and propofol are reported to be safe).

II. COMPARATIVE PHYSIOCHEMICAL AND CLINICAL PHARMACOLOGIC PROPERTIES

A. Barbiturates

1. Thiopental and thiamylal are thiobarbiturates with similar potency (adult induction dose is 3 to 5 mg/kg iv) and pharmacologic profile. Methohexital is an oxybarbiturate with a greater potency (adult induction dose is 1.5 mg/kg iv) than the thiobarbiturates and is associated with a high incidence of myoclonic-like muscle tremors and other signs of excitatory activity (hiccoughing).

   a. These drugs are provided as racemic mixtures that are alkaline (thiopental 2.5% has a pH >9) and will precipitate when added to acidic solutions (Ringer's lactate).

   b. Geriatric patients require a 30 to 40% reduction in the usual adult dose because of a decrease of the volume of the central compartment and slowed redistribution of thiopental from the vessel-rich tissues to lean muscle.

   c. Thiopental is seldom used to maintain anesthesia because of its long context-sensitive half-time and prolonged recovery period.

   d. Accidental intra-arterial injection of barbiturates may result in formation of crystals in arterioles and capillaries causing intense vasoconstriction, thrombosis, and even tissue necrosis (treat with intra-arterial administration of papaverine and lidocaine, brachial plexus block, heparin).

2. Methohexital is metabolized in the liver to inactive metabolites more rapidly than thiopental.

3. Barbiturates produce a maximum decrease in $CMRO_2$ (55%) when the EEG becomes isoelectric (associated with a decrease in CBF and ICP).

   a. An isoelectric EEG can be maintained with a thiopental infusion rate of 4 to 6 mg/kg/hr iv.

   b. Although barbiturate therapy is widely used to control ICP after brain injury, the results of outcome studies are no better than with other aggressive forms of cerebral antihypertensive therapy.
   c. Barbiturates have no place in the therapy following resuscitation of a cardiac arrest patient.
   d. Barbiturates may improve the brain's tolerance to incomplete ischemia and may be used for cerebroprotection during carotid endarterectomy, profound controlled hypotension, or cardiopulmonary bypass (moderate degrees of hypothermia [33°C to 34°C] may provide superior neuroprotection without prolonging the recovery phase).
   e. Barbiturates possess potent anticonvulsant activity (methohexital produces epileptogenic effects in patients with psychomotor epilepsy).
4. Barbiturates cause dose-dependent depression of ventilation (bronchospasm and laryngospasm are usually the result of airway manipulation in the presence of inadequate anesthesia).
5. Cardiovascular effects of barbiturates include decreases in blood pressure (decreased venous return due to peripheral pooling and direct myocardial depression) and a compensatory increase in heart rate.
6. Hypotension is exaggerated in the presence of hypovolemia.

B. **Propofol**
1. As an alkylphenol compound this drug is virtually insoluble in water, requiring its preparation in an egg-lecithin emulsion as a 1% (10 mg/mL) solution.
   a. An alternative propofol formulation containing sodium metabisulfite (rather than disodium edetate) as an antimicrobial is associated with less pain on injection. The concern regarding use of this formulation in sulphite-allergic patients does not seem to be a clinically important problem.
   b. Ampofol is a lower-lipid formulation of propofol and the increased free fraction of propofol leads to increased pain with injection into small veins.
   c. Aquavan is a water-soluble pro-drug that is rapidly metabolized in the circulation to release propofol. Onset is slower but recovery is similar to propofol.

2. Propofol is rapidly cleared from the central compartment by hepatic metabolism and the context-sensitive half-time for continuous intravenous infusions (up to 8 hours) is <40 minutes (emergence and awakening are prompt and complete after even prolonged infusions).
   a. Hepatic metabolism is prompt to inactive water-soluble metabolites that are eliminated by the kidneys.
   b. The clearance rate (1.5 to 2.2 L/min) exceeds hepatic blood flow, suggesting that an extrahepatic route of elimination (lungs) also contributes to its clearance (important during anhepatic phase of liver transplantation).
3. The induction dose in adults is 1.5 to 2.5 mg/kg iv and the recommended intravenous infusion rate for hypnosis is 100 to 200 μg/kg/min and 25 to 75 μg/kg/min for sedation.
   a. Pain on injection occurs in a high proportion of patients when injected into small hand veins but can be minimized by injection into larger veins or by prior administration of 1% lidocaine.
   b. Propofol may produce a subjective feeling of well-being and euphoria and may have abuse potential as a result of these effects.
4. Propofol decreases $CMRO_2$, CBF, and ICP, but the associated decrease in systemic blood pressure may also significantly decrease cerebral perfusion pressure.
   a. Cortical EEG changes produced by propofol resemble thiopental.
   b. A neuroprotective effect may reflect antioxidant properties.
   c. Induction of anesthesia with propofol is occasionally accompanied by excitatory motor activity (nonepileptic myoclonia).
   d. This drug is an anticonvulsant (duration of seizure activity following electroconvulsive therapy is shorter with propofol than methohexital) and is effective in terminating status epilepticus.
5. Propofol produces dose-dependent depression of ventilation (apnea occurs in 25 to 35% of patients after induction of anesthesia).
   a. Bronchodilatation may occur in patients with chronic obstructive pulmonary disease.

    b. Hypoxic pulmonary vasoconstriction is not inhibited by propofol.

  6. Propofol produces greater cardiovascular depressant effects than thiopental, reflecting decreased systemic vascular resistance (arterial and venous dilation) and direct myocardial depressant effects.

  7. Propofol appears to possess antiemetic properties that contribute to a low incidence of emetic sequelae after propofol anesthesia (subanesthetic doses [10 to 20 mg] may be used to treat nausea and emesis in the early postoperative period). Postulated antiemetic mechanisms include an antidopaminergic activity and a depressant effect on the chemoreceptor trigger zone and vagal nuclei.

  8. Propofol decreases the pruritus associated with neuraxial opioids.

  9. Propofol does not trigger malignant hyperthermia and may be considered the induction drug of choice in patients susceptible to malignant hyperthermia.

C. Benzodiazepines

  1. The benzodiazepines of primary interest to anesthesiologists are diazepam, lorazepam, midazolam, and the antagonist flumazenil.

    a. These drugs are primarily used as preoperative medication and adjuvant drugs because of their anxiolytic, sedative, and amnestic properties.

    b. Diazepam and lorazepam are insoluble in water and their formulation contains proplene glycol, a tissue irritant that causes pain on injection and venous irritation.

    c. Midazolam is a water-soluble benzodiazepine that produces minimal irritation after intravenous or intramuscular injection. When exposed to physiologic pH, an intramolecular rearrangement occurs that changes the physiocochemical properties of midazolam such that it becomes more lipid soluble.

  2. Benzodiazepines undergo hepatic metabolism via oxidation and glucuronide conjugation (oxidation reactions are susceptible to hepatic dysfunction and coadministration of other drugs such as H2-receptor antagonists).

    a. The hepatic clearance rate of midazolam is 5 times greater than lorazepam and 10 times greater than diazepam.

   b. Diazepam is metabolized to active metabolites, which can prolong its residual sedative effects.
   c. Lorazepam is directly conjugated glucuronic acid to form pharmacologically inactive metabolites, while the primary metabolite of midazolam (1-hydroxymethylmidazolam) has some CNS depressant activity.
   d. The context-sensitive half-times for diazepam and lorazepam are very long; therefore, only midazolam should be used for continuous infusion.
3. Benzodiazepines decrease $CMRO_2$ and CBF analogous to the barbiturates and propofol, but these drugs have not been shown to possess neuroprotective activity in humans.
   a. In contrast to other compounds, midazolam is unable to produce an isoelectric EEG.
   b. Like the other sedative–hypnotic drugs, the benzodiazepines are potent anticonvulsants that are commonly used to treat status epilepticus.
4. Benzodiazepines produce dose-dependent depression of ventilation that is enhanced in patients with chronic respiratory disease, and synergistic depressant effects occur when benzodiazepines are co-administered with opioids.
5. Both midazolam and diazepam produce decreases in systemic vascular resistance and systemic blood pressure (accentuated with hypovolemia) when large doses are administered for induction of anesthesia, but a ceiling effect appears to exist above which little further change in arterial pressure occurs.
6. Short-acting intravenous sedatives are characterized by water-soluble benzodiazepines with full agonist activity and a higher plasma clearance rate compared with midazolam.
7. In contrast to all other sedative–hypnotic drugs, there is a specific antagonist for benzodiazepines (flumazenil has a high affinity for CNS benzodiazepine receptors but possesses minimal intrinsic activity).
   a. Flumazenil acts as a competitive antagonist in the presence of benzodiazepine agonist compounds.
   b. Recurrence of the CNS effects of benzodiazepines may occur after a single dose of flumazenil (rapidly metabolized in the liver with an elimination half-time of about 1 hour) as a result of

residual effects of the more slowly eliminated agonist.
- c. In general, 45 to 90 minutes of antagonism can be expected following flumazenil (1 to 3 mg iv) (sustained effects require repeated doses or continuous infusion).

D. Etomidate
1. Etomidate is a carboxylated imidazole (only the dextro isomer possesses anesthetic activity) that is structurally unrelated to any other intravenous anesthetic but, like midazolam (which also contains an imidazole nucleus), undergoes an intramolecular rearrangement at physiologic pH, resulting in a closed ring structure with enhanced lipid solubility.
   - a. This drug is formulated with propylene glycol contributing to a high incidence of pain on injection and occasional venoirritation.
   - b. The standard induction dose of etomidate (0.2 to 0.4 mg/kg iv) produces a rapid onset of anesthesia (myoclonic movements common owing to an alteration in the balance of inhibitory and excitatory influence on the thalamocortical tract) and emergence is prompt (extensive ester hydrolysis in the liver forming inactive water-soluble metabolites).
2. Analogous to the barbiturates, etomidate decreases $CMRO_2$, CBF, and ICP, but the hemodynamic stability associated with etomidate will maintain adequate cerebral perfusion pressure.
   - a. An inhibitory effect on adrenocortical synthetic function (single dose inhibits 11-β-hydroxylase for 5 to 8 hours) limits its clinical usefulness for long-term treatment of increased ICP.
   - b. Although an anticonvulsant effective in terminating status epilepticus, etomidate is also capable of evoking EEG evidence of seizure activity in attempts to identify seizure foci.
   - c. Etomidate produces a significant increase in the amplitude of somatosensory-evoked potentials and can be used to facilitate the interpretation of somatosensory-evoked potentials when the signal quality is poor.
3. Etomidate causes minimal depression of ventilation and cardiovascular function (may be recommended

for induction of anesthesia in poor-risk patients with cardiopulmonary disease) and does not release histamine (acceptable drug for use in patients with reactive airway disease).

4. Etomidate is associated with a high incidence and vomiting especially if combined with an opioid.

5. Etomidate may inhibit platelet function and prolong bleeding time.

E. Ketamine

1. Ketamine is an acrylcyclohexilamine that is structurally related to phencyclidine.

   a. The commercially available preparation is a racemic mixture, although the S+ isomer possesses more potent anesthetic and analgesic properties reflecting its fourfold greater affinity at the binding sites on the NMDA receptor. Hepatic biotransformation of the S+ isomer is more rapid contributing to a faster return of cognitive function. Both isomers possess similar cardiovascular-stimulating properties and the incidence of dreaming is similar with the S+ isomer and the racemic mixture.

   b. Ketamine produces dose-dependent CNS depression leading to a so-called dissociative anesthetic state characterized by profound analgesia and amnesia. Low-dose ketamine (75 to 200 μg/kg/min iv) produces opioid-sparing effects when administered as an adjuvant during general anesthesia.

   c. Induction of anesthesia can be accomplished with 1 to 2 mg/kg iv (4 to 8 mg/kg iv) producing an effect that lasts 10 to 20 minutes, although recovery to full orientation may require an additional 60 to 90 minutes.

   d. Subanesthetic doses of ketamine (0.1 to 0.5 mg/kg iv) produce analgesic effects. A low-dose infusion of ketamine (4 μg/kg/min iv) is equivalent to morphine (2 mg/hr iv) for production of postoperative analgesia.

2. Ketamine is extensively metabolized in the liver to norketamine, which is one-third to one-fifth as potent as the parent compound.

3. Psychomimetic reactions during the recovery period from ketamine anesthesia are less likely in patients

also treated with benzodiazepines, barbiturates, or propofol.

4. Ketamine increases $CMRO_2$, CBF, and ICP (minimized by hyperventilation of the lungs and pretreatment with benzodiazepines).

5. Ketamine can activate epileptogenic foci in patients with known seizure disorders but otherwise appears to possess anticonvulsant activity.

6. Ketamine is often recommended for induction of anesthesia in patients with asthma because of its ability to produce bronchodilation.

   a. Depression of ventilation is minimal in clinically relevant doses.

   b. Increased oral secretions can contribute to the development of laryngospasm.

7. Ketamine has prominent cardiovascular-stimulating effects (increased blood pressure, heart rate, pulmonary artery pressure) most likely because of direct stimulation of the sympathetic nervous system (possibly undesirable in patients with coronary artery disease).

   a. Ketamine has intrinsic myocardial depressant properties, which may only become apparent in the seriously ill patient with depleted catecholamine.

   b. Ketamine can reduce the magnitude of redistribution hypothermia owing to its peripheral arteriolar vasoconstriction.

8. The anesthetic and analgesic potency of S(+)-ketamine is 3 times greater than R(−)-ketamine and twice that of the racemic mixture.

III. CLINICAL USES OF INTRAVENOUS ANESTHETICS

A. Use of Intravenous Anesthetics as Induction Agents
(Table 13-5)

1. Propofol has become the intravenous drug of choice for outpatients undergoing ambulatory surgery.

2. Clinical use of midazolam (often combined with other injected drugs), etomidate (cardiac stability), and ketamine (hypovolemic patients) is restricted to specific situations where their unique pharmacologic profiles offer advantages over other available intravenous anesthetics.

TABLE 13-5
INDUCTION CHARACTERISTICS AND DOSAGE REQUIREMENTS FOR INTRAVENOUS ANESTHETIC DRUGS

Drug	Induction dose (mg/kg)	Onset (sec)	Duration (min)	Excitatory activity	Pain on injection	Heart rate	Blood pressure
Thiopental	3–6	<30	5–10	+	0/+	+	–
Methohexital	1–3	<30	5–10	++	+	++	–
Propofol	1.5–2.5	15–45	5–10	0	++	0/–	–
Midazolam	0.2–0.4	30–90	10–30	0	0	0	0/–
Diazepam	0.3–0.6	45–90	15–30	0	+++	0	0/–
Lorazepam	0.03–0.06	60–120	60–120	0	+++	0	0/–
Etomidate	0.2–0.3	15–45	13–12	+++	++	0	0
Ketamine	1–2	45–60	10–20	+	0	+	++

0 = no change; + = increase; – = decrease.

TABLE 13-6

FACTORS THAT INFLUENCE INTRAVENOUS DRUG
DOSE REQUIREMENTS

Concomitant use of adjunctive drugs
Type of operation (superficial, intra-abdominal)
Patient age
Preexisting diseases (hepatic, renal, cardiac)
Intraoperative interventions (laryngoscopy, skin incision)

B. Use of Intravenous Drugs for Maintenance of Anesthesia

1. The availability of intravenous drugs with more rapid onset and shorter recovery profiles, as well as easier-to-use infusion delivery systems, has facilitated the maintenance of anesthesia with continuous infusion of intravenous drugs (total intravenous anesthetic [TIVA] techniques) producing an anesthetic state that compares favorably with volatile anesthetics.

2. The optimal intravenous dose range is influenced by many factors (Table 13-6).

3. Clinical signs of depth of anesthesia such as skeletal muscle tone, ventilation, blood pressure, and heart rate may be obscured by adjuvant drugs.

   a. Analysis of the spontaneous EEG (bispectral index [BIS], patient state index [PSI], or response entropy [RE]) may provide useful information regarding anesthetic (hypnotic) depth.

   b. The BIS can improve titration of both intravenous and inhaled anesthetics thus facilitating the recovery process.

4. When using constant-rate intravenous infusions, 4 to 5.5 times may be required to achieve a steady-state anesthetic concentration (offset with an initial loading [primary] dose) (Fig. 13-4).

   a. Rapid, short-acting, sedative–hypnotics and opioids are better suited for continuous administration techniques because they can be more precisely titrated to meet the unique and changing needs of the individual patient.

   b. Context-sensitive half-time is more appropriate in choosing drugs for continuous intravenous administration (Fig. 13-5).

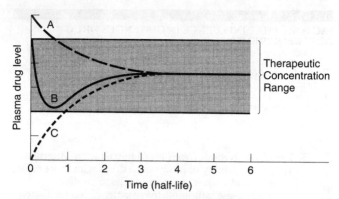

FIGURE 13-4. Simulated drug level curves when a constant infusion is administered following a full dose (*curve A*), a smaller loading dose (*curve B*), and no loading dose (*curve C*).

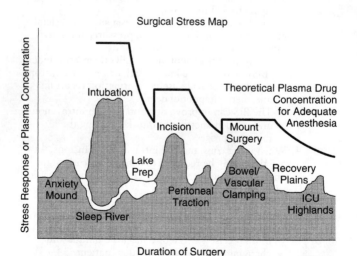

FIGURE 13-5. Context-sensitive half-time values as a function of infusion duration for intravenous anesthetics. The context-sensitive half-times for thiopental and diazepam are significantly longer compared with etomidate, propofol, and midazolam with an increasing infusion duration.

    c. None of the currently available intravenous drugs can provide for a complete anesthetic state without producing prolonged recovery times and undesirable side effects (administer combinations of drugs to achieve hypnosis, amnesia, analgesia, and hemodynamic stability).

C. Use of Intravenous Anesthetics for Sedation. The use of sedative–hypnotic drugs as part of a monitored anesthesia care technique in combination with local anesthetics and to provide sedation for the management of patients in the intensive care unit is becoming increasingly popular.

CHAPTER 14 ■ OPIOIDS

Opioid is an all-inclusive term that describes drugs (natural and synthetic) and endogenous peptides that bind to morphine receptors (Coda BA: Opioids. In Barash PG, Cullen BF, Stoelting RK [eds]: *Clinical Anesthesia*, pp 353–383. Philadelphia, Lippincott Williams & Wilkins, 2006). This term includes drugs that are agonists, agonist–antagonists, and antagonists. Opiate is often used interchangeably with opioid but historically designates only drugs derived from opium (morphine, codeine). Narcotic is a nonspecific designation applicable to any drug that produces sleep.

I. ENDOGENOUS OPIOIDS AND OPIOID RECEPTORS (Table 14-1)

A. Most currently used opioids (morphine, fentanyl) are highly selective for μ-opioid receptors.

B. All opioid receptors appear to be coupled to G proteins, which regulate the activity of adenylate cyclase and subsequent ion channel conduction characteristics.

C. All of the endogenous opioids are derived from prohormones, and each of these precursors is encoded by a separate gene. Synthesis of endorphins is from a prohormone principally located in the anterior pituitary.

II. PHARMACOKINETICS AND PHARMACODYNAMICS

A. **Physicochemical properties** of opioids influence both pharmacokinetics and pharmacodynamics (Table 14-2).

1. To reach its sites of action (receptors on neuronal cell membranes in the central nervous system [CNS]), an opioid must cross the blood-brain barrier.

a. The ability of opioids to cross the blood-brain barrier depends on properties such as molecular size, ionization, lipid solubility, and protein binding.

TABLE 14-1

CLASSIFICATION OF OPIOID RECEPTORS AND ACTIONS

Receptor	Analgesia	Respiratory	Gastrointestinal	Endocrine	Other
μ	Peripheral		Slowed gastric emptying Antidiarrheal		Pruritus Skeletal muscle rigidity ?Urinary retention Cardiovascular effects
μ_1	Supraspinal				
μ_2	Spinal	Depression		Prolactin release	
K	Peripheral		Slowed gastric emptying	Decreased ADH release	Sedation
K_1	Spinal				
K_2	?				
K_3	Supraspinal	?Depression			
∂	Peripheral		Slowed gastric emptying	?Growth hormone release	?Urinary retention
∂_1	Spinal		Antidiarrheal		Dopamine turnover
∂_2	Supraspinal				Miosis Nausea and vomiting
Unknown receptor subtype					

ADH = antidiuretic hormone.

TABLE 14-2

PHYSICOCHEMICAL CHARACTERISTICS AND PHARMACOKINETICS OF COMMONLY USED OPIOID AGONISTS

Parameter	Morphine	Meperidine	Fentanyl	Sufentanil	Alfentanil	Remifentanil
pKa	7.9	8.5	8.4	8.0	6.5	7.3
Nonionized (pH 7.4) (%)	23	7	8.5	20	89	58
Protein binding (%)	35	70	84	93	92	66–93
Clearance (mL/min)	1050	1020	1530	900	238	3000
Volume of distribution (steady state, L)	224	305	335	123	27	2.5–30
Elimination half-time (hr)	1.7–3.3	3–5	3.1–6.6	2.2–4.6	1.4–1.5	0.17–0.33

   b. The degree of ionization depends on the pKa of
      the opioid and the pH of the tissue (nonionized
      drugs are 1,000 to 10,000 times more lipid
      soluble than the ionized form).
   2. The major plasma proteins to which opioids bind
      are albumin and α-1 acid glycoprotein.
B. **Biotransformation** and **excretion** are the principal
   mechanisms for elimination of opioids.
   1. Opioids are metabolized in the liver (conjugation,
      oxidative, and reductive reactions) or hydrolyzed in
      the plasma (unique for remifentanil).
   2. With the exception of the N-dealkylated metabolite
      of meperidine, and the 6- and possibly
      3-glucuronides of morphine, opioid metabolites are
      generally inactive.
   3. Opioid metabolites and, to a lesser extent, parent
      compounds are excreted by the kidneys. The biliary
      system and gastrointestinal tract are less important
      routes of opioid excretion.

III. MORPHINE

A. Morphine mimics the effects of endogenous opioids by
   acting as an agonist at μ-1 and μ-2 opioid receptors
   throughout the body and is considered the agonist to
   which other μ agonists are compared (Tables 14-3 and
   14-4).
B. **Analgesia.** Opioids are administered primarily for their
   analgesic effect. Morphine analgesia results from
   complex interactions at a number of discrete sites in the
   brain, spinal cord, and under certain conditions,
   peripheral tissues, and involves both μ-1 and μ-2
   opioid effects.
   1. Supraspinal opioid analgesia originates in the
      periacqueductal gray matter, the locus ceruleus, and
      nuclei within the medulla and primarily involves
      μ_1-opioid receptors.
   2. At the spinal cord level, morphine acts
      presynaptically on primary afferent nociceptors to
      decrease the release of substance P and also
      hyperpolarizes interneurons in the substantia
      gelatinosa of the dorsal spinal cord to decrease
      afferent transmission of nociceptive impulses. Spinal
      morphine analgesia is mediated by μ_2 opioid
      receptors.

TABLE 14-3
RELATIVE POTENCIES AND PLASMA CONCENTRATIONS FOR VARIOUS OPIOID EFFECTS

Effect	Morphine	Meperidine	Fentanyl	Sufentanil	Alfentanil	Remifentanil
Relative potencies	1	0.1	100	500–1,000	10–20	
Analgesic dose (mg)	10	100	0.1	0.01–0.02	0.5–1.5	
Minimum effective analgesic concentration (ng/mL)	10–15	200	0.6	0.03	15	
Moderate to strong analgesia (ng/mL)	20–50	400–600	1.5–5.1	0.05–0.11	40–80	
Decrease MAC 50% (ng/mL)	NA	>500	0.5–2	0.145	200	1.3
Surgical analgesia with 70% nitrous oxide (ng/mL)	NA	NA	15–25	NA	300–500	
Depression of ventilation threshold (ng/mL)	25	200	1	0.02–0.04	50–100	
Ventilatory response to carbon dioxide decreased 50% (ng/mL)	50	NA	1.5–3	0.04	120–350	2.1–2.9
Apnea (ng/mL)	NA	NA	7–22	NA	300–600	
Unconsciousness (not reliably achieved with opioids alone) (ng/mL)	NA	Seizures	15–20	NA	500–1500	

NA = not available.

TABLE 14-4
EFFECTS OF OPIOID AGONISTS[a]

Central Nervous System (Brain and Spinal Cord)
Analgesia
Sedation
Euphoria
Depression of ventilation (increased $PaCO_2$ [decreased ventilatory response to carbon dioxide because of brainstem depression] and decreased breathing rate and minute ventilation)
Nausea and vomiting (stimulation of the chemoreceptor trigger zone especially in ambulatory patients, high doses of opioids depress the vomiting center and may overcome the chemoreceptor trigger zone stimulating effect)
Pruritus
Miosis (diagnostic of opioid administration)
Depressed cough reflex
Skeletal muscle rigidity
Myoclonus (may be confused with seizures)

Gastrointestinal Tract
Slowed gastric emptying
Increased tone of the common bile duct and sphincter of Oddi (reversed by nitroglycerin [angina too], naloxone [not angina]; can prevent visualization of contrast material in the duodenum resulting in the erroneous conclusion that the common bile duct is blocked by a stone)

Genitourinary Tract
Urinary retention

Endocrine System
Antidiuretic hormone release

Autonomic Nervous System
Arterial and venous vasodilation (orthostatic hypotension)
Bradycardia (Sympatholytic and parasympathomimetic mechanisms)

Histamine Release (morphine and meperidine probably not mediated by opioid receptors)

[a] Similar for all opioid agonists but magnitude of effect of equianalgesic doses may differ.

3. Peripheral analgesia produced by morphine is most likely because of activation of opioid receptors on primary afferent neurons, which occurs only when inflammation is present.
4. The minimum effective analgesic concentration of morphine for postoperative pain relief is 10 to 15 ng/mL (more likely to be maintained by

patient-controlled analgesia than by intermittent intravenous or intramuscular injections) (see Table 14-3).

C. **Effect on Minimum Alveolar Concentration (MAC) of Volatile Anesthetics**
   1. The μ agonists are used extensively in conjunction with nitrous oxide with or without a volatile anesthetic to produce "balanced anesthesia."
   2. Morphine (1 mg/kg iv) administered with 60% inhaled nitrous oxide blocks the adrenergic response to surgical skin incision in 50% of patients (MAC-BAR).
   3. Neuraxial morphine may also decrease MAC.

D. **Other CNS Effects**
   1. Morphine can produce sedation as well as cognitive and fine motor impairment, even at plasma concentrations commonly achieved during management moderate to severe pain.

E. **Respiratory Depression**
   1. Morphine and other μ agonists produce dose-dependent ventilatory depression primarily by decreasing the responsiveness of the medullary respiratory center to carbon dioxide.
   2. Frequent periods of oxygen desaturation associated with obstructive apnea, paradoxic breathing, and slow respiratory rate may occur in patients receiving morphine infusions for postoperative analgesia. Sleep apnea increases the risk of morphine-induced respiratory depression

F. **Cardiovascular Effects**
   1. In doses typically used for pain management or as part of balanced anesthesia, morphine has little effect on blood pressure or heart rate and cardiac rhythm in the supine normovolemic patient.
   2. Large doses may produce peripheral vasodilation (central sympatholytic activity) especially in patients with high sympathetic nervous system tone (congestive heart failure, severe trauma). Hypotension may reflect sympatholysis.
   3. Morphine does not suppress myocardial contractility but does produce bradycardia probably by both sympatholytic and parasympathomimetic mechanisms. In clinical anesthesia practice, opioids are often used for cardiac surgery to prevent

tachycardia and decrease myocardial oxygen demand.

4. Morphine does not directly affect cerebral circulation as long as drug-induced depression of ventilation with retention of carbon dioxide (would produce cerebral vasodilation) is prevented by mechanical support of breathing.

G. **Disposition Kinetics.** Following intramuscular morphine administration, peak plasma concentration is seen at 20 minutes.

H. Morphine's major metabolic pathway is conjugation in the liver to morphine-3-glucuronide (M3G) and morphine-6-glucuronide (M6G). The importance of extrahepatic sites of glucuronidation (kidneys, lungs, gastrointestinal tract) in humans is unknown.

1. M6G possesses significant μ-receptor affinity and potent antinociceptive activity.

2. Sensitivity of renal failure patients to morphine may reflect the dependence of M6G on renal excretion.

I. **Dosage and Administration of Morphine**

1. Morphine crosses the blood-brain barrier relatively slowly because of its hydrophilicity.

2. Because of its delayed onset of action, morphine can be more difficult to titrate as an anesthetic supplement than the more rapidly acting opioids.

IV. MEPERIDINE

A. **Analgesia and Effect on MAC of Volatile Anesthetics**

1. Meperidine's analgesic potency is about one-tenth that of morphine's and is most likely mediated by μ-opioid receptor activation.

2. Unlike morphine, meperidine plasma concentrations correlate with analgesic effects (see Table 14-3).

3. Meperidine is unique among the opioids in also possessing a **weak local anesthetic** properly (useful for neuraxial administration).

B. **Side effects** resemble morphine (Table 14-4).

1. High doses of meperidine are associated with central nervous system (CNS) excitement (seizures) and decreased myocardial contractility (hypotension).

2. The increase in common bile duct pressure occurs to a lesser extent than with equianalgesic doses of morphine and fentanyl.

C. **Shivering.** Meperidine (25 to 50 mg iv) is effective in decreasing postoperative shivering, whereas equianalgesic doses of morphine and fentanyl are not effective. The observation that drugs other than opioids (clonidine, serotonin antagonists, propofol, physostigmine) reduce postoperative shivering suggests that a nonopioid mechanism may be involved.

D. **Disposition Kinetics** (see Table 14-2)
   1. Absorption after intramuscular administration to postoperative patients is variable with peak plasma concentration occurring between 5 and 110 minutes.
   2. Meperidine is metabolized mainly in the liver by N-demethylation to form normeperidine, the principal metabolite, and by hydrolysis to form meperidinic acid.
   3. **Active Metabolites.** Normeperidine has pharmacologic activity and can produce signs of CNS excitation (daily doses >1,000 mg increase the risk of seizures).

E. **Dosage and Administration of Meperidine** (see Table 14-3)

V. METHADONE

A. Methadone is a synthetic μ-opioid receptor agonist that possesses a long elimination half-time (most often used for long-term pain management (10 mg similar to morphine) and in treatment of abstinence syndrome).

B. **Side effects** are similar in magnitude and frequency to those of morphine.

C. **Disposition Kinetics.** Methadone is well absorbed after oral administration and reaches peak plasma concentration at 4 hours after oral administration.

D. **Dosage and Administration of Methadone.** Patients with significant pain have no depression of respiration or level of consciousness.

VI. FENTANYL

A. Fentanyl and its related μ-opioid receptor analogs sufentanil and alfentanil are the most frequently used opioids in clinical practice. The clinical potency of fentanyl is 50 to 100 times that of morphine, and there is a direct relationship between plasma concentrations and analgesia (see Table 14-3).

B. **Effect on MAC of Volatile Anesthetics and Use in Anesthesia**
   1. Plasma fentanyl concentrations decrease rapidly after a single intravenous injection so the magnitude of MAC reduction will vary depending on time after fentanyl administration (computer-assisted continuous infusion provides a constant plasma concentration and associated decrease in anesthetic requirements).
   2. Combining opioids with propofol rather than an inhaled anesthetic can produce general anesthesia (total intravenous anesthesia). Plasma concentrations of fentanyl and propofol that prevent responses to skin incision in 50% of patients have been determined.
   3. Fentanyl has been used as the sole drug for anesthesia (50 to 150 μg/kg iv or a stable plasma concentration in the range of 20 to 30 ng/mL) because hemodynamic stability is desirable for patients with heart disease.
      a. High doses of opioids when administered rapidly intravenously can produce skeletal muscle rigidity.
      b. Combining opioids with other depressant drugs (nitrous oxide, benzodiazepines) changes the stable hemodynamic profile of the opioid alone and hypotension can occur.
C. **Other CNS Effects**
   1. The effects of fentanyl on intracranial pressure (ICP) are inconsistent with some reports showing an increase and others no change.
   2. Fentanyl has been associated with seizure-like movements (most likely myoclonus), but seizure activity is not present on the electroencephalogram.
   3. Fentanyl-induced **pruritus** often presents as facial itching but can be generalized (similar with sufentanil and alfentanil).
D. **Respiratory Depression**
   1. Peak depression of ventilation occurs in about 5 minutes and parallels the plasma concentration and intensity of analgesia (see Table 14-3).
   2. The magnitude of respiratory depression can be greatly increased when fentanyl is administered with another sedative drug such as a benzodiazepine.

E. **Airway Reflexes**
  1. Like volatile anesthetics, opioids depress airway reflexes elicited in response to laryngeal stimulation (placement of a laryngeal mask airway [LMA]).
  2. Cough is the laryngeal reflex most vulnerable to depression by fentanyl.
F. **Cardiovascular and Endocrine Effects**
  1. In clinical practice, high-dose fentanyl administration is associated with remarkable hemodynamic stability (combination with other anesthetic drugs can result in cardiovascular depression).
  2. Hypertension in response to median sternotomy is the most common hemodynamic disturbance during high-dose fentanyl anesthesia.
  3. Unlike morphine and meperidine, which induce hypotension, at least in part by histamine release, high-dose fentanyl is not associated with significant histamine release.
G. **Smooth Muscle and Gastrointestinal Effects.** Fentanyl, like morphine and meperidine, increases common bile duct pressure. Fentanyl can cause nausea and vomiting, especially in ambulatory patients, and can delay gastric emptying.
H. **Disposition Kinetics** (see Table 14-2)
  1. Fentanyl's high lipid solubility allows it to cross biologic membranes rapidly (rapid onset) followed by redistribution to inactive tissue sites such as skeletal muscle and fat (short duration). High doses or prolonged administration of fentanyl can saturate redistribution sites converting this drug to a long-acting opioid.
  2. Clearance of fentanyl is primarily by hepatic metabolism (*N*-dealkylation to norfentanyl and hydroxylation of both the parent compound and norfentanyl).
  3. A patient with respiratory acidosis will have a higher proportion of unbound (active) fentanyl.
I. **Dosage and Administration of Fentanyl** (see Table 14-3)
  1. Fentanyl can be used as a sedative/analgesic premedication when given a short time prior to induction of anesthesia (25 to 50 μg iv or transmucosal delivery system for pediatric and adult patients). Respiratory depression can occur,

emphasizing the need to monitor patients treated with these doses of fentanyl.

2. Fentanyl is commonly used as an adjunct to induction drugs to blunt the hemodynamic response to laryngoscopy and tracheal intubation. Because fentanyl's peak effect lags behind the peak plasma concentration by 3 to 5 minutes, fentanyl should be administered about 3 minutes before initiating laryngoscopy.

3. Perhaps the most common use of fentanyl and its derivatives is as an analgesic component of balanced general anesthesia (0.5 to 2.5 μg/kg iv as dictated by the intensity of the surgical stimulus or 2 to 10 μg/kg/hr as a continuous infusion).

4. High-dose fentanyl (50 to 150 μg/kg iv) may be used as the sole anesthetic for cardiac surgery (may not provide total amnesia in healthy patients).

5. Fentanyl has been used as an analgesic in the management of acute and chronic pain. Both transdermal and transmucosal fentanyl delivery systems are effective for relief of cancer pain.

VII. SUFENTANIL

A. Sufentanil is a highly selective and potent (10 to 15 times that of fentanyl) μ-opioid receptor agonist that equilibrates rapidly between blood and brain.

B. **Effect on MAC of Volatile Anesthetics and Use in Anesthesia**
   1. Sufentanil, like other opioids, produces a dose-dependent decrease in the MAC of volatile anesthetics.
   2. In clinical practice, sufentanil is used as a component of balanced anesthesia and in high doses (10 to 30 μg/kg iv) for cardiac surgery (like fentanyl does not completely block the hemodynamic response to noxious stimuli).

C. **Other CNS effects** resemble fentanyl.

D. **Respiratory depression** resembles other μ-opioid receptor agonists and can be especially marked in the presence of inhaled anesthetics.

E. **Disposition Kinetics** (see Table 14-2)
   1. Sufentanil is a highly lipid soluble and has pharmacokinetic properties that resemble fentanyl. Because of its lower degree of ionization at

physiologic pH and higher degree of plasma protein binding, its volume of distribution is somewhat smaller and its elimination half-time shorter than that of fentanyl. Obesity may increase the volume of distribution and prolong the elimination half-time of sufentanil.

2. Clearance of sufentanil (like fentanyl) is rapid primarily by hepatic metabolism (*N*-dealkylation and *O*-demethylation).

F. **Dosage and Administration of Sufentanil** (see Table 14-3)

1. Sufentanil (like fentanyl) is most often used as a component of balanced anesthesia or in high doses for cardiac surgery (up to 50 μg/kg iv).

2. Doses in the range of 0.3 to 1 μg/kg iv given 1 to 3 minutes before laryngoscopy can be expected to blunt hemodynamic responses to tracheal intubation.

3. For maintenance of balanced anesthesia, sufentanil can be administered in intermittent doses (0.1 to 0.5 μg/kg iv) or as a continuous infusion (0.3 to 1 μg/kg/hr iv).

VIII. ALFENTANIL

A. Alfentanil is a μ-opioid receptor agonist with a potency approximately 10 times that of morphine and one-fourth to one-tenth that of fentanyl. In contrast to fentanyl and sufentanil, the duration of even very large doses of alfentanil is brief, necessitating its administration by continuous infusion if a sustained effect is desired.

B. **Nausea and Vomiting.** Clinical comparisons between alfentanil and sufentanil or fentanyl and nitrous oxide reveal a similar incidence of nausea and vomiting.

C. **Disposition Kinetics** (see Table 14-2)

1. Alfentanil pharmacokinetics differ from fentanyl and sufentanil with respect to pK (alfentanil 6.8 and all other opioids above 7.4). This results in 90% of unbound plasma alfentanil being unionized at a plasma pH of 7.4. This property, together with moderate lipid solubility, enables alfentanil to cross the blood-brain barrier rapidly (blood-brain equilibration half-time 1.1 minutes

versus >6 minutes for fentanyl and sufentanil) and accounts for its rapid onset of action.

2. Alfentanil has a smaller volume of distribution than fentanyl, which is a result of its lower lipid solubility and high protein binding (about 92%, mostly to α-1 acid glycoprotein).

3. Plasma alfentanil concentrations decrease rapidly (90% of an administered dose has left the plasma by 30 minutes) because of rapid distribution to tissues. After a single intravenous dose, redistribution will be the most important mechanism for recovery, but after a very large dose, repeated small doses, or a continuous infusion, elimination will be a more important determinant of the duration of alfentanil's effects.

4. Clearance of alfentanil is only half that of fentanyl but because its volume of distribution is four times smaller than fentanyl's, more alfentanil is available to the liver for metabolism (cirrhosis slows elimination of alfentanil). Alfentanil undergoes N-dealkylation and O-demethylation in the liver to form inactive metabolites.

D. **Dosage and Administration of Alfentanil** (see Table 14-3)

1. Because of its rapid onset of action, alfentanil has been used for the induction of anesthesia (120 μg/kg iv produces unconsciousness in 2 to 2.5 minutes).

2. Rapid blood-brain equilibration time permits administration of alfentanil (30 μg/kg iv) 60 to 90 seconds before initiation of direct laryngoscopy in an attempt to blunt circulatory responses to tracheal intubation.

3. Alfentanil is used as a continuous infusion (25 to 100 μg/kg/hr iv) with nitrous oxide or a propofol infusion.

IX. REMIFENTANIL

A. Remifentanil is an ultrashort-acting μ-receptor opioid agonist that is unique among the opioids in that it contains a methyl ester side chain that is susceptible to hydrolysis by blood and tissue esterases (ultrashort acting as a result of metabolism rather than redistribution).

B. **Analgesia** produced by remifentanil 1.5 μg/kg iv and alfentanil 32 μg/kg iv is similar in magnitude and duration (about 10 minutes).

C. **Effect on MAC of Volatile Anesthetics and Use in Anesthesia**

1. The rapid onset and brief duration of action of remifentanil suggest that this opioid may be suitable for induction of anesthesia, yet a high incidence of skeletal muscle rigidity and purposeless movements have been described. At doses >1 μg/kg iv, there is a brief increase in blood pressure and heart rate but histamine release does not occur.

2. Recovery from remifentanil is rapid with return of spontaneous ventilation in 2 to 5 minutes, but the disadvantage is that patients may require analgesics soon after remifentanil is discontinued.

3. The rapid onset and brief duration of remifentanil make this opioid suitable for combination with other injected drugs (propofol) to provide total intravenous anesthesia.

4. Remifentanil produces dose-dependent nausea and vomiting similar to other short-acting μ-opioid agonists.

5. Remifentanil is frequently administered with propofol to provide total intravenous anesthesia (fixed infusion rates or computer-controlled systems that provide target plasma concentrations).

6. As with other opioids, higher rates of respiratory depression occur when propofol is combined with remifentanil.

D. **Disposition Kinetics** (see Table 14-2)

1. The key structural feature of remifentanil is the ester side chain that is susceptible to hydrolysis by blood and tissue esterases resulting in rapid metabolism (elimination half-time 10 to 20 minutes).

2. Because the short duration of action is because of metabolism rather than redistribution, remifentanil should be less likely to accumulate with repeated dosing or prolonged infusion.

3. Pharmacokinetic parameters of remifentanil are unchanged by hepatic or renal disease. Nevertheless, patients with hepatic disease appear to be more sensitive to remifentanil-induced respiratory depression.

4. Advanced age is associated with a decrease in clearance and volume of distribution of remifentanil as well as an increase in potency.

E. **Dosage and Administration of Remifentanil.** Because of its short duration of action, remifentanil is best administered as a continuous intravenous infusion in combination with another anesthetic drug to produce general anesthesia.

F. **Induction Dosage, Intubation, and Laryngeal Mask Airway (LMA) Placement**

1. The most common remifentanil-based regimen for anesthetic induction and laryngoscopy consists of remifentanil 0.5 to 1 μg/kg/ iv administered over 60 seconds plus propofol 1 to 2 mg/kg iv followed by remifentanil infusion of 0.25 to 0.5 μg/kg/min (with or without midazolam premedication)

2. Patients may experience moderate to severe postoperative pain reflecting the short duration of action of remifentanil. Continuing the remifentanil infusion at a lower infusion rate may prevent this problem.

G. **Monitored Anesthesia Care (MAC)**

1. Remifentanil can be used as an adjunct for sedation or analgesia during regional anesthesia (0.5 to 1.0 μg/kg/min iv), for block placement (retrobulbar block preceded by remifentanil 1.0 μg/kg iv 90 seconds before the block), and as part of monitored anesthetic care (colonoscopy).

2. The dose requirement for remifentanil for sedation and analgesia is decreased when the opioid is combined with midazolam (as much as 50%) or propofol.

3. The risk of excessive depression of ventilation or development of chest rigidity following a bolus dose of remifentanil can be minimized by injecting the dose over 30 seconds.

X. PARTIAL AGONISTS AND MIXED AGONIST–ANTAGONISTS (Table 14-5)

A. The partial agonist and mixed agonist–antagonist opioids are synthetic or semisynthetic compounds that are structurally related to morphine.

1. These drugs are characterized by binding activity at multiple opioid receptors and differential effects

TABLE 14-5
RECEPTOR EFFECTS AND RELATIVE POTENCIES OF OPIOID AGONISTS–ANTAGONISTS

Drug	μ Receptor	K Receptor	Relative potency[a]	Analgesic dose (mg)
Nalbuphine	Partial agonist	Partial agonist	11	10
Butorphanol	Partial agonist	Partial agonist	15	2–3
Buprenorphine	Partial agonist	?Antagonist	30	0.3

[a] Morphine is 1.

   (agonist, partial agonist, antagonist) at each
   receptor type.
   2. The major clinical use of these drugs is the provision
      of postoperative analgesia, but they have also been
      used for intraoperative sedation, as adjuncts during
      general anesthesia, and to antagonize some of the
      effects of μ-receptor agonists.
B. **Nalbuphine**
   1. The modest ability of this drug to decrease MAC
      (8 versus 65% for morphine) suggests that
      nalbuphine may not be a useful adjunct for general
      anesthesia.
   2. Analgesia (mediated by K and μ receptors) and
      associated depression of ventilation (mediated by
      μ receptors) produced by nalbuphine have a
      ceiling effect. Nalbuphine has been used to
      antagonize the ventilatory depressant effects of
      μ agonists while still providing analgesia by
      K receptor stimulation.
C. **Butorphanol**
   1. This drug has partial agonist activity at μ- and
      K-opioid receptors (similar to nalbuphine).
      Compared to nalbuphine and similar drugs,
      butorphenol has a pronounced **sedative** effect,
      which is probably mediated by K receptors.
   2. Increases in intrabiliary pressure do not occur, and
      this drug may be effective in treatment of
      postoperative shivering.
   3. Butorphanol is indicated for sedation as well as
      treatment of moderate to severe postoperative pain.

D. **Buprenorphine**
   1. Buprenorphine is a highly lipid-soluble thebaine derivative that is 25 to 50 times more potent than morphine. Slow dissociation from μ receptors can lead to prolonged effects that are not easily antagonized by naloxone.
   2. Unlike nalbuphine and butorphanol, buprenphine does not seem to possess agonist activity at K receptors (may act as an antagonist at these receptors).

XI. OPIOID ANTAGONISTS (NALOXONE AND NALTREXONE)

A. **Naloxone** is a pure antagonist at μ, K, *and* ∂-opioid receptors.
   1. In clinical practice, naloxone is administered to antagonize opioid-induced respiratory depression and sedation.
   2. Because opioid antagonists will reverse all opioid effects, including analgesia, naloxone should be carefully titrated (20 to 40 μg iv produces peak effects in 1 to 2 minutes) to avoid producing sudden, severe pain in postoperative patients.
      a. Sudden, complete antagonism of opioid effects can cause hypertension, tachycardia, ventricular cardiac dysrhythmias, and pulmonary edema.
      b. Pulmonary edema can occur in the absence of heart disease and is thought to reflect centrally mediated catecholamine release causing acute pulmonary hypertension.
      c. Naloxone will precipitate opioid withdrawal symptoms in opioid-dependent individuals.
   3. Because naloxone has a short duration of action (1 to 4 hours), depression of ventilation may recur if large systemic doses of opioids and/or long-acting opioid agonists or neuraxial opioids have been administered. When prolonged depression of ventilation is anticipated, an initial loading dose of naloxone followed by a continuous intravenous infusion (3 to 10 μg/kg/hr) can be used.
B. **Naltrexone** is a long-acting oral antagonist of opioid effects.

TABLE 14-6
CLINICAL USES OF OPIOIDS
Premedication
Induction of anesthesia (sole drug or adjuvant)
Blunt hemodynamic responses to noxious stimulation (alfentanil most rapid blood-brain equilibration time)
Intraoperative analgesia
Postoperative pain relief (patient-controlled analgesia, neuraxial, parenteral)
Adjuvant to facilitate mechanical ventilation and tolerance to tracheal tube

XII. USE OF OPIOIDS IN CLINICAL ANESTHESIA
(Tables 14-6 and 14-7)

A. Opioids are used alone or in combination with other drugs, such as sedatives or anticholinergics, as pharmacologic preoperative medication.

B. Intraoperatively, opioids are administered as components of balanced anesthesia or alone in high doses.

1. Fentanyl and its derivatives sufentanil and alfentanil are the opioids most often used as supplements to general anesthesia (more easily titrated than morphine because of their rapid onset of action).

2. Important pharmacokinetic differences among opioids include volumes of distribution and intercompartmental (distributional) and central (elimination) clearances.

3. The major pharmacodynamic differences among these opioids are potency and equilibration time between the plasma and the site of drug effect (brain-blood equilibration times are more rapid with alfentanil [and remifentanil] than with fentanyl or sufentanil).

4. The rate of recovery after a continuous infusion of any drug including opioids will depend on the duration of the infusion as well as the magnitude of decline that is required (Fig. 14-1).

XIII. CONTEXT-SENSITIVE HALF-TIME

A. The time required for the drug concentration in the central compartment (circulation) to decrease 50% and

TABLE 14-7

DOSAGE FOR OPIOID AGONISTS IN ELECTIVE SURGERY IN ADULTS

Anesthetic phase	Fentanyl	Sufentanil	Alfentanil	Remifentanil
Premedication (μg)	25–50	2–5	250–500	
Induction				
With hypnotic (μg/kg)	1.5–5	0.1–1	10–50	0.5–1.0 or 0.25–0.5 μg/kg/min
With 60–70% N20 (μg/kg)	8–23	1.3–2.8		2.5 or 2 μg/kg/min
High dose opioid (μg/kg)	50	10–30	120	
Maintenance				
Balanced anesthesia				
Intermittent bolus (μg)	25–100	5–20	250–500	25–50
Infusion (μg/kg/min)	0.033	0.005–0.015	0.5–1.5	0.25–0.5
High dose opioid (μg/kg/min)	0.5	2.5–10	1.0–3.0	
Transition to PACU[a] (μg/kg/min)				0.05–0.15
Monitored Anesthesia Care				
Intermittent bolus (μg/kg)	12.5–50	2.5–10	125–250	12.5–25
Infusion (μg/kg/min)				0.01–0.02

[a]PACU = postanesthesia care unit.

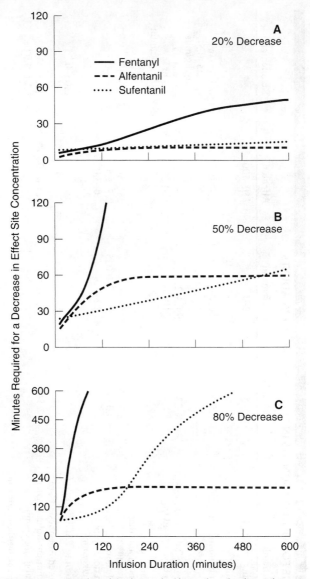

FIGURE 14-1. Overlay of the fentanyl, alfentanil, and sufentanil recovery curves describing the time required for decreases of 20% (**A**), 50% (**B**), and 80% (**C**) from the maintained intraoperative effect site concentration after termination of the infusion.

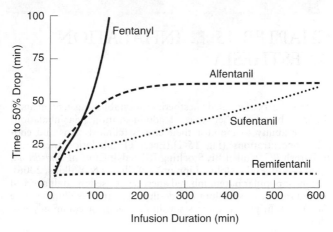

FIGURE 14-2. A simulation of the time necessary to achieve a 50% decrease in drug concentration in the blood after variable-length intravenous infusions of opioids.

the influence of duration of the intravenous infusion on this time is defined as the context-sensitive half-time (Fig. 14-2).

B. Context-sensitive half-time curves are theoretical predictions based on computer models. It is not known if a decrement of 50% provides the most clinically useful description of the rate of offset of opioid effects.

CHAPTER 15 ■ INHALATION ANESTHESIA

The popularity of inhaled anesthetics for establishing general anesthesia is based on their ease of administration (via inhalation) and the ability to monitor their effects (clinical signs and end-tidal concentrations) (Fig. 15-1) (Ebert TJ: Inhalation anesthesia. In Barash PG, Cullen BF, Stoelting RK [eds]: *Clinical Anesthesia*, pp 384–420. Philadelphia, Lippincott Williams & Wilkins, 2006). The most popular potent inhaled anesthetics used in adult surgical procedures are sevoflurane, desflurane, and isoflurane (see Fig. 15-1). In pediatric cases sevoflurane is most commonly employed.

I. HISTORY

A. The volatile anesthetics in early clinical use consisted of flammable gases, including diethyl ether and cyclopropane. Advances in fluorine chemistry and subsequent fluorine substitutions for other halogens on the ether molecule lowered the boiling point, increased stability, decreased flammability, and generally decreased toxicity.
   1. Halothane was synthesized in 1951 and introduced into clinical practice in 1956 rapidly becoming the most popular inhaled anesthetic (lack of flammability, lower solubility, and potency permitted more rapid induction of anesthesia, more pleasant to inhale, and less nausea and vomiting). The principal disadvantages of halothane were its ability to sensitize the myocardium to catecholamines and the subsequent recognition of halothane hepatitis.
   2. Between 1959 and 1966, Terrel and colleagues at Ohio Medical Products synthesized more than 700 halogenated compounds. The 347th compound was enflurane, the 469th compound was isoflurane, and the 653rd compound was desflurane (introduced into clinical practice in 1993).
   3. Another new compound described in the early 1970s by Wallin and colleagues at Travenol

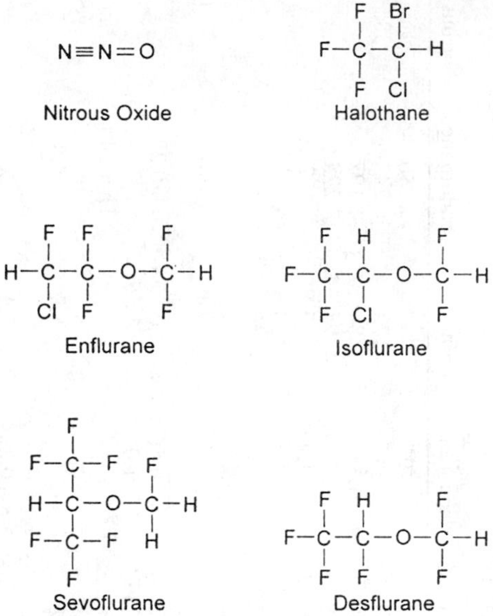

FIGURE 15-1. Chemical structure of inhaled anesthetics. Halothane is an alkane, whereas all the other volatile anesthetics are ether derivatives. Isoflurane, enflurane, and desflurane are methyl ethyl ether derivatives and sevoflurane is a methyl isopropyl ether. Isoflurane and enflurane are isomers and desflurane differs from isoflurane in the substitution of a fluorine for a chlorine atom.

Laboratories was a fluorinated isopropyl ether that was introduced into clinical practice in 1995 as sevoflurane.

B. The most important differences of the newer inhaled anesthetics (sevoflurane and desflurane compared with isoflurane) are their lower blood and tissue solubility, which allows rapid induction and prompt recovery necessary for ambulatory anesthesia (Table 15-1 and 15-2).

II. PHARMACOKINETIC PRINCIPLES

A. Drug pharmacology is classically divided into pharmacodynamics (what the body does to a drug) and pharmacokinetics (what the drug does to the body).

TABLE 15-1

PHYSIOCHEMICAL PROPERTIES OF VOLATILE ANESTHETICS

	Sevoflurane	Desflurane	Isoflurane	Enflurane	Halothane	Nitrous oxide
Boiling point (°C)	59	24	49	57	50	−88
Vapor pressure at 20°C (mm Hg)	157	669	238	172	243	38,770
Molecular weight (g)	200	168	184	184	197	44
Oil:gas partition coefficient	47	19	91	97	224	1.4
Blood:gas partition coefficient	0.65	0.42	1.46	1.9	2.50	0.46
Brain:blood solubility	1.7	1.3	1.6	1.4	1.9	1.1
Fat:blood solubility	47.5	27.2	44.9	36	51.1	2.3
Muscle:blood solubility	3.1	2.0	2.9	1.7	3.4	1.2
MAC in oxygen, 30–60 yr, at 37°C, PB760 (%)	1.8	6.6	1.17	1.63	0.75	104
MAC in 60–70% nitrous oxide	0.66	2.38	0.56	0.57	0.29	
MAC, >65 yr (%)	1.45	5.17	1.0	1.55	0.64	
Preservative	no	yes	no	no	Thymol	no
Stable in moist carbon	no	yes	yes	yes	no	yes
Flammability (%) (in 70% nitrous oxide and 30% oxygen)	10	17	7	5.8	4.8	
Recovered as metabolites (%)	2–5	0.02	0.2	2.4	20	

TABLE 15-2
TISSUE GROUPS AND PHARMACOKINETICS

Group	% Body Mass	% Cardiac output	Perfusion (mL/min/100 g)
Vessel rich	10	75	75
Muscle	50	19	3
Fat	20	6	3

Drug pharmacokinetics has four phases (absorption [uptake], distribution, metabolism, and excretion [elimination]).

B. **Unique Features of Inhaled Anesthetics**
  1. Inhaled anesthetics are unique with respect to their speed of action, their existence as gases (technically nitrous oxide is the only gas, whereas others are vapors of volatile liquids), and their administration via the lungs.
  2. Speed, gaseous state, and the lung route of administration combine to form the major beneficial feature of inhaled anesthetics, which is the ability to decrease plasma concentrations as easily and rapidly as they are increased.

C. **Physical Characteristics of Inhaled Anesthetics**
  1. The goal of delivering inhaled anesthetics is to produce the anesthetic state by establishing a specific concentration (partial pressure) in the central nervous system (CNS). This is achieved by establishing the desired partial pressure in the lungs that ultimately equilibrates with the brain and spinal cord.
  2. At equilibrium the CNS partial pressure equals the blood partial pressure, which equals alveolar partial pressure.

D. **Anesthetic Transfer: Machine to Central Nervous System**
  1. Anesthetics follow a multistep route from the anesthesia machine to the patient (and back) (Table 15-3).

E. **Uptake and Distribution**
  1. A common way to assess anesthetic uptake is to follow the ratio of the of alveola anesthetic concentration (F_A) to the inspired

TABLE 15-3

FACTORS THAT INCREASE OR DECREASE THE RATE
OF RISE OF F_A/F_I

Increase	Decrease	
Low blood solubility	High blood solubility	The lower the blood:gas solubility, the faster the rise in F_A/F_I
Low cardiac output	High cardiac output	The lower the cardiac output, the faster the rise in the F_A/F_I
High minute ventilation	Low minute ventilation	The higher the minute ventilation, the faster the rise in F_A/F_I
High pulmonary arterial to venous blood partial pressure	Low pulmonary arterial to venous blood partial pressure	At the beginning of induction, the pulmonary to venous blood partial pressure gradient is zero but rises rapidly and F_A/F_I increases rapidly. Later, during induction and maintenance, the pulmonary venous blood partial pressure rises more slowly so F_A/F_{IA} rises more slowly

      anesthetic concentration (F_I) over time (F_A/F_I)
      (Fig. 15-2).

   2. Factors that increase or decrease the rate of rise of
      F_A/F_I will determine the speed of induction of
      anesthesia (see Fig. 15-2 and Table 15-3).

  F. **Overpressurization and Concentration Effect**
   1. Overpressurization (delivering a higher F_I than the
      F_A actually desired for the patient) is analogous to
      an intravenous bolus and thus speeds the induction
      of anesthesia.

   2. Concentration effect (the greater the F_I of an inhaled
      anesthetic, the more rapid is the rate of rise of the
      F_A/F_I) is a method to speed the induction of
      anesthesia (Fig. 15-3).

  G. **Second Gas Effect**
   1. A special case of the concentration effect is admin-
      istration of two gases simultaneously (nitrous oxide
      and a potent volatile anesthetic) in which the high
      volume uptake of nitrous oxide increases the FA (con-
      centrates) of the volatile anesthetic (see Fig. 15-3).

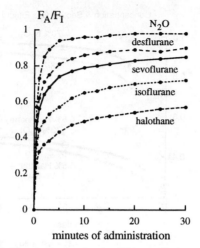

FIGURE 15-2. The rise in the alveolar (FA) anesthetic concentration toward the inspired (FI) is most rapid with the least soluble anesthetics, nitrous oxide, desflurane, and sevoflurane, and intermediate with the more soluble anesthetics, isoflurane and halothane. After 10 to 15 minutes of administration (about three time constants) the slope of the curve decreases, reflecting saturation of vessel-rich group tissues and subsequent decreased uptake of the inhaled anesthetic.

H. **Ventilation Effects**
1. Inhaled anesthetics with a low blood solubility have a rapid rate of rise in the F_A/F_I with induction of anesthesia such that there is little room to improve this rate of rise by increasing or decreasing ventilation (see Fig. 15-2).
2. To the extent that inhaled anesthetics depress ventilation with an increasing F_I, alveolar ventilation will decrease and so will the rate of rise of F_A/F_I (negative feedback that results in apnea and may prevent an overdose).

I. **Perfusion Effects**
1. As with ventilation, cardiac output does not greatly affect the rate of rise of the F_A/F_I for poorly soluble anesthetics.
2. Cardiovascular depression caused by a high F_I results in depression of anesthetic uptake from the lungs and increases the rate of rise of F_A/F_I (positive

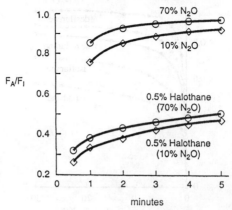

Concentration & Second Gas Effects

FIGURE 15-3. The concentration effect is demonstrated in the top half of the graph in which 70% nitrous oxide produces a more rapid rise in the F_A/F_I ratio of nitrous oxide than does administration of 10% nitrous oxide. The second gas effect is demonstrated in the lower graphs in which the F_A/F_I ratio for halothane rises more rapidly when administered with 70% nitrous oxide than with 10% nitrous oxide.

feedback that may result in profound cardiovascular depression).

J. Exhalation and Recovery
   1. Recovery from anesthesia, like induction of anesthesia, depends on the drug's solubility (primary determinant of the rate of decrease in FA), ventilation, and cardiac output (Fig. 15-4).
   2. The "reservoir" of anesthetic in the body at the conclusion of anesthesia is determined by the solubility of the inhaled anesthetic and the dose and duration of the drug's administration (can slow the rate of decrease in the FA).
   3. Pharmacokinetic differences between recovery and induction of anesthesia include the absence of overpressurization (cannot give less than zero) during recovery and the presence of tissue anesthetic concentrations present at the start of recovery (tissue concentration zero at start of induction of anesthesia).

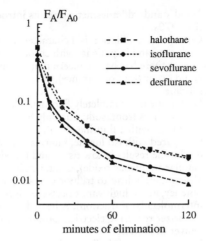

FIGURE 15-4. Elimination of anesthetic gases is defined as the ratio of end-tidal anesthetic concentration (F_A) to the last F_A during administration and immediately before beginning elimination (F_{A0}). During the 120-minute period after ending anesthetic delivery, the elimination of sevoflurane and desflurane is 2 to 2.5 times faster than isoflurane or halothane.

III. CLINICAL OVERVIEW OF CURRENT INHALED ANESTHETICS (see Table 15-1 and Fig. 15-1)

A. Halothane
1. Halothane is a halogenated ethane derivative that possesses intermediate blood solubility and is relatively nonpungent, and therefore, can be inhaled via the face mask.
2. In humans, halothane has been associated with an immune-mediated hepatitis, sensitization to epinephrine resulting in cardiac dysrhythmias, and bradycardia in pediatric patients.

B. Enflurane
1. Enflurane is a halogenated methyl ethyl ether that is an isomer of isoflurane.
2. Seizure-like activity may accompany administration of high concentrations of enflurane and fluoride is a result of this drug's metabolism.

C. Isoflurane
1. Isoflurane is a halogenated methyl ethyl ether that has a high degree of stability and has become the

"gold standard" anesthetic since its introduction in the 1970s.

2. Coronary vasodilation is a characteristic of isoflurane and in patients with coronary artery disease there has been concern that coronary steal could occur (rare occurrence).

D. **Desflurane**

1. Desflurane is a completely fluorinated methyl ethyl ether (differs from isoflurane only by replacement of a chlorine with a fluorine atom).

2. Compared with isoflurane, fluorination of desflurane results in low tissue and blood solubility (similar to nitrous oxide), greater stability (near absent metabolism to trifluoroacetate), loss of potency, and a high vapor pressure (decreased intermolecular attraction). A heated and pressurized vaporizer requiring electrical power is necessary to deliver desflurane.

3. Disadvantages of desflurane include its pungency (cannot be administered by face mask to an awake patient), transient sympathetic nervous system stimulation when F_I is abruptly increased, and degradation to carbon monoxide when exposed to dry carbon dioxide absorbents (more so than isoflurane).

E. **Sevoflurane**

1. Sevoflurane is completely fluorinated methyl isopropyl ether with a vapor pressure similar to isoflurane and it can be used in a conventional vaporizer.

2. Compared with isoflurane, sevoflurane is less soluble in blood and tissues (resembles desflurane), is less potent, and lacks coronary artery vasodilating properties.

3. Sevoflurane has minimal odor and pungency (useful for mask induction of anesthesia) and is a potent bronchodilator.

4. Similar to enflurane, the metabolism of sevoflurane results in fluoride, but unlike enflurane this has not been associated with renal concentrating defects.

5. Unlike other volatile anesthetics, sevoflurane is not metabolized to trifluoroacetate but rather to hexafluoroisopropanol that does not stimulate formation of antibodies and immune-mediated hepatitis.

6. Sevoflurane does not decompose to carbon monoxide on to dry carbon dioxide absorbents but rather is degraded to a vinyl halide (compound A), which is a dose-dependent nephrotoxin in rats. Renal injury has not been shown to occur in patients even when fresh gas flows are 1 L/min or less.

F. **Xenon**
1. This inert gas has many characteristics of an "ideal" inhaled anesthetic (blood gas partition coefficient 0.14, provides some analgesia, nonpungent, does not produce myocardial depression).
2. The principal disadvantages of xenon are its expense (difficult to obtain) and high MAC (71%) value.

G. **Nitrous Oxide**
1. Nitrous oxide is a sweet-smelling, nonflammable gas of low potency and limited blood and tissue solubility that is most often administered as an adjuvant in combination with other volatile anesthetics or opioids.
2. Controversy surrounding the use of nitrous oxide is related to its unclear role in postoperative nausea and vomiting, its potential toxicity related to inactivation of vitamin B12, its effects on embryonic development, and its adverse effects related to its absorption into air-filled cavities and bubbles (compliant spaces such as a pneumothorax expand and noncompliant spaces such as the middle ear experience increased pressure).
   a. Inhalation of 75% nitrous oxide can expand a pneumothorax to double its size in 10 minutes.
   b. Accumulation of nitrous oxide in the middle ear can diminish hearing postoperatively.

IV. NEUROPHARMACOLOGY OF INHALED ANESTHETICS

A. The mechanism of anesthesia (a state in which the brain is incapable of self-awareness or recall) is not known.
B. **Minimum Alveolar Concentration (MAC)**
1. MAC is the F_A of an anesthetic at 1 atmosphere and 37°C that prevents movement in response to a surgical stimulus in 50% of patients (analogous to an ED50 for injected drugs) (Table 15-1). Clinical experience is that 1.2 to 1.3 MAC consistently prevents patient movement during surgical

TABLE 15-4

FACTORS THAT INFLUENCE (INCREASE OR DECREASE) MAC

Increase
  Increased central neurotransmitter levels (monoamine oxidase
    inhibitors, acute dextroamphetamine administration,
    cocaine, ephedrine, levodopa)
  Hyperthermia
  Chronic ethanol abuse
  Hypernatremia

Decrease
  Increasing age
  Metabolic acidosis
  Hypoxia (PaO$_2$ <38 mm Hg)
  Induced hypotension (MAP <50 mm Hg)
  Decreased central neurotransmitter levels (α-methyldopa,
    reserpine)
  α-2 agonists
  Hypothermia
  Hyponatremia
  Lithium
  Hypoosmolality
  Pregnancy
  Acute ethanol administration
  Ketamine
  Lidocaine
  Opioids
  Opioid agonist–antagonist analgesics
  Barbiturates
  Diazepam
  Hydroxyzine
  delta-9-tetrahydrocannabinol
  Verapamil
  Anemia (<4.3 mL oxygen/dL blood)

stimulation. While these MAC levels do not
absolutely ensure the defining criteria for brain
anesthesia (the absence of self-awareness and recall),
it is unlikely for a patient to be aware of or to recall
the surgical incision at these anesthetic
concentrations unless other conditions exist such
that MAC is increased in that patient (Table 15-4).
Self-awareness and recall are prevented by 0.4 to
0.5 MAC.

2. Standard MAC values are roughly additive (0.5
   MAC of a volatile anesthetic and 0.5 MAC of

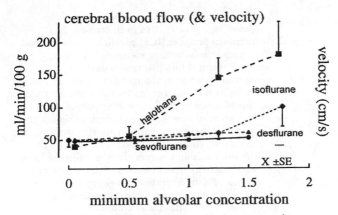

FIGURE 15-5. Cerebral blood flow measured in the presence of normocapnia and in the absence of surgical stimulation in volunteers. At light levels of anesthesia, halothane, but not isoflurane, sevoflurane, or desflurane, increased cerebral blood flow. Isoflurane increased cerebral blood flow at 1.6 MAC.

nitrous oxide is equivalent to 1 MAC of the volatile anesthetic).

3. A variety of factors may increase or decrease MAC (see Table 15-4).

C. **Other Alterations in Neurophysiology**

1. Currently used volatile anesthetics have qualitatively similar effects on cerebral metabolic rate, the electroencephalogram, cerebral blood flow, and cerebral blood flow autoregulation.

   a. Halothane is the most potent cerebral vasodilator of the currently used volatile anesthetics (Fig. 15-5). The dose-dependent increase in cerebral blood flow caused by volatile anesthetics occurs despite concomitant decreases in cerebral metabolic rate (uncoupling).

   b. High concentrations of sevoflurane (1.5 to 2.0 MAC), a sudden increase in cerebral sevoflurane concentrations, and hypocapnia can trigger EEG abnormalities that often are associated with increases in heart rate (raises questions as to the use of sevoflurane in patients with epilepsy).

   c. Because volatile anesthetics are direct vasodilators they are considered to diminish autoregulation in a dose-dependent fashion (halothane greater than isoflurane).

2. **Intracranial pressure (ICP)** parallels cerebral blood flow such that halothane increases ICP to the greatest extent (brain protrusion during craniotomy), whereas changes during administration of isoflurane, desflurane, and sevoflurane are mild.

   a. Introduction of desflurane after propofol induction of anesthesia may result in significant increases in heart rate, mean arterial pressure, and middle cerebral artery blood flow velocity that are not noted in patients given sevoflurane (may reflect airway irritant effects of desflurane rather than a specific alteration in neurophysiology).

   b. Increases in ICP may be slightly greater in the presence of desflurane as compared with sevoflurane and isoflurane.

   c. Any of the potent inhaled agents may be used with neurosurgical procedures in the presence of the appropriate dose and adjunctive and compensatory therapies. However, patients with traumatic head injuries, increased ICP or space-occupying brain lesions are probably better served with isoflurane, sevoflurane, and possibly desflurane.

3. Data on the effects of nitrous oxide on cerebral blood flow (CBF) and ICP are conflicting and there may be an associated antineuroprotective effect of this agent (consider avoiding in surgical cases in which there is a high likelihood of increased ICP or significant cerebral ischemia).

V. THE CIRCULATORY SYSTEM

A. Hemodynamics

1. Volatile anesthetics produced dose-dependent and similar decreases in systemic blood pressure (Fig. 15-6). Halothane decreases blood pressure primarily by decreasing cardiac output, whereas the other volatile anesthetics decrease blood pressure primarily by decreasing systemic vascular resistance while cardiac output is maintained (Fig. 15-7).

2. In volunteers, sevoflurane and halothane up to about 1 MAC results in minimal changes in heart rate, whereas isoflurane is associated with an increase of

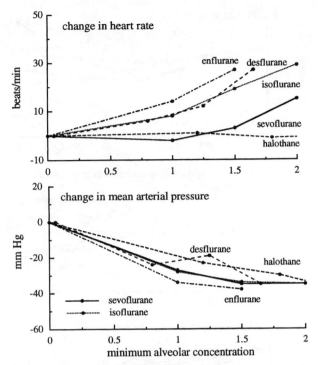

FIGURE 15-6. Heart rate and systemic blood pressure changes (from awake baseline) in volunteers receiving general anesthesia with a volatile anesthetic. Halothane and sevoflurane produced little change in heart rate at less than 1.5 MAC. All anesthetics caused similar decreases in blood pressure.

10 to 15 beats/min (see Fig. 15-6). At anesthetic levels >1 MAC, desflurane has been associated with an increase in heart rate similar to isoflurane.

a. Rapid increases in the delivered concentration of desflurane (and to a lesser extent of isoflurane) can transiently increase heart rate and systemic blood pressure.

b. Administration of an opioid blunts the heart rate responses evoked by volatile anesthetics, including those responses associated with abrupt

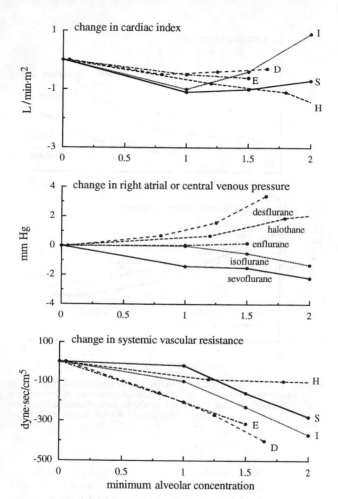

FIGURE 15-7. Cardiac index, systemic vascular resistance, and central venous pressure changes from awake baseline in volunteers receiving general anesthesia with a volatile anesthetic. Increases in central venous pressure in the presence of halothane may reflect myocardial depression, whereas increases in the presence of desflurane are more likely a result of venoconstriction.

increases in the delivered concentration of volatile drug.

B. **Myocardial contractility** is decreased in a dose-dependent manner with halothane having a greater depressant effect than isoflurane, desflurane, and sevoflurane.

C. Nitrous oxide is associated with increased sympathetic nervous system activity when administered alone or in combination with other volatile anesthetics.

D. **Coronary steal** has not been confirmed to occur with isoflurane, desflurane, or sevoflurane concentrations up to 1.5 MAC.

E. **Myocardial ischemia and cardiac outcome** seem more related to events that alter myocardial oxygen delivery and demand and not the specific anesthetic drug selected.

F. **Cardioprotection from Volatile Anesthetics**
   1. Volatile anesthetics mimic ischemic preconditioning and initiate a cascade of intracellular events resulting in myocardial protection against ischemia and reperfusion injury that last beyond elimination of the anesthetic.
   2. It is likely that anesthetic cardioprotection lessens myocardial damage (based on troponin levels) during cardiac surgery with or without cardiopulmonary bypass.
   3. Sulfonylurea oral hyperglycemic drugs close KATP channels and abolish anesthetic preconditioning. Hyperglycemia also prevents preconditioning so insulin therapy should be started when oral agents are discontinued preoperatively.

G. **Autonomic Nervous System**
   1. Isoflurane, desflurane, and sevoflurane produce similar dose-dependent depression of reflex control of sympathetic nervous system outflow.
   2. Desflurane is unique in evoking increased sympathetic nervous system outflow (paralleled by increased plasma concentrations of catecholamine) when the delivered concentration of this drug is abruptly increased (Fig. 15-8).

VI. THE PULMONARY SYSTEM

A. All volatile anesthetics decrease tidal volume but have lesser effects on decreasing minute ventilation because

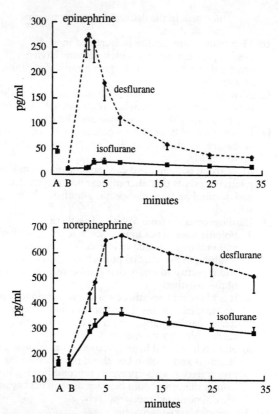

FIGURE 15-8. Stress hormone responses to a rapid increase in anesthetic concentration from 4 to 12% inspired. Data are mean ± SE. A = awake; B = value after 32 minutes of 0.55 MAC. Time represents minutes after initiation of increased anesthetic concentration.

of an offsetting response to increase breathing frequency (Fig. 15-9). The increase in resting $PaCO_2$ as an index of depression of ventilation is somewhat offset by surgical stimulation (Fig. 15-10).

B. **Ventilatory Mechanics.** Functional residual capacity is decreased during general anesthesia (decreased intercostal muscle tone, alterations in diaphragm position, changes in thoracic blood volume).

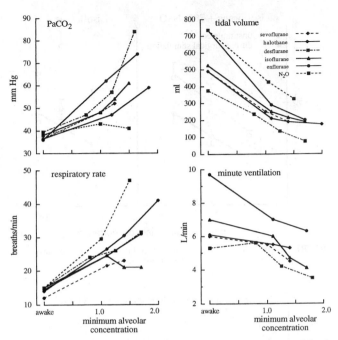

FIGURE 15-9. Comparison of mean changes in resting $PaCO_2$, tidal volume, respiratory rate, and minute ventilation in patients receiving an inhaled anesthetic.

C. **Response to Carbon Dioxide and Hypoxemia**
   1. All of the inhaled anesthetics produce a dose-dependent depression in the ventilatory response to hypercarbia (Fig. 15-11).
   2. Even subanesthetic concentrations of volatile anesthetics (0.1 MAC) produce depression of chemoreceptors responsible for the ventilatory response to hypoxia.
D. **Bronchiolar Smooth Muscle Tone**
   1. Bronchoconstriction during anesthesia is most likely a result of mechanical stimulation of the airway in the presence of minimal concentrations of inhaled anesthetics. This response is enhanced in patients with reactive airway disease.

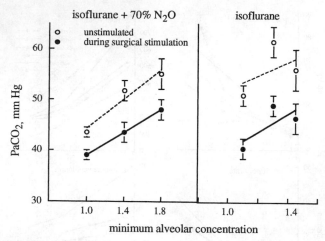

FIGURE 15-10. The effect of surgical stimulation on the ventilatory depression produced by isoflurane with or without nitrous oxide.

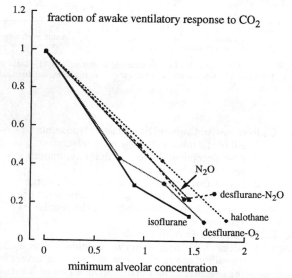

FIGURE 15-11. All inhaled anesthetics produce similar dose-dependent decreases in the ventilatory response to carbon dioxide.

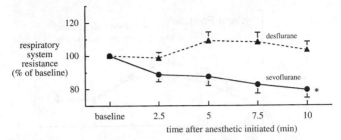

FIGURE 15-12. Changes in airway resistance before (baseline) and following tracheal intubation were significantly different in the presence of sevoflurane compared with desflurane. (Adapted from Goff MJ, Arain SR, Ficke DJ *et al*: Absence of bronchodilation during desflurane anesthesia: A comparison to sevoflurane and thiopental. Anesthesiology 93:404, 2000.)

    2. Volatile anesthetics relax airway smooth muscle by directly depressing smooth muscle contractility and indirectly by inhibiting the reflex neural pathways. Airway resistance increases more with desflurane than sevoflurane (Fig. 15-12).

  E. Pulmonary Vascular Resistance
    1. The pulmonary vasodilator action of volatile anesthetics is minimal. The effect of nitrous oxide on pulmonary vascular resistance may be exaggerated in patients with resting pulmonary hypertension.
    2. All inhaled anesthetics inhibit hypoxic pulmonary vasoconstriction in animals. Nevertheless, in patients undergoing one-lung ventilation during thoracic surgery, minimal effects on PaO_2 and intrapulmonary shunt fraction occur regardless of the volatile anesthetic being administered (Fig. 15-13).

VII. HEPATIC EFFECTS

  A. Halothane-associated liver damage may be mild and transient (nonspecific mechanism) or life threatening (immune mechanism).
  B. Ether-based anesthetics (isoflurane, desflurane, sevoflurane) maintain or increase hepatic artery blood flow while decreasing or not changing portal vein blood flow. This contrasts with halothane where decreases in portal vein blood flow are not

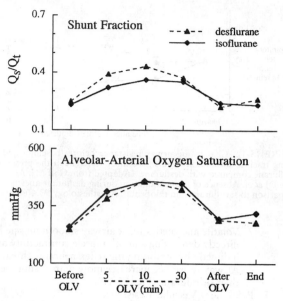

FIGURE 15-13. Shunt fraction (top panel) and alveolar-arterial oxygen gradient (bottom panel) before, during, and after one-lung ventilation (OLV) in patients anesthetized with desflurane or isoflurane. (Adapted from Pagel PS, Fu JL, Damask MC *et al*: Desflurane and isoflurane produce similar alterations in systemic and pulmonary hemodynamics and arterial oxygenation in patients undergoing one-lung ventilation during thoracotomy. Anesth Analg 87:800, 1998.)

compensated by increases in hepatic artery blood flow (selective hepatic artery vasoconstriction) (Fig. 15-14).

VIII. NEUROMUSCULAR SYSTEM AND MALIGNANT HYPERTHERMIA

A. Compared to the alkane halothane, the ether-derived fluorinated anesthetics produce about twofold greater skeletal muscle relaxation (postsynaptic effect at the neuromuscular junction).

  1. Although the mechanism of this potentiation is not entirely clear, it appears to be largely a result of a postsynaptic effect at the nicotinic acetylcholine receptors located at the neuromuscular junction

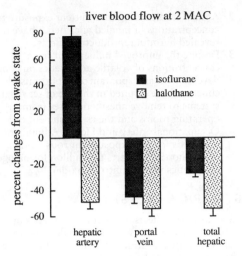

FIGURE 15-14. Changes (%, mean ≠ SE) in hepatic blood flow during administration of isoflurane or halothane.

(volatile anesthetics act synergistically with neuromuscular blocking drugs to enhance their action).

B. All volatile anesthetics serve as triggers for malignant hyperthermia (halothane greatest and desflurane least), whereas nitrous oxide is only a weak trigger.

IX. GENETIC EFFECTS

A. The Ames test (identifies chemicals that act as mutagens and carcinogens) is negative for all the inhaled anesthetics although metabolites of halothane may be positive.

B. Virtually every volatile anesthetic has been shown to be teratogenic in animal studies but none has been shown to be teratogenic in humans.

1. There has been ongoing concern about the incidence of spontaneous abortions in operating room personnel chronically exposed to trace concentrations of inhaled anesthetics, especially nitrous oxide (inhibits vitamin B12-dependent enzymes).

2. Animal studies using intermittent exposure to trace concentrations of inhaled anesthetics have not revealed harmful reproductive effects.
3. Despite the unproved influence of trace concentrations of volatile anesthetics on congenital development and spontaneous abortions, these concerns have resulted in the use of scavenging systems to remove anesthetic gases from the operating rooms and the establishment of Occupational Safety and Health Administration standards for gas exposure (nitrous oxide 25 parts per million and 2 parts per million for halogenated anesthetics without nitrous oxide).

X. OBSTETRIC EFFECTS

A. Similar to the effects of volatile anesthetics on vascular smooth muscle, a dose-dependent decrease in uterine smooth muscle contractility and blood flow occurs, which appears to be similar for the volatile anesthetics.
B. Uterine relaxation can be troubling at concentrations of volatile anesthetics >1 MAC.

XI. ANESTHETIC DEGRADATION BY CARBON DIOXIDE ABSORBERS

A. Carbon dioxide absorbents contain potassium hydroxide or sodium hydroxide, which degrade volatile anesthetics (soda lime less than barium hydroxide lime, which contains more potassium).
  1. Halothane and sevoflurane are degraded to haloalkenes, which are nephrotoxic in rats.
  2. Desflurane and isoflurane are degraded only by dehydrated carbon dioxide absorbents to carbon monoxide.
  3. Novel carbon dioxide absorbents have reduced or eliminated sodium and potassium hydroxide content and contain primarily calcium hydroxide. These carbon dioxide absorbents are chemically unreactive with all the volatile anesthetics and thus prevent the degradation of these compounds to compound A and carbon monoxide (Fig. 15-15).
B. Compound A
  1. Sevoflurane undergoes base-catalyzed degradation in carbon dioxide absorbents to form a vinyl ether

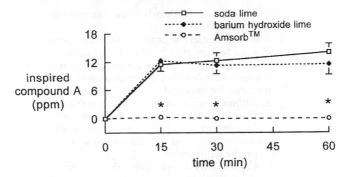

FIGURE 15-15. Compound A levels produced from three carbon dioxide absorbents during 1 MAC sevoflurane anesthesia delivered at a fresh gas flow of 1 L/min (mean ≠ SE). * $P<0.05$ versus soda lime and barium hydroxide lime. (Adapted from Kharasch ED, Hoffman GM, Thorning D *et al*: Role of the renal cysteine conjugate β-lyase pathway in inhaled compound A nephrotoxicity in rats. Anesthesiology 88:1624, 1998.)

designated as compound A. The production of compound A is enhanced in low flow or closed-circuit breathing systems and by warm or very dry carbon dioxide absorbents.

2. There are species differences in the threshold for compound A–induced nephrotoxicity (β-lyase-dependent metabolism pathway for compound A breakdown to cysteine-s conjugates is less in humans than rats). There is a high probability that renal injury in patients receiving sevoflurane does not occur regardless of the fresh gas flow rate.

C. Carbon Monoxide and Heat

1. Carbon dioxide absorbents degrade sevoflurane, desflurane, and isoflurane to carbon monoxide when carbon dioxide absorbent has become desiccated (water content below 5%).
   a. The degradation is the result of an exothermic reaction of the anesthetics with the absorbent.
   b. Instances of carbon monoxide poisoning have occurred in situations where the carbon dioxide absorbent has been presumably desiccated because an anesthetic machine has been left on with a high fresh gas flow passing through the

carbon dioxide absorbent over an extended period of time.

2. Although desflurane produces the most carbon monoxide with anhydrous carbon dioxide absorbents, the reaction with sevoflurane produces the most heat (exothermic reaction with the potential for fires and patient injuries).

   a. Although sevoflurane is not flammable at less than 11%, formaldehyde, methanol, and formate may result from degradation at high temperatures and in combination with oxygen can be flammable.

   b. Carbon dioxide absorbents that do not contain strong bases do not degrade anesthetics (to either compound A or carbon monoxide) and they should reduce exothermic reactions (adoption of these absorbents into clinical practice seems prudent).

XII. ANESTHETIC METABOLISM

A. **Fluoride-Induced Nephrotoxicity.** Despite the potential for relatively high plasma levels of fluoride following prolonged exposure to sevoflurane and enflurane, the minimal amount renal defluorination of these drugs may explain the relative absence of renal concentrating effects.

B. **Hepatic Injury from Metabolism: Halothane Hepatitis**

1. An oxidative metabolite of halothane may bind to liver cytochromes and act as a hapten (neoantigens) and induce an immune reaction (Fig. 15-16).

2. The metabolic pathway involving cytochrome P450 leading to the formation of neoantigens is identical for halothane, enflurane, isoflurane, and desflurane, introducing the possibility for cross-sensitization between all these anesthetics. The antigenic load will be determined by the magnitude of metabolism (halothane > isoflurane > desflurane).

3. Immunologic memory resulting in hepatitis after an initial exposure to halothane is prolonged (at least 28 years).

   a. Cross-sensitivity may occur in which exposure to one fluorinated anesthetic (exception sevoflurane) can sensitize patients to a second but different anesthetic.

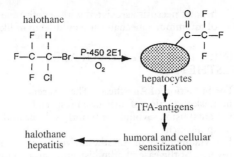

FIGURE 15-16. Halothane is metabolized to a trifluoroacetylated metabolite (TFA) adduct that binds to liver proteins. In susceptible patients, this adduct (altered protein) is seen as nonself (neoantigen), generating an immune response (production of antibodies). Subsequent exposure to halothane may result in hepatotoxicity. A similar process may occur in genetically susceptible patients after exposure to other fluorinated anesthetics (enflurane, isoflurane, desflurane) that also generate a TFA adduct.

    b. Autoantibodies have been identified in 10% of health care workers chronically exposed to low levels of anesthetics in the operating room.

   4. Sevoflurane is not metabolized to a trifluoroacetyl halide but rather to hexafluoroisopropanol that does not serve as a neoantigen (Fig. 15-17). Fulminant

FIGURE 15-17. Pathway for oxidative metabolism of sevoflurane.

hepatic necrosis associated with sevoflurane because of an immune mechanism would seem unlikely.

XIII. CLINICAL UTILITY OF VOLATILE ANESTHETICS

A. **For Induction of Anesthesia.** There is renewed interest in mask induction of anesthesia (especially pediatric patients) using sevoflurane (poorly soluble and nonpungent).

B. **For Maintenance of Anesthesia.** Volatile anesthetics because of the ease of administration and ability to adjust (titrate) the dose remain the most popular drugs for maintenance of anesthesia.

XIV. PHARMACOECONOMICS AND VALUE-BASED DECISIONS

A. In the current environment of cost containment, clinicians are constantly being pressured to use less expensive anesthetic agents, including antiemetics, neuromuscular blocking drugs, and volatile anesthetics.

B. Factors involved in value-based decisions include efficacy of the drug (all volatile anesthetics similar in efficacy) and side effects (halothane hepatic toxicity and cardiac sensitization offset its low cost).

1. The need for rescue medications to treat nausea and vomiting after volatile anesthesia needs to be weighed in any cost analysis.

2. Reducing the fresh gas flow of sevoflurane and desflurane can half the cost/MAC hour of these more expensive anesthetics without compromising their speed and effectiveness.

CHAPTER 16 ■
NEUROMUSCULAR BLOCKING AGENTS

The introduction of muscle relaxants (neuromuscular blocking drugs, NMBDs) into clinical practice more than 60 years ago is an important milestone in the history of anesthesia (Donati F, Bevan DR: Neuromuscular blocking drugs. In Barash PG, Cullen BF, Stoelting RK [eds]: *Clinical Anesthesia*, pp 421–452. Philadelphia, Lippincott Williams & Wilkins, 2006). In addition to providing immobility and better surgical conditions, NMBDs improve intubating conditions. As it is important to provide adequate anesthesia while a patient is totally or partially paralyzed, it is also essential to make sure that the effects of NMBDs have worn off or are reversed before the patient regains consciousness. With the introduction of shorter acting NMBDs, it was thought that reversal of blockade could be omitted. However, residual paralysis is still a problem and the threshold for complete neuromuscular recovery is not considered to be a train-of-four (TOF) of 0.9 rather than 0.7.

I. PHYSIOLOGY AND PHARMACOLOGY

   A. The process of skeletal muscle contraction originates at the neuromuscular junction (NMJ) with the release of acetylcholine (ACh). Anatomically, the NMJ is the synapse between the presynaptic membrane of the motor nerve ending and the postsynaptic membrane of the skeletal muscle fiber (Fig. 16-1).
   B. **Release of acetylcholine** into the synaptic cleft occurs when an action potential arrives at the nerve terminal.
   C. **Postsynaptic Events**
      1. Activation of the postsynaptic nicotinic receptor requires simultaneous occupation of the receptor's two *alpha subunits* by ACh (Fig. 16-2). Skeletal muscle contraction occurs when ACh-induced changes in the muscle cell's transmembrane permeability results in inward movement of sodium sufficient to decrease intracellular negativity (depolarization) and causes an action potential.

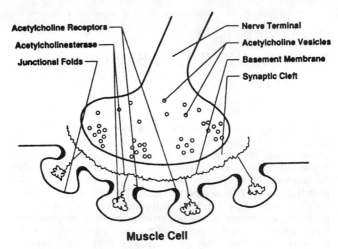

FIGURE 16-1. Diagram of the neuromuscular junction.

2. Propagation of the action potential initiates release of calcium from the sarcoplasmic reticulum, where activation of myosin adenosine triphosphate leads to excitation-contraction coupling of the myofilaments.
3. ACh is hydrolyzed (milliseconds to prevent prolonged depolarization) by acetylcholinesterase

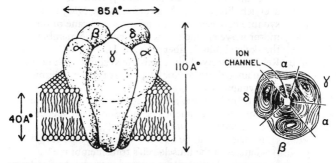

FIGURE 16-2. The nicotinic acetylcholine receptor consists of five glyco-protein subunits arranged to form an ion channel. The *alpha* subunits carry a recognition site for agonists and antagonists.

(true cholinesterase) to choline (reused for synthesis of new ACh) and acetate.

D. **Presynaptic Events**
   1. The release of ACh normally decreases during high-frequency stimulation under physiologic conditions because the pool of readily releasable ACh becomes depleted faster than it can be replenished. In the presence of muscle relaxants this decreased release of ACh produces a progressive decrease in skeletal muscle response (fade) with each stimulus.
   2. Fade is an important property of nondepolarizing neuromuscular blockade and is useful for monitoring purposes.

II. NEUROMUSCULAR BLOCKING AGENTS
(Table 16-1)

A. **Pharmacological Characteristics of Neuromuscular Blocking Agents.** The effect of NMBDs is measured as the depression of adductor muscle contraction (twitch) following electrical stimulation of the ulnar nerve.
B. **Potency** is determined by constructing the dose-response curves, which describe the relationship between twitch depression and dose.
   1. The ED95 is a clinically relevant value that corresponds to 95% block of single twitch (half the patients will reach 95% block and half will be less).
C. **Onset time** or time to maximum blockade can be shortened if the dose is increased (2 × ED95).
D. **Duration of action** is the time from injection of the NMBD to return of 25% twitch height (comparisons are usually made at 2 × ED95). Categories of NMBDs may be based on the duration of action.
E. **Recovery index** is the time interval between 25 and 75% twitch height (reflects speed of recovery once return of twitch is manifest). The adductor pollicis is the most commonly monitored muscle for determining onset and duration of action of NMBDs.

III. DEPOLARIZING BLOCKING DRUGS: SUCCINYLCHOLINE (SCh).
Succinylcholine remains a useful muscle relaxant because of its ultrarapid-onset and short-duration neuromuscular blocking properties that

TABLE 16-1

DEFINITION OF NEUROMUSCULAR BLOCKING DRUGS
ACCORDING TO ONSET AND DURATION OF BLOCK AT
ADDUCTOR POLLICIS

Onset to Maximum Block

Ultrarapid (<1 min)	Succinylcholine
Rapid (1–2 min)	Rocuronium
Intermediate (2–4 min)	Atracurium
	Mivacurium
	Vecuronium
	Pancuronium
Long (>4 min)	Cisatracurium
	Doxacurium

Duration to 25% Recovery of T1

Ultrashort (<8 min)	Succinylcholine
Short (8–20 min)	Mivacurium
Intermediate (20–50 min)	Atracurium
	Cisatracurium
	Rocuronium
	Vecuronium
Long (>50 min)	Doxacurium
	Pancuronium

cannot be duplicated by any of the available
nondepolarizing muscle relaxants.

A. **Neuromuscular Effects.** SCh binds to postsynaptic
   nicotinic receptors where it exhibits ACh-like activity.
   SCh also binds to extrajunctional receptors and
   presynaptic receptors.
   1. The net effect of SCh-induced depolarization is
      uncoordinated skeletal muscle activity that
      manifests clinically as fasciculations.
   2. SCh predictably increases masseter muscle tone
      (may be responsible for poor intubating conditions)
      and masseter muscle spasm may be associated with
      malignant hyperthermia. It is likely that increased
      masseter muscle tone is mediated by Ach receptors
      because it is blocked by nondepolarizing drugs.
   3. Nonparalyzing doses of nondepolarizing drugs
      (pretreatment) block visible evidence of
      SCh-induced depolarization, suggesting that
      presynaptic receptors are principally involved in the
      production of fasciculations.

TABLE 16-2

CHARACTERISTICS OF PHASE I DEPOLARIZING BLOCKADE

Decreased twitch amplitude
Absence of fade with continuous (tetanic) stimulation
Similar decreases in the amplitude of all twitches in the train-of-four (ratio >0.7)
Absence of post-tetanic potentiation
Antagonism by nondepolarizing muscle relaxants
Augmentation by anticholinesterase drugs

   4. The blocking effect of SCh at the NMJ is probably because of desensitization (prolonged exposure to an agonist leads to a state characterized by a lack of responsiveness of the receptors).
B. **Characteristics of Depolarizing Blockade**
   1. SCh initially produces features characterized as Phase I block (Table 16-2).
   2. Phase II block develops after prolonged exposure to SCh or high doses of SCh and has characteristics of a nondepolarizing neuromuscular blockade (Table 16-3). The onset of Phase II block coincides with the appearance of tachyphylaxis to the effects of SCh.
C. **Pharmacology of Succinylcholine**
   1. SCh is rapidly hydrolyzed (elimination half-time estimated to be 2 to 4 minutes) by plasma cholinesterase (pseudocholinesterase) to choline and succinylmonocholine (about 1/20 the neuromuscular blocking properties of the parent drug).
   2. The ED95 of SCh in the presence of opioid–nitrous oxide anesthesia is 0.30 to 0.35 mg/kg.

TABLE 16-3

CHARACTERISTICS OF NONDEPOLARIZING NEUROMUSCULAR BLOCKADE

Decreased twitch amplitude
Fade with continuous (tetanic) stimulation
Train-of-four ratio <0.7
Post-tetanic potentiation
Absence of fasciculations
Antagonism by anticholinesterase drugs
Augmentation by other nondepolarizing muscle relaxants

3. The onset of neuromuscular blocking effect is usually within 1 minute following high doses of SCh (1 to 2 mg/kg iv), and the time until full recovery of the electromyographic response is 10 to 12 minutes after a dose of 1 mg/kg iv.

4. A small proportion of patients (1:1,500 to 1:3,000) have a genetically determined (atypical plasma cholinesterase) inability to metabolize SCh (1 to 1.5 mg/kg iv lasts 3 to 6 hours).

D. **Side Effects** (Table 16-4)

E. **Clinical Uses**

1. The principal indication for SCh is to facilitate tracheal intubation (1 mg/kg iv is the usual dose, increased to 1.5 to 2.0 mg/kg iv if pretreatment is used).

2. The use of SCh in children is limited largely because of concerns about triggering hyperkalemia in young boys with unrecognized muscular dystrophy and the occasional triggering of malignant hyperthermia in the pediatric age group.

TABLE 16-4

SIDE EFFECTS OF SUCCINYLCHOLINE

Bradycardia (especially in children; more likely in adults with second dose)

Allergic reactions

Fasciculations

Muscle pains (relationship to fasciculations not conclusively established)

Increased intragastric pressure (offset by even greater increase in lower esophageal sphincter pressure)

Increased intraocular pressure (a result of cycloplegic action of succinylcholine and not reliably blunted by pretreatment)

Increased intracranial pressure (small effect and of questionable clinical significance)

Transient increase in plasma potassium concentration (normal increase 0.5–1.0 mEq/L is enhanced by denervation injuries, burns, extensive trauma, unrecognized muscular dystrophy in male children)

Trigger for malignant hyperthermia (masseter muscle spasm may be an early sign)

Prolonged response in presence of atypical cholinesterase or drug-induced inhibition of plasma cholinesterase activity (neostigmine but not edrophonium)

TABLE 16-5

TYPICAL PHARMACOKINETIC DATA FOR NONDEPOLARIZING MUSCLE RELAXANTS

	Volume of distribution (L/kg)	Clearance (mL/kg/min)	Elimination half-time (min)
Short-duration drugs			
Mivacurium			
cis-trans	0.05	46	2.0
trans-trans	0.05	29	2.4
cis-cis	0.18	7	30
Intermediate-duration drugs			
Atracurium	0.14	5.5	20
Cisatracurium	0.12	5	23
Rocuronium	0.3	3	90
Vecuronium	0.4	5	70
Long-duration drugs			
Doxacurium	0.2	2.5	95
Pancuronium	0.3	1.8	140

IV. NONDEPOLARIZING DRUGS. Nondepolarizing neuromuscular blocking drugs bind to postsynaptic receptors (must bind to one of the α subunits) in a competitive fashion to produce neuromuscular blockade.

   A. Characteristics of Nondepolarizing Blockade (see Table 16-3)

   B. Pharmacokinetics (Table 16-5)

   1. The pharmacokinetic variables derived from measurements of plasma concentrations of nondepolarizing muscle relaxants depend on the dose administered, the sampling schedule used, and the accuracy of the assay.
   2. All nondepolarizing muscle relaxants have a volume of distribution that is approximately equal to extracellular fluid volume.

   C. Onset and Duration of Action (Table 16-6)

   1. Although peak plasma concentrations of nondepolarizing muscle relaxants occur within 1 to 2 minutes of injection, the onset of maximum blockade is reached only after 2 to 7 minutes,

TABLE 16-6

COMPARATIVE PHARMACOLOGY OF NONDEPOLARIZING
MUSCLE RELAXANTS

	ED95 (mg/kg) (min)	Onset time (min)	Duration to 25% recovery (min)	Recovery index (25–75% recovery) (min)
Short-duration drugs				
Mivacurium	0.08	3–4	15–20	7–10
Intermediate-duration drugs				
Atracurium	0.2–0.25	3–4	35–45	10–15
Cisatracurium	0.05	5–7	35–45	12–15
Rocuronium	0.3	1.5–3	30–40	8–12
Vecuronium	0.05	3–4	35–45	10–15
Long-duration drugs				
Doxacurium	0.025	5–10	40–120	30–40
Pancuronium	0.07	2–4	60–120	30–40

reflecting the time required for drug transfer
between plasma and neuromuscular junction.

2. The duration of action of nondepolarizing drugs is
determined by the time required for plasma
concentrations to decrease below a critical level.

D. **Individual Nondepolarizing Relaxants** (Tables 16-5,
16-6, 16-7, and 16-8)

1. **Atracurium** is an intermediate-acting
benzylisoquinolinium-type nondepolarizing
neuromuscular blocking drug.

a. **Metabolism** is by ester hydrolysis (accounts for
an estimated two-thirds of the drug's metabolism)
and Hofmann elimination (nonenzymatic
degradation at body temperature and pH). A
metabolite of atracurium, laudanosine is a
cerebral stimulant, but it is unlikely that this is
clinically significant with the usual clinical doses
of atracurium administered.

b. **Hypotension and tachycardia** may accompany
high doses of atracurium (>2 × ED95), reflecting
dose-related histamine release (attenuated by

TABLE 16-7

AUTONOMIC AND HISTAMINE-RELEASING EFFECTS OF MUSCLE RELAXANTS

	Nicotinic receptors at autonomic ganglia	Cardiac muscarinic receptors	Histamine release
Succinylcholine	Stimulates	Stimulates	Rare
Mivacurium	No effect	No effect	Minimal
Atracurium	No effect	No effect	Minimal
Cisatracurium	No effect	No effect	0
Rocuronium	No effect	No effect	0
Vecuronium	No effect	No effect	0
Doxacurium	No effect	No effect	0
Pancuronium	No effect	No effect	0

injection of the muscle relaxant over 1 to 3 minutes).

   c. **Dose requirements** are similar in all age groups, presumably reflecting the absence of atracurium's dependence on renal or hepatic clearance mechanisms. The dose of atracurium, as for all nondepolarizing drugs, should be decreased on a mg/kg basis to reflect lean body mass.

2. **Cisatracurium** is an intermediate-acting benzylisoquinolinium-type neuromuscular blocking drug.

   a. As one of the ten isomers of atracurium, this drug resembles atracurium in onset, duration of action, rate of recovery, and clearance mechanisms (Hofmann elimination rendering both drugs independent of hepatic and renal function). Cisatracurium does not undergo significant hydrolysis by nonspecific plasma esterases.

   b. The metabolites of cisatracurium include laudanosine (peak plasma concentrations are about fivefold less than present with atracurium) and monoquaternary acrylate. These metabolites are not active at the NMJ.

   c. In contrast to atracurium, cisatracurium is more potent (ED95 0.05 mg/kg), devoid of histamine-releasing properties even at high doses (8 × ED95), and lacks cardiovascular effects.

TABLE 16-8

MECHANISMS FOR CLEARANCE OF NONDEPOLARIZING MUSCLE RELAXANTS

	Renal excretion (% unchanged)	Biliary excretion (% unchanged)	Hepatic degradation (% unchanged)	Hydrolysis in plasma
Mivacurium	Insignificant	Insignificant	Insignificant	Enzymatic
Atracurium	Insignificant	Insignificant	?	Spontaneous enzymatic
Cisatracurium	Insignificant	Insignificant	?	Spontaneous
Rocuronium	10–25	50–70	10–20	0
Vecuronium	15–25	40–75	20–30	0
Doxacurium	70	30	?	0
Pancuronium	80	5–10	10–40	0

    d. Neuromuscular block is easily maintained at a stable level by continuous infusion of cisatracurium at a constant rate and does not diminish over time. The rate of recovery is independent of the dose of cisatracurium or the duration of administration presumably reflecting independence of its clearance mechanisms from hepatic and renal function.

    e. Recovery from drug-induced neuromuscular blockade can be facilitated by administration of an anticholinesterase drug.

3. Doxacurium is a long-acting nondepolarizing muscle relaxant that is devoid of histamine-releasing or cardiovascular side effects.

4. GW280430A is a nondepolarizing drug whose main degradation pathway involves cysteine in the plasma and is independent of plasma cholinesterase. At doses required for tracheal intubation (0.4 to 0.6 mg/kg iv), onset at the adductor pollicis is 1.5 minutes and duration to 25% first twitch recovery is 8 to 10 minutes.

5. Mivacurium is a short-acting nondepolarizing neuromuscular blocking drug (mixture of three isomers) that is hydrolyzed by plasma cholinesterase (more slowly than SCh and a prolonged duration of action is predictable in patients with atypical cholinesterase).

    a. Following administration of 0.25 mg/kg iv, the onset of mivacurium's blocking effects is about 90 seconds. Recovery to 95% twitch height occurs in about 30 minutes. Rapid spontaneous recovery suggests that pharmacologic antagonism may be unnecessary.

    b. The cardiovascular response to mivacurium is minimal at doses up to $2 \times ED95$ (rapid intravenous injection of $3 \times ED95$ may evoke sufficient histamine release to transiently decrease mean arterial pressure by about 15%).

    c. The effect of anticholinesterase drugs is additive (no evidence that the potential antagonist-induced inhibition of plasma cholinesterase occurs) to the rate of spontaneous recovery from mivacurium.

6. **Pancuronium** is a long-acting nondepolarizing neuromuscular blocking drug with a steroid structure but lacking any endocrine effects.
   a. The drug is metabolized to a 3-OH compound that has one-half the neuromuscular blocking activity of the parent compound.
   b. Pancuronium is associated with modest (usually <15%) increases in heart rate, blood pressure, and cardiac output.
   c. Pancuronium does not release histamine.
   d. The use of pancuronium to provide muscle relaxation may offer some advantage over the use of cardiovascularly neutral muscle relaxants in patients anesthetized with high doses of opioids.
   e. Continued popularity of pancuronium compared with newer and more expensive short- and intermediate-acting nondepolarizing neuromuscular blocking drugs is dependent on cost. Generic pancuronium is the least expensive muscle relaxant to provide neuromuscular blockade for long operations (>2 hours), but its routine use in these situations may result in an increased incidence of postoperative skeletal muscle weakness.
   f. Pancuronium neuromuscular blockade is more difficult to reverse than that of the intermediate-acting nondepolarizing neuromuscular blocking drugs.
7. **Rapacuronium** is an aminosteroid neuromuscular blocking drug that produces intubating conditions in 60 seconds following administration of 1.5 mg/kg iv with spontaneous recovery to a train-of-four ratio of 0.7 in 35 minutes. It was withdrawn in 2001 because of rare, but severe cases of bronchospasm after intubation.
8. **Rocuronium** is an aminosteroid neuromuscular blocking drug that has a more rapid onset (intubating conditions 60 seconds following 1 mg/kg iv resemble SCh 1 mg/kg iv) but similar duration of action as vecuronium and similar pharmacokinetic characteristics.
   a. As for other short- and intermediate-acting nondepolarizing muscle relaxants, the onset of

action of rocuronium is more rapid at the diaphragm and laryngeal muscle than at the adductor pollicis, and about twice as much drug is required to produce the same degree of paralysis.

b. Hemodynamic changes or release of histamine does not follow administration of even high doses (4 × ED95) of rocuronium.

9. **Vecuronium** is an intermediate-acting aminosteroid nondepolarizing neuromuscular blocking drug that is devoid of histamine-releasing or cardiovascular side effects.

a. Vecuronium is a monoquaternary ammonium compound produced by demethylation of the pancuronium molecule. This demethylation decreases the ACh-like characteristics of the molecule and increases its lipophilicity, which encourages hepatic uptake.

b. Vecuronium undergoes spontaneous deacetylation. The most potent of the resulting metabolites, 3-OH vecuronium, has about 60% of the activity of vecuronium, is excreted by the kidneys, and may contribute to prolonged paralysis (incriminated in prolonged weakness following chronic use to maintain patients on mechanical ventilation).

c. Vecuronium is less potent and has a shorter duration of action in men than women probably as a result of a decrease in the volume of distribution, which results in increased plasma concentrations in women.

d. Accidental mixing of vecuronium and thiopental in the intravenous tubing may form a precipitate of barbituric acid and obstruct the intravenous cannula.

e. The cardiovascular neutrality and intermediated duration of action make vecuronium a suitable drug for use in patients with ischemic heart disease or those undergoing short ambulatory surgery.

V. DRUG INTERACTIONS (Table 16-9)

VI. ALTERED RESPONSES TO NEUROMUSCULAR BLOCKING AGENTS (Table 16-10)

TABLE 16-9
DRUG INTERACTIONS INVOLVING MUSCLE RELAXANTS

Volatile anesthetics (dose-dependent potentiation of all muscle
relaxants; impact on initial dose of muscle relaxant may be
greater with sevoflurane or desflurane, reflecting rapid
equilibration of these poorly soluble drugs)

Local anesthetics (potentiate effects of all muscle relaxants)

Nondepolarizing muscle relaxants (depending on combination
produce synergistic or additive effects; clinical significance
doubtful)

Nondepolarizing–depolarizing muscle relaxants (response depends
on sequence; nondepolarizer before SCh interferes with SCh
blockade; nondepolarizer after SCh is potentiated)

Antibiotics (aminoglycosides and polymyxins most likely to
potentiate muscle relaxants)

Anticonvulsants (resistance to nondepolarizing muscle relaxants)

VII. MONITORING NEUROMUSCULAR BLOCKADE

A. Why Monitor? The margin of safety is narrow because
blockade occurs over a narrow range of receptor
occupancy. Furthermore, there is considerable
interindividual variability in response to the same dose
of neuromuscular blocking drug. To test the function of
the NMJ, a peripheral nerve (ulnar nerve or the facial
nerve) is electrically stimulated with a peripheral nerve

TABLE 16-10
ALTERED RESPONSES TO NEUROMUSCULAR BLOCKING AGENTS

Intensive care unit (enthusiasm for liberal use of neuromuscular
blockings agents has waned because of myopathy)

Myasthenia gravis (usually resistant to SCh and highly sensitive to
nondepolarizing muscle relaxants)

Myotonia (sustained contracture in response to SCh; normal
response to nondepolarizing muscle relaxants)

Muscular dystrophy (SCh contraindicated)

Neurologic diseases (isolated reports of hyperkalemia in response
to SCh)

Hemiplegia/paraplegia (hyperkalemia in response to SCh;
resistant to nondepolarizing muscle relaxants)

Burn injury (hyperkalemia in response to SCh; resistant to effects
of nondepolarizing muscle relaxants)

TABLE 16-11

ASSESSMENT OF THE ADEQUACY OF ANTAGONISM OF
NEUROMUSCULAR BLOCKADE

Responses to electrical stimulation of a peripheral nerve (ulnar,
   facial)
Head lift for 5 seconds
Tongue protrusion
Tongue depressor
Hand grip strength
Maximum negative inspiratory pressure (> minus 25 cm H_2O)

   stimulator, and the response of the skeletal muscle is
   assessed.
   B. **Stimulator Characteristics.** The response of the nerve to
      electrical stimulation depends on three factors: the
      current applied, the duration of the current, and the
      position of the electrodes.
   C. **Monitoring Modalities** (Table 16-11)
   D. **Recording the Response**
      1. **Visual and tactile evaluation** is the easiest and least
         expensive way to assess the response to electrical
         stimulation applied to a peripheral nerve. The
         disadvantage of this technique is the subjective
         nature of its interpretation.
      2. **Measurement of force** using a force transducer
         provides accurate assessment of the response elicited
         by electrical stimulation of a peripheral nerve.
      3. **Electromyography** measures the electrical rather
         than mechanical response of the skeletal muscle.
   E. **Choice of Muscle**
      1. The **adductor pollicis** supplied by the ulnar nerve is
         the most common skeletal muscle monitored
         clinically. This muscle is relatively sensitive to
         nondepolarizing muscle relaxants, and during
         recovery it is blocked more than some respiratory
         muscles such as the diaphragm and laryngeal
         adductors.
      2. There seem to be important differences in the
         responses of muscles innervated by the facial nerve
         (stimulated 2 to 3 cm posterior to the lateral border
         of the orbit) around the eye.
         a. The response of the orbicularis oculi over the
            eyelid is similar to the adductor pollicis.

      b. The response of the eyebrow (corrugator supercilii) parallels the laryngeal adductors (onset more rapid and recovery sooner than at the adductor pollicis). This response is useful for predicting intubating conditions.

F. Clinical Application

  1. Monitoring Onset. After induction of anesthesia, the intensity of neuromuscular blockade must be assessed to determine the time for tracheal intubation (maximum relaxation of laryngeal and respiratory muscles). Single-twitch stimulation is often used to monitor the onset of neuromuscular blockade.

  2. Surgical relaxation is usually adequate when fewer than two or three visible twitches of the train-of-four are observed in response to stimulation of the adductor pollicis muscle.

  3. Monitoring recovery is useful in determining whether spontaneous recovery has progressed to a degree that allows reversal drugs to be given (preferably four twitches visible) and to assess the effect of these drugs (supplement with other clinical observations) (see Table 16-11).

    a. Traditionally, a train-of-four ratio of 0.7 has been considered to be the threshold below which residual weakness of the respiratory muscles could be present. Evidence suggests, however, that significant weakness and impairment of swallowing may be present at a train-of-four ratio of 0.9.

    b. A sustained head lift test may not guarantee full skeletal muscle recovery.

    c. The upper airway muscles used to retain a tongue depressor between the teeth are very sensitive to residual effects of muscle relaxants.

  4. Factors Affecting the Monitoring of Neuromuscular Blockade

    a. If the monitored hand is cold, the degree of paralysis will appear to be increased.

    b. If the monitored limb is characterized by nerve damage (stroke, spinal cord transection, peripheral nerve trauma), there is inherent resistance to the effects of muscle relaxants, and the degree of skeletal muscle paralysis will be underestimated.

VIII. ANTAGONISM OF NEUROMUSCULAR BLOCKADE

A. **Anticholinesterase Pharmacology.** The pharmacologic principle involved in drug-enhanced antagonism of muscle relaxants is the decrease of the effect of competitive blocking drugs by increasing the concentration of ACh at the NMJ.

1. **Inhibition of acetylcholinesterase** by anticholinesterase drugs (neostigmine, pyridostigmine, edrophonium) results in an increase in the amount of ACh that reaches the receptor.

2. Anticholinesterase drugs may also have presynaptic effects.

3. **Potency** ratios are difficult to determine because the slopes of the edrophonium and neostigmine dose-response curves are not parallel.

4. The **pharmacokinetics** of anticholinesterase drugs reflect the dependence of these drugs on renal clearance (Table 16-12).

5. **Pharmacodynamics.** The onset of action of edrophonium to peak effect (1 to 2 minutes) is much more rapid than that of neostigmine (7 to 11 minutes) or pyridostigmine (15 to 20 minutes).

   a. Recovery of neuromuscular activity reflects spontaneous recovery plus augmented (accelerated) recovery induced by the anticholinesterase drug.

   b. **Recurarization** should not be expected as long as the duration of the anticholinesterase drug exceeds that of the muscle relaxant.

B. **Factors Affecting Reversal** (Table 16-13)

1. The dose of anticholinesterase drug selected and the time to effective recovery are directly related to the intensity of blockade at the time of reversal (Table 16-14).

   a. Neostigmine is more effective than edrophonium or pyridostigmine in antagonizing intense neuromuscular blockade.

   b. Because of the ceiling effect, there is little benefit in administering more than 0.7 mg/kg of neostigmine.

2. The overall rate of recovery (spontaneous plus drug enhanced) is more rapid from atracurium or vecuronium than from pancuronium.

TABLE 16-12

PHARMACOKINETICS OF ANTICHOLINESTERASE DRUGS

	Patient status	Volume of distribution (L/kg)	Clearance (mL/kg/mn)	Elimination half-time (min)
Neostigmine	Normal	0.7	9.2	177
	Renal failure	1.6	7.8	181
Edrophonium	Normal	1.1	9.6	110
	Renal failure	0.7	2.7	206
Pyridostigmine	Normal	1.1	8.6	112
	Renal failure	1.0	2.1	379

TABLE 16-13

FACTORS AFFECTING REVERSAL

Block intensity (time to drug-augmented recovery is directly
  proportional to intensity of blockade present at the time of
  antagonism, see Table 16-14)
Anticholinesterase dose
Muscle relaxant administered
Age
Renal failure
Acid-base balance (impairment of antagonism by acidosis is difficult
  to document)

Furthermore, the doses of antagonist drugs required
to produce the same degree of antagonism are
greater after the long-acting than the
intermediate-acting and short-acting muscle
relaxants.

  3. Recovery of neuromuscular activity occurs more
     rapidly with lower doses of anticholinesterase drugs
     in infants and children than in adults.

C. **Cardiovascular Effects**
  1. Anticholinesterase drugs evoke profound vagal
     stimulation that can be prevented by concomitant
     administration of an anticholinergic drug.
  2. Because of its rapid onset (1 minute), atropine is
     appropriate for use in combination with
     edrophonium, whereas glycopyrrolate (onset 2 to
     3 minutes) may be more suitable for use with
     neostigmine or pyridostigmine.

TABLE 16-14

**RECOMMENDED DOSES OF ANTICHOLINESTERASE DRUGS
AND ANTICHOLINERGIC DRUGS BASED ON
TRAIN-OF-FOUR STIMULATION**

Visible	Fade	Anticholinesterase	Dose (mg/kg/iv)	Anticholinergic dose(μg/kg iv)
<2	++++	Neostigmine	0.07	Glycopyrrolate 7 or atropine 15
3–4	+++	Neostigmine	0.04	Glycopyrrolate 7 or atropine 15
4	++	Edrophonium	0.5	Atropine 7
4	+/–	Edrophonium	0.25	Atropine 7

3. Atropine requirements are less when combined with edrophonium (7 to 10 mg/kg iv) than with neostigmine (15 to 20 mg/kg iv).
D. **Other cholinergic effects** of anticholinesterase drugs include increased salivation, enhanced bowel motility (concern about increase in bowel anastomatic leakage), and an alleged increased incidence of nausea and vomiting after ambulatory surgery.

CHAPTER 17 ■ LOCAL ANESTHETICS

Local anesthetics block the generation, propagation, and oscillations of electrical impulses in electrically excitable tissue. (Liu SS, Joseph RS: Local anesthetics. In Barash PG, Cullen BF, Stoelting, RK [eds]: *Clinical Anesthesia*, pp 453–471. Philadelphia, Lippincott Williams & Wilkins, 2006). Use of local anesthetics in clinical anesthesia is varied and includes direct injection into tissues, topical application, and intravenous administration to produce clinical effects at varied locations including the central neuraxis, peripheral nerves, mucosa, skin, heart, and airway.

I. MECHANISM OF ACTION OF LOCAL ANESTHETICS

A. Anatomy of Nerves

1. Peripheral nerves are mixed nerves containing afferent and efferent fibers that may be myelinated (all nerves with a diameter >1 μm) or unmyelinated (all nerves with a diameter <1 μm).

2. Individual nerves are gathered into fascicles and surrounded by perineurium composed of connective tissue.

3. Protective layers around myelinated and unmyelinated nerve fibers presents a substantial barrier to the entry of local anesthetics.

4. Nerve fibers are classified by diameter, conduction velocity, presence or absence of myelin, and function (Table 17-1). In general, myelination and increasing nerve fiber diameter result in increased conduction velocity.

B. Electrophysiology of Neural Conduction

1. Ionic disequilibrium across semipermeable membranes is the basis for neuronal resting potentials and for the potential energy needed to initiate and maintain electrical impulses.

2. The resting potential of neural membranes averages -60 to -70 mV with the interior being negative to the exterior (maintained by a potassium ion gradient with

TABLE 17-1
CLASSIFICATION OF NERVE FIBERS

Classification	Diameter (μ)	Myelin	Conduction (m/sec)	Location	Function
A-alpha	6–22	+	30–120	Afferents/efferents for muscles and joints	Motor
A-beta					Proprioception
A-gamma	3–6	+	15–35	Efferent to muscle spindle	Muscle tone
A-delta	1–4	+	5–25	Afferent sensory nerve	Pain
					Touch
					Temperature
B	<3	+	3–15	Preganglionic sympathetic	Autonomic function
C	0.3–1.3	–	0.7–1.3	Postganglionic sympathetic	Autonomic function
				Afferent sensory nerve	Pain
					Temperature

a 10-fold greater concentration of potassium ion within the cell).

3. In contrast to the dependence of the resting membrane potential on potassium disequilibrium, generation of the action potential is primarily a result of activation of voltage-gated sodium channels.

4. Repolarization after action potential generation and propagation is because of increasing equilibrium of internal and external sodium ions, a time-controlled decrease in sodium conductance, and a voltage-controlled increase in potassium conductance.

C. **Molecular Mechanisms of Action of Local Anesthetics**

1. The mechanism of action of local anesthetics is best explained by direct interaction with the sodium channel (modulated receptor theory).

2. Local anesthetics may act on the sodium channel either by modification of the lipid membrane surrounding it or by direct interaction with its protein structure.

3. Sodium channel blockade results in attenuation of neural action potential formation and propagation.

D. **Mechanism of Blockade of Peripheral Nerves**

1. Local anesthetics block peripheral nerve function through several mechanisms including sodium channel blockade and resulting attenuation of neural action potential formation and propagation.

2. Differential sensory block (loss of temperature sensation followed by loss of sharp pain and then light touch) is observed clinically.

   a. This sequence of sensory blockade has been erroneously assumed to reflect increased susceptibility of unmyelinated (C) fibers conducting temperature compared with myelinated (A) fibers conducting touch.

   b. Explanation is more complex and depends on length of nerve fiber exposed to the local anesthetic, frequency of membrane stimulation, and specific local anesthetic. In this regard small nerve fibers require a shorter length (<1 cm) exposed to local anesthetic for block to occur than do large fibers.

E. **Mechanism of Blockade of Central Neuraxis**

1. Local anesthetics can exert ion channel block (sodium, potassium, calcium channels) in the dorsal horn.

2. In addition to blockade of ion channels, local anesthetics can influence analgesic pathways and postsynaptic effects of nociceptive neurotransmitters.

II. PHARMACOLOGY AND PHARMACODYNAMICS

A. **Chemical Properties and Relationship to Activity and Potency**
   1. Clinically used local anesthetics consist of a lipid-soluble, substituted benzene ring linked to an amine group via an alkyl chain containing either an amide or **ester** linkage.
   2. The type of linkage separates the local anesthetics into either aminoamides, metabolized in the liver, or aminoesters, metabolized in the liver or by plasma cholinesterase.
   3. All clinically used local anesthetics are weak bases that can exist as either the lipid-soluble, neutral form or as the charged, hydrophilic form. The combination of pH and pKa of the local anesthetic determines how much of the compound exists in each form (Table 17-2).
   4. Increased lipid solubility of the local anesthetic results in increased penetration of the drug into the myelin and other lipid-soluble compartments and results in a slowed rate of onset of action.
   5. Protein binding influences activity of local anesthetics because only the unbound form is pharmacologically active.
   6. Stereoisomers of local anesthetics appear to have potentially different effects on anesthetic potency, pharmacokinetics, and systemic toxicity.

B. **Tachyphylaxis and Local Anesthetics**
   1. Tachyphylaxis to local anesthetics following repeated injection of the same dose of local anesthetic leads to decreasing efficacy (has been described after central neuraxial blocks and peripheral nerve blocks).
   2. Tachyphylaxis to local anesthetics is influenced by the dosing interval (short dosing intervals that do not permit pain to occur are not associated with tachyphylaxis).

C. **Additives to Increase Local Anesthetic Activity** (Table 17-3)

TABLE 17-2

PHYSIOCHEMICAL PROPERTIES OF CLINICALLY USED LOCAL ANESTHETICS

Local anesthetic	pKa	% Ionized (at pH 7.4)	Partition coefficient (lipid solubility)	% Protein binding
Amides				
Bupivacaine[a]	8.1	83	3420	95
Etridocaine	7.7	66	7317	94
Lidocaine	7.9	76	366	64
Mepivacaine	7.6	61	130	77
Prilocaine	7.9	76	129	55
Ropivacaine	8.1	83	775	94
Esters				
Chloroprocaine	8.7	95	810	n/a
Procaine	8.9	97	100	6
Tetracaine	8.5	93	5822	94

[a]Levo-bupivacaine is the same as bupivacaine.

TABLE 17-3
EFFECTS OF ADDITION OF EPINEPHRINE TO LOCAL ANESTHETICS

	Increase duration	Decrease blood levels (%)	Dose/concentration of epinephrine
Nerve Block			
Bupivacaine	Inconsistent	10–20	1:200,000
Lidocaine	Yes	20–30	1:200,000
Mepivacaine	Yes	20–30	1:200,000
Ropivacaine	Doubtful	0	1:200,000
Epidural			
Bupivacaine	Inconsistent	10–20	1:300,000–1:200,000
levo-bupivacaine	Inconsistent	10	1:200,000–1:400,000
Chloroprocaine	Yes		1:200,000
Lidocaine	Yes	20–30	1:600,000–1:200,000
Mepivacaine	Yes	20–30	1:200,000
Ropivacaine	Doubtful	0	1:200,000
Spinal			
Bupivacaine	Inconsistent		
Lidocaine	Yes		0.2 mg
Tetracaine	Yes		0.2 mg

1. **Epinephrine** added to the local anesthetic solution may prolong the local anesthetic block, increase the intensity of the block, and decrease systemic absorption of the local anesthetic.
   a. Vasoconstrictive effects produced by epinephrine augment local anesthetics by antagonizing inherent vasodilating effects of local anesthetics decreasing systemic absorption and intraneural clearance, and perhaps by redistribution of intraneural local anesthetic.
   b. Analgesic effects of epinephrine via interaction with *a*-2 adrenergic receptors in the spinal cord and brain may play a role in the effects of epinephrine added to the local anesthetic solution.
   c. The effectiveness of epinephrine depends on the local anesthetic administered, the type of regional block performed, and the amount of epinephrine added to the local anesthetic solution.
2. **Opioids** added to the local anesthetic solution placed into the epidural or subarachnoid space result in synergistic analgesia and anesthesia without increasing the risk of toxicity.
   a. Peripheral opioid receptors make coadministration of local anesthetic and opioid into intra-articular and peri-incisional sites effective.
   b. Coadministration of local anesthetic and opioids is of no value in enhancing the effects of a peripheral nerve block.
3. **α-2 adrenergic agonists** such as clonidine produce synergistic analgesia via supraspinal and spinal adrenergic receptors. Clonidine also has direct inhibitory effects on peripheral nerve conduction (A and C nerve fibers).

III. PHARMACOKINETICS OF LOCAL ANESTHETICS (Tables 17-4 and 17-5)

A. Clearance of local anesthetics from neural tissue and from the body govern both duration of effect and potential toxicity.
   1. Systemic toxicity is primarily dependent on blood levels of the local anesthetic.

TABLE 17-4

TYPICAL PEAK PLASMA CONCENTRATIONS (CMAX) AFTER REGIONAL ANESTHETICS

Local anesthetic/technique	Dose (mg)	Peak plasma concentration (μg/ml)	Time to peak plasma concentration (min)	Toxic plasma concentration (μg/mL)
Bupivacaine				
Brachial plexus	150	1.0	20	3
Celiac plexus	100	1.5	17	
Epidural	150	1.26	20	
Intercostal	140	0.90	30	
Lumbar sympathetic	52.5	0.49	24	
Sciatic/Femoral	400	1.89	15	
levo-bupivacaine				
Epidural	75	0.36	50	4
Brachial plexus	250	1.2	55	
Lidocaine				
Brachial plexus	400	4.0	25	5
Epidural	400	4.27	20	
Intercostal	400	6.8	15	
Mepivacaine				
Brachial plexus	500	3.68	24	5
Epidural	500	4.95	16	
Intercostal	500	8.06	9	
Sciatic/Femoral	500	3.59	31	
Ropivacaine				
Brachial plexus	190	1.3	53	4
Epidural	150	1.07	40	
Intercostal	140	1.10	21	

TABLE 17-5

PHARMACOKINETIC PARAMETERS OF LOCAL
ANESTHETICS

Local anesthetic	Volume of distribution at steady state (VDss) (L/kg)	Clearance (L/kg/hr)	Elimination half-time (hr)
Bupivacaine	1.02	0.41	3.5
levo-bupivacaine	0.78	0.32	2.6
Chloroprocaine	0.50	2.96	0.11
Etidocaine	1.9	1.05	2.6
Lidocaine	1.3	0.85	1.6
Mepivacaine	1.2	0.67	1.9
Prilocaine	2.73	2.03	1.6
Procaine	0.93	5.62	0.14
Ropivacaine	0.84	0.63	1.9

2. In general, local anesthetics with decreased systemic absorption have a greater margin of safety in clinical use.
B. **Systemic Absorption** (Table 17-6)
C. **Distribution**
   1. Regional distribution of local anesthetics following systemic absorption is dependent on organ blood flow, partition coefficient of the local anesthetic between compartments, and protein binding.
   2. The end organs of main concern for toxicity are the cardiovascular and the central nervous system (CNS).
D. **Elimination**
   1. Clearance of aminoester local anesthetics is primarily dependent on clearance by cholinesterase.

TABLE 17-6

DETERMINANTS OF THE RATE AND EXTENT OF SYSTEMIC
ABSORPTION OF LOCAL ANESTHETICS

Site of injection (intercostal > caudal > brachial plexus > sciatic/femoral)
Dose
Physiochemical properties (lipid solubility, protein binding)
Addition of epinephrine

      2. Clearance of aminoamide local anesthetics is dependent on hepatic extraction.

E. **Clinical Pharmacokinetics**

      1. The primary benefit of a knowledge of the systemic pharmacokinetics of local anesthetics is the ability to predict Cmax after the drugs are administered, and thus reduce the likelihood of administration of toxic doses.

      2. Pharmacokinetics are difficult to predict in any given circumstance because both physical and pathophysiologic characteristics will affect individual pharmacokinetics.

IV. CLINICAL USE OF LOCAL ANESTHETICS
(Tables 17-7 and 17-8)

V. TOXICITY OF LOCAL ANESTHETICS

A. **Central Nervous System Toxicity**

      1. Local anesthetics readily cross the blood-brain barrier and generalized CNS toxicity may occur from systemic absorption or direct vascular injection.

      2. Development of CNS toxicity is more likely with certain local anesthetics (Table 17-9) and the signs of generalized CNS toxicity as a result of local anesthetics are dose-dependent (Table 17-10).

      3. Factors that increase CNS toxicity include decreased protein binding, acidosis, vasoconstriction, and hyperdynamic circulation because of epinephrine added to the local anesthetic solution.

      4. Factors that decrease CNS toxicity include drugs (barbiturates, benzodiazepines) and decreased

---

TABLE 17-7

CLINICAL USE OF LOCAL ANESTHETICS

Regional anesthesia and analgesia
Intravenous regional anesthesia
Peripheral nerve blocks (single injection or continuous infusion)
Topical
Blunt responses to tracheal intubation

systemic absorption because of epinephrine added to the local anesthetic solution.

5. The incidence of CNS toxicity with epidural injection of local anesthetics is estimated to be 3/10,000 and for peripheral nerve blocks 11/10,000.

B. **Cardiovascular Toxicity**

1. In general, much greater doses of local anesthetics are required to produce cardiovascular toxicity than CNS toxicity (see Table 17-10).

   a. Use of single-optical isomer (*S/L*) preparations of ropivacaine and levo-bupivacaine may improve the safety profile for long-lasting regional anesthesia.

   b. Reduced potential for cardiotoxicity is likely because of reduced affinity for brain and myocardial tissue by the single isomer preparation.

   c. In addition to the stereoselectivity, the larger butyl side chain in bupivacaine may also have more of a cardiodepressant effect as opposed to the propyl side chain of ropivacaine.

2. Cardiovascular toxicity produced by less lipid-soluble and potent local anesthetics such as lidocaine (hypotension, bradycardia, arterial hypoxemia) are different from that produced by more potent and lipid-soluble anesthetics such as bupivacaine (sudden cardiovascular collapse because of ventricular cardiac dysrhythmias that are resistant to resuscitation).

3. All local anesthetics block the cardiac conduction system via a dose-dependent block of sodium channels.

4. Bupivacaine cardiotoxicity compared to that of lidocaine is enhanced by this drug's stronger binding affinity to resting and inactivated sodium channels.

5. Local anesthetics bind to sodium channels during systole and dissociate during diastole.

   a. Bupivacaine dissociates more slowly from sodium channels during cardiac diastole than lidocaine.

   b. Bupivacaine dissociates so slowly that the duration of diastole at heart rates between 60 and 180 beats/min does not allow enough time for complete recovery of sodium channels and bupivacaine conduction block increases.

TABLE 17-8
CLINICAL PROFILE OF LOCAL ANESTHETICS

Local anesthetic	Concentration (%)	Clinical use	Onset	Duration (hr)	Recommended maximum single dose (mg)
Amides					
Bupivacaine (levobupivacaine)	0.25	Infiltration	Fast	2–8	175/225 + epinephrine
	0.25–0.5	Peripheral nerve block	Slow	4–12	175/225 + epinephrine
	0.5–0.75	Epidural anesthesia	Moderate	2–5	175/225 + epinephrine
	0.5–0.75	Spinal anesthesia	Fast	1–4	20
Lidocaine	0.5–1	Infiltration	Fast	2–8	300/500 + epinephrine
	0.25–0.5	Intravenous regional	Fast	0.5–1	300
	1–1.5	Peripheral nerve block	Fast	1–3	300/500 + epinephrine
	1.5–2	Epidural anesthesia	Fast	1–2	300/500 + epinephrine
	1.5–2	Spinal anesthesia	Fast	0.5–1	100
	4	Topical	Fast	0.5–1	300
Mepivacaine	0.5–1	Infiltration	Fast	1–4	400/500 + epinephrine
	1–1.5	Peripheral nerve block	Fast	2–4	400/500 + epinephrine
	1.5–2	Epidural anesthesia	Fast	1–3	400/500 + epinephrine
	2–4	Spinal anesthesia	Fast	1–2	100

Drug	Technique	Concentration (%)	Onset	Duration (h)	Maximum dose (mg)
Prilocaine	Infiltration	0.5–1	Fast	1–2	600
	Intravenous regional	0.25–0.5	Fast	0.5–1	600
	Peripheral nerve block	1.5–2	Fast	1.5–3	600
	Epidural	2–3	Fast	1–3	600
Ropivacaine	Infiltration	0.2–0.5	Fast	2–6	200
	Peripheral nerve block	0.5–1	Slow	5–8	250
	Epidural anesthesia	0.5–1	Moderate	2–6	200
Mixture					
Lidocaine + prilociane	Skin topical	2.5/2.5	Slow	3–5	20 g
Esters					
Benzocaine	Skin topical	up to 20%	Fast	0.5–1	200
Chloroprocaine	Infiltration	1	Fast	0.5–1	800/1,000 + epinephrine
	Peripheral nerve block	2	Fast	0.5–1	800/1,000 + epinephrine
	Epidural anesthesia	2–3	Fast	0.5–1	800/1,000 + epinephrine
Cocaine	Topical	4–10	Fast	0.5–1	150
Procaine	Spinal anesthesia	10	Fast	0.5–1	1,000
Tetracaine	Topical	2	Fast	0.5–1	20
	Spinal anesthesia	0.5	Fast	2–6	20

TABLE 17-9
CENTRAL NERVOUS SYSTEM (CNS) AND CARDIOVASCULAR
(CVS) TOXICITY

Local anesthetic	Relative potency for CNS toxicity	Ratio of dose needed for CVS:CNS toxicity
Bupivacaine	4.0	2.0
levo-bupivacaine	2.9	2.0
Chloroprocaine	0.3	3.7
Etidocaine	2.0	4.4
Lidocaine	1.0	7.1
Mepivcaine	1.4	7.1
Prilocaine	1.2	3.1
Procaine	0.3	3.7
Ropivacaine	2.9	2
Tetracaine	2.0	

      c. Lidocaine fully dissociates from sodium channels
      during diastole and little accumulation of
      conduction block occurs.
    6. Bupivacaine may inhibit cyclic adenosine
    monophosphate (cAMP) production, suggesting that
    large doses of epinephrine (resuscitative effects
    modulated by cAMP) may be needed during
    resuscitations from bupivacaine overdose.
C. Treatment of Systemic Toxicity from Local Anesthetics
  (Table 17-11)
    1. The best method to avoid systemic toxicity from local
    anesthetics is through prevention (frequent syringe

TABLE 17-10
DOSE-DEPENDENT SYSTEMIC EFFECTS OF LIDOCAINE

Plasma concentration (μg/mL)	Effect
1–5	Analgesia
5–10	Light-headedness
	Tinnitus
	Numbness of tongue
10–15	Seizures
	Unconsciousness
15–25	Coma
	Respiratory arrest
>25	Cardiovascular depression

TABLE 17-11
TREATMENT OF SYSTEMIC TOXICITY AS A RESULT OF LOCAL ANESTHETICS

Stop injection of local anesthetic
Administer supplemental oxygen
Support ventilation
Tracheal intubation and control ventilation if necessary
Suppress seizure activity (thiopental, midazolam, propofol)
Treat ventricular dysrhythmias (electrical cardioversion, epinephrine, vasopressin, amiodarone, consider 20% lipid solutions to remove bupivacaine from its sites of action)

aspirations, use of a small local anesthetic test dose [3 mL], and slow injection or fractionation of the dose of local anesthetic).
2. Treatment of systemic toxicity is primarily supportive.

D. **Neural Toxicity of Local Anesthetics**
1. Although all clinically used local anesthetics can cause concentration-dependent nerve fiber damage in peripheral nerves when used in high concentrations, it is believed that clinically used concentrations are safe for peripheral nerves.
2. Compared with peripheral nerves, the spinal cord and nerve roots are more prone to injury.
   a. Lidocaine and tetracaine may be especially neurotoxic in a concentration-dependent fashion and this neurotoxicity could theoretically occur with clinically used concentrations.
   b. Despite laboratory findings that all local anesthetics can cause neurotoxicity, spinal administration of local anesthetics in patients have not manifested a neurotoxic potential.

E. **Transient Neurologic Symptoms (TNS) After Spinal Anesthesia**
1. TNS (pain or sensory abnormalities in the lower back and extremities) occur after all local anesthetics used for spinal anesthesia (Table 17-12).
2. Increased risk of TNS is associated with lidocaine, the lithotomy position, and ambulatory anesthesia but not the baricity of the solution or the dose of local anesthetic.
3. The potential neurological etiology of this syndrome coupled with known concentration-dependent toxicity

TABLE 17-12

INCIDENCE OF TRANSIENT NEUROLOGIC SYMPTOMS (TNS) AFTER SPINAL ANESTHESIA

Local anesthetic	Concentration	Type of surgery	Approximate incidence of TNS
Lidocaine	2%–5%	Lithotomy position	30%–36%
	2%–5%	Knee arthroscopy	18%–22%
	0.5%	Knee arthroscopy	17%
	2%–5%	Mixed supine position	4%–8%
Mepivacaine	1.5%–4%	Mixed	23%
Procaine	10%	Knee arthroscopy	6%
Bupivacaine	0.5%–0.75%	Mixed	1%
levo–bupivacaine	0.5%	Mixed	1%
Prilocaine	2%–5%	Mixed	1%
Ropivacaine	0.5%–0.75%	Mixed	1%

of lidocaine has led to concerns over a neurotoxic etiology for TNS from spinal lidocaine (Table 17-13).
   4. Preservative-free 2-chloroprocaine provides an anesthetic profile similar to lidocaine without TNS
   F. **Myotoxicity of Local Anesthetics.** Local anesthetics have the potential for myotoxicity in clinically applicable concentrations (dysregulation of intracellular calcium concentrations).

TABLE 17-13

POSSIBLE ETIOLOGIES OF TRANSIENT NEUROLOGIC SYMPTOMS

Concentration dependent neurotoxicity (?)
Patient positioning
Early ambulation
Needle trauma
Neural ischemia
Pooling secondary to maldistribution

G. **Allergic Reactions to Local Anesthetics**
   1. True allergic reactions to local anesthetics, especially aminoamides, are rare.
   2. Increased allergenic potential with ester local anesthetics may be because of metabolism to para-aminobenzoic acid, which is a known antigen.
   3. Preservatives such as methylparaben and metabisulfite can also provoke an allergic response.

CHAPTER 18 ■ PREOPERATIVE EVALUATION AND MANAGEMENT

I. **INTRODUCTION.** The goals of preoperative evaluation are to reduce patient risk and the morbidity of surgery, as well as to promote efficiency and reduce costs (Hata TM, Moyers JR: Preoperative evaluation and management. In Barash PG, Cullen BF, Stoelting RK [eds]: *Clinical Anesthesia*, pp 475–501. Philadelphia, Lippincott Williams & Wilkins, 2006).

   A. The Joint Commission for the Accreditation of Healthcare Organizations (JCAHO) requires that all patients receive a preoperative anesthetic evaluation.

   B. The American Society of Anesthesiologists (ASA) has approved Basic Standards for Pre-anesthetic Care, which outlines the minimum requirements for a preoperative evaluation.

   C. Conducting a preoperative evaluation is based on the premise that it will modify patient care and improve outcome.

   1. Based on the history and physical examination, the appropriate laboratory tests and preoperative consultations should be obtained.

   2. Guided by the history and physical examination, the anesthesiologist should choose the appropriate anesthetic and care plan.

II. **CHANGING CONCEPTS IN PREOPERATIVE EVALUATION**

   A. The first time the anesthesiologist performing the anesthetic sees the patient may be just prior to anesthesia and surgery (seen previously by others in a preoperative evaluation clinic).

   B. Information technology has helped the anesthesiologist in previewing the upcoming patients that will be anesthetized (preoperative questionnaires and computer-driven programs).

III. APPROACH TO THE HEALTHY PATIENT

A. The preoperative evaluation form is the basis for formulating the best anesthetic plan tailored to the patient. It should aid the anesthesiologist in identifying potential complications, as well as serve as a medicolegal document (information obtained needs to be complete, concise, and legible).

B. The approach to the patient should always begin with a thorough history and physical examination (may be sufficient without additional routine laboratory tests).

1. The indication for the surgical procedure may also have implications on other aspects of perioperative management.

   a. Small bowel obstruction has implications regarding the risk of aspiration and the need for a rapid sequence induction.

   b. The extent of a lung resection will dictate the need for further pulmonary testing and perioperative monitoring.

   c. Patients undergoing carotid endarterectomy may require a more extensive neurologic examination, as well as testing to rule out coronary artery disease.

2. The ability to review previous anesthetic records is helpful in detecting the presence of a difficult airway, a history of malignant hyperthermia, and the individual's response to surgical stress and specific anesthetics.

3. The patient should be questioned regarding any previous difficulty with anesthesia or other family members having difficulty with anesthesia (history relating an "allergy" to anesthesia should make one suspicious for malignant hyperthermia).

4. The history should include a complete list of medications, including over-the-counter and herbal products, in order to define a preoperative medication regimen, anticipate potential drug interactions, and provide clues to underlying disease.

C. Systems Approach

1. Airway

   a. Evaluation of the airway involves determination of the thyromental distance, the ability to flex the base of the neck and extend the head, and

TABLE 18-1

AIRWAY CLASSIFICATION SYSTEM

Class	Direct visualization	Laryngoscopic view (patient seated)
I	Soft palate, fauces, uvula, pillars	Entire glottic opening
II	Soft palate, fauces, uvula	Posterior commissure
III	Soft palate, uvular base	Tip of epiglottis
IV	Hard palate only	No glottal structures

    examination of the oral cavity including dentition.

    b. The Mallampati classification has become the standard for assessing the relationship of the tongue size relative to the oral cavity although by itself the Mallampati classification has a low positive predictive value in identifying patients who are difficult to intubate (Table 18-1).

    c. In appropriate patients, the presence of pain or symptoms of cervical cord compression on movement should be assessed. In other instances, radiographic examination may be required.

  2. **Pulmonary** (Table 18-2)

  3. **Cardiovascular System** (Table 18-3)

  4. **Neurologic System.** The patient's ability to answer health history questions practically ensures a normal mental status (exclude the presence of increased intracranial pressure, cerebrovascular disease, seizure history, preexisting neuromuscular disease, or nerve injuries).

  5. **Endocrine System.** Each patient should be screened for endocrine diseases (diabetes mellitus, adrenal cortical suppression) that may affect the perioperative course

IV. EVALUATION OF THE PATIENT WITH KNOWN SYSTEMIC DISEASE

  A. **Cardiac Disease**

    1. The goals are to define risk, determine which patients will benefit from further testing, form an appropriate anesthetic plan, and identify patients

TABLE 18-2

SCREENING EVALUATION FOR THE PULMONARY SYSTEM

History
Tobacco use
Shortness of breath
Cough
Wheezing
Stridor
Snoring or sleep apnea
Recent history of an upper respiratory tract infection

Physical Examination
Respiratory rate
Chest excursion
Use of accessory muscles
Nail color
Ability to walk or carry on conversation without dyspnea
Auscultation to detect decreased breath sounds, wheezing, stridor, rales

who will benefit from perioperative beta-blockade, intervention therapy, or even surgery (Table 18-4).

2. Independent predictors of complications in the Goldman risk index include high-risk type of surgery, history of ischemic heart disease, history of congestive heart failure, history of cerebrovascular disease, preoperative treatment with insulin, and preoperative serum creatinine >2.0 mg/dL.

TABLE 18-3

SCREENING EVALUATION FOR THE CARDIOVASCULAR SYSTEM

Uncontrolled hypertension
Unstable cardiac disease
  Myocardial ischemia (unstable angina)
  Congestive heart failure
  Valvular heart disease (aortic stenosis, mitral valve prolapse)
  Cardiac dysrhythmias
Auscultation of the heart (murmur radiating to the carotids)
Bruits over the carotid arteries
Peripheral pulses

TABLE 18-4

AMERICAN SOCIETY OF ANESTHESIOLOGISTS (ASA)
PHYSICAL STATUS CLASSIFICATION

Status	Disease state
ASA Class 1	No organic, physiologic, biochemical, or psychiatric disturbance
ASA Class 2	Mild to moderate systemic disturbance that may not be related to the reason for surgery
ASA Class 3	Severe systemic disturbance that may or may not be related to the reason for surgery
ASA Class 4	Severe systemic disturbance that is life threatening with or without surgery
ASA Class 5	Moribund patient who has little chance of survival but is submitted to surgery as a last resort (resuscitative effort)
Emergency operation (E)	

3. The presence of unstable angina has been associated with a high perioperative risk of myocardial infarction (MI).
4. The presence of congestive heart failure preoperatively is associated with an increased incidence of perioperative cardiac morbidity.
5. The importance of the intervening time interval between an acute MI and elective surgery (traditionally 6 months or longer) may no longer be valid in the current era of interventional therapy (Table 18-5).

B. Patients with Coronary Artery Disease (CAD)
  1. For those patients without overt symptoms or history, the probability of CAD varies with the type and number of atherosclerotic risk factors present (peripheral arterial disease diabetes mellitus [autonomic neuropathy, the best predictor of silent CAD], hypertension [left ventricular hypertrophy], atherosclerosis associated with tobacco use, hypercholesterolemia).
    a. Although there has been a suggestion in the literature that a case should be delayed if the diastolic pressure is greater than 110 mm Hg, the

TABLE 18-5

CLINICAL PREDICTORS OF INCREASED PERIOPERATIVE
CARDIOVASCULAR RISK (MYOCARDIAL INFARCTION,
CONGESTIVE HEART FAILURE)

Major
Unstable coronary syndromes
  Recent myocardial infarction
  Unstable or severe angina
  Decompensated congestive heart failure
Significant arrhythmias
  High-grade atrioventricular block
  Symptomatic ventricular arrhythmias
  Supraventricular arrhythmias with uncontrolled ventricular rate
Severe valvular disease

Intermediate
Mild angina pectoris
Prior myocardial infarction by history or pathological Q waves
Compensated or prior congestive heart failure
Diabetes mellitus

Minor
Advanced age
Abnormal ECG (left ventricular hypertrophy, left bundle-branch
  block, ST-T abnormalities)
Rhythm other than sinus (atrial fibrillation)
Low functional capacity (inability to climb one flight of stairs with
  a bag of groceries)
History of stroke
Uncontrolled systemic hypertension

    study often quoted as the basis for this
    determination demonstrated no major morbidity
    in that small group of patients.
  b. Other authors state that there is little association
    between blood pressures of less than 180 mm Hg
    systolic or 110 mm Hg diastolic and
    postoperative outcomes (such patients are
    prone to perioperative myocardial ischemia,
    ventricular dysrhythmias, and lability in blood
    pressure).
C. Importance of Surgical Procedure (Table 18-6)
  1. The surgical procedure influences the scope of
    preoperative evaluation required by determining the
    potential range of physiologic flux during the
    perioperative period.

TABLE 18-6
CARDIAC RISK STRATIFICATION FOR NONCARDIAC SURGICAL PROCEDURES

HIGH (reported cardiac risk often >5%)
Emergent major operations, particularly in the elderly
Aortic and other major vascular
Peripheral vascular
Anticipated prolonged surgical procedures associated with large fluid shifts and/or blood loss

INTERMEDIATE (reported cardiac risk generally <5%)
Carotid endarterectomy
Head and neck
Intraperitoneal and intrathoracic
Orthopedic
Prostate

LOW (reported cardiac risk generally <1%)
Endoscopic procedures
Superficial procedures
Cataract
Breast

- a. Peripheral procedures performed as ambulatory surgery are associated with an extremely low incidence of morbidity and mortality.
- b. High-risk procedures include major vascular, abdominal, thoracic, and orthopedic surgery.
- D. Importance of Exercise Tolerance
  1. Exercise tolerance is one of the most important determinants of perioperative risk and the need for further testing and invasive monitoring.
  2. An excellent exercise tolerance, even in patients with stable angina, suggests that the myocardium can be stressed without failing.
     - a. If a patient can walk a mile without becoming short of breath, the probability of extensive coronary artery disease is small.
     - b. If patients experience dyspnea associated with chest pain during minimal exertion, the probability of extensive coronary artery disease is high (associated with greater perioperative risk).
  2. There is good evidence to suggest that minimal additional testing is necessary if the patient is able to describe a good exercise tolerance.

V. INDICATIONS FOR FURTHER CARDIAC TESTING (Fig. 18-1).

No preoperative cardiovascular testing should be performed if the results will not change perioperative management.

A. Cardiovascular Tests

1. **Electrocardiogram**
   a. Abnormal Q waves in high-risk patients are highly suggestive of a past MI (estimated that approximately 30% of MIs occur without symptoms and can only be detected on routine electrocardiograms).
   b. The presence of Q waves on a preoperative electrocardiogram in a high-risk patient, regardless of symptoms, should alert the anesthesiologist to the increased perioperative risk and the possibility of active ischemia.
   c. Current recommendations include the need for a preoperative electrocardiogram in the presence of systemic vascular disease (those patients with hypertension or peripheral vascular disease), for males over 40 years of age and for females over 50.

2. **Noninvasive Cardiovascular Testing**
   a. The exercise electrocardiogram represents the most cost-effective and least invasive method for detecting ischemia.
   b. Pharmacologic stress thallium imaging is useful in those patients who are unable to exercise.
   c. Dopamine can be used to increase myocardial oxygen demand, by increasing heart rate and blood pressure, in those patients who cannot exercise.
   d. The ambulatory electrocardiogram (Holter monitoring) provides a means of continuously monitoring the electrocardiogram for significant ST segment changes preoperatively.
   e. Stress echocardiography may be of value in evaluating patients with suspected CAD.
   f. Dobutamine echocardiography has been found to have one of the best predictive values.

3. **Assessment of Ventricular and Valvular Function**
   a. Both echocardiography and radionuclide angiography can assess cardiac ejection fraction

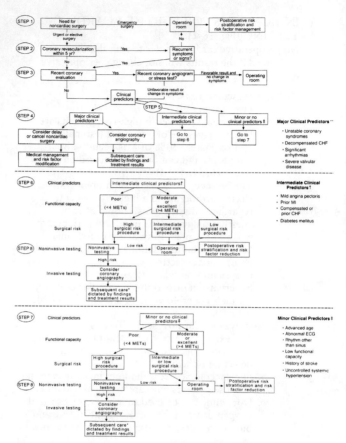

FIGURE 18-1. The American Heart Association/American College of Cardiology Task Force on Perioperative Evaluation of Cardiac Patients Undergoing Noncardiac Surgery has proposed an algorithm for decisions regarding the need for further evaluation. (Adapted with permission from Eagle K, Brundage B, Chaitman B *et al:* Guidelines for perioperative cardiovascular evaluation of noncardiac surgery. A report of the American Heart Association/American College of Cardiology Task Force on Assessment of Diagnostic and Therapeutic Cardiovascular Procedures. Circulation 93:1278, 1996.)

at rest and under stress, but echocardiography is less invasive and is also able to assess regional wall motion abnormalities, wall thickness, valvular function, and valve area.

b. Aortic stenosis has been associated with a poor prognosis in noncardiac surgical patients, and knowledge of valvular lesions may modify perioperative hemodynamic therapy.

4. **Coronary angiography** is the best method for defining coronary anatomy (narrowing of the left main coronary artery may be associated with a greater perioperative risk).

B. **Perioperative Coronary Interventions**

1. In some patients scheduled for high-risk surgery, long-term survival may be enhanced by revascularization (translumimal coronary angioplasty, coronary stent placement).

VI. APPROACH TO THE PATIENT WITH PULMONARY DISEASE

A. The site and type of surgery (thoracic and upper abdominal surgery) are the strongest predictors of pulmonary complications.

1. Diaphragmatic dysfunction occurs despite adequate analgesia and is theorized to reflect phrenic nerve inhibition.

2. Duration of anesthesia is a well-established risk factor for postoperative pulmonary complications, with morbidity rates increasing after 2 to 3 hours.

B. **Patient-Related Factors**

1. Preoperative evaluation of patients with preexisting pulmonary disease should include assessment of the type and severity of disease, as well as its reversibility.

2. Inquiries are made with respect to exercise intolerance, chronic cough, or unexplained dyspnea.

3. On physical examination, findings of wheezing, rhonchi, decreased breath sounds, dullness to percussion, and a prolonged expiratory phase are important.

4. **Tobacco** is an important risk factor, but one that usually cannot be influenced.

a. Cessation of smoking for 2 days can decrease carboxyhemoglobin levels, abolish the nicotine effects, and improve mucous clearance but smoking cessation for at least 8 weeks is necessary to reduce the rate of postoperative pulmonary complications.

5. **Asthma**

   a. Frequent use of bronchodilators, hospitalizations for asthma, and the requirement for systemic steroids are all indicators of the severity of the disease.

   b. After an episode of asthma, airway hyperreactivity may persist for several weeks.

   c. The possibility of adrenal insufficiency is also a concern in those patients who have received more than a "burst and taper" of steroids in the previous 6 months.

VII. ENDOCRINE DISEASE

A. Diabetics have an increased risk of CAD, perioperative MI, hypertension, and congestive heart failure.

   1. Administration of perioperative beta-blockers should be considered in diabetic patients with CAD to help limit perioperative myocardial ischemia.

   2. Significant renal disease develops commonly in diabetics, many times necessitating chronic dialysis.

   3. Peripheral and autonomic nervous system neuropathies are common in diabetics.

B. There is consensus that for patients taking corticosteroids for long periods that perioperative steroid supplementation is indicated to cover the stresses of anesthesia and surgery.

VIII. OTHER ORGAN SYSTEMS

A. Renal disease has important implications for fluid and electrolyte management, as well as metabolism of drugs.

B. Liver disease is associated with altered protein binding and volume of distribution of drugs, as well as coagulation abnormalities (may influence the choice of regional anesthesia).

C. Musculoskeletal disorders have been associated with an increased risk of malignant hyperthermia.
D. Osteoarthritis may result in difficulty exposing the glottic opening for tracheal intubation or difficulty in positioning for a regional anesthetic.

IX. PERIOPERATIVE LABORATORY TESTING

A. **The Value of Preoperative Testing: Normal Values**
   1. The vast majority of tests only increase or decrease the probability of disease.
   2. To determine the clinical relevance, a test must be interpreted within the context of the clinical situation (high incidence of false-positives when performing tests in normal patients).
B. **The Value of Preoperative Testing: Bayesian Analysis.** If a test is used in a population with a very low prevalence of disease, a positive result is frequently a false-positive.
C. **Risks and Costs Versus Benefits** (Table 18-6)
   1. The use of medical testing is associated with significant cost, both in real dollars and in potential harm.
   2. Even if testing better defines a disease state, the risks of any intervention based on the results may outweigh the benefit.
D. **Recommended Laboratory Testing** (Table 18-7)
   1. **Complete Blood Count and Hemoglobin Concentration**
      a. The current recommendations of the National Blood Resource Education Committee is that a hemoglobin of 7 g/dL is acceptable in patients without systemic disease.
      b. In patients with systemic disease, signs of inadequate systemic oxygen delivery (tachycardia, tachypnea) are an indication for transfusion.
   2. **Electrolytes**
      a. The only consensus is the lack of need for routine testing in asymptomatic adults, although a creatinine and glucose has been recommended in older patients.
      b. In patients with systemic diseases or on medications that affect the kidneys, a BUN and creatinine are indicated.

TABLE 18-7
RECOMMENDED LABORATORY TESTING

Blood Count
Neonates
Physiologic age ≥75 yr
Class C procedure
Malignancy
Renal disease
Tobacco use
Anticoagulant use

Electrolytes
Renal disease
Diabetes
Diuretic, digoxin, or steroid use
CNS disease

Blood Glucose
Physiologic age ≥75 yr
Class C procedure
Diabetes
Steroid use
CNS disease

ECG
Physiologic age ≥75 yr
Class C procedure
Cardiovascular disease
Pulmonary disease
Radiation Therapy
Diabetes
Digoxin use
CNS disease

Coagulation Studies
Chemotherapy
Hepatic disease
Bleeding disorder
Anticoagulants

BUN/Creatinine
Physiologic age ≥75 yr
Class C procedure
Cardiovascular disease
Renal disease
Diabetes
Direct or digoxin use
CNS disease

Liver Function Tests
Hepatic disease
Hepatitis exposure
Malnutrition

Chest X-ray
Physiologic age ≥75 yr
Cardiovascular disease
Pulmonary disease
Malignancy
Radiation Therapy
Tobacco ≥20 pack years

Pregnancy Test
Possible pregnancy

Albumin
Malnutrition
Physiologic age ≥75 yr
Class C procedure

3. **Coagulation Studies**
   a. Abnormal laboratory studies in the absence of clinical abnormalities will rarely lead to perioperative problems.
   b. A prothrombin and partial thromboplastin time analysis is indicated in the presence of previous bleeding disorders (following injuries, after tooth extraction or surgical procedures, and in patients with known or suspected liver disease, malabsorption or malnutrition, and on certain

medications such as antibiotics and chemotherapeutic agents).

4. **Pregnancy Testing.** Current practice varies dramatically among centers and anesthesiologists, and may be a function of the population served with regard to the need to routinely test those women with a negative pregnancy history.

5. **Chest X-Rays**
   a. A preoperative chest x-ray can identify abnormalities that may lead to either delay or cancellation of the planned surgical procedure or modification of perioperative care.
   b. Routine testing in the population without risk factors can lead to more harm than benefit.
   c. A preoperative chest x-ray is indicated in patients with a history or clinical evidence of active pulmonary disease, and *may* be indicated routinely only in patients with advanced age.

6. **Pulmonary function tests** can be divided into spirometry and an arterial blood gas.
   a. With the advent of the pulse oximeter, the use of preoperative arterial blood gas sampling has become less important.
   b. A normal serum bicarbonate will virtually exclude the diagnosis of CO_2 retention.

X. PREOPERATIVE MEDICATION consists of
psychological preparation and pharmacologic preparation of patients before surgery. Ideally, all patients should enter the preoperative period free from apprehension, sedated but easily arousable, and fully cooperative.

A. **Psychological preparation** is provided by the preoperative visit and interview with patients and family members serving as a nonpharmacologic antidote to apprehension (Table 18-8).

B. **Pharmacologic Preparation**
   1. Drugs selected for preoperative medication are administered orally with up to 150 mL of water 1 to 2 hours before the anticipated induction of anesthesia. Drugs may be administered intramuscularly if the oral route of administration is judged to be not effective or possible. Alternatively,

---
TABLE 18-8

AREAS TO BE DISCUSSED DURING A PREOPERATIVE INTERVIEW

Review medical history with patient
  Coexisting diseases
  Chronic drug therapy
  Prior anesthetic experience
Describe anesthetic techniques available and associated risks
Review planned preoperative medication and time of scheduled surgery
Describe what to expect on arrival in the operating room
Describe anticipated duration of surgery and expected time to return to room
Describe methods available to manage postoperative pain
  Patient-controlled analgesia
  Neuraxial opioids

---

   drugs may be administered intravenously in the immediate preoperative period.
2. **Various Goals for Pharmacologic Premedication** (Table 18-9)
3. **Determinant of Drug Choice and Dose** (Table 18-10)
4. Several classes of drugs are available to facilitate achievement of the desired individual goals for pharmacologic premedication (Table 18-11).
5. There is no best drug or drug combination for preoperative medication.

TABLE 18-9

GOALS FOR PREOPERATIVE MEDICATION

Relief of anxiety
Sedation
Amnesia
Analgesia
Drying of airway secretions
Prevention of autonomic reflex responses
Reduction of gastric fluid volume and increased pH
Antiemetic effects
Reduction of anesthetic requirements
Facilitation of smooth induction of anesthesia
Prophylaxis against allergic reactions

TABLE 18-10
DETERMINANT OF DRUG CHOICE AND DOSE

Patient age and weight
ASA physical status classification
Level of anxiety
Tolerance for depressant drugs
Prior adverse experiences with premedication
Drug allergies
Elective versus emergency surgery
Inpatient versus outpatient

    a. The choice may be influenced by tradition and the anesthesiologist's previous experience.
    b. Timing of drug delivery is as important as drug selection.
  6. Ideally, the specific drugs selected are based on the goals of premedication balanced against potential

TABLE 18-11
DRUGS USED FOR PHARMACOLOGIC PREMEDICATION

Drug	Route of administration	Adult dose (mg)
Diazepam	oral	5–20
Lorazepam	oral, im	1–4
Midazolam	oral (children)	0.5 mg/kg
	im	3–5
	iv	1–2.5
Morphine	im	5–15
Meperidine	im	50–150
Fentanyl	iv	0.05–0.150
	transmucosal	5–20 μg/kg
Promethazine	im	25–50
Diphenhydramine	oral, im	25–75
Cimetidine	oral, im, iv	150–300
Ranitidine	oral	50–200
Famotidine	oral	20–40
Metoclopramide	oral, im, iv	5–20
Atropine or scopolamine	im, iv	0.3–0.6
Glycopyrrolate	im, iv	0.1–0.3
Antacids	oral	10–30 mL

undesirable effects these drugs may produce. It is important to recognize that some patients may not need (elderly) or should not receive (decreased level of consciousness, intracranial hypertension, severe pulmonary disease, profound hypovolemia) depressant drugs for preoperative medication.

7. **Benzodiazepines** act on specific brain receptors (gamma-aminobutyric acid) to produce selective anti-anxiety effects at doses that do not produce excessive sedation, depression of ventilation, or adverse cardiac effects.

   a. **Diazepam** produces a peak effect 30 to 60 minutes after oral administration. Because diazepam is insoluble in water and must be dissolved in organic solvents, pain may occur with intramuscular or intravenous injection.

   b. **Lorazepam** produces intense amnesia, but sedation and prolonged duration of action detract from its use for short surgical procedures or in outpatients. Peak effects after oral administration may not occur for 2 to 4 hours.

   c. **Midazolam** has replaced diazepam in its use for preoperative medication and conscious sedation. An oral form of midazolam is particularly useful for preoperative medication in children. The incidence of side effects after administration of midazolam is low, although depression of ventilation and sedation may be greater than expected especially in elderly patients or when the drug is combined with other central nervous system depressants. The onset after intravenous administration of midazolam is in 1 to 2 minutes and recovery occurs rapidly, reflecting this drug's poor lipid solubility and rapid distribution to peripheral receptors compared with diazepam. Furthermore, the metabolites of midazolam are not likely to be pharmacologically active. For all these reasons, midazolam usually should be administered within 1 hour of induction of anesthesia.

8. **Opioids** are used for preoperative medication when there is a need to provide analgesia, as before institution of a regional anesthetic or when patients have pain owing to their surgical disease. Anesthesiologists often use a combination of an

TABLE 18-12

SIDE EFFECTS OF OPIOIDS AS USED FOR PHARMACOLOGIC PREMEDICATION

Depression of ventilation
Nausea and vomiting
Synergistic effects especially when administered with
    benzodiazepines
Orthostatic hypotension
Delayed gastric emptying
Pruritus
Choledochoduodenal sphincter spasm

opioid, benzodiazepine, and scopolamine for preoperative medication of patients who are likely to be unusually apprehensive, as before cardiac surgery or cancer surgery. Administration of opioids has the potential to produce multiple side effects, which may be exaggerated when other depressant drugs are also included in the preoperative medication (Table 18-12).

a. **Morphine** produces peak effects within 45 to 90 minutes after intramuscular injection. Inclusion of morphine in the preoperative medication decreases the likelihood that undesirable increases in heart rate will accompany surgical stimulation.

b. **Meperidine** is often administered in combination with promethazine. Peak effects after intramuscular injection of meperidine may be unpredictable.

c. **Fentanyl** (75 to 125 times more potent than morphine as an analgesic) may be administered intravenously to provide a rapid onset of preoperative analgesia. Oral transmucosal fentanyl may be an option to relieve anxiety and provide pain relief in children (high incidence of nausea and vomiting) and adults.

C. **Gastric Fluid pH and Volume**

1. Despite the predictable presence of acidic fluid in the stomach at the time of induction of anesthesia, clinically significant pulmonary aspiration of gastric fluid is rare in healthy patients undergoing elective surgery. The American Society of Anesthesiologists

TABLE 18-13

SUMMARY OF FASTING RECOMMENDATIONS TO REDUCE
THE RISK OF PULMONARY ASPIRATION[a]

Ingested material	Minimum fasting period (applied to all ages)
Clear liquids (water, fruit juice without pulp, carbonated beverages, clear tea, black coffee)	2 hr
Breast milk	4 hr
Infant formula	6 hr
Nonhuman milk	6 hr
Light meal (toast and clear liquids)	6 hr

[a]Applies only to healthy patients who are undergoing elective procedures and are not intended for women in labor. Following these guidelines does not guarantee complete gastric emptying.

has adopted guidelines for preoperative fasting (Table 18-13).

  a. Maintenance of a patent airway is more important than routine pharmacologic prophylaxis in otherwise healthy patients undergoing elective surgery.

  b. Ingestion of clear fluids in the 2 hours preceding the induction of anesthesia does not increase gastric fluid volume. Patients who are permitted to ingest clear fluids preoperatively are more comfortable than those who have been fasted. Under no circumstances are solid foods permitted in the period preceding induction of anesthesia for elective surgery.

  2. **Drugs Used to Decrease Gastric Fluid Volume and Increase Gastric Fluid pH** (Table 18-14)

D. **Antiemetics** may be administered in the preoperative or intraoperative period as prophylaxis against postoperative nausea and vomiting, especially in patients considered to be at increased risk for this complication (prior history of vomiting, obese, ophthalmologic or gynecologic surgery) (Table 18-15).

E. **Anticholinergics**

  1. Routine inclusion of anticholinergics as part of the pharmacologic premedication is not mandatory but rather should be individualized based on a patient's

TABLE 18-14

DRUGS USED TO DECREASE GASTRIC FLUID VOLUME AND INCREASE GASTRIC FLUID pH

Anticholinergics (do not reliably increase gastric fluid pH at clinical doses and may relax the lower esophageal sphincter, making gastroesophageal reflux more likely)

H2-receptor antagonists (not 100% effective in increasing gastric fluid pH)

Cimetidine (inhibits mixed-function oxidase enzyme systems and decreases hepatic blood flow, which may prolong the elimination half-life of some drugs)

Ranitidine (more potent and longer lasting than cimetidine)

Famotidine (longest duration of action of all H2-receptor antagonists)

Antacids (nonparticulate antacids recommended to decrease the risk of pulmonary reaction if antacid inhaled; in contrast to H2-receptor antagonists, there is no lag time before gastric fluid pH is increased)

Omeprazole (increases gastric fluid pH by blocking secretion of hydrogen ions by parietal cells)

Gastrokinetic agents

Metoclopramide (onset in 30–60 minutes after oral administration and 3–5 minutes after intravenous administration; gastric emptying effects may be offset by opioids, anticholinergics, or antacids)

needs and the pharmacology of the anticholinergic (Table 18-16).
2. **Indications for Anticholinergics** (Table 18-17)
3. **Side Effects of Anticholinergic Drugs** (Table 18-18)
F. **Alpha-2 Adrenergic Agonists**

TABLE 18-15

ANTIEMETICS USED TO PREVENT OR TREAT POSTOPERATIVE NAUSEA AND VOMITING

Droperidol (sedation and dysphoria may be side effects; inexpensive, use limited by rare risk of prolongation of the QTc interval)

Metoclopramide (?)

Transdermal scopolamine patch (apply several hours before induction of anesthesia)

Ondansetron or granisetron

TABLE 18-16

COMPARATIVE EFFECTS OF ANTICHOLINERGICS[a]

	Atropine	Scopolamine	Glycopyrrolate
Antisialagogue effect	+	+ + +	+ +
Sedative and amnesic effects	+	+ + +	0
Central nervous system toxicity	+	+ +	0
Relaxation of gastroesophageal sphincter	+ +	+ +	+ +
Mydriasis and cycloplegia	+	+ +	0
Increased heart rate	+ + +	+	+ +

[a]Intravenous administration.
0 = none; + = mild; + + = moderate; + + + = marked.

TABLE 18-17

INDICATIONS FOR ANTICHOLINERGICS

Antisialagogue effect (not necessary when regional anesthesia planned)
Sedation and amnesia (decrease doses in elderly patients; scopolamine most effective)
Vagolytic action (intramuscular administration not as effective as intravenous injection just before the anticipated vagal stimulus)

TABLE 18-18

SIDE EFFECTS OF ANTICHOLINERGIC DRUGS

Central nervous system toxicity (restlessness and confusion especially in elderly patients; unlikely with glycopyrrolate because it crosses the brain barrier minimally)
Relaxation of the lower esophageal sphincter (may not be clinically significant)
Mydriasis and cycloplegia (continue miotic eye drops in patients with glaucoma)
Increased physiologic dead space
Drying of airway secretions
Interference with sweating (an important consideration in febrile patients, especially children)
Increased heart rate (unlikely after intramuscular administration)

TABLE 18-19

OTHER DRUGS GIVEN WITH PREOPERATIVE MEDICATION

Beta-blockers (patients with known or suspected coronary artery disease may be protected)

Antibiotics (may potentiate neuromuscular blocking drugs)

Steroids (history of hypoadrenocorticism or treatment of nonadrenal diseases)

Insulin

1. Clonidine (5 mg/kg orally as preoperative medication) produces sedation, decreases anesthetic requirements for inhaled and injected drugs, and attenuates the sympathetic nervous system response (hypertension, tachycardia, catecholamine release) to tracheal intubation.
2. Dexmedetomidine is a more selective α-adrenergic agonist than clonidine that has also been used for preoperative medication.
3. Side effects (hypotension, bradycardia, dry mouth) limit the usefulness of these drugs for preoperative medication.

G. **Other Drugs Given with Preoperative Medication** (Table 18-19)

H. **Differences in Preoperative Medication Between Pediatric and Adult Patients**

1. Children differ from adults with regard to preoperative medication in terms of (1) psychological preparation, (2) greater use of oral medications, and (3) more frequent use of anticholinergics to reduce vagal activity.
2. **Psychological Factors in Pediatric Patients**
   a. Age is probably the most important factor in the success of a preoperative visit and interview.
   b. Children who do not ask questions or appear disinterested during the preoperative interview may be masking a high level of anxiety.
   c. Some children wish to take an active part in the induction of anesthesia. In this regard, it may be helpful to have the parents accompany these children to the operating room.
2. **Differences in Pharmacologic Preparation**
   a. Use of pharmacologic premedication in children after 6 months of age is controversial and has not

294 Preparing for Anesthesia

been proven to decrease unwanted psychological outcomes. More important in avoiding long-lasting psychological problems is a pleasant induction of anesthesia.

b. Oral administration (often midazolam in a flavored liquid) is preferred to intramuscular injections in children.

c. Easily induced vagal reflexes in response to airway manipulation is the reason that some anesthesiologists prefer to administer atropine intramuscularly or intravenously just before the induction of anesthesia.

CHAPTER 19 ■ ANESTHESIA FOR PATIENTS WITH RARE AND COEXISTING DISEASES

Knowledge of the pathophysiology of coexisting diseases and an understanding of the implications of concomitant drug therapy are important for the management of anesthesia for an individual patient (Dierdorf SF, Walton JS: Anesthesia for patients with rare coexisting diseases. In Barash PG, Cullen BF, Stoelting RK [eds]: *Clinical Anesthesia*, pp 502–528. Philadelphia, Lippincott Williams & Wilkins, 2006). In many instances, the nature of the coexisting disease has more impact on the management of anesthesia than does the actual surgical procedure. A variety of rare disorders may influence the selection and conduct of anesthesia (Table 19-1).

I. MUSCULAR DYSTROPHY

A. The muscular dystrophies are characterized by a progressive but variable rate of loss of skeletal muscle function. Cardiac and smooth muscle function are also affected.

B. **Duchenne's Muscular Dystrophy**

1. This is the most severe form of muscular dystrophy and is produced by a genetic abnormality resulting in lack of production of muscle protein, dystrophin, an important component of the skeleton of the muscle membrane.

2. The genetic defect is sex linked (manifests only in males), symptoms manifest between 2 and 5 years of age (creatine kinase may be increased before symptoms appear). Death is usually secondary to congestive heart failure or pneumonia.

   a. Axial skeletal muscle imbalance produces **kyphoscoliosis**, which often requires surgical correction.

   b. Involvement of cardiac muscle is reflected by a progressive loss of the R-wave amplitude on the lateral precordial leads of the electrocardiogram. Routine echocardiography can provide important information about cardiac function. Progressive

TABLE 19-1

COEXISTING DISEASES THAT INFLUENCE ANESTHESIA MANAGEMENT

Musculoskeletal
Muscular dystrophy
Myotonic dystrophy
Myasthenia gravis
Myasthenic syndrome
Familial periodic paralysis
Guillain-Barré syndrome

Central Nervous System
Multiple sclerosis
Epilepsy
Parkinson's disease
Alzheimer's disease
Amyotrophic lateral sclerosis
Creutzfeldt-Jakob disease

Anemias
Nutritional deficiency
Hemolytic
Hemoglobinopathies
Thalassemias

Collagen Vascular
Rheumatoid arthritis
Systemic lupus erythematosus
Scleroderma
Polymyositis

Skin
Epidermolysis bullosa
Pemphigus

loss of myocardial tissue results in cardiomyopathy, ventricular dysrhythmias, and mitral regurgitation.
  c. Degeneration of respiratory muscles (reflected by spirometry) results in an ineffective cough with retention of secretions and pneumonia.
  d. Smooth muscle involvement causes intestinal tract hypomotility, delayed gastric emptying, and gastroparesis.
3. **Management of Anesthesia**
  a. Reports of cardiac arrest suggest that these patients are more sensitive to the cardiac depressant effects of anesthetic drugs.

      b. Succinylcholine should not be administered to these patients in view of reports of hyperkalemia in young male patients with unrecognized muscular dystrophy.

      c. Sevoflurane is a less potent stimulus for release of calcium from the sarcoplasmic reticulum and may be the preferred volatile anesthetic for patients with Duchenne's muscular dystrophy.

      d. Susceptibility to malignant hyperthermia is unpredictable.

      e. Nondepolarizing neuromuscular blocking drugs may be administered although the response may be variable and prolonged (response to mivacurium is normal).

      f. Degeneration of gastrointestinal smooth muscle with hypomotility of the intestinal tract and delayed gastric emptying in conjunction with impaired swallowing mechanisms may increase the risk of perioperative aspiration.

II. THE MYOTONIAS

A. Delayed relaxation of skeletal muscle after voluntary contraction is the common feature of all myotonias. Myotonia is caused by abnormal ion channel activity, and drugs that depress sodium influx into the cell and delay return of membrane excitability (quinine) may relax myotonic contracture.

B. **Myotonic Dystrophy (Steinert's Disease)**

    1. This is an autosomally dominant inherited disorder characterized by delayed relaxation of skeletal muscles after voluntary contraction.

      a. Cardiac dysrhythmias and atrioventricular heart block reflect degeneration of cardiac conduction muscle before that of contractile muscle. Other cardiac abnormalities associated with myotonic dystrophy include mitral valve proplase, left ventricular diastolic dysfunction, and cardiac failure.

      b. Weakness of respiratory muscles diminishes the effectiveness of cough and may lead to pneumonia.

    2. **Management of anesthesia**

      a. Succinylcholine produces myotonia and should not be administered to these patients. The response of these patients to nondepolarizing muscle relaxants

TABLE 19-2
CLINICAL FEATURES OF FAMILIAL PERIODIC PARALYSIS

Hypokalemic
Calcium channel defect
Potassium level <3 mEq/L during symptoms
Precipitating factors
   Large glucose meals
   Strenuous exercise
   Glucose-insulin infusions
   Stress
   Hypothermia
Other features
   Chronic myopathy with aging

Hyperkalemic
Sodium channel defect
Potassium level normal or >5.5 mEq/L during symptoms
Precipitating factors
   Rest after exercise
   Potassium infusions
   Metabolic acidosis
   Hypothermia
Other features
   Skeletal muscle weakness may be localized to tongue and eyelids

seems normal. An anticholinesterase may precipitate myotonia, thus supporting the issue of short- and intermediate-acting muscle relaxants.

  b. Patients with myotonia are very sensitive to the ventilatory depressant effects of opioids, barbiturates, benzodiazepines, and volatile anesthetics.

  c. Skeletal muscle weakness and myotonia are exacerbated in pregnancy.

C. **Familial Periodic Paralysis** (Table 19-2)

  1. These diseases have been reclassified as skeletal muscle channelopathies. Intermittent but acute episodes of skeletal muscle weakness or paralysis occur in the presence of hypokalemia or hyperkalemia.

  2. **Management of Anesthesia**

    a. The primary goal of the perioperative management of patients with both forms of periodic paralysis is the maintenance of normal potassium levels and avoidance of events that precipitate muscle weakness (alkalosis owing to hyperventilation, carbohydrate loads, hypothermia).

    b. Short-acting muscle relaxants are preferred and the response should be monitored with a peripheral nerve stimulator. Succinylcholine is avoided because it may enhance potassium release from skeletal muscle cells.

    c. The electrocardiogram should be monitored for evidence of hypokalemia and associated cardiac dysrhythmias (measure serum potassium concentration during prolonged operations).

    d. After surgery adequate skeletal muscle strength must be confirmed before mechanical ventilation of the lungs is discontinued.

D. **Myasthenia gravis** is an autoimmune disease with antibodies directed against the nicotinic acetylcholine receptor or other muscle membrane proteins (Table 19-3). The majority of patients have abnormalities of the thymus (thymoma, thymic hyperplasia, thymic atrophy).

  1. The clinical hallmark of myasthenia gravis is skeletal muscle weakness (increased by repetitive muscle use) with periods of exacerbation and remission.

    a. Neonatal myasthenia begins 12 to 48 hours after birth and reflects transplacental passage of antiacetylcholine antibodies.

    b. Focal myocarditis and atrioventricular heart block may be present.

  2. **Treatment** includes administration of anticholinesterase drugs, thymectomy, corticosteroids, and immunosuppressants. Underdosage with anticholinesterase drugs results in skeletal muscle weakness, whereas overdosage leads to a "cholinergic crisis."

  3. **Management of Anesthesia**

    a. The primary concern is the potential interaction between the disease, treatment of the disease, and neuromuscular blocking drugs. The uncontrolled or poorly controlled myasthenic patient is exquisitely sensitive to even small (defasiculating) doses of nondepolarizing muscle relaxants.

    b. The variability in response to different muscle relaxants warrants careful monitoring with a peripheral nerve stimulator and its correlation with clinical signs of recovery from neuromuscular blockade. Short- or intermediate-acting nondepolarizing muscle relaxants are usually recommended.

TABLE 19-3
SUMMARY OF THE DIFFERENT PRESENTATIONS OF MYASTHENIA GRAVIS

	Etiology	Onset (y)	Gender	Thymus	Course
Neonatal myasthenia	Passage of antibodies from myasthenic mother across the placenta	Neonatal	Both sexes	Normal	Transient
Congenital myasthenia	Congenital end-plate pathology, genetic, autosomal recessive pattern of inheritance	0–2	Male > female	Normal	Nonfluctuating, compatible with long survival
Juvenile myasthenia	Autoimmune disorder	2–20	Female > male (4:1)	Hyperplasia	Slowly progressive, tendency to relapse and remission
Adult myasthenia	Autoimmune disorder	20–40	Female > male	Hyperplasia > thymoma	Maximum severity within 3–5 y
Elderly myasthenia	Autoimmune disorder	>40	Male > female	Thymoma (benign or locally invasive)	Rapid progress, higher mortality

TABLE 19-4

FEATURES OF MYASTHENIA GRAVIS ASSOCIATED WITH THE NEED TO PROVIDE POSTOPERATIVE MECHANICAL VENTILATION OF THE LUNGS

Duration of myasthenia gravis >6 years
History of chronic obstructive pulmonary disease
Treatment with daily pyridostigmine doses >750 mg
Preoperative vital capacity <2.9 L

c. Risk factors have been identified that increase the likelihood of the need for postoperative mechanical support of ventilation (Table 19-4).

E. **Myasthenic Syndrome (Lambert-Eaton Syndrome)**
   1. The myasthenic syndrome is a disorder of neuromuscular transmission associated with carcinomas, particularly small-cell carcinoma of the lung (suspected in patients undergoing diagnostic procedures, such as diagnostic bronchoscopy, mediastinoscopy, or exploratory thoracotomy for possible cancer) (Table 19-5).
   2. Administration of aminopyridines (potassium channel blockers, which increase the release of acetylcholine) is the most effective pharmacologic treatment.
   3. These patients are sensitive to the effects of both depolarizing and nondepolarizing muscle relaxants.

F. **Guillain-Barré syndrome** is an autoimmune disease triggered by bacterial or viral infection.
   1. This syndrome is characterized by the acute or subacute onset of skeletal muscle weakness or paralysis of the legs, which spreads cephalad and may result in difficulty swallowing and impaired ventilation from paralysis of intercostal muscles.
      a. The most serious immediate problem is hypoventilation (measure vital capacity frequently and if decreases to <15 to 20 mL/kg, mechanical ventilation of the lungs is indicated).
      b. **Autonomic nervous system** dysfunction may be associated with wide fluctuations in blood pressure (physical stimulation may precipitate hypertension), tachycardia, cardiac dysrhythmias, and cardiac arrest.
   2. **Management of Anesthesia**
      a. Compensatory cardiovascular responses may be absent (autonomic nervous system dysfunction),

TABLE 19-5
COMPARISON OF MYASTHENIA GRAVIS AND MYASTHENIC SYNDROME

	Myasthenia gravis	Myasthenic syndrome
Manifestations	Extraocular, bulbar, and facial muscle weakness	Proximal limb weakness (legs > arms)
	Fatigue with exercise	Exercise improves strength
	Muscle pain uncommon	Muscle pain common
	Reflexes normal or decreased	Reflexes absent
Gender	Female > male	Male > female
Coexisting pathology	Thymoma	Cancer (especially small-cancer of the lung)
Response to muscle relaxants	Resistant to succinylcholine and sensitive to nondepolarizing muscle relaxants	Sensitive to succinylcholine and nondepolarizing muscle relaxants
	Poor response to anticholinesterases	Poor response to anticholinesterases

resulting in significant hypotension secondary to postural changes, blood loss, or positive airway pressure. Conversely, stimuli such as laryngoscopy and tracheal intubation may produce hypertension and tachycardia.

b. Succinylcholine is not recommended because drug-induced potassium release may result in hyperkalemia and cardiac arrest. The response to nondepolarizing muscle relaxants ranges from sensitivity to resistance.

III. CENTRAL NERVOUS SYSTEM DISEASES

A. Multiple Sclerosis

1. This disease is characterized by multiple sites of demyelination in the brain and spinal cord (visual disturbances, limb weakness, paresthesias).

2. It is difficult to determine the efficacy of treatment modalities because of the disease's natural history of exacerbations and remissions.
3. **Management of Anesthesia.** The effect of anesthesia and surgery on the course of multiple sclerosis is controversial.
    a. Regional and general anesthesia have been reported to exacerbate or have no effect on multiple sclerosis. Factors other than anesthesia such as infection, emotional stress, and hyperpyrexia may contribute to an increased risk of perioperative exacerbation.
    b. A neurological examination before anesthesia and surgery is helpful to document coexisting neurologic deficits.
    c. Patients being treated with corticosteroids may require perioperative supplementation, and immunosuppressants can produce cardiotoxicity and subclinical cardiac dysfunction.
    d. Autonomic nervous system dysfunction caused by multiple sclerosis may produce exaggerated hypotensive effects in response to volatile anesthetics.
    e. Respiratory muscle weakness and dysfunction may increase the likelihood of the need for postoperative mechanical ventilation.
B. **Epilepsy** (Table 19-6)
    1. A seizure results from the excessive discharge of large numbers of neurons that become depolarized in an asynchronous fashion.
        a. The sudden onset of seizures in a young to middle-aged adult arouses the suspicion of focal brain disease (tumor), whereas onset after 60 years of age is usually secondary to cerebrovascular disease.
        b. The onset of seizures requires a thorough neurologic evaluation to determine the etiology (advanced neuroimaging techniques).
    2. **Management of Anesthesia**
        a. Anticonvulsant medications should be maintained throughout the perioperative period (Table 19-7).
        b. An anesthetic technique that does not increase the likelihood of seizure activity is often selected (avoid enflurane and possibly ketamine and methohexital). Isoflurane, sevoflurane, and desflurane produce

TABLE 19-6

CLASSIFICATION OF SEIZURES

Localization-Related Epilepsies and Seizures
Idiopathic
  Benign childhood epilepsy
  Childhood epilepsy with occipital paroxysms

Generalized Epilepsies
Idiopathic
  Absence epilepsy (childhood or juvenile)
  Benign neonatal convulsions
  Myoclonic epilepsy (neonatal or juvenile)
  Grand mal seizures on awakening
Idiopathic and/or symptomatic
  West's syndrome
  Lennox-Gestaut syndrome
  Myoclonic-astatic seizures
  Myoclonic absences
Symptomatic
  Nonspecific etiology

Undetermined Epilepsies and Syndromes (Generalized and Focal)
Neonatal seizures
Severe myoclonic epilepsy of infancy
Acquired epileptic aphasia

Special Syndromes
Febrile seizures
Alcohol-related seizures

a dose-dependent depression of EEG activity, and propofol may increase the seizure threshold. Reported seizure activity after administration of opioids may reflect myoclonic activity.

  C. **Parkinson's disease** is a degenerative disease of the central nervous system caused by the loss of dopaminergic fibers in the basal ganglia of the brain (occurs in 1% of population over 60 years of age).
    1. Typical clinical features are secondary to depletion of dopamine from basal ganglia (Table 19-8).
    2. Treatment protocols involve combinations of drugs designed to increase dopamine levels in the brain while blunting the peripheral effects of dopamine.
      a. The combination of levodopa and carbidopa (blocks peripheral conversion of levodopa to dopamine) is the most frequent treatment.

TABLE 19-7
ANTICONVULSANT DRUGS

Drug	Seizure type	Therapeutic blood level (μg/mL)	Side effects
Phenobarbital	Generalized	15–35	Sedation Increased drug metabolism
Valproate	Generalized Absence	50–100	Pancreatitis Hepatic dysfunction Thrombocytopenia
Felbamate	Generalized Partial		Insomnia Ataxia Nausea
Phenytoin	Generalized Partial	10–20	Gingival hyperplasia Dermatitis Resistance to nondepolarizing muscle relaxants
Carbamazepine	Generalized Partial	6–12	Cardiotoxicity Hepatitis Resistance to nondepolarizing muscle relaxants
Lamotrigine	Generalized Partial	2–16	Rash Stevens-Johnson syndrome
Topiramate	Generalized Partial	4–10	
Gabapentin	Generalized Partial	4–16	Fatigue Somnolence
Primidone	Generalized Partial	6–12	Nausea Ataxia
Clonazepam	Absence	0.01–0.07	Ataxia
Ethosuximide	Absence	40–100	Leukopenia Erythema multiforme
Levetiracetam	Generalized Partial	5–45	Dizziness Headache
Oxycarbazepine	Partial	10–35	Hyponatremia Diplopia Somnolence
Tiagabine	Partial		Tremor Depression
Zonisamide	Generalized Partial	10–40	Anorexia Decreased cognition

---

TABLE 19-8

CLINICAL FEATURES OF PARKINSON'S DISEASE

Increases in spontaneous movements
Cogwheel rigidity of the extremities (shuffling gait, stooped
  posture)
Facial immobility
Rhythmic tremor at rest
Seborrhea
Sialorrhea
Orthostatic hypotension
Bladder dysfunction
Diaphragmatic spasm
Oculogyric crises
Mental depression

---

  b. Side effects of levodopa include depletion of
     myocardial norepinephrine stores, peripheral
     vasoconstriction, hypovolemia, and orthostatic
     hypotension.
  c. Surgical pallidotomy (local anesthesia) is a new
     alternative to medical therapy.
 3. **Management of anesthesia**
  a. Drugs that may antagonize the effects of dopamine
     in the central nervous system (droperidol,
     metoclopramide, alfentanil[?]) should be avoided.
  b. Levodopa has a brief half-life, and interruption of
     therapy for >6 to 12 hours can result in skeletal
     muscle rigidity that interferes with ventilation.
  c. The success with the use of selegiline for the
     treatment of parkinsonism increases the likelihood
     of having to anesthetize a patient who is receiving a
     monoamine oxidase B inhibitor (avoid meperidine).
  d. **Autonomic dysfunction** is common, manifesting as
     esophageal dysfunction (risk of aspiration) and
     orthostatic hypotension (exaggerated decreases in
     blood pressure in response to volatile anesthetics).
  e. Postoperatively, these patients may develop mental
     confusion.
 D. **Alzheimer's Disease**
 1. Alzheimer's disease is responsible for 50 to 60% of
    the cases of dementia (intellectual and cognitive
    deterioration that impairs social function) that affect
    a large proportion of the population older than
    70 years.

2. Management of Anesthesia

a. Sedative drugs for preoperative medication could result in further mental confusion.

b. Anesthetics known to result in prompt postoperative recovery may be advantageous by permitting a more rapid return to the patient's preoperative state.

c. If an anticholinergic drug is required, glycopyrrolate, which does not easily cross the blood-brain barrier, is preferable to scopolamine or atropine.

d. Patients receiving cholinesterase inhibitors may have a prolonged response to succinylcholine and mivacurium.

IV. ANEMIAS (Table 19-9)

A. In an otherwise healthy person, symptoms do not develop from anemia until the hemoglobin level decreases below 7 g/dL (physiologic compensation includes increased blood volume and cardiac output and decreased blood viscosity). There is no universally accepted hemoglobin level that mandates blood transfusion. The patient's

---

TABLE 19-9

TYPES OF ANEMIA

Nutritional
Iron deficiency
Vitamin B12 deficiency
Folic acid deficiency
Chronic illness

Hemolytic
Spherocytosis
Glucose-6-phosphate dehydrogenase deficiency (triggered by drugs including phenacetin, isoniazid, and methylene blue)
Immune-mediated
Drug-induced ABO incompatibility

Genetic
Hemoglobin S (sickle cell)
Thalassemias
   Thalassemia major (Cooley's anemia)
   Thalassemia intermedia
   Thalassemia minor

physiologic status and coexisting diseases must be
factored into a highly subjective decision.

B. **Nutritional Deficiency Anemia**
1. **Iron deficiency anemia** may be an absolute deficiency
because of decreased oral intake of iron or a relative
deficiency of iron caused by a rapid turnover of red
blood cells (chronic blood loss, hemolysis). Severe iron
deficiency produces microcytic anemia and can result
in thrombocytopenia and neurologic abnormalities.
2. **Vitamin B12 deficiency** results in megaloblastic
anemia and nervous system dysfunction (peripheral
neuropathy secondary to degeneration of the lateral
and posterior columns of the spinal cord manifesting
as symmetric paraesthesias with loss of proprioception and vibratory sensation especially in the lower
extremities). Prolonged exposure to nitrous oxide
(inactivates the vitamin B12 component of methionine
synthetase) results in megaloblastic anemia and
neurologic changes similar to those that occur in
pernicious anemia.
3. **Folic acid deficiency** (alcoholism, pregnancy,
malabsorption [phenytoin, methotrexate]) results in
megaloblastic anemia, but peripheral neuropathy is
not as common as with vitamin B12 deficiency.

C. **Hemolytic anemias** reflect premature destruction (before
120 days) of red blood cells.

D. **Hemoglobinopathies (Sickle Cell Disease)**
1. Sickle cell trait is present in 8 to 10% of blacks and 1
in 400 blacks has sickle cell anemia (hemoglobin S
[HbS] is a variant of normal hemoglobin [valine for
glutamic acid] that produces structural changes in red
blood cells when it deoxygenates).
   a. Lower oxygen tension (PaO_2 < 50 mm Hg) and
   acidosis (decreased tissue blood flow) may induce
   sickling.
   b. The definitive diagnosis of sickle-cell disease is
   made with hemoglobin electrophoresis.
2. **Clinical manifestations** (Table 19-10)
3. **Treatment**
   a. Maintenance of systemic oxygenation and
   hydration to ensure good tissue perfusion are
   essential.
   b. Pain management is important during a
   vaso-occlusive crisis (venous thrombosis results in
   infarction and severe pain).

TABLE 19-10

CLINICAL MANIFESTATIONS OF SICKLE CELL DISEASE

System	Clinical manifestations
Hematologic	Hemolytic anemia (hemoglobin 7–8 g/dL)
	Aplastic anemia
Spleen	Infarction
	Hyposplenism
	Splenic sequestration
Central nervous system	Stroke
	Hemorrhage
	Aneurysms
	Meningitis
Musculoskeletal	Painful episodes
	Bone marrow hyperplasia
	Avascular necrosis (hip, shoulder)
	Osteomyelitis
	Bone infarcts
Cardiac	Cardiomegaly
Renal	Papillary necrosis
	Glomerular sclerosis
	Renal failure
Pulmonary	Acute chest syndrome
	Pulmonary infarction
	Fibrosis
	Asthma
	Pulmonary hypertension
	Thromboembolism
	Pneumonia
Genitourinary	Priapism
	Infection
Hepatobiliary	Right upper quadrant syndrome
	Hepatitis
	Cirrhosis
	Cholelithiasis
	Cholestasis
	Jaundice
Immune system	Immunosuppression
Psychosocial	Depression
	Anxiety
	Substance abuse

4. **Management of anesthesia**
   a. Supplemental oxygen is recommended during and after regional and general anesthesia.
   b. Circulatory stasis can be prevented with hydration and anticipation of intraoperative blood loss so as to avoid acute hypovolemia.
   c. Normothermia is desirable because hyperthermia increases the rate of gel formation and hypothermia produces vasoconstriction that impairs organ blood flow.
   d. The use of a tourniquet or preoperative transfusion is controversial.
   e. Hemoglobin and hematocrit should be measured preoperatively and adequate oxygen carrying capacity maintained by transfusion to keep the hematocrit near 30% and reduce the concentration of hemoglobins S to 30 to 40% (accomplish with exchange transfusions).
   f. Drugs commonly used for anesthesia do not have any significant effects on the sickling process assuming arterial hypoxemia, vascular stasis, and reduced cardiac output are avoided. Regional anesthesia has been successfully utilized for surgery, labor and delivery, and pain management.

V. COLLAGEN VASCULAR DISEASES (Table 19-11)

A. **Rheumatoid arthritis** is a chronic inflammatory disease characterized by symmetric and significant polyarthropathy (hands and wrists first, cervical spine as reflected by magnetic resonance imaging) and systemic involvement (Table 19-12).
   1. A large number of drugs have been used for the treatment of rheumatoid arthritis, and side effects are common (Table 19-13).
   2. **Management of Anesthesia**
      a. The joint effects of rheumatoid arthritis (temporomandibular joints, cervical spine, cricoarytenoid joints) can render direct laryngoscopy and tracheal intubation difficult.
      b. **Atlantoaxial instability** is relatively common, and flexion of the neck may compress the spinal cord.
      c. The need for postoperative ventilatory support should be anticipated if severe restrictive pulmonary disease is present.

TABLE 19-11

COLLAGEN VASCULAR DISEASES

Rheumatoid Arthritis

Lupus
Systemic lupus erythematosus
Drug-induced lupus
Discoid lupus

Scleroderma
Progressive systemic sclerosis
CREST syndrome (Calcinosis Raynaud's phenomenon, esophageal dysfunction, sclerodactyly, telangiectasis)
Focal scleroderma

Polymyositis
Dermatomyositis

Overlap Syndromes

    d. Restriction of joint mobility necessitates careful positioning to minimize the risk of neurovascular compression.

B. Systemic lupus erythematosus is an autoimmune disease with diverse clinical (polyarthritis, dermatitis, renal failure, pericarditis, pulmonary hypertension) and immunologic manifestations.

    1. Drug-induced systemic lupus erythematosus (phenytoin, hydralazine, isoniazid) is usually mild and resolves within 4 weeks of discontinuation of the drug.

    2. Management of anesthesia is influenced by disease-induced organ dysfunction and drugs used in treatment.

        a. Renal dysfunction is common and necessitates preoperative evaluation.

        b. Laryngeal involvement may manifest postoperatively as laryngeal edema and/or stridor.

        c. Supplemental steroids may be necessary in patients being treated with corticosteroids.

C. Scleroderma is an autoimmune collagen vascular disease affecting the skin (thickened and swollen), joints, and visceral organs (pulmonary interstitial fibrosis and impaired diffusing capacity, pericardial effusion, renal dysfunction, decreased gastrointestinal motility).

    1. Raynaud's phenomenon occurs in 95% of patients.

TABLE 19-12

EXTRA-ARTICULAR MANIFESTATIONS OF RHEUMATOID ARTHRITIS

Skin
Raynaud's phenomenon
Digital necrosis

Eyes
Scleritis
Corneal ulceration

Lungs
Pleural effusion
Pulmonary fibrosis

Heart
Pericarditis
Cardiac tamponade
Coronary arteritis
Aortic insufficiency

Kidneys
Interstitial fibrosis
Glomerulonephritis
Amyloid deposition

Peripheral Nervous System
Compression syndromes
Mononeuritis

Central Nervous System
Dural nodules
Necrotizing vasculitis

Liver
Hepatitis

Blood
Anemia
Leukopenia

2. **Management of anesthesia** is influenced by the degree of organ dysfunction error.
   a. The risk for aspiration pneumonitis during induction of anesthesia may be increased because of the high incidence of gastroesophageal reflux.
   b. Tracheal intubation may be difficult as fibrotic and taut skin can hinder active and passive opening of the mouth and severely restrict mobility of the temporomandibular joint.

TABLE 19-13

ADVERSE EFFECTS OF DRUGS USED TO TREAT COLLAGEN
VASCULAR DISEASES

Drug	Side effects
Immunosuppressants	
Methotrexate	Hepatotoxicity, anemia, leukopenia
Azathioprine	Biliary stasis, leukopenia
Cyclosporine	Renal dysfunction, hypertension, hypomagnesemia
Cyclophosphamide	Leukopenia, hemorrhagic cystitis, inhibition of pseudocholinesterase
Leflunomide	Hepatotoxicity, weight loss, hypertension
TNF Antagonists	
Etanercept	Bacterial infections, tuberculosis
Infliximab	Lymphoma, heart failure
Adalimumab	
Interleukin-1 Antagonists	
Anakinra	Infection, skin irritation
Corticosteroids	Hypertension, fluid retention, osteoporosis, infection
Aspirin	Platelet dysfunction, peptic ulcer, hepatic dysfunction, hypersensitivity
NSAIDs	Peptic ulcer, hypertension, hyperglycemia, leukopenia
COX-2 Inhibitors	Renal dysfunction
Gold	Aplastic anemia, dermatitis, nephritis
Antimalarials	Myopathy, retinopathy
Penicillamine	Glomerulonephritis, myasthenia, aplastic anemia

    c. Chronic arterial hypoxemia may reflect restrictive lung disease and impaired oxygen diffusion.

    d. Venous access may be difficult.

    e. Skeletal muscle involvement may increase the sensitivity to muscle relaxants.

  D. **Polymyositis/dermatomyositis** is a noninfectious inflammatory myopathy (dermatomyositis when characteristic erythematous rash over the face, neck, and upper chest are present).

    1. Altered cellular immunity is supported by the development of cancer in 10 to 20% of patients with this disorder.

2. Aspiration pneumonitis (dysphagia and gastroesophageal reflux) is a common complication.
3. The most effective treatment is with corticosteroids.
4. **Management of Anesthesia**
   a. Tracheal intubation may be difficult in patients with restricted joint mobility.
   b. Despite the theoretical potential for succinylcholine to produce hyperkalemia in these patients, there is no evidence that this occurs.
   c. It should be anticipated that considerable individual variation will occur in response to nondepolarizing muscle relaxants.

VI. SKIN DISORDERS

A. **Epidermolysis bullosa** is characterized by abnormal collagen that is insufficient for anchoring skin layers to each other (laryngeal involvement is rare).
   1. Pressure applied perpendicular to the skin is less likely to produce separation of skin layers (intradermal fluid accumulation and bullae formation) than are lateral shearing forces.
   2. **Management of anesthesia** is based on avoidance of trauma to skin and mucous membranes from adhesive tape, blood pressure cuffs, tourniquets, and adhesive electrodes.
      a. Lubrication of the face mask is useful for decreasing trauma to the face.
      b. Use of upper airway instruments and passage of an esophageal stethoscope should be avoided. The safety of tracheal intubation has been established for patients with the dystrophic form of this disease.
      c. Ketamine is useful anesthesia for superficial surgical procedures.
B. **Pemphigus** is an autoimmune vesiculobullous disease that involves skin and mucous membranes. Oral lesions are common, and corticosteroids are effective in therapy.

CHAPTER 20 ■ MALIGNANT HYPERTHERMIA AND OTHER PHARMACOGENETIC DISORDERS

Certain inherited disorders are enhanced or instigated by drugs administered by anesthesiologists (Rosenberg H, Brandom BW, Sambuughin N, Fletcher JE: Malignant hyperthermia and other pharmacogenetic disorders. In Barash PG, Cullen BF, Stoelting RK [eds]: *Clinical Anesthesia*, pp 529–556. Philadelphia, Lippincott Williams & Wilkins, 2006).

I. **MALIGNANT HYPERTHERMIA.** Molecular biologic techniques are used to identify genes associated with malignant hyperthermia susceptibility.

A. **Clinical Presentation**
   1. Malignant hyperthermia is a hypermetabolic disorder of skeletal muscle that may or may not have an inherited component.
   2. An important pathophysiologic process in this disorder is intracellular hypercalcemia, which activates metabolic pathways, resulting in adenosine triphosphate depletion, acidosis, membrane destruction, and cell death.

B. **Classic Malignant Hyperthermia**
   1. The first manifestations of this syndrome most often occur in the operating room but can also occur within the first few hours of recovery from anesthesia (Table 20-1).
   2. Succinylcholine may accelerate the onset of malignant hyperthermia (entire course over 5 to 10 minutes) in some patients, whereas in others a volatile anesthetic plus succinylcholine is necessary to trigger the response. Some susceptible patients may develop malignant hyperthermia despite multiple prior uneventful exposures to triggering drugs.
   3. Even with successful treatment, patients with malignant hyperthermia are at risk for myoglobinuric renal failure and disseminated intravascular coagulation. Creatine phosphokinase levels may exceed

TABLE 20-1
MANIFESTATIONS OF MALIGNANT HYPERTHERMIA
Hypercarbia (reflects hypermetabolism and is responsible for many of the signs of sympathetic nervous system stimulation; may be masked by hyperventilation of the patient's lungs)
Tachycardia
Tachypnea
Temperature increase (1°C–2°C increase every 5 minutes)
Hypertension
Cardiac dysrhythmias
Acidosis
Arterial hypoxemia
Hyperkalemia
Skeletal muscle activity
Myoglobinuria

20,000 U in the first 12 to 24 hours. Recrudescence of the syndrome may occur in the first 24 to 36 hours.

C. **Masseter Muscle Rigidity**
   1. The differential diagnosis when rigidity of jaw muscles develops after the administration of succinylcholine (peripheral nerve stimulator shows flaccid paralysis) includes susceptibility to malignant hyperthermia (muscle biopsy testing has shown that about 50% of patients [peak incidence in those 8 to 12 years of age] who experience masseter muscle rigidity are also susceptible to malignant hyperthermia) (Table 20-2).
   2. The need to administer dantrolene following an episode of masseter muscle rigidity is unclear (malignant hyperthermia is more likely if masseter muscle rigidity is also accompanied by chest or limb rigidity).
   3. Recovery is usually uneventful following masseter muscle rigidity if the anesthetic is immediately

TABLE 20-2
EVENTS THAT MIMIC MASSETER SPASM
Inadequate dose of succinylcholine
Inadequate time for onset of action of succinylcholine
Temporomandibular joint dysfunction
Myotonic syndrome

discontinued and the patient is allowed to awaken. Nevertheless, creatine phosphokinase elevation (>20,000 U virtually confirms the diagnosis of malignant hyperthermia susceptibility) and myoglobinuria are usually present within 4 to 12 hours. Patients should be observed for 12 to 24 hours, and some recommend prophylactic administration of dantrolene (1 to 2 mg/kg iv).

4. An alternative to canceling elective surgery when masseter muscle rigidity occurs is continuing the anesthetic with nontriggering drugs and monitoring with capnography. This assumes that dantrolene is immediately available and the anesthesiologist is comfortable with managing malignant hyperthermia should it occur.

5. Pediatric anesthesiologists may avoid the use of succinylcholine except on specific indications based on the observation that masseter muscle rigidity has occurred only in association with administration of this muscle relaxant.

D. **Late Onset of Malignant Hyperthermia and Myoglobinuria.** Tachycardia, tachypnea, hypertension, dysrhythmias, and myoglobinuria in the early postoperative period may signal impending malignant hyperthermia.

E. **Myodystrophies Exacerbated by Anesthesia: Relation to Malignant Hyperthermia**

1. Patients suffering from muscular dystrophy (Duchenne or Beckers) are at risk for development of hyperkalemic cardiac arrest after administration of succinylcholine.

2. Central cord disease is a congenital myopathy characterized by muscle weakness and malignant hyperthermia susceptibility.

F. **Syndromes with a Clinical Resemblance to Malignant Hyperthermia** (Table 20-3)

G. **Neuroleptic Malignant Syndrome and Other Drug-Induced Hyperthermic Reactions**

1. Neuroleptic malignant syndrome may mimic malignant hyperthermia (dantrolene may be effective). Unlike malignant hyperthermia, this syndrome is associated with prolonged drug therapy with psychoactive drugs (phenothiazines or haloperidol) or sudden withdrawal of drugs used to treat Parkinson's disease. Bromocriptine (a dopamine agonist) is useful

318   *Preparing for Anesthesia*

TABLE 20-3

SYNDROMES WITH A CLINICAL RESEMBLANCE TO MALIGNANT HYPERTHERMIA

Pheochromocytoma
Sepsis
Hypoxic encephalopathy
Mitochondrial myopathies
Periodic paralyses (hypokalemic and hyperkalemic)

in treatment, suggesting that this syndrome may reflect depletion of central nervous system dopamine stores by psychoactive drugs.

    a. From an anesthesiologist's point of view, it is best to treat patients with neuroleptic malignant syndrome as though they are susceptible to malignant hyperthermia.

    b. The recommendation is to conduct electroconvulsive therapy without the use of succinylcholine or other triggering drugs.

  2. Similar signs have been observed in some patients taking serotonin uptake inhibitors.

H. Drugs That Trigger Malignant Hyperthermia (Table 20-4)

TABLE 20-4

DRUGS THAT MAY OR MAY NOT TRIGGER MALIGNANT HYPERTHERMIA

Unsafe Drugs	
Succinylcholine	Volatile anesthetics
Safe Drugs	
Antibiotics	Antihistamines
Antipyretics	Vasoactive drugs
Barbiturates	Benzodiazepines
Droperidol	Ketamine (inherent circulatory effects may mimic malignant hyperthermia)
Local anesthetics	Nitrous oxide
Opioids	Propranolol
Propofol	Nondepolarizing neuromuscular blocking drugs

I. **Incidence and Epidemiology**
 1. A better understanding of the prevalence of malignant hyperthermia is being provided by use of molecular genetics for the diagnosis of malignant hyperthermia susceptibility.
 2. Although the incidence of reported cases of malignant hyperthermia has increased, the mortality rate from malignant hyperthermia has declined (under 5%), reflecting both a greater awareness of the syndrome and earlier diagnosis followed by better treatment.

J. **Inheritance of Malignant Hyperthermia**
 1. The inheritance of malignant hyperthermia in humans has been described as autosomal dominant with variable penetrance.
 2. It is estimated that 50% of the children of malignant hyperthermia-susceptible parents are at risk for this disorder. Relatives of malignant hyperthermia-susceptible individuals who also have an increased creatine phosphokinase level have a >80% chance of being susceptible.

K. **Diagnostic Tests for Malignant Hyperthermia**
 1. **Halothane–Caffeine Contracture Test**
     a. Although several tests have been described, this test remains the standard.
     b. Skeletal muscle biopsy specimens (usually vastus lateralis) are bathed in a solution containing 1.5 to 3% halothane plus caffeine or, alternatively, either drug alone. A response indicative of malignant hyperthermia susceptibility is based on a previously established contracture threshold.
 2. **Other Contracture Tests**
     a. **Ryanodine.** This test was based on the premise that a defect in the ryanodine receptor (calcium release channel of skeletal muscle) was the only cause of malignant hyperthermia that would afford maximum specificity (premise no longer valid).
     b. **4-Chloro-m-cresol** is a potent activator of ryanodine receptor-mediated calcium release. Contractures occur in 100% of skeletal muscles from patients who are malignant hyperthermia susceptible.
 3. **Pitfalls in the Contracture Test**
     a. Because of the variation in the presentation of malignant hyperthermia it may not be possible to achieve agreement on the status of a patient based

on clinical history. A clinical grading scale is used to evaluate the clinical episode (Table 20-5).

b. Malignant hyperthermia trigger agents are avoided if a patient has a positive contracture test.

4. **Tests with More Limited Usefulness in Malignant Hyperthermia Diagnosis**

   a. Use of resting CK levels for screening for malignant hyperthermia is neither sensitive nor specific but there is a relationship between postoperative CK levels associated with masseter muscle rigidity and the probability of a positive contracture test.

   b. Elevated CK levels may be useful in identifying family members to be referred for contracture testing and in identifying malignant hyperthermia

TABLE 20-5

CRITERIA USED IN THE MALIGNANT HYPERTHERMIA GRADING SCALE

Process I: Muscle Rigidity	
Generalized rigidity	15
Masseter rigidity	15
Process II: Myonecrosis	
Elevated CK >20,000 (SCh)	15
Elevated CK >20,000 (no SCh)	15
Cola colored urine	10
Myoglobin in urine >60 μg/L	5
Blood/serum K >6 mEq/L	3
Process III: Respiratory Acidosis	
PetCO2 >55 with CV	15
PaCO2 >60 with CV	15
PetCO2 >60 with SV	15
Inappropriate hypercarbia	15
Inappropriate tachypnea	10
Process IV: Temperature Increase	
Rapid increase in temperature	15
Inappropriate temperature >38.8°C in the perioperative period	10
Process V: Cardiac Involvement	
Inappropriate tachycardia	3
Ventricular tachycardia or ventricular fibrillation	3

CK, creatine kinase; SCh, succinylcholine; K, potassium; Pet, end-tidal; CV, controlled ventilation; SV, spontaneous ventilation.

> in children too young to undergo contracture testing.

   5. **Molecular Genetic Testing for Malignant Hyperthermia Susceptibility**
      a. Multiple mutations on the RYR1 gene and mutations in other genes have been shown to be causal for malignant hyperthermia.
      b. Ultimately, genetic testing is likely to replace more invasive diagnostic tests.
      c. The presence of a ryanodine mutation predicts malignant hyperthermia susceptibility.

L. **Treatment of Malignant Hyperthermia.** Malignant hyperthermia is a treatable disorder that should have a mortality near zero when recognized early and treated promptly. All institutions in which anesthetic drugs are administered (hospitals, ambulatory surgery facilities, doctors' offices) should have **dantrolene** available (36 ampules [720 mg]) and an established management plan (see inside back cover for Malignant Hyperthermia Protocol).

   1. **Acute Episode** (Table 20-6)

TABLE 20-6

MANAGEMENT OF THE ACUTE EPISODE OF MALIGNANT HYPERTHERMIA

Discontinue inhaled anesthetics and succinylcholine

Hyperventilate the lungs with oxygen at 10 L/min (hastens purging of residual anesthetic gases)

Utilize Ambu bag and E cylinder (do not spend time replacing anesthesia machine)

Administer dantrolene (2.5 mg/kg iv) with repeated doses (2–3 mg/kg often sufficient but may require >10 mg/kg) based on $Paco_2$, heart rate, and body temperature

Place bladder catheter (each 20 mg of dantrolene contains 300 mg of mannitol)

Treat persistent acidosis with sodium bicarbonate (1–2 mEq/kg iv)

Control body temperature (gastric lavage, external ice packs until 38°C)

Monitor with capnography (best clinical measurement to guide therapy) and arterial blood gases

Be prepared to treat hyperkalemia (glucose, insulin, hyperventilation, calcium) and cardiac dysrhythmias (avoid verapamil, lidocaine acceptable)

TABLE 20-7

MANAGEMENT OF MALIGNANT HYPERTHERMIA AFTER THE ACUTE EPISODE

Continue dantrolene (1–2 mg/kg iv) every 6 hours for at least 24–36 hours
Anticipate complications
    Recrudescence
    Disseminated intravascular coagulation
    Myoglobinuric renal failure
    Skeletal muscle weakness
    Electrolyte abnormalities

2. **Management After the Acute Episode** (Table 20-7)
3. **Dantrolene**
   a. This drug acts in skeletal muscle cells to decrease intracellular levels of calcium most likely by decreasing sarcoplasmic reticulum release or inhibiting excitation-contracture coupling at the transverse tubular level.
   b. **Therapeutic levels** of dantrolene (2.5 mg/mL) usually persist for 4 to 6 hours after an intravenous dose of 2.5 mg/kg (reason to supplement every 4 hours).
   c. **Prophylaxis** for malignant hyperthermia should be carried out with intravenous or oral dantrolene (5 mg/kg).
4. **Management of the Patient Susceptible to Malignant Hyperthermia** (Table 20-8)
   a. There have been no deaths from malignant hyperthermia in previously diagnosed malignant hyperthermia-susceptible patients when the anesthesiologist was prospectively aware of the problem. This information is useful to allay the patient's preoperative anxiety.
   b. Dantrolene need not be repeated after the anesthetic is terminated if there were no signs of malignant hyperthermia during surgery.
   c. In a malignant hyperthermia-susceptible parturient, an acceptable approach to management of routine labor is epidural analgesia without dantrolene pretreatment and close monitoring of vital signs. If general anesthesia is necessary for delivery, an acceptable approach is to administer dantrolene

TABLE 20-8

MANAGEMENT OF MALIGNANT HYPERTHERMIA-SUSCEPTIBLE PATIENTS

Standard preoperative medication

Dantrolene (2.5 mg/kg iv) 15–30 minutes before induction of anesthesia

Clean anesthesia machine (disposable circuit, new soda lime, drain vaporizers, oxygen flow 10 L/min for 20 minutes to flush system)

Modern anesthesia work stations are larger than traditional anesthesia machines (flush for 30 minutes at 10 L/min)

Capnography (increased end-tidal carbon dioxide concentration is the earliest sign of malignant hyperthermia)

Monitor body temperature

Use nontriggering drugs and techniques (regional if possible)

Observe closely postoperatively (routine administration of dantrolene not indicated in absence of signs of malignant hyperthermia)

Rehydration (decreases chance that fever as a result of dehydration will occur)

intravenously and use nontriggering drugs. No adverse fetal effects of dantrolene have been observed.

II. DISORDERS OF PLASMA CHOLINESTERASE

A. Succinylcholine-Related Apnea

1. Hydrolysis of succinylcholine by plasma cholinesterase is slowed to absent in patients with inherited alterations on the gene locus responsible for production of this enzyme by the liver (Table 20-9).

   a. When there is a question about the rate of hydrolysis of succinylcholine, the plasma cholinesterase activity as well as dibucaine and fluoride numbers should be measured.

   b. Patients who are homozygous for atypical cholinesterase enzyme should wear Medic-Alert bracelets indicating that succinylcholine will result in prolonged apnea (often longer than 2 hours).

2. Depression of plasma cholinesterase activity in the absence of atypical genotypes can be seen following

TABLE 20-9
GENOTYPES FOR PLASMA CHOLINESTERASE ENZYME

Genotype	Dibucaine number	Fluoride number	Cholinesterase activity	Response to succinylcholine	Incidence
EuEu	78–86	55–65	Normal	Normal	96%
EaEa	18–26	16–32	Decreased	Greatly prolonged	1 in 2,000
EuEa	51–70	38–55	Intermediate	Slightly prolonged	1 in 25
EuEf	74–80	47–48	Intermediate	Slightly prolonged	1 in 200
EfEa	49–59	25–33	Intermediate	Greatly prolonged	1 in 20,000
EfEs	63	26	Decreased	Moderately prolonged	1 in 150,000

TABLE 20-10
CAUSES OF CHANGES IN CHOLINESTERASE ACTIVITY

Inherited
Cholinesterase variants (silent gene, C5 variant)

Physiologic
Decreases in last trimester of pregnancy
Decreases in newborn

Acquired decreases
Liver disease
Cancer
Debilitating diseases
Collagen diseases
Uremia
Malnutrition
Myxedema

Acquired increases
Obesity
Alcoholism
Thyrotoxicosis
Nephrosis
Psoriasis
Electroshock therapy

Drugs
Echothiophate iodide
Anticholinesterases
Chlorpromazine
Cyclophosphamide
Monoamine oxidase inhibitors
Pancuronium
Contraceptives
Organophosphate insecticides
Hexaflurenium

Other causes of decreased activity
Plasmapheresis
Extracorporeal circulation
Tetanus
Radiation therapy
Burns

administration of anticholinesterase drugs or plasmapheresis and in the presence of advanced liver disease (Table 20-10). This usually results in only moderate prolongation of succinylcholine-induced skeletal muscle paralysis (rarely longer than 30 minutes).

3. Treatment of Succinylcholine Apnea
   a. The safest course of treatment after the patient fails to breathe spontaneously within 10 to 15 minutes after succinylcholine administration is to continue mechanical ventilation of the lungs until adequate skeletal muscle strength has returned.
   b. The use of anticholinesterase drugs in treating succinylcholine apnea is controversial.

B. Plasma Cholinesterase Abnormalities and the Metabolism of Local Anesthetics
   1. Ester local anesthetics are metabolized by plasma cholinesterase.
   2. Despite the theoretical argument that the action of these drugs might be prolonged, there is evidence that the response of homozygous atypical patients is usually normal.

C. Mivacurium Disposition and Plasma Cholinesterase. Prolonged skeletal muscle paralysis may follow administration of this nondepolarizing muscle relaxant to patients with atypical cholinesterase enzyme, emphasizing its dependence on hydrolysis by plasma cholinesterase.

III. PORPHYRIAS

A. These inherited defects of heme synthesis can mimic surgical diseases and can be provoked by administration of certain drugs (Table 20-11).

B. Management of Patients with Porphyria
   1. Triggering drugs (barbiturates, perhaps benzodiazepines and ketamine) are avoided. Nontriggering drugs include propofol, nitrous oxide, volatile anesthetics, opioids, and muscle relaxants. Regional anesthesia may be avoided to prevent

TABLE 20-11

MANIFESTATIONS OF PORPHYRIA

Abdominal pain	Fever
Vomiting	Confusion
Tachycardia	Seizures
Hypertension	Somnolence
Neuropathy	

confusion should neurologic changes occur postoperatively.

2. Glucose infusions are important in prevention (starvation can induce an attack) and treatment of porphyria.

IV. GLYCOGEN STORAGE DISEASES

A. These inherited diseases are characterized by dysfunction of one of the many enzymes involved in glucose metabolism.

B. Associated problems that may influence anesthetic management include hypoglycemia, acidosis, and cardiac and hepatic dysfunction.

V. OTHER INHERITED DISORDERS

A. **Osteogenesis imperfecta** occurs in approximately 1 in 50,000 births. Minor trauma can lead to fractures, and airway management may be difficult because of cervical spine involvement. Inhalation anesthetics have been administered to many of these patients without complications of malignant hyperthermia.

B. **Prader-Willi syndrome** is characterized by hypotonia (airway management and response to muscle relaxants), hypoglycemia, and obesity.

C. **Riley-Day syndrome (familial dysautonomia)** is characterized by denervation supersensitivity (vasopressors), dysphagia (aspiration), no sensitivity to pain, postural hypotension, and impaired body temperature control.

CHAPTER 21 ■ DELIVERY SYSTEMS FOR INHALED ANESTHETICS

An understanding of the components of the anesthesia system (machine, vaporizers, ventilator, circuit) is important for the safe practice of anesthesia (Brockwell RC, Andrews JJ: Delivery systems for inhaled anesthetics. In Barash PG, Cullen BF, Stoelting RK [eds]: *Clinical Anesthesia*, pp 557–594. Philadelphia, Lippincott Williams & Wilkins, 2006).

I. ANESTHESIA MACHINE

A. Anesthesia machines have evolved from simple pneumatic devices to complex integrated computer-controlled multisystem workstations.

B. **Standards for Anesthesia Machines and Workstations**
   1. These standards provide guidelines to manufacturers regarding minimum performance, design characteristics, and safety requirements for anesthesia machines.
   2. To comply with the American Society for Testing and Materials Standards, newly manufactured workstations must have monitors to measure specific parameters and possess a prioritized alarm system (Table 21-1).

C. **Checking Your Anesthesia Workstation.** A complete anesthesia apparatus checkout procedure must be performed each day prior to the first use of the anesthesia workstation ("machine check list") (Appendix A) (Table 21-2).

II. ANESTHESIA WORKSTATION PNEUMATICS

A. **The Anatomy of an Anesthesia Workstation** (Fig. 21-1)
   1. Gases such as oxygen (O_2), nitrous oxide (N_2O), and air are usually supplied from a central pipeline with cylinders on the machine as a backup. The pipeline source is usually at 50 psig (pounds per square inch gauge). A full O_2 cylinder contains only

TABLE 21-1

AMERICAN SOCIETY FOR TESTING AND MATERIALS STANDARDS FOR MANUFACTURED WORKSTATIONS

Parameters Monitored
Continuous breathing system pressure
Exhaled CO_2 concentration
Anesthetic vapor concentration
Inspired O_2 concentration
O_2 supply pressure
Arterial hemoglobin oxygen saturation
Arterial blood pressure
Continuous electrocardiogram

Prioritized Alarms System
High, medium, and low categories
Alarms automatically or manually enabled

gas, and the tank pressure decreases linearly from a maximum of about 2200 psig as it is consumed. N_2O is compressed to a liquid in tanks and maintains a pressure of 745 psig until all the liquid is dissipated.

2. A **fail-safe** valve is located downstream from the N_2O supply source and serves as an interface between the O_2 and N_2O supply sources. This valve shuts off or proportionally decreases the supply of N_2O if the oxygen supply decreases.

TABLE 21-2

CHECKING YOUR ANESTHESIA WORKSTATION

Oxygen analyzer calibration (evaluates integrity of low-pressure circuit, only machine monitor that detects problems downstream from the flow control valves)
Low-pressure circuit leak test (checks integrity of the anesthesia machine from flow control valves to the common outlet; leaks in the low-pressure circuit may cause hypoxia and awareness)
Circle system test (evaluates integrity of system from common gas outlet to the Y-piece)
Leak test (close pop-off valve, occlude the Y-piece, and pressurize the circuit to 30 cm H_2O using the oxygen flush valve)
Flow test (confirms integrity of unidirectional valves; perform by disconnecting the Y-piece and breathing through each corrugated tube individually)

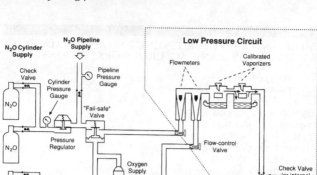

FIGURE 21-1. Schematic diagram of a generic two-gas anesthesia machine.

3. **Regulators** downstream from the O_2 supply source adjust the pressure to about 14 psig before entering the flowmeter assembly.

4. **Flow control valves** separate the intermediate-pressure circuit from the low-pressure circuit (that part of the machine that is downstream from the flow control valves). The operator regulates flow entering the low-pressure circuit by adjusting the flow control valves. After leaving the flow tubes, the mixture of gases travels through a common manifold and may be directed to a calibrated vaporizer.

5. A one-way check valve located between the vaporizer and common gas outlet prevents back flow into the vaporizer during positive-pressure ventilation.

6. The oxygen flush connection joins the mixed-gas pipeline between the one-way check valve and the machine outlet. When the oxygen flush valve is activated the pipeline oxygen pressure is reflected in the common gas outlet.

B. **Pipeline Supply Source.** Most hospitals have a central piping system to deliver medical gases such as O_2, N_2O, and air to the operating room at appropriate pressures in order for the anesthesia workstation to function properly.

C. **Flowmeter assemblies** precisely measure gas flow to the common gas outlet. Depending on the setting of the flow control valve, gases flow through variable orifice tapered tubes at a rate indicated by the position of a float indicator in relation to a calibrated scale.

   1. At low flow rates, the viscosity of the gas is dominant in determining flow, whereas density is dominant at high flow rates.

   2. Safety features include use of standardized colors for each gas, an O_2 flowmeter dial that is distinct from the others, and positioning of the O_2 flowmeter immediately proximal to the common gas outlet to minimize the chance of delivery of hypoxic mixtures in the event of leaks in the flowmeter assembly.

   3. **Problems with Flowmeters**

      a. **Leaks** are hazardous as flowmeters are located downstream from all machine safety devices except the oxygen analyzer. The use of electronic flowmeters and the removal of conventional glass flow tubes help eliminate this potential source of leak and potential for delivery of hypoxic gas mixtures (minimized if oxygen flowmeter is located downstream from all other flowmeters).

      b. **Inaccuracy** of flow measurement can occur (dirt or static electricity cause a float to stick).

      c. **Ambiguous scale** in which operator reads the float position beside an adjacent but erroneous scale (minimize by etching scale into tube).

D. **Dilution of Inspired Oxygen Concentration by Volatile Inhaled Anesthetic**

   1. Concentrations of less-potent volatile anesthetics (maximum desflurane dial setting 18%) when added to the inhaled gases downstream from flowmeters and proportioning system can result in a gas/vapor mixture that contains an inspired O_2 concentration that is <21%.

III. VARIABLE BYPASS VAPORIZERS

A. The Datex-Ohmeda Tec 4, 5, and 7 and the North American Draeger Vapor 19n and 20n are classified as variable bypass (method for regulating output concentration), flow-over, temperature-compensated, agent-specific (keyed filling devices), out-of-breathing circuit vaporizers.

 1. Basic Operating Principles
  a. As gas flow enters the vaporizer's inlet, the setting of the concentration dial determines the ratio of flow that goes through the bypass chamber and through the vaporizing chamber. The gas diverted to the vaporizing chamber flows over the liquid anesthetic and becomes saturated with vapor.
  b. The amount of gas diverted into the vaporizing chamber is primarily a function of the anesthetic vapor pressure. A temperature-compensating device helps maintain a constant vaporizer output over a wide range of temperatures.

 2. Safety Features (Table 21-3)
 3. Hazards (Table 21-4)

B. The Datex-Ohmeda Tec 6 vaporizer for desflurane is an electrically heated, pressurized device specifically designed to deliver desflurane.

 1. Desflurane boils at 22.8°C and its vapor pressure is three to four times that of other contemporary inhaled anesthetics.
 2. Desflurane's high volatility and moderate potency precluded its use with contemporary variable bypass vaporizers.

TABLE 21-3

SAFETY FEATURES OF VARIABLE BYPASS VAPORIZERS

Agent specific (keyed filling devices)

Filler port placed at maximum safe liquid level (prevents overfilling)

Secured to vaporizer manifold (prevents tipping and spillage of liquid anesthetic into the bypass chamber and delivery of an overdose)

Interlock system (prevents delivery of more than one volatile anesthetic simultaneously)

TABLE 21-4

HAZARDS ASSOCIATED WITH VARIABLE BYPASS VAPORIZERS

Misfilling
Contamination of volatile agent added to vaporizer
Tipping (unlikely if properly mounted on manifold)
Overfilling
Underfilling
Simultaneous inhaled anesthetic administration (unlikely with newer machines)
Leaks (loose filler cap the most common cause; risk of patient awareness)
Internal ferrous components a risk in MRI suite

    3. **Factors That Influence Vaporizer Output**
       a. **Varied altitudes** will influence the output of this vaporizer that is unlike contemporary variable bypass vaporizers, which deliver a relatively constant partial pressure of anesthetic at varied ambient pressures. At a given concentration dial setting, the Tec 6 provides a lower partial pressure of the anesthetic as altitude increases. For example, at 2,000 m elevation the concentration dial setting of the Tec 6 must be increased from 10 to 12.5% to deliver the same partial pressure as at sea level.
       b. **Carrier gas composition.** Vaporizer output approximates the dial setting when O_2 is the carrier gas. At low flow rates using N_2O as the carrier gas (decreased viscosity compared with O_2), vaporizer output is approximately 20% less than the dial setting.
    4. **Safety features.** The agent-specific filler cap of the desflurane bottle prevents its use with traditional vaporizers.
    5. The Datex-Ohmeda Aladin Cassette Vaporizer is an electronically controlled vaporizer designed to deliver five different (halothane, isoflurane, enflurane, sevoflurane, desflurane) inhaled anesthetics.

IV. ANESTHETIC CIRCUITS

  A. An anesthetic circuit is interposed between the anesthesia machine, common gas outlet, and the

patient. The function of the circuit is to deliver
anesthetic gases and O_2 to a patient and to remove
exhaled carbon dioxide (CO_2).

B. Mapleson Systems
   1. In 1954 Mapleson described and analyzed five
      different semiclosed anesthetic systems (Mapleson
      Systems A-E) in which the amount of CO_2
      rebreathing associated with each system is
      multifactorial (Table 21-5) (Fig. 21-2).
   2. The **Bain circuit** is a modification of the Mapleson
      D circuit, in which fresh gas flow is delivered at the
      end nearest the patient through a small inner tube
      located within the larger corrugated tubing (see
      Fig. 21-2).
   3. The advantages of all these systems are that they are
      lightweight and convenient. The main disadvantage
      is that high fresh gas flows are required.

C. Circle Breathing Systems
   1. Technological changes in the traditional circle
      breathing system include application of single-circuit
      piston-type ventilators and use of new spirometry
      devices that are located at the Y-connector instead of
      at the traditional location on the expiratory circuit
      limb.
   2. **The Traditional Circle Breathing System.** The circle
      system (fresh gas inflow, inspiratory and expiratory
      unidirectional valves, inspiratory and expiratory
      corrugated tubing, Y-piece connector, overflow or

TABLE 21-5

VARIABLES THAT DETERMINE THE AMOUNT OF CO_2 REBREATHING ASSOCIATED WITH MAPLESON SYSTEMS

Fresh gas inflow rate
Minute ventilation
Mode of ventilation (spontaneous or controlled)
Tidal volume
Breathing rate
Inspiratory/expiratory ratio
Duration of expiratory pause
Peak inspiratory flow rate
Volume of reservoir tube
Volume of breathing bag
Ventilation by mask or tracheal tube
CO_2 sampling site

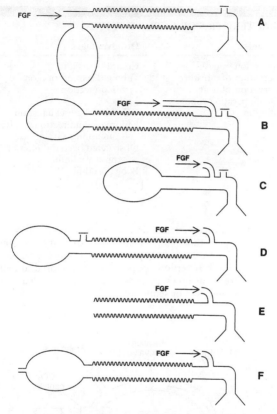

FIGURE 21-2. Schematic diagram of a Bain circuit.

pop-off valve, reservoir bag, and a canister containing a CO_2 absorbent) is the most popular breathing system in the United States (Table 21-6) (Fig. 21-3).

a. The unidirectional valves are placed so that gases flow in only one direction and through the CO_2 absorber (see Fig. 21-3).

b. If the valves are functioning properly, the only dead space in the system is between the Y-piece and the patient.

TABLE 21-6
CHARACTERISTICS OF A CIRCLE SYSTEM

Advantages	Disadvantages
Conservation of gases	Complex design
Conservation of moisture	Tubing disconnection or
Conservation of heat	misconnection
Minimal operating room	Leaks
pollution	CO_2 absorbent exhaustion
	Failure of unidirectional valves
	(rebreathing, circuit occlusion)
	Obstructed bacterial filter in
	expiratory limb
	Poor portability

3. A **closed system** exists when the fresh gas flow equals that being consumed by the patient (about 300 mL/min of O_2 plus uptake of anesthetic gases) and the overflow (pop-off) valve is closed. If high fresh gas flows are used, the system is called semiclosed or semiopen.

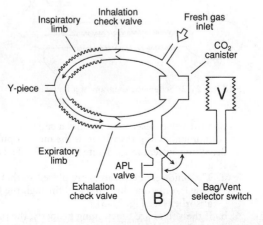

FIGURE 21-3. Components of the circle system. APL = adjustable pressure-limiting valve or "pop-off" valve.

D. **Carbon Dioxide Absorbents**
   1. Undesirable chemical reactions between desiccated Baralyme (no longer clinically available) include exothermic reactions with sevoflurane (fires in the breathing system), production of carbon monoxide (desflurane) and compound A (sevoflurane).
   2. **Chemistry of Absorbents**
      a. Available formulations of carbon dioxide absorbents include soda lime and calcium hydroxide lime (Amsorb).
      b. Advantages of calcium hydroxide is the lack of strong bases (sodium and potassium hydroxide), absence of undesirable chemical reactions and formation of heat, compound A, and carbon monoxide.
      c. Absorption of CO_2 is accomplished in a circle system by a chemical reaction that results in water and heat as byproducts (Table 21-7).
   3. **Absorptive Capacity**
      a. The maximum amount of carbon dioxide that can be absorbed by soda lime is 26 L of CO_2 per 100 g of absorbent.
      b. The absorptive capacity of calcium hydroxide is less (10.2 L of CO_2 per 100 g of absorbent).
   4. **Indicators**
      a. Ethyl violet is the pH indicator added to soda lime that changes from colorless to violet in color when the pH of the absorbent decreases as a result of carbon dioxide absorption.
      b. Prolonged exposure of ethyl violet to fluorescent lights can produce photodeactivation of the dye (absorbent appears white even though it may have a reduced pH and its absorptive capacity has been exhausted). Indicators are placed in the CO_2 absorbent where they change color when the absorbent is exhausted.

TABLE 21-7

CHEMICAL REACTION OF CO_2 WITH SODA LIME

$CO_2 + H_2O \rightarrow H_2CO_3$
$H_2CO_3 + 2NaOH(KOH) \rightarrow Na_2CO_3(K_2CO_3) + 2H_2O + heat$
$Na_2CO_3(K_2CO_3) + Ca(OH)_2 \rightarrow CaCO_3 + 2NaOH(KOH)$

TABLE 21-8

INTERACTIONS OF INHALED ANESTHETICS WITH
ABSORBENTS

Sevoflurane and formation of compound A
Formation of carbon monoxide (increased carboxyhemoglobin,
 formation greatest with desflurane and least with sevoflurane)
Fires in the breathing circuit (desiccated Baralyme and
 sevoflurane)

V. INTERACTIONS OF INHALED ANESTHETICS WITH ABSORBENTS (Table 21-8). The likelihood of adverse chemical reactions between carbon dioxide absorbents and volatile anesthetics is minimized by avoiding the use of desiccated carbon dioxide absorbents that contain strong bases.

VI. ANESTHESIA VENTILATORS

A. Classification
  1. Ventilators can be classified according to their power source (electricity and/or compressed gas), drive mechanism (pneumatically driven), and cycling mechanism (time cycled, pressure cycled).
  2. Bellows Classification
     a. The direction of the bellows movement during the expiratory phase determines the bellows classification.
     b. Ascending (standing) bellows ascend during the expiratory phase whereas descending (hanging) bellows descend during the expiratory phase.
     c. Ascending bellows will not fill if a total disconnection occurs while a descending bellows ventilator will continue its up and down movement despite a patient disconnection (driving gas pushes bellows up during the inspiratory phase).
     d. An essential safety feature of any anesthesia workstation that utilizes a descending bellows is an integrated CO_2 apnea alarm that cannot be disabled while the ventilator is in use.
B. Problems and Hazards (Table 21-9)

TABLE 21-9
HAZARDS ASSOCIATED WITH VENTILATORS

Accidental disconnection
Delivery of excessive pressure
Leaks in bellows
Erroneous connection of tubing to anesthetic circuit
Failure of the ventilator relief valve
Failure of the driving mechanism

VII. ANESTHESIA WORKSTATION VARIATIONS

A. **The Datex-Ohmeda S/5 ADU** eliminates gas flow tubes and conventional anesthesia vaporizors in exchange for a computer screen with digital fresh gas flow scales and a built-in Aladin Cassette vaporizer system.
   1. Entry of the fresh gas inflow on the patient side of the inspiratory valve is more efficient in delivering fresh gas flow to the patient and preferentially eliminating exhaled gases.
   2. This arrangement is less likely to result in desiccation of the carbon dioxide absorbent.
B. **The Draeger Medical Narkomed 6000 Series and Fabius GS** is characterized by the absence of flow tubes and glowing electronic fresh gas flow indicators.
   1. Fresh gas decoupling decreases the risk of barotrauma (fresh gas coming into the system from the patient is isolated while the ventilator exhaust valve is closed) and volutrauma.
   2. A disadvantage of the anesthesia circle systems that utilize fresh gas decoupling is the possibility of entraining room air into the patient gas circuit (high-priority audible and visual alarms are needed to notify the user that fresh gas flow is inadequate and room air is being entrained).

VIII. SCAVENGING SYSTEMS

A. Scavenging systems are designed to collect and subsequently vent gases from operating rooms.
B. These systems minimize operating room pollution but increase the complexity of the anesthesia system (Table 21-10).

TABLE 21-10
HAZARDS INTRODUCED BY SCAVENGING SYSTEMS

Transmission of excessive positive pressure to the breathing system (obstruction of scavenging pathways)

Application of excessive negative pressure to the breathing system (relief valve or port becomes obstructed)

Loss of means of monitoring (conceals odor of excessive anesthetic concentration)

C. The two major causes of waste gas contamination in the operating room are the anesthetic technique (failure to discontinue gas delivery from the anesthesia machine at the conclusion of anesthesia, poorly fitting face mask, flushing the breathing circuit) and equipment (leaks).

CHAPTER 22 ■ AIRWAY MANAGEMENT

Techniques of difficult airway management are influenced by expanded application of supraglottic airways (SGAs) and nonirritating inhalation agents (Rosenblatt WH: Airway management. In Barash PG, Cullen BF, Stoelting RK [eds]: *Clinical Anesthesia*, pp 595–642. Philadelphia, Lippincott Williams & Wilkins, 2006). Routine patient evaluations often fail to detect difficult airways but this has become less of a problem as SGA use proliferates and new means of intubation are adopted. Airway difficulties and mismanagement are the cause of a significant proportion of adverse anesthetic outcomes. Perioperative airway management includes a (1) thorough airway history and physical examination, (2) management plan for use of an SGA (face mask, laryngeal mask airway [LMA]), (3) management plan for intubation and extubation techniques, and (4) an alternative plan should emergencies arise.

I. AIRWAY ANATOMY

A. The term "airway" refers to the upper airway consisting of the nasal and oral cavities, pharynx, larynx, trachea, and principal bronchi.

1. The laryngeal skeleton consists of nine cartilages (three paired and three unpaired) that together house the vocal folds that extend in the anterior-posterior plane from the thyroid cartilage to the laryngeal cartilages.

2. The larynx is innervated by two branches of the vagus nerve—superior laryngeal nerve and recurrent laryngeal nerve.

   a. Recurrent laryngeal nerve supplies all the intrinsic muscles of the larynx with the exception of the cricothyroid muscle.

   b. Vocal cord dysfunction accompanies trauma to these nerves. Unilateral nerve injury is unlikely to impair airway function but the protective role of the larynx in preventing aspiration may be compromised.

3. Cricothyroid membrane covers the cricothyroid space (about 9 mm).

4. Cricoid cartilage is at the base of the larynx and is suspended by the underside of the cricothyroid membrane.
5. Trachea in adults measures about 15 cm and is supported circumferentially by 17 to 18 C-shaped cartilages with a posterior membranous aspect overlying the esophagus.
   a. The first tracheal ring is anterior to the sixth cervical vertebra.
   b. The trachea ends at the fifth thoracic vertebra (carina) where it bifurcates into the right and left bronchi. The right mainstem bronchus is larger than the left and deviates from the plane of the trachea at a less acute angle (aspirated materials as well as a deeply placed tracheal tube are more likely to enter the right than left bronchus).

B. **Patient History and Physical Exam**
   1. Preoperative evaluation of the patient should elicit a thorough history of airway-related untoward events as well as related airway symptoms (obstructive sleep apnea, chipped teeth, dysphagia, stridor, cervical spine pain or limited range of motion, temporomandibular joint pain, or dysfunction).
   2. Physical findings that may indicate subsequent difficult airway management include a short muscular neck with full dentition, a receding mandible, protruding maxillary central incisor teeth, decreased mobility at the temporomandibular joints, a long high arched palate, and increased alveolar-mental distance.
   3. No common index for difficult airway prediction has proven to be both sensitive and specific (Table 22-1).
      a. Mallampati classification (based on tongue size in the intraoral cavity) is determined with the patient seated and head in neutral position and the mouth opened as widely as possible and the tongue protruded. The extent to which the base of the tongue is able to mask the visibility of the pharyngeal structures is the basis of classifying the airway as Mallampati I (uvula fully visible) to IV (only hard palate is visible). The practical value of this classification is its ease of application, but this index (like most others) has not proven to be sensitive or specific (many false-positives) in identifying patients who may be difficult to

TABLE 22-1

SENSITIVITY AND SPECIFICITY OF PREOPERATIVE
FINDINGS FOR DIFFICULT AIRWAY MANAGEMENT

	Sensitivity (%)	Specificity (%)	Positive Predictive Value[a]
Mouth opening (<4cm)	26.3	94.8	25
Thromental distance (<6cm)	7	99.2	38.5
Mallampati Class III	44.7	89.0	21
Neck movement <80 degrees	10.4	99.4	29.5
Inability to prognath	16.5	95.8	20.6
Body weight >110 kg	11.1	94.6	11.8
History of difficult intubation	4.5	99.9	69.0

[a] For finding of a grade III/IV view on direct laryngoscopy.

       intubate, or the ease of using supraglottic
ventilatory devices (LMA, fiberoptic brochoscope).
  b. The multivariate index (MI) assigns relative weights
to each exam finding (thyromental distance, mouth
opening, Mallampati score, head and neck
movement, ability to prognath). Compared to the
Mallampati classification, the MI has an improved
positive predictive value and specificity.

II. CLINICAL MANAGEMENT OF THE AIRWAY

A. Preoxygenation
  1. This procedure entails the replacement of the lung's
nitrogen volume ("denitrogenation") with oxygen to
provide a reservoir for diffusion of oxygen into the
alveolar capillary bed after the onset of apnea (as
associated with direct laryngoscopy for tracheal
intubation).
    a. Breathing room air will result in desaturation to
<90% after about 2 minutes of apnea.
    b. Breathing oxygen for 5 minutes will maintain
oxyhemoglobin saturation at 90% for about
6 minutes. As an alternative to breathing oxygen
for 5 minutes, the patient may take four vital
capacity breaths of oxygen over 30 seconds (or
eight vital capacity breaths over 60 seconds).

2. Alveolar carbon dioxide increases during any period of apnea independent of preoxygenation.

B. **Support of the Airway with the Induction of Anesthesia**

1. With the induction of anesthesia and the onset of apnea, ventilation and oxygenation are supported by the anesthesiologist using traditional methods (face mask, tracheal tube) or newer supralaryngeal airway support devices (LMA).

2. **The anesthesia face mask** is the most ubiquitous device used to deliver anesthetic gases and oxygen as well as to ventilate a patient who has been rendered apneic. Appropriate positioning of the patient's head and neck ("sniffing position") is paramount to successful mask ventilation.

   a. After induction of anesthesia, the face mask is held firmly on the patient's face with downward pressure on the mask applied by the anesthesiologist's thumb and first/second fingers with concurrent upward displacement of the mandible with the other fingers (known as a jaw thrust), which raises the soft tissues of the anterior airway off the pharyngeal wall and allows for improved ventilation.

   b. In patients who are obese, edentulous, or with beards, two hands may be required to ensure a tight-fitting face mask (when two hands are required a second operator is needed).

   c. In the presence of normal lung compliance the lung inflation pressure should not exceed 20 to 25 cm H_2O.

   d. If more pressure is required it may be prudent to consider other devices to aid in the creation of a patent upper airway (oral airway, a nasal airway, LMA) to create an artificial passage between the roof of the mouth, tongue, and posterior pharyngeal wall.

   e. Oral airways may provoke coughing, vomiting, and/or laryngospasm when placed into the pharynx of a semiconscious patient.

C. **Supraglottic Airways**

1. **Laryngeal mask airway** is composed of a small "mask" designed to sit in the hypopharynx with an aperture overlying the laryngeal inlet. The rim of the mask is comprised of an inflatable silicone cuff that fills the hypopharyngeal space, creating a seal that

allows positive-pressure ventilation with up to 20 cm H_2O pressure.

2. **The LMA and Gastroesophageal Reflux**
   a. The predominant clinical perception is that the LMA does not protect against pulmonary aspiration.
   b. The risk of it is minimal in patients at low risk of aspiration although the incidence of gastroesophageal reflux may be increased compared to the use of a face mask.

3. **LMA and Positive-Pressure Ventilation.** Contrary to the initial impression, positive-pressure ventilation can be safely accomplished with the LMA (limit airway pressures to 20 cm H_2O).

4. **The LMA and Bronchospasm.** As a supraglottic airway, the LMA appears to be well suited for patients with a history of bronchial asthma.

5. **LMA removal** should occur when the patient is deeply anesthetized or after protective upper airway reflexes have returned.

6. **Contraindications to LMA Use** (Table 22-2)

7. **LMA Use Complications** (Table 22-3)

D. **The LMA Proseal** (Table 22-4)

E. **The laryngeal tube** consists of a single-lumen tube with an approximately 130° midshaft angle and two (distal and proximal) low-pressure cuffs. When inserted correctly, the distal cuff seals the oral and nasal pharynx. Ventilation (spontaneous or positive pressure) occurs via the midcuff orifice.

TABLE 22-2

CONTRAINDICATIONS TO USE OF THE LARYNGEAL MASK AIRWAY

Risk of pulmonary aspiration of gastric contents ("full stomach" patient)
Hiatal hernia with significant gastroesophageal reflux
Morbid obesity
Intestinal obstruction
Delayed gastric emptying
Poor pulmonary compliance
Increased airway resistance
Glottic or subglottic airway obstruction
Limited mouth opening (<1.5 mm)

TABLE 22-3

COMPLICATIONS WITH USE OF THE LARYNGEAL MASK AIRWAY

Gastroesophageal reflux and aspiration
Laryngospasm
Coughing
Bronchospasm
Sore throat (less than tracheal intubation)
Transient changes in vocal cord function (possibly related to cuff overinflation during prolonged procedures)
Nerve injury (recurrent laryngeal, hypoglossal, lingual), LMA cuff pressure should not exceed 60 cm H_2O
Nitrous oxide may diffuse into cuff and increase pressure

F. **The Cobra pharyngeal laryngeal airway** is a disposable supralaryngneal device with a single lumen that terminates in a widened distal end. A fiberscope and/or tracheal tube may be passed through this device.

G. **Tracheal Intubation**
   1. **Routine Laryngoscopy.** Repeated attempts at tracheal intubation often result in edema and bleeding of the anterior upper airway structures hindering subsequent attempts at visualization and causing increased airway obstruction.

TABLE 22-4

FEATURES OF THE LMA PROSEAL

Feature	Clinical Impact
Gastric drain	Position confirmation
	Active gastric emptying
	Passive gastric emptying
	Protection from gastric content aspiration
Posterior cuff	Increased seal pressure
Bite block	Prevents patient biting obstruction
Wire-reinforced airway barrel	Reduced overall size
	Decreased ability to tracheally intubate
Large barrel/bite block configuration	First attempt insertion less successful than LMA classic
	Confers rotational stability
	Size choice—size down from LMA classic

2. **Direct Laryngoscopy.** Successful laryngoscopy involves the distortion of the normal anatomic planes of the supralaryngeal airway to produce a line of direct visualization ("sniff position of the patient's head") from the operator's eyes to the larynx (requires alignment of the oral, pharyngeal, and laryngeal axes) (Fig. 22-1).
   a. Lateral external pressure over the larynx may be applied in an attempt to improve the view of the laryngoscopist.
   b. The mouth can be opened by hyperextension of the atlanto-occipital joint using the laryngoscopist's hand placed under the patient's occiput or by application of downward pressure on the chin.
3. **Use of the Laryngoscope Blade** (Fig. 22-2)
   a. The laryngoscope blade is inserted into the right side of the patient's mouth (care taken not to compress the upper lip against the teeth or to rotate the blade on the upper incisors) and advanced toward the epiglottis as the tongue is displaced to the left.
   b. The Macintosh blade tip is advanced into the vallecula, whereas the Miller blade is advanced until it is positioned beneath the epiglottis while the laryngoscopist's arm and shoulder lifts in an anterior and caudad direction.
   c. The view of the larynx may be complete, partial, or not possible (Fig. 22-3).
   d. The tracheal tube is inserted with the right hand and passed through the vocal folds to a depth of at least 2 cm after the disappearance of the tracheal tube cuff past the vocal folds (represents midtrachea, which corresponds to the 21- and 23-cm external marking on the tracheal tube at the teeth for the typical adult woman and man, respectively).
   e. The gold standard for confirmation that the tube has been placed in the trachea is sustained detection of exhaled carbon dioxide as measured with capnography.
4. **NPO Status and Rapid-Sequence Induction.** In the rapid-sequence induction of anesthesia the intravenous administration of an induction drug is followed by a rapidly acting neuromuscular blocking drug. Direct laryngoscopy and tracheal intubation

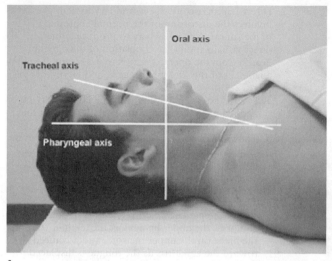

A

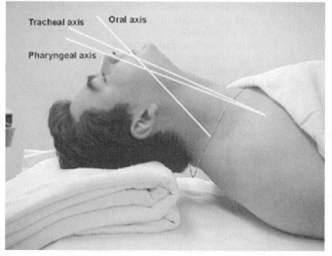

B

FIGURE 22-1. With the patient supine and no head support, the oral, pharyngeal, and tracheal axes do not overlap (**A**). The "sniff" position maximally overlaps the three axes (**B**).

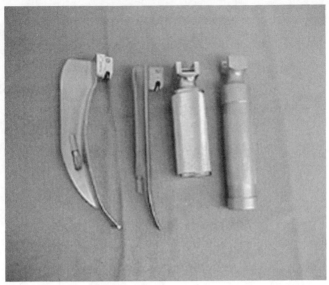

FIGURE 22-2. Macintosh (*curved*) and Miller (*straight*) laryngoscope blades and small and regular-sized handles.

are performed as soon as muscle relaxation is confirmed.

5. **The Intubating Laryngeal Mask Airway.** Blind fiberoptic aide, stylet-guided, and laryngoscopy-directed intubation via the LMA can be accomplished in adults and children.

   a. A limiting factor is the size of the tracheal tube that may be passed through the airway.

   b. **LMA-Fastrach** can accommodate up to an 8-mm cuffed tracheal tube and is indicated for routine elective intubation and for anticipated and unanticipated difficult intubation.

6. **Extubation of the trachea** is often performed after the return of consciousness (follow simple commands) and spontaneous ventilation (resolution of neuromuscular blockade). The patient who presented with a "difficult airway" at the time of induction of anesthesia must also be considered a "difficult extubation" at the time of extubation.

350 *Preparing for Anesthesia*

A

FIGURE 22-3. The Cormack and Lehane laryngeal view scoring system. **A.** Grade 1, visualization of the entire glottic aperture. **B.** Grade 2, visualization of only the posterior aspects of the glottic aperture. **C.** Grade 3, visualization of the tip of the epiglottis. **D.** Grade 4, visualization of no more than the soft palate.

a. **Laryngospasm** is a possible cause of airway compromise following tracheal extubation (treat by administration of oxygen with continuous positive airway pressure and if necessary the use of a small dose of a rapidly acting muscle relaxant). Negative-pressure pulmonary edema may result from airway obstruction in a patient who develops laryngospasm and who continues to create negative intrathoracic pressure as a result of voluntary respiratory effort.

b. **Approach to the difficult extubation.** When there is a suspicion that a patient may have difficulty with

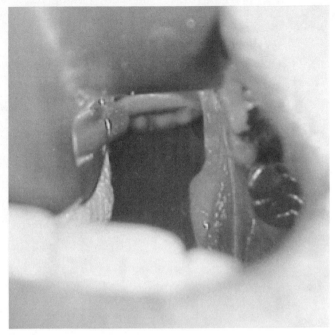

B

FIGURE 22-3. (*Continued*)

oxygenation or ventilation after tracheal
extubation, the clinician may choose from a variety
of management strategies (standby reintubation
equipment, placement of a guide for reintubation
and/or oxygenation).

III. THE DIFFICULT AIRWAY

A. The Difficult Airway Algorithm (Fig. 22-4)

1. A difficult airway is defined as the situation in which a
   conventionally trained anesthesiologist experiences
   difficulty with mask ventilation (unassisted
   anesthesiologist unable to maintain SpO_2 >90%
   using 100% oxygen) and/or inability to place a
   tracheal tube with conventional laryngoscopy

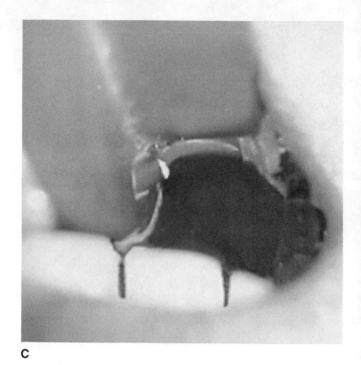

C

FIGURE 22-3. (*Continued*)

(more than three attempts or more than
10 minutes).

2. The incidence of failed tracheal intubation is
   estimated to be 0.05 to 0.35% and the incidence of
   failed intubation plus inability to achieve mask
   ventilation is estimated to be 0.01 to 0.03%.

3. Even if the patient's oxygen saturation remains
   adequate during unsuccessful attempts at tracheal
   intubation, it is prudent to limit the number of
   attempts to three because significant soft tissue trauma
   can result from multiple laryngoscopies. At this stage,
   the clinician may consider alternatives to direct
   laryngoscopy and tracheal intubation that include
   fiberoptic laryngoscopy, use of an LMA, or

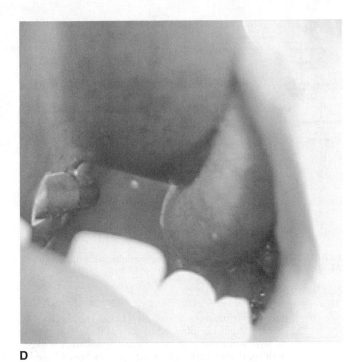

D

FIGURE 22-3. (*Continued*)

establishment of a surgical airway. In some instances, it may be best to allow the patient to resume spontaneous ventilation and awaken.

B. Awake Airway Management

1. Awake airway management (LMA, fiberoptic intubation) is indicated if after a thorough airway examination or a review of previous anesthetics, the ability to safely control ventilation and oxygenation, without the risk of pulmonary aspiration, is in question.

2. Important to the success of awake intubation techniques is administration of drugs to reduce anxiety and secretions.

3. Local anesthetics are a cornerstone of awake airway techniques (topical lidocaine, benzocaine spray,

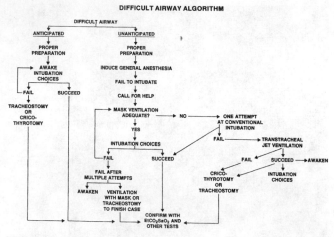

FIGURE 22-4. The American Society of Anesthesiologists' Difficult Airway Algorithm.

phenylephrine, oxymatazolone). Local anesthetic therapy should be directed to the nasal cavity/nasopharynx (cotton-tipped applicators soaked with local anesthetic solution), pharynx base of the tongue (aerosolized local anesthetic solution or voluntary "swish and swallow," superior laryngeal nerve block), and the larynx/trachea (transtracheal injection of local anesthetic solution).

C. Use of the Fiberoptic Bronchoscope in Airway Management
   1. The fiberoptic bronchoscope has proven to be the most versatile tool to the anesthesiologist dealing with the awake or unconscious patient who is or appears to be difficult to intubate.
   2. Use of the Fiberoptic Bronchoscope
      a. A variety of intubation airways are available and designed to provide a clear visual path from the oral aperture to the pharynx, keep the bronchoscope in the midline, prevent the patient from biting the insertion cord, and provide a clear airway for the spontaneously or mask-ventilated patients.

     b. After successful navigation through the supraglottic airway, the endoscopist visualizes the vocal folds. Once the larynx is entered, a landmark is selected (carina) to serve as an identifying landmark as the tracheal tube is advanced.

     c. An estimated 20 to 30% of tracheal tube advancements are accompanied by "hang up."

D. Video-Macintosh laryngoscope consists of a conventional appearing laryngoscope and a fiberoptic cable that enters the handle where the camera elements are housed. The video image is displayed and the operator or second operator directs the tube into position.

E. Retrograde wire intubation is performed with the patient in a sitting position by percutaneous placement of an 18-gauge catheter through the cricothyroid membrane, a radiographic guide wire placed through the catheter until it appears in the mouth, and a 7.0 tracheal tube placed over the wire and guided into the trachea.

F. Use of Esophageal Tracheal Combitube

    1. The tube is inserted blindly and the oropharyngeal balloon and distal cuff balloon are inflated.

    2. In the majority of patients tube placement results in an esophageal position and ventilation occurs via this lumen's hypopharyngeal perforations.

    3. Advantages include rapid airway control, airway protection from regurgitation, easy use by an inexperienced operator, no need to visualize the glottic opening, and ability to maintain the neck in a neutral position.

G. The LMA in the Failed Airway

    1. It is estimated that 1 in 10,000 patients cannot be ventilated by mask and cannot be intubated by traditional means, whereas it is estimated that 1 in 800,000 patients cannot be managed with an LMA.

    2. The major disadvantage of the LMA is the lack of mechanical protection from regurgitation and aspiration.

H. Minimally Invasive Transtracheal Procedures

    1. Cricothyrotomy is the procedure of choice in emergency situations.

    2. Percutaneous transtracheal jet ventilation is a form of cricothyrotomy that is an option in the "cannot ventilate/cannot intubate" situation (Table 22-5).

TABLE 22-5

PERCUTANEOUS TRANSTRACHEAL JET VENTILATION

Intravenous catheter (12, 14, 16 gauge) is attached to syringe (5 mL or larger) that is empty or partially filled with saline (alternatively a commercially available "Emergency Cricothyroidotomy Catheter" set is available).

Larynx is stabilized by the anesthesiologist's nondominant hand and the catheter needle is advanced through the caudad one-third of the cricothyroid membrane.

Constant aspiration on the syringe plunger is applied and free aspiration of air confirms entrance into the trachea.

Catheter is advanced into the trachea.

Oxygen source is attached (fresh gas outlet of anesthesia machine is acceptable by placing a cuffed tracheal tube into the barrel of a 5- to 10-mL syringe to engage the catheter while the 15-mm adapter of the tracheal tube is fitted into the fresh gas outlet of the anesthesia machine.

Manual closure of the mouth and nose may be needed during insufflation but not exhalation.

CHAPTER 23 ■ PATIENT POSITIONING

Positioning of a patient for a surgical procedure is frequently a compromise between what the anesthetized patient can tolerate (structurally and physiologically) and what the surgical team requires for anatomic access (Warner MA: Patient positioning. In Barash PG, Cullen BF, Stoelting RK [eds]: *Clinical Anesthesia*, pp 643–667. Philadelphia, Lippincott Williams & Wilkins, 2006). There is a lack of solid scientific information on basic mechanisms of position-related complications. Notations about positions used during anesthesia and surgery, as well as brief comments about special protective measures such as eye care and pressure-point padding, are useful information to include on the anesthesia record.

I. DORSAL DECUBITUS POSITIONS

A. **Physiology**
  1. **Circulatory.** In patients in the supine position, the influence of gravity on the vascular system is minimal.
     a. Intravascular pressures change by 2 mm Hg for every 2.5 cm that a given site varies in vertical height above or below the reference point at the heart. This is the reason to place transducers at the level of vital organs to be perfused (heart or brain).
     b. Head-down tilt (Trendelenburg position) increases cerebral venous pressure and intracranial pressure. Venous congestion and resultant edema may cause a "compartment syndrome" in areas within the head as vessels and nerves are squeezed as they traverse small bony spaces.
  2. **Respiratory.** Movement of abdominal viscera toward or away from the diaphragm in association with the head-up or head-down position influences the effectiveness of spontaneous ventilation.
B. **Variations of the Dorsal Decubitus Positions** (Table 23-1)
C. **Complications of the Dorsal Decubitus Positions** (Table 23-2)
D. **Brachial Plexus and Upper Extremity Injuries** (Table 23-3)

TABLE 23-1
DORSAL DECUBITUS POSITIONS

Supine

Horizontal (arms are padded and restrained alongside the trunk or abducted on padded arm boards; does not place hips and knees in a neutral position resulting in discomfort for awake patients)

Contour (arms as for horizontal position; slightly flex hip and knees; good for routine use)

Frog leg (lower extremities bent at hips and soles of feet together; permits access to the perineum and vagina for the surgeon standing at the side of the patient's abdomen)

Lithotomy

Standard (lower extremities flexed at hips and knees and simultaneously elevated to expose the perineum; at the end of surgery both legs are lowered together to minimize torsion stress on the lumbar spine)

Exaggerated (stresses the lumbar spine and restricts ventilation because of abdominal compression by the thighs)

Head-Down Tilt (avoid in patients with intracranial pathology)

Trendelenburg position (30 to 45 degrees head-down, which may necessitate shoulder braces placed over the acromioclavicular joint to prevent cephalad movement of the patient; risk of brachial plexus injury if shoulder braces improperly placed)

1. **Ulnar neuropathy** is characterized by an occurrence predominately in men (70 to 90%), high frequency of contralateral nerve dysfunction (suggests many patients have asymptomatic but abnormal ulnar nerves prior to their anesthetics), and appearance of symptoms often delayed (48 hours) after the surgical procedure.

TABLE 23-2
COMPLICATIONS OF DORSAL DECUBITUS POSITIONS

Postural hypotension (most common complication of head-up position; lower legs simultaneously from lithotomy position if patient is hypovolemic)

Pressure alopecia (use padded head supports)

Pressure-point reactions (heels, elbows, sacrum; protects against skin and soft tissue compression and ischemia but no evidence beneficial in reducing peripheral neuropathies in the perioperative period)

TABLE 23-3
BRACHIAL PLEXUS AND UPPER EXTREMITY INJURIES

Brachial plexus neuropathy (most likely if the head is turned away from an excessively abducted arm; may be associated with first rib fracture during median sternotomy)

Long thoracic nerve dysfunction (winging of the scapula reflecting serratus anterior muscle dysfunction, consider viral origin)

Radial nerve compression (vertical bar of screen forces nerve against the humerus; wrist drop)

Ulnar nerve compression (trauma occurs as the nerve passes behind medial epicondyle of the humerus; sensory loss of the fifth finger and lateral border of the fourth finger)

Lumbar backache (ligamentous relaxation during anesthesia; lithotomy position worsens pain because of a herniated intervertebral disk)

Compartment syndrome (characterized by systemic hypotension and impaired perfusion pressure to legs that is augmented by elevation of the extremities; decompressive fasciotomies necessary to relieve increased tissue pressure)

2. Elbow flexion (>110 degrees) can cause ulnar nerve damage by compression of the nerve by the aponeurosis of the flexor carpi ulnaris muscle and cubital retinaculum. Conversely, in some patients the roof of the cubital is poorly formed such that the ulnar nerve subluxes over the medial epicondyle of the humerus during elbow flexion producing recurrent mechanical trauma.

3. External compression in the absence of elbow flexion may occur within the condylar groove or distal to the medial epicondyle where the nerve and its associated artery are relatively superficial.

4. Anatomic differences between men and women (tubercle of the coronoid process is approximately 1.5 times larger in men, less adipose tissue over the medial aspect of the elbow in men, thicker flexor cubital retinaculum in men) may explain the higher incidence of ulnar nerve neuropathy in men.

5. The time of recognition of digital anesthesia associated with ulnar nerve dysfunction may be important in establishing the origin of the postoperative syndrome.

   a. If ulnar hypesthesia or anesthesia is noted promptly after the end of anesthesia (in the postanesthesia care unit) it is likely to be associated with events that occurred during anesthesia and surgery.

b. If recognition is delayed for many hours, the likelihood of cause shifts to postoperative events despite accepted methods of padding and positioning during the intraoperative period.

c. Opioids may mask dysthesia and pain postoperatively but not loss of sensation as a result of nerve dysfunction. It may be helpful to assess ulnar nerve function and record these observations before discharging patients from the postanesthesia care unit.

II. LATERAL DECUBITUS POSITIONS

A. **Physiology**

1. **Circulatory.** In the low-pressure pulmonary circuit, there is overperfusion of the dependent lung and relative hypoperfusion of the lung that is positioned superiorly.

   a. A small support should be placed just caudad to the down-side axilla ("axillary roll" is a misnomer as it should not be placed in the axilla) so as to lift the thorax enough to relieve pressure on the axillary neurovascular bundle and prevent decreased blood flow to the hand.

   b. This support has not been proven to decrease the frequency of ischemia, nerve damage, or compartment syndrome to the down-side upper

---

TABLE 23-4

LATERAL DECUBITUS POSITIONS

Standard (Horizontal) Lateral Position
Flex the down-side thigh and knee, pillows placed between the legs and under the head to maintain alignment of the cervical and thoracic spines

Flexed Lateral Positions
Lateral jackknife (down-side iliac crest is over the table hinge to allow stretch of the up-side flank; venous pooling occurs in the legs)
Kidney (elevated table rest under the iliac crest further increases lateral flexion to expose kidney; venous pooling and ventilation-to-perfusion mismatch may occur)

TABLE 23-5

COMPLICATIONS OF LATERAL DECUBITUS POSITIONS

Damage to the eyes and/or ears (avoid pressure)
Neck injury (lateral flexion is a risk, especially in arthritic patients)
Suprascapular nerve injury (placement of a pad caudad to the
   dependent axilla prevents circumduction of the nerve; injury
   manifests as diffuse shoulder pain)
Long thoracic nerve dysfunction may reflect lateral flexion of the
   neck and stretch of the nerve

---

       extremity but it may decrease postoperative
       shoulder discomfort.
   c. Dependent venous pooling is minimized by
       compressive wrappings applied to the legs and
       thighs.
  2. Respiratory. Ventilation tends to be directed to the
       more compliant superiorly positioned lung, resulting
       in hyperventilation of this underperfused lung and
       hypoventilation of the overperfused dependent lung.
 B. **Variations of the Lateral Decubitus Positions** (Table 23-4)
 C. **Complications of the Lateral Decubitus Positions**
   (Table 23-5)

III. VENTRAL DECUBITUS (PRONE) POSITIONS

 A. **Physiology**
  1. Circulatory. Pressure on compressed viscera is
       transmitted to mesenteric and paravertebral vessels,
       resulting in increased venous bleeding.
  2. Respiratory. Compressed abdominal viscera force the
       diaphragm cephalad. Support provided by pads under
       the shoulder girdle and pelvis allow the abdomen to
       hang free, thus minimizing loss of functional residual
       capacity and obstruction to venous return.
 B. **Variations of the Ventral Decubitus Positions** (Table 23-6)
 C. **Complications of the Ventral Decubitus Positions** (Table
   23-7)
  1. Blindness following nonocular surgery may reflect
       compromise of oxygen delivery to elements of the
       visual pathway and include ischemic optic neuropathy,
       retinal artery occlusion, and cortical blindness.
  2. Blindness following spinal surgery that is unrelated to
       external compression on the globe has been associated
       with prolonged surgery in the prone position that may

TABLE 23-6

VENTRAL DECUBITUS POSITIONS

Full prone (use supportive pads under the abdomen)
Prone jackknife
Kneeling

> be accompanied by intraoperative anemia
> (hemoglobin concentrations <8 g/dL) and
> intraoperative hypotension. Venous congestion in the
> head associated with the prone position may also be a
> contributing factor.

IV. HEAD-ELEVATED POSITIONS

A. The sitting position permits improved surgical exposure
for operations involving the posterior fossa and cervical
spine.
1. Mean arterial pressure should be measured at the level
of the circle of Willis (transducer placed at the level of
the external ear canal) because this site is an accurate
reflection of the perfusion pressure to the brain.
2. Compressive wraps about the legs decrease pooling of
blood in the lower extremities.
B. Complications of the Head-Elevated Positions
(Table 23-8)

V. PERIOPERATIVE PERIPHERAL NEUROPATHIES

A. **Prevention** (Table 23-9)

TABLE 23-7

COMPLICATIONS OF VENTRAL DECUBITUS POSITIONS

Eyes and ears (avoid pressure; consider use of protective goggles)
Blindness
Neck injury (an arthritic neck may be best managed in the sagittal
plane; head rotation may decrease carotid and vertebral blood
flows)
Brachial plexus injuries
Thoracic outlet syndrome (may be useful to ask patients
preoperatively if they are able to sleep with their arms elevated
overhead)
Breast injuries
Impaired venous return (use supportive pads under the abdomen)

TABLE 23-8

COMPLICATIONS OF THE SITTING POSITION

Postural hypotension (normal compensatory reflexes are inhibited by anesthesia)

Air embolus (potential increases with the degree of elevation or the operative site above the heart air can pass through a probe patent foramen ovale if right atrial pressure exceeds left atrial pressure)

Pneumocephalus

Ocular compression

Edema of the face and tongue

Midcervical tetraplegia

Sciatic nerve injury

B. Practical Considerations
   1. Padding Exposed Peripheral Nerves
      a. Many types of padding are available to protect exposed peripheral nerves. There are no data to suggest that one material is more effective than another or that any padding is better than no padding.
      b. The goal is to position and pad exposed peripheral nerves to prevent their stretch beyond normally tolerated limits while awake, avoid direct compression of peripheral nerves if possible, and distribute over as large an area as possible any compressive forces that must be placed on the peripheral nerve.
   2. Prolonged Duration in One Position
      a. Prolonged duration in the lithotomy position increases the risk of lower extremity neuropathy.
      b. It may be prudent to limit as much as practical the time spent in a single position. However, intermittent movement of the limbs or head during the intraoperative period may increase the risk of other problems including moving an extremity into a suboptimal position.
C. Course of Action for the Patient with a Neuropathy
   1. Is the Neuropathy Sensory or Motor?
      a. Sensory symptoms are usually transient (many resolve in first 5 days). Typically, the patient is reassured and advised to avoid postures that might compress or stretch the involved nerve. If

TABLE 23-9

SUMMARY OF AMERICAN SOCIETY OF ANESTHESIOLOGISTS' ADVISORY ON PREVENTION OF PERIPHERAL NEUROPATHIES

Preoperative Assessment
When appropriate it is helpful to determine if patients can comfortably tolerate the position required for the planned operation.

Upper Extremity Positioning
Arm abduction should be limited to 90 degrees in supine patients.
Arms should be positioned to decrease pressure on the postcondylar groove of the humerus (tucked at side in a neutral forearm position or abducted on arm boards in either a neutral or supinated forearm position).

Lower Extremity Positioning
Lithotomy positions may stretch the sciatic nerve.
Prolonged pressure on the peroneal nerve at the fibular head should be avoided.

Protective Padding
Padded armboards may decrease the risk of upper extremity neuropathy.
Padding at the elbow and at the fibular head may decrease the risk of neuropathies.

Equipment
Properly functioning automatic blood pressure cuffs on the upper arms do not affect the risk of neuropathies.
Shoulder braces in steep head-down positions may increase the risk of brachial plexus neuropathies.

Postoperative Assessment
Assessment of extremity nerve function may lead to early recognition of peripheral neuropathies.

Documentation
Charting specific positioning actions during the care of the patient may result in improvements of care.

symptoms persist a consultation with a neurologist may be indicated.
b. If the neuropathy has a motor component a neurologist should be consulted promptly because electromyographic studies may be needed to assess the location of any acute lesion as well as to determine the presence of any chronic abnormalities such as in the contralateral but asymptomatic extremity.

CHAPTER 24 ■ MONITORING THE ANESTHETIZED PATIENT

Monitoring represents the process by which anesthesiologists recognize and evaluate potential physiologic problems by identifying prognostic trends in patients in a timely manner (Murphy GS, Vender JS: Monitoring the anesthetized patient. In Barash PG, Cullen BF, Stoelting RK [eds]: *Clinical Anesthesia*, pp 668–687. Philadelphia, Lippincott Williams & Wilkins, 2006). Effective monitoring decreases the potential for poor outcomes that may follow anesthesia by identifying derangements before they result in serious or irreversible injury. Monitoring devices increase the specificity and precision of clinical judgments. Standards for Basic Anesthesia Monitoring have been adopted by the American Society of Anesthesiologists (see Appendix).

I. INSPIRATORY AND EXPIRED GAS MONITORING

A. The concentration of oxygen in the anesthetic circuit must be measured. Manufacturers of gas machines place oxygen sensors on the inspired limb of the anesthesia circuit to ensure that hypoxic gas mixtures are not delivered to patients. Monitoring inspired oxygen concentration does not guarantee the adequacy of arterial oxygenation.

B. **Monitoring of Expired Gases**
1. Monitoring of expiratory CO_2 (end-tidal CO_2 or $PETCO_2$) has evolved as an important physiologic and safety procedure for **identifying placement** of the endotracheal tube (does not confirm placement above the carina) and for **assessing variables** such as ventilation ($PaCO_2$), rebreathing, cardiac output, distribution of blood flow, and metabolic activity.
2. **Capnometry** is the measurement and numeric representation of the CO_2 concentration (mm Hg).
   a. **Capnogram** is a continuous concentration-time display of the CO_2 concentration (divided into four distinct phases) sampled at the patient's airway during ventilation (Fig. 24-1).

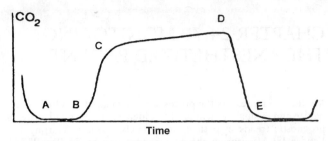

FIGURE 24-1. The capnogram is divided into four distinct phases. The first phase (A-B) represents the initial stage of expiration (gas from anatomic dead space) and is usually devoid of CO_2. At point B, CO_2-containing gas is present at the sampling site and a sharp upstroke (B-C) is seen in the capnogram. Phase C-D represents the ventilation-weighted average concentration of CO_2 in alveolar gas. Point D is the highest value and is designated the end-tidal CO_2 concentration. At point D, the patient begins to inspire CO_2-free gas, and there is a steep downstroke (D-E) back to baseline. Normally, unless rebreathing of CO_2 occurs, the baseline approaches zero.

    b. Capnography is the continuous monitoring of the patient's capnogram.
  3. The end-tidal CO_2 concentration provides a clinical estimate of the $PaCO_2$, assuming ventilation and perfusion in the lungs are appropriately matched (normal gradient is 5 to 10 mm Hg) and no sampling errors occur during measurement (sidestream analyzers can dilute a patient's tidal breath with fresh gas, especially when tidal volume is small, as in the young patient; loose connections and system leaks also dilute end-tidal CO_2).
    a. Dead space (ventilation without perfusion) and a resulting increase in the difference between the $PaCO_2$ and the end-tidal CO_2 (dead space gases containing little or no CO_2 greatly dilute the end-tidal CO_2 concentration) may reflect hypoperfusion states, chronic obstructive pulmonary disease, and embolic phenomena (thrombus, air).
    b. Shunt (perfusion without ventilation) causes minimal changes in the gradient between $PaCO_2$ and end-tidal CO_2.
  4. Capnography has decreased the potential for unrecognized accidental esophageal intubation.

TABLE 24-1

EXPLANATION FOR CHANGES IN THE END-TIDAL CO_2 CONCENTRATION

Increases	Decreases
Hypoventilation	Hyperventilation
Hyperthermia	Hypothermia
Sepsis	Hypoperfusion
Malignant hyperthermia	Pulmonary embolism
Rebreathing	Slowed metabolism
Increased skeletal muscle activity	

    a. Because the esophageal or gastric gas concentration is primarily composed of inspired gas, it should contain exceedingly small amounts of CO_2. After an accidental esophageal intubation, the first one or two "breaths" may contain some CO_2, but the concentration should approach zero after four or five "breaths."

    b. A continuous stable CO_2 waveform ensures the presence of alveolar ventilation (tube in the trachea) but does not necessarily indicate that the endotracheal tube is properly positioned above the carina.

5. Common etiologies of gradual increases or decreases in end-tidal CO_2 reflect changes in CO_2 production or changes in CO_2 elimination (Table 24-1).

6. A sudden decrease in end-tidal CO_2 to near zero requires a rapid assessment of possible causes (Table 24-2).

7. The adequacy of cardiopulmonary resuscitation can be assessed by capnography, as reflected by a

TABLE 24-2

EXPLANATIONS FOR ABRUPT DECREASES IN THE END-TIDAL CO_2 CONCENTRATION

Malposition of tracheal tube into the pharynx or esophagus
Disruption of airway integrity (disconnection or obstruction)
Disruption of sampling line
Pulmonary embolism
Low cardiac output
Cardiac arrest

TABLE 24-3

INFORMATION DERIVED FROM THE CAPNOGRAM WAVEFORM

Slow Rate of Rise of Upstroke
Chronic obstructive pulmonary disease
Acute airway obstruction

Normally Shaped but Increased End-Tidal CO_2 Concentration
Alveolar hypoventilation
Increased CO_2 production

Transient Increases in End-Tidal CO_2 Concentration
Tourniquet release/aortic unclamping
Administration of bicarbonate
Insufflation of CO_2 during laparoscopy

Failure of the Baseline to Return to Zero
Rebreathing

reappearance or an increase in end-tidal CO_2 with
restoration of pulmonary blood flow.

8. The size and shape of the capnogram waveform can
be informative (Table 24-3).

C. **Multiple Expired Gas Analysis**

1. Intraoperative breath-by-breath analysis of
respiratory (O_2, CO_2, N_2) and anesthetic gases is
achieved by mass spectrometry or Raman
spectroscopy (RASCAL is an instrument using this
technology).

2. Many critical events can be detected by analysis of
respiratory and anesthetic gases (Table 24-4).

3. Nitrogen monitoring provides quantification of
washout during preoxygenation. A sudden increase
in the N_2 concentration in the exhaled gas indicates
either introduction of air from leaks in the
anesthesia delivery system or venous air embolism.

II. OXYGENATION MONITORING

A. **Pulse oximetry** (measurement of the peripheral O_2
saturation of hemoglobin [SpO_2] on a continual basis)
is the **standard of care for measuring oxygenation**
during anesthesia and in the postanesthesia care unit.

1. Overwhelming evidence supports the capability of
pulse oximetry for detecting desaturation before it is
clinically apparent.

TABLE 24-4

GAS ANALYSIS AND THE DETECTION OF CRITICAL EVENTS

Event	Monitored Gas
Error in gas delivery system	Oxygen
	Carbon dioxide
	Nitrogen
	Inhaled anesthetic
Anesthesia machine malfunction	Oxygen
	Carbon dioxide
	Nitrogen
	Inhaled anesthetic
Disconnection	Carbon dioxide
	Oxygen
	Inhaled anesthetic
Vaporizer malfunction or contamination	Volatile anaesthetic
Anesthesia circuit leaks	Nitrogen
	Carbon dioxide
Tracheal tube cuff leaks	Nitrogen
	Carbon dioxide
Poor mask fit	Nitrogen
	Carbon dioxide
Air embolism	Nitrogen
	Carbon dioxide
Hypoventilation	Carbon dioxide
Airway obstruction	Carbon dioxide
Malignant hyperthermia	Carbon dioxide
Circuit hypoxia	Oxygen

2. No definitive data demonstrate a decrease in morbidity and mortality associated with the use of pulse oximetry.

B. Pulse oximetry combines the use of plethysmography and spectrophotometric analysis (light-emitting diodes are sources of two wavelengths of light that are passed through an arterial bed represented by a finger or ear lobe).

1. Absorption of specific wavelengths of light relative to the ratio of oxyhemoglobin (pulsatile signal) is transmitted to a photodetector to calculate SpO_2 on a noninvasive, continuous basis.

a. The absence of a pulsatile waveform limits the ability of a pulse oximeter to calculate the SpO_2.

b. A relationship exists between hemoglobin saturation and oxygen tension (mm Hg) as

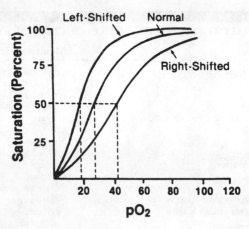

FIGURE 24-2. The relationship between arterial hemoglobin saturation with oxygen (%) and PO_2 is represented by the sigmoid-shaped oxyhemoglobin dissociation curve.

        depicted by the oxyhemoglobin dissociation curve (Fig. 24-2).

    c. The SpO_2 measured by pulse oximetry is not the same as the arterial saturation (SaO_2) measured by a laboratory co-oximeter. In clinical circumstances where other hemoglobin moieties are present in low concentrations (methemoglobin, carboxyhemoglobin), the SpO_2 value is higher than the SaO_2 reported by the blood gas laboratory.

  2. Many factors may influence the accuracy or ability of the pulse oximeter to calculate SpO_2 (Table 24-5).

III. BLOOD PRESSURE MONITORING

  A. Intraoperative measurement and recording of arterial blood pressure (at least every 5 minutes) are important indicators of the adequacy of circulation.

    1. Changes in systolic blood pressure correlate with changes in myocardial oxygen requirements.

    2. Changes in diastolic blood pressure reflect coronary perfusion pressure.

TABLE 24-5

FACTORS THAT INFLUENCE ACCURACY OF PULSE OXIMETRY

Absence of a Pulsatile Waveform
Hypothermia
Hypotension
Altered vascular resistance (vasoactive drugs)

Factitiously High SpO$_2$
Increased carboxyhemoglobin concentration
Increased methemoglobin concentration (SpO$_2$ tends to be 85% regardless of the actual SaO$_2$ or PaO$_2$)

Motion
Awake patient
Shivering

Extraneous Light Sources

Factitiously Low SpO$_2$
Methylene blue
Fingernail polish

3. Mean arterial pressure represents the "hydrostatic force" that powers diffusion and filtration functions. Mean arterial pressure (P) is often used in conjunction with resistance (R) when estimating cardiac output or tissue perfusion (Q). Rearranged, this equation becomes $Q = P/R$.

B. **Indirect Measurement of Arterial Blood Pressure**

1. The simplest method of blood pressure determination estimates systolic blood pressure by palpating the return of the arterial pulse or Doppler sounds while an occluding cuff is deflated.

2. **Auscultation** of Korotkoff sounds (result from turbulent flow within an artery in response to the mechanical deformation from the blood pressure cuff) is a common method of blood pressure measurement.

   a. Systolic blood pressure is considered to be equivalent to the appearance of the first Korotkoff sound, whereas disappearance of the sounds or a muffled tone is considered to be equivalent to the diastolic blood pressure. Mean arterial pressure is calculated as the diastolic blood pressure plus one-third of the pulse

TABLE 24-6

MECHANICAL ERRORS ASSOCIATED WITH AUSCULTATORY MEASUREMENT OF BLOOD PRESSURE

Falsely High Estimates of Blood Pressure
Cuff too small (bladder width should approximate 40% of the circumference of the extremity)
Cuff applied too loosely
Uneven compression of the underlying artery
Extremity is below heart level

Falsely Low Estimates of Blood Pressure
Cuff too large
Cuff deflation at a rate more rapid than 3 mm Hg per second
Extremity is above heart level

pressure (systolic blood pressure minus diastolic blood pressure).
   b. The detection of sound changes is subjective, requires pulsatile flow (unreliable during low flow), and is prone to mechanical errors (Table 24-6).
3. **Automated oscillometry** has replaced auscultatory and palpatory techniques for routine intraoperative blood pressure monitoring.
   a. Oscillometry accurately measures systolic blood pressure, diastolic blood pressure, and mean arterial pressure (discrepancy with centrally placed arterial line <5 mm Hg).
   b. A variety of cuff sizes makes it possible to use oscillometry in all age groups.
   c. **Complications** may accompany repeated inflations of automatically cycled blood pressure cuffs placed on the upper extremity (Table 24-7).
C. **Invasive Measurement of Vascular (Arterial Blood) Pressure**
   1. Indwelling arterial cannulation not only offers anesthesiologists the opportunity to monitor beat-to-beat changes in arterial blood pressure but also provides vascular access for arterial blood sampling.
   2. Intra-arterial measurement of blood pressure is subject to many sources of error based on the physical properties of fluid motion and the performance of the catheter-transducer-amplification

TABLE 24-7

PROBLEMS ASSOCIATED WITH NONINVASIVE AUTOMATIC CYCLED CUFF-BASED

Blood Pressure Monitoring Systems
Edema of the extremity
Petechiae formation
Ulnar neuropathy (apply encircling cuff proximal to the ulnar
groove)
Interference with timing of intravenous drug administration when
access site is located in the same extremity as monitoring system
Hydrostatic effect (correct by adding or subtracting 0.7 mm Hg
for every centimeter the cuff is above or below the level of the
heart)

system used to sense, process, and display the
pressure pulse wave. Ideally, the catheter and
tubings are stiff, the volume of fluid in the
connecting tubing is small, the number of
stopcocks is limited, and the connecting tubing
length is not excessive.

3. Because many therapeutic decisions are based on
changes in arterial blood pressure, it is imperative
that anesthesiologists understand the physical
limitations imposed by fluid-filled pressure
transducer systems.

   a. In clinical practice, underdamped
   catheter–transducer systems tend to overestimate
   systolic blood pressure by 15 to 30 mm Hg and
   to amplify artifact ("catheter whip").

   b. Air bubbles cause overdamping and
   underestimation of systolic blood pressure.

   c. Mean arterial pressure is accurately measured
   even in the presence of overdamping or
   underdamping.

   d. In clinical practice, it is sufficient to calibrate the
   transducer to atmospheric pressure, usually with
   the transducer located at the level of the right
   atrium.

4. **Arterial Cannulation**

   a. The radial artery remains the most popular site
   for cannulation because of its accessibility and
   the presence of a collateral blood supply
   (Fig. 24-3).

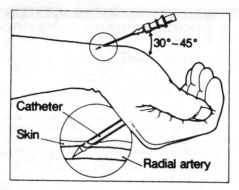

FIGURE 24-3. Technique for radial artery cannulation.

    b. The prognostic value of the Allen test in assessing the adequacy of the ulnar collateral circulation has not been confirmed.

5. Complications of Invasive Arterial Monitoring (Table 24-8)

    a. Traumatic cannulation has been associated with median nerve dysfunction, hematoma formation, and thrombosis.

    b. Abnormal radial artery blood flow following the removal of an arterial catheter (nontapered 20- to 22-gauge Teflon catheter recommended) occurs frequently (presumably because of radial artery thrombosis), with normalization of blood flow usually occurring in 3 to 70 days.

6. Direct arterial pressure monitoring requires constant vigilance and correlation of the measured blood pressure with other clinical parameters before therapeutic interventions are initiated.

    a. Sudden increases or decreases in blood pressure may represent a hydrostatic error because the position of the transducer was not adjusted following changes in the position of the operating room table.

    b. A sudden decrease in blood pressure may be caused by a damped tracing because the arterial catheter is partially occluded or kinked.

TABLE 24-8

CANNULATION SITE FOR DIRECT ARTERIAL BLOOD
PRESSURE MONITORING

Site	Clinical Points
Radial artery	Preferred cannulation site
	Ischemia most likely reflects arterial thrombosis
	Aneurysm formation
	Arteriovenous fistula formation
	Infection
	Fluid overload in neonates from continuous flush techniques (3–6 mL/hr)
Ulnar artery	Complications similar to those of radial artery
	Principal source of blood flow to the hand
Brachial artery	Insertion site medial to biceps tendon
	Median nerve damage
Axillary artery	Insertion site at junction of pectoralis major and deltoid muscles
Femoral artery	Easy access in low-flow states
	Potential for local and retroperitoneal hemorrhage
	Catheter with increased length preferred
Dorsalis pedis artery	Collateral circulation via posterior tibial artery
	Higher systolic blood pressure

    c. Before initiating therapy based on a change in blood pressure, the calibration of the transducer system and the patency of the arterial cannula should be verified.

IV. CENTRAL VENOUS AND PULMONARY ARTERY MONITORING

  A. The **right internal jugular vein** is preferred as an access site (Table 24-9 and Figs. 24-4, 24-5, and 24-6).

  B. **Central Venous Pressure Monitoring**

    1. Central venous pressure is essentially equivalent to right atrial pressure, and the normal waveform consists of three peaks (a, c, and v waves) and two descents (x, y) (Table 24-10 and Fig. 24-7).

    2. The possibility of venous air embolism is decreased by positioning the patient in a head-down position during placement or removal of the central venous catheter.

TABLE 24-9
CENTRAL VENOUS PRESSURE CANNULATION SITES

Site	Advantages	Disadvantages
Right internal jugular vein	Accessible from head of operating room table Predictable anatomy High success rate in both adults and children Good landmarks	Carotid artery puncture Trauma to the brachial plexus Pneumothorax
Left internal jugular vein	Same as for right internal	Damage to thoracic duct Difficulty in maneuvering catheter through the jugular-subclavian junction Carotid artery puncture and embolization of the left dominant cerebral hemisphere
External jugular vein	Superficial location Safety	Lower success rate Kinks at subclavian vein
Subclavian vein	Accessible Good landmarks	Pneumothorax Hemothorax Chylothorax Pleural effusion
Antecubital vein	Few complications	Lowest success rate Thrombosis Thrombophlebitis
Femoral vein	High success rate	Catheter sepsis Thrombophlebitis

3. Central venous catheter placement is an important source of nosocomial infection and sepsis. This emphasizes the importance of sterile technique during catheter placement and of the application of appropriate dressings (Table 24-11).

C. **Pulmonary Artery Monitoring**

1. **Indications** for placement of a pulmonary artery catheter are broadly defined (measure intracardiac pressures, thermodilution cardiac output, and mixed venous oxygen saturations; calculate derived hemodynamic indices). The measured and derived information is used to help define the clinical

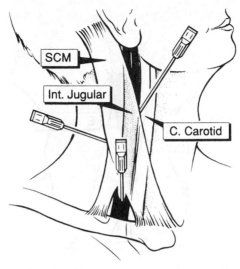

FIGURE 24-4. Three anatomic approaches for placement of a catheter in the internal jugular vein. The patient is placed head-down with the head turned away from the intended venipuncture site. A 22-gauge locator needle may be inserted initially to identify the vein and thus minimize the likelihood of accidental carotid artery puncture when placing the larger needle. Return of desaturated blood or transduction of the catheter (venous pressure) confirms entry into the internal jugular vein.

problem, monitor the progression of hemodynamic dysfunction, and guide the response to therapy.
  a. Pulmonary artery catheter monitoring may decrease perioperative complications if its use is tailored to the clinical condition of the patient as it changes with time.
  b. The American Society of Anesthesiologists has developed Practice Guidelines for Pulmonary Artery Catheterization.
2. Correct placement of the pulmonary artery catheter is most often guided by observing changes in vascular waveforms (Fig. 24-8).
3. Pulmonary capillary wedge pressure is used to indirectly assess left ventricular end-diastolic volume by reflecting changes in left ventricular end-diastolic pressure. Right-sided filling pressures often are poor

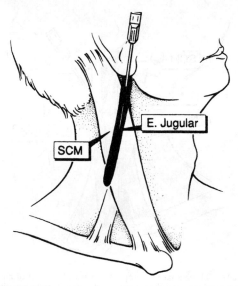

FIGURE 24-5. Placement of a catheter in the external jugular vein.

    indicators of left ventricular filling, either as absolute numbers or in terms of direction of change in response to therapy.

  4. Factors affecting the accuracy of pulmonary artery catheter data (Table 24-12).

  5. Adverse Effects of Pulmonary Artery Catheter Monitoring (Tables 24-13 and 24-14)

D. Mixed Venous Oximetry

  1. Advances in fiberoptic technology have led to the development of pulmonary artery catheters that can continuously measure **mixed venous** oxygen saturation (SvO_2).

  2. SvO_2 varies directly with cardiac output, hemoglobin concentration, and SaO_2 and inversely with minute oxygen consumption.

    a. When all other variables are constant, SvO_2 reflects corresponding changes in cardiac output.

    b. The normal SvO_2 is 75% and anaerobic metabolism occurs when SvO_2 is <30%.

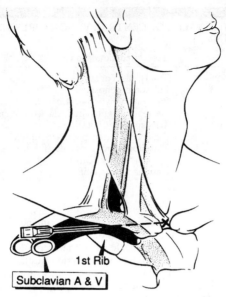

FIGURE 24-6. Placement of a catheter (infraclavicular approach) in the subclavian vein. The patient is placed head-down with the head turned away from the intended venipuncture site. Placing a roll between the scapulas opens the space between the clavicle and first rib. The needle is inserted 1 cm below the midpoint of the clavicle and advanced toward the anesthesiologist's finger in the suprasternal notch, keeping close to the posterior surface of the clavicle. Return of desaturated blood or transduction of the catheter (venous pressure) confirms entry into the subclavian vein.

V. INDICATOR DILUTION APPLICATIONS

A. **Thermodilution cardiac output determination** is the most widely used adaptation of the indicator dilution principle. Cooled 5% dextrose or 0.9% saline is injected into the proximal (central venous) port of a thermodilution pulmonary artery catheter, and a thermistor in the distal end of the catheter records the decrease in temperature between the two points, which is proportional to blood flow or cardiac output.

B. Comparison studies suggest that either room temperature or an iced injectate can be used, but the

TABLE 24-10

DIAGNOSTIC VALUE OF CENTRAL VENOUS PRESSURE WAVEFORMS

Waveform	Associated Conditions
Large a waves	Tricuspid stenosis
	Pulmonic stenosis
	Pulmonary hypertension
	Decreased right ventricular compliance
Large v waves	Tricuspid regurgitation
	Right ventricular papillary muscle ischemia and/or right ventricular failure
	Constrictive pericarditis
	Cardiac tamponade

iced injectate produces a more exacting curve with a better signal-to-noise ratio.

1. When properly performed (maintaining consistency of injection volume and injection rate), thermodilution cardiac output measurements correlate with direct Fick's and dye dilution determinations.
2. False high thermodilution cardiac output determinations occur when the injectate volume is too small (incomplete filling of syringe, leaks) or

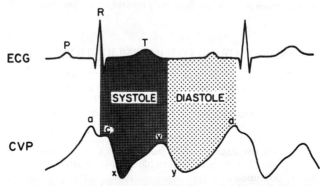

FIGURE 24-7. Central venous pressure (CVP) waveforms in relation to electrical events on the electrocardiogram (ECG).

TABLE 24-11

COMPLICATIONS COMMON TO ALL CENTRAL VENOUS PRESSURE CATHETER PLACEMENT TECHNIQUES

Accidental arterial puncture (hematoma, false aneurysm, arteriovenous fistula)
Poor positioning of catheter during placement (vascular or cardiac chamber perforation, cardiac dysrhythmias)
Injury to surrounding structures
Clot and fibrinous sleeve formation
Thrombosis of the vein (embolus)
Catheter-related sepsis (guidelines for prevention of catheter-related infections developed by the Centers for Disease Control and Prevention)
Bleeding

when a thrombus insulates the pulmonary artery catheter thermistor.

3. Alterations in right-sided cardiac output vary during inhalation and exhalation, such that thermodilution cardiac output measurements made with injection

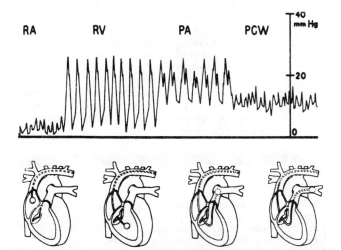

FIGURE 24-8. Pressure tracing observed during flotation of a pulmonary artery catheter through the right atrium (RA), right ventricle (RV), pulmonary artery (PA), and into a pulmonary capillary wedge (PCW) position.

TABLE 24-12

FACTORS AFFECTING THE ACCURACY OF PULMONARY ARTERY CATHETER DATA

Pulmonary vascular resistance (any increase [disease or drug-induced] alters the relationship between pulmonary capillary wedge pressure and pulmonary artery end-diastolic pressure).

Alveolar–pulmonary artery pressure relationships (flow-directed pulmonary artery catheters usually advance to gravity-dependent areas of highest pulmonary blood flow; confirm location of catheter by a lateral chest x-ray).

Intracardiac factors (mitral stenosis interferes with validity of left atrial pressure as a reflection of left ventricular end-diastolic pressure; decreased left ventricular compliance interferes with the validity of pulmonary capillary wedge pressure as a reflection of left ventricular end-diastolic pressure).

timed to peak inspiration and end-expiration have less variability.

4. Repetition of injections should be delayed for at least 90 seconds to allow for a steady thermal environment.
   a. In clinical practice, triplicate determinations are averaged to increase accuracy (differences <15% are not of clinical significance).
   b. It is important to consider sources of error in measurement of thermodilution cardiac outputs before initiating changes in clinical treatment based on this measurement.
5. **Clinical Benefits of Pulmonary Artery Monitoring.** Perioperative outcomes have been reported to be improved, worsened, or unchanged by pulmonary artery catheter useage.

TABLE 24-13

COMPLICATIONS OF PULMONARY ARTERY CATHETER PASSAGE

Cardiac dysrhythmias (most common complication, usually transient)
Catheter knotting, kinking, or coiling
Cardiac valve damage
Heart block
Perforation of pulmonary artery, right atrium, or right ventricle
Trauma to right ventricular endocardium

TABLE 24-14

COMPLICATIONS OF PULMONARY ARTERY CATHETER
PRESENCE

Thrombosis	Pulmonary infarction
Pulmonary artery rupture	Thrombocytopenia
Sepsis/infection	Cardiac valve damage
Endocarditis	Thromboembolism
Balloon rupture	Cardiac dysrhythmias
Trauma to right ventricular endocardium	

VI. NONINVASIVE TECHNIQUES FOR CARDIAC OUTPUT.

Techniques include impedance plethysmography, Doppler ultrasonography, and arterial pulse contour analysis (area under the systolic portion of the arterial pulse waveform).

VII. TRANSESOPHAGEAL ECHOCARDIOGRAPHY

A. Transesophageal echocardiography (TEE) appears to offer distinct advantages over other monitors of cardiovascular function and can provide the anesthesiologist with unique diagnostic information in the operating room.
   1. Modern TEE machines offer a number of imaging techniques (M-mode, two-dimensional mode, pulsed wave Doppler, continuous flow Doppler, color flow Doppler).
   2. Blood flow toward the transducer is coded red and flow away from the transducer is coded blue. Rapidly accelerating or turbulent flow is coded green.
B. Monitoring applications for TEE in the perioperative period are described according to practice guidelines published by the American Society of Anesthesiologists and the Society of Cardiovascular Anesthesiologists (Table 24-15).
   1. TEE is used extensively as a motor of ventricular function.
      a. Preload is determined by measuring the end-diastolic area (more accurate estimate of left-ventricular preload than is data obtained from a pulmonary artery catheter).

TABLE 24-15

INDICATIONS FOR PERIOPERATIVE TRANSESOPHAGEAL ECHOCARDIOGRAPHY

Category I Indications (Supported by Strongest Clinical Evidence and Expert Consensus)

Intraoperative evaluation of acute hemodynamic disturbances

Intraoperative cardiac valve repair

Intraoperative congenital heart surgery

Intraoperative repair of hypertrophic obstructive cardiomyopathy

Preoperative use in patients with suspected thoracic aortic aneurysms

Intensive care unit evaluation of patients with unexplained hemodynamic disturbances

Category II Indications (Supported by Weaker Clinical Evidence and Expert Consensus)

Perioperative use in patients with increased risk of myocardial ischemia or infarction

Perioperative use in patients with increased risk of hemodynamic disturbances

Intraoperative assessment of valve replacement

Intraoperative detection of foreign bodies or air emboli

Intraoperative assessment of cardiac trauma

Intraoperative evaluation of pericardial effusions

Intraoperative evaluation of anastomotic sites during heart and/or lung transplantation

Monitoring placement and function of assist devices

Category III Indications (Little Current Scientific or Expert Support)

Intraoperative evaluation of myocardial perfusion, coronary artery anatomy, graft patency

Intraoperative monitoring for emboli during orthopedics procedures

Intraoperative evaluation of pleuropulmonary diseases

Monitoring placement of intra-aortic balloon pumps, automatic implantable cardiac defibrillators, or pulmonary artery catheters

   b. **Intracardiac filling pressures** estimated by TEE correlate well with data obtained from a pulmonary artery catheter.

   c. **Left ventricular contractility** can be estimated by calculation of the **ejection fraction** (left ventricular end-diastolic area minus left ventricular end-systolic area), stroke volume (Doppler flow velocity times the area through which the flow occurs), and cardiac output (stroke volume times heart rate).

    d. Myocardial ischemia is manifest as wall motion abnormalities within seconds on the TEE and before changes occur on the electrocardiogram or in data collected from the pulmonary artery catheter.

  2. TEE is the only intraoperative monitor that provides information on the structure and function of the mitral, aortic, tricuspid, and pulmonic valves.

  3. TEE may be used to determine the etiology of acute hypotension in the perioperative period (left ventricular dysfunction, hypovolemia, peripheral vasodilation, pericardial, pulmonary embolism, aortic dissection).

C. TEE is moderately invasive and may be associated with major complications (esophageal trauma, cardiac dysrhythmias, hemodynamic instability). Most complications have been observed in awake patients and some complications may be less frequent in anesthetized patients.

VIII. MONITORING NEUROLOGIC FUNCTION

A. Intracranial Pressure Monitoring

  1. Intracranial pressure (normal <15 mm Hg) can be monitored by insertion of a subarachnoid bolt (Richmond bolt), insertion of a ventricular catheter, insertion of an epidural transducer, or placement of a fiberoptic sensor in the epidural space. Each of these techniques is invasive and requires a burr hole.

  2. An acute increase in cerebral blood volume may result in a sustained increase of 50 to 100 mm Hg in the intracranial pressure (plateau wave, a wave).

B. Electroencephalogram

  1. Spontaneous electrical activity of pyramidal cells located in the outer cerebral cortex is responsible for the electroencephalogram.

    a. The electrical signal is difficult to measure and evaluate accurately in the operating room because of low voltages (10 to 100 mV, which is 1,000 times less than the electrical signal that results in the electrocardiogram) and the variation in frequencies (1 to 30 Hz) recorded from scalp electrodes.

    b. During periods of ischemia or when the patient is under general anesthesia, electroencephalographic activity generally decreases in both amplitude and frequency.

    c. Generation of electroencephalographic activity is responsible for approximately 50% of the total oxygen consumption of the cerebral cortex.

2. Electroencephalographic monitoring has been advocated for the intraoperative detection of cerebral ischemia during deliberate hypotension or during carotid endarterectomy, for the intraoperative or perioperative assessment of pharmacologic interventions, for the identification of epileptic foci, and for the assessment of coma or brain death.

3. **Processing electroencephalographic data.** Instruments are available to process electroencephalographic data to create a graphic display (compressed spectral analysis) so as to improve the ability of clinicians to interpret changes and evaluate trends.

    a. The bispectral index (BIS) is a variable derived from the electroencephalogram that is a measure of the hypnotic effect (depth of consciousness) of injected and inhaled anesthetic drugs. The range of values for the BIS is 0 to 100 with values <60 appearing to predict the absence of consciousness.

    b. The BIS does not appear to be reliable in predicting movement in response to a noxious stimulus (motor responses may be mediated by subcortical structures that are not measured by the BIS monitor).

    c. Clinical studies have demonstrated that BIS can predict the level of sedation, loss of consciousness, and the probability of recall.

    d. The use of the BIS monitor can facilitate faster emergence and improved recovery from general anesthesia by allowing more precise titration of the anesthetic effect.

4. Other monitoring systems have been developed that process the EEG in order to quantify the depth of anesthesia.

    a. Patient State Index (PSI) records the EEG from the anterior and posterior scalp. PSI values (0 to 100) correlate with the level of consciousness.

       b. Narcotrend classifies the EEG into 14 stages (A is awake and F1 is isoelectric).

C. Evoked Potential Monitoring

    1. Evoked potentials represent a small electrical signal generated in neural pathways following periodic neural stimulation (reflects the functional integrity of the brainstem, visual, or peripheral neural pathways).

       a. In the cortex and subcortex, the evoked potential signals are much smaller than the background electroencephalogram, such that computer signal averaging and filtering are used to remove the random background electrical activity.

       b. The average evoked response is then displayed as a plot of voltage over time.

       c. Anesthetic drugs, blood pressure changes, and temperature changes may interfere with interpretation and assessment of evoked potentials in the intraoperative period.

    2. Three sensory pathways are commonly used intraoperatively to monitor neural function (Table 24-16).

    3. **Motor evoked potentials** provide a means of assessing descending motor pathways (transcranial electrical stimulation or direct spinal cord stimulation) that function independently from sensory pathways.

    4. Monitoring **facial nerve function** is commonly performed during procedures within the posterior fossa. Although facial nerve function is insensitive to anesthetic influences, muscle relaxants need to be limited to allow adequate monitoring conditions.

IX. TEMPERATURE MONITORING

A. The potential for accidental heat loss or the risk of triggering malignant hyperthermia requires the continued observation of temperature changes.

B. Perioperative hypothermia commonly results from anesthetic-induced inhibition of thermoregulation as well as a cold ambient environment in the operating room and heat loss owing to surgical exposure of tissues.

    1. Anesthetized patients often behave like poikilotherms until core temperature approaches a new set point for thermoregulation.

388 *Preparing for Anesthesia*

TABLE 24-16

SENSORY PATHWAYS AVAILABLE FOR EVOKED POTENTIAL MONITORING

Brainstem Auditory Evoked Responses
Produced by stimulation of the cochlea using pulsed sound
Assess auditory pathway (ear and brainstem)
Useful for monitoring comatose patients or those undergoing surgical procedures on the cerebellopontine angle, floor of fourth ventricle, or cranial nerves V, VII, or VIII
May remain normal despite severe cortical dysfunction and deep anesthesia
Commercially available monitor accurately reflects the depth of anesthesia

Visual Evoked Potentials
Produced by flashing light to stimulate the retina
Assess integrity of the visual pathways
Useful for monitoring procedures on the visual system; during resection of pituitary tumors, and during procedures in the vicinity of the optic tracts (anterior cerebral artery aneurysms)
Very sensitive to depressant effects of anesthetics

Somatosensory Evoked Potentials
Produced by stimulation of a peripheral nerve (median, ulnar, common, peroneal, posterior tibial) using low-current electrical impulses
Useful for monitoring cerebral function and ischemia associated with cerebral procedures and hemorrhage; spinal cord function during instrumentation of the spine or during thoracoabdominal vascular surgery
Injury or ischemia to the spinal cord manifests as decreased amplitude and increased latency of the evoked potential tracing
Does not monitor function of motor pathways

---

   2. Those patients at greatest risk for perioperative hypothermia include the elderly, burn patients, neonates, and patients with spinal cord injuries.
   C. **Perioperative hyperthermia** occurs rarely, and potential explanations other than malignant hyperthermia include exposure to endogenous pyrogens, increases in metabolic rate secondary to thyrotoxicosis or pheochromocytoma and anticholinergic blockade of sweating.
   D. Central temperature is customarily measured using temperature probes placed in the nasopharynx, esophagus, blood (pulmonary artery catheter), bladder, or rectum.

1. During routine noncardiac surgery, temperature differences between these sites are small.
2. During and following cardiopulmonary bypass or deliberate hypothermia, gradients between these sites are predictable.
   a. During cooling in anesthetized patients, changes in rectal temperature often lag behind changes in central (core) temperature.
   b. During rewarming, probe locations residing in regions of high blood flow often reflect blood temperature rather than central temperature, emphasizing that the adequacy of rewarming is best judged by measuring temperature at more than one location.

CHAPTER 25 ■ EPIDURAL AND SPINAL ANESTHESIA

Spinal anesthesia and epidural anesthesia have been shown to blunt the "stress response" to surgery, decrease intraoperative blood loss, lower the incidence of postoperative thromboembolic events, possibly decrease morbidity in high-risk surgical patients, and serve as a useful method to extend analgesia into the postoperative period (Bernards CM: Epidural and spinal anesthesia. In Barash PG, Cullen BF, Stoelting RK [eds]: *Clinical Anesthesia*, pp 691–717. Philadelphia, Lippincott Williams & Wilkins, 2006). Spinal and epidural techniques extend analgesia into the postoperative period and provide better analgesia than can be achieved with parenteral opioids.

I. ANATOMY

A. Proficiency in spinal and epidural anesthesia requires a thorough understanding of the anatomy of the spine and spinal cord.

B. **Vertebrae**

1. The spine consists of 7 cervical, 12 thoracic, 5 lumbar, 5 fused sacral, 5 fused coccygeal vertebrae.

2. With the exception of C1 (lacks a body or spinous process), the vertebrae consist of a body anteriorly, two pedicles that project posteriorly from the body, and two lamina that connect the pedicles to form the vertebral canal, which contains the spinal cord, spinal nerves, and epidural space (Fig. 25-1).

3. The laminae give rise to the transverse processes, which project laterally, and the spinous process, which projects posteriorly (see Fig. 25-1).

4. The fifth sacral vertebra is not fused posteriorly, giving rise to a variably shaped opening known as the sacral hiatus (opening into the sacral canal, which is the caudal termination of the epidural space). Sacral cornu are bony prominences on either side to the hiatus and aid in identifying it.

5. Identifying individual vertebrae is important for correctly locating the desired interspace for

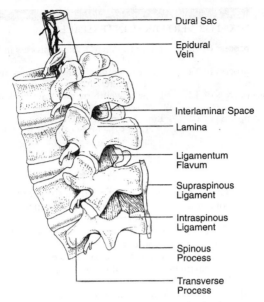

FIGURE 25-1. Anatomy of the vertebral column.

performance of epidural and spinal anesthesia (Table 25-1).

C. **Ligaments**
   1. The vertebral bodies are stabilized by five ligaments that increase in size between the cervical and lumbar vertebrae (see Fig. 25-1).
   2. The **ligamentum flavum** is thickest in the midline (3 to 5 mm at L2–3) and also farthest from the spinal meninges in the midline (4 to 6 mm at L2–3). As a result, midline insertion of an epidural needle is least likely to result in accidental meningeal puncture.

D. **Epidural Space**
   1. The epidural space lies between the spinal meninges and the sides of the vertebral canal. It is bounded cranially by the foramen magnum, caudally by the sacrococcygeal ligament (sacral hiatus), and posteriorly by the ligamentum flavum and vertebral pedicles.

TABLE 25-1

LANDMARKS FOR VERTEBRAL INTERSPACES

Spinous process of C7	First prominent spinous process in back of neck
Spinous process of T1	Most prominent spinous process and immediately follows C7
Spinous process of T12	Palpate twelfth rib and trace back to its attachment of T12
Spinous process of L5	Line drawn between the iliac crests crosses the body of L5 or the L4–5 interspace

2. The epidural space is not a closed space but communicates with the paravertebral space via the intervertebral foramina.
3. The epidural space is composed of a series of discontinuous compartments, which become continuous when the potential space separating the compartments is opened up by injection of air or liquid.
4. The most ubiquitous material in the epidural space is fat.
5. Veins are present principally in the anterior and lateral portions of the epidural space with few, if any, veins present in the posterior epidural space (see Fig. 25-1). These veins anastomose freely with extradural veins (pelvic veins, azygous system, intracranial veins).

E. **Epidural fat** has important effects on the pharmacology of epidurally and intrathecally administered opioids and local anesthetics.
1. Lipid solubility results in opioid sequestration in epidural fat with associated decreases in bioavailability.
2. Transfer of opioid from the epidural space to intrathecal space is greatest with poorly lipid soluble morphine and least for the highly lipid soluble opioids, fentanyl and sufentanil.

F. **Meninges**
1. **Dura mater** is the outermost and thickest meningeal tissue that begins at the foramen magnum (fuses with the periosteum of the skull forming the cephalad border of the epidural space) and ends at

approximately S2 where it fuses with the filum terminale. The dura mater extends laterally along the spinal nerve roots and becomes continuous with the connective tissue of the epineurium at approximately the level of the intervertebral foramina.

a. The presence of a midline connective tissue band (plica medianis dorsalis) running from the dura mater to the ligamentum flavum is controversial but may be invoked as an explanation for unilateral epidural block.

b. The subdural space is a potential space between the dura mater and arachnoid mater. Drug intended for either the epidural space or the subarachnoid space may be accidentally injected into this space.

2. **Arachnoid Mater**

a. The arachnoid mater is an avascular membrane that serves as the principal physiologic barrier for drugs moving between the epidural space and the subarachnoid space.

b. The **subarachnoid space** lies between the arachnoid mater and pia mater and contains cerebrospinal fluid (CSF). The spinal CSF is in continuity with the cranial CSF and provides an avenue for drugs in the spinal CSF to reach the brain. Spinal nerve roots and rootlets run in the subarachnoid space.

3. **Pia mater** is adherent to the spinal cord.

G. **Spinal Cord**

1. In the adult, the caudad tip of the spinal cord typically ends at the level of L1 (extends to L3 in 10% of adults).

2. The spinal cord gives rise to 31 pairs of spinal nerves, each composed of an anterior motor root and a posterior sensory root.

a. **Dermatome** is the skin area innervated by a given spinal nerve (Fig. 25-2).

b. The intermediolateral gray matter of T1 to L12 contains the cell bodies of the preganglionic sympathetic neurons. These sympathetic neurons travel with the corresponding spinal nerve to a point just beyond the intervertebral foramen where they exit to join the sympathetic chain ganglia.

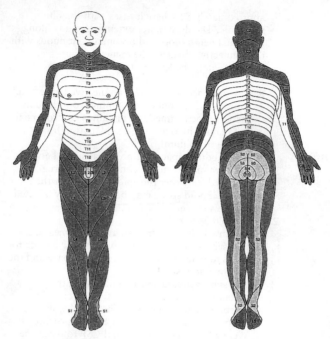

FIGURE 25-2. Human sensory dermatomes.

    c. Because the spinal cord ends between L1 and L2, the thoracic, lumbar, and sacral nerve roots travel increasingly longer distances in the subarachnoid space (cauda equina) to reach the intervertebral foramen through which they exit.

II. TECHNIQUE

  A. Spinal and epidural anesthesia should be performed only after appropriate monitors are applied in a setting where equipment for airway management and resuscitation is immediately available.

  B. Needles

    1. Spinal and epidural needles are named for the design of their tips ("pencil point," beveled tip with cutting edge) (Fig. 25-3).

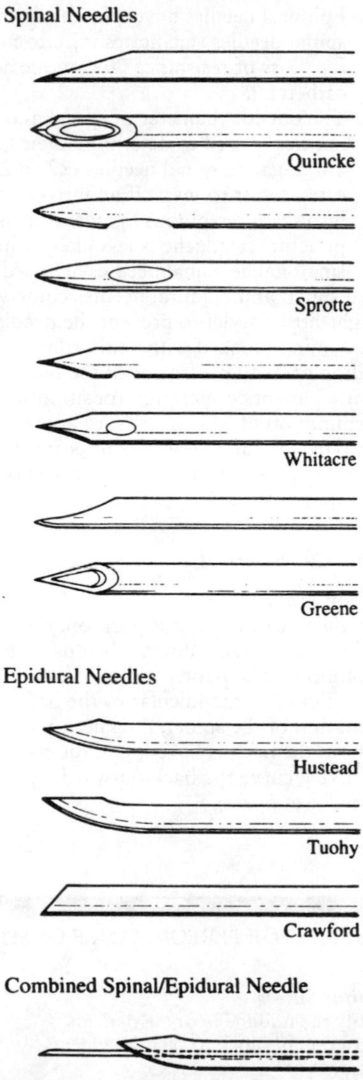

Spinal Needles

Quincke

Sprotte

Whitacre

Greene

Epidural Needles

Hustead

Tuohy

Crawford

Combined Spinal/Epidural Needle

FIGURE 25-3. Examples of commercially available spinal and epidural needles. Needles are distinguished by the design of their tips.

      a. Epidural needles have a larger diameter than spinal needles (facilitates injection of air or fluid for "loss of resistance" technique and passage of catheters).

      b. The outside diameter of spinal and epidural needles is used to determine their gauge. Large-gauge spinal needles (22 to 29 gauge) are often easier to insert if an introducer (inserted into the interspinous ligament) is used. Postdural puncture headache is less likely when small-gauge spinal needles are used.

   2. All spinal and epidural needles come with a tight-fitting stylet to prevent the needle from becoming plugged with skin or fat.

C. **Sedation** prior to placement of the block is limited because patient cooperation (positioning, determination of level of sensory anesthesia, occurrence of paresthesias) is important. After the anesthesia is established, the patient may be sedated as deemed appropriate.

III. SPINAL ANESTHESIA

A. **Position** (Table 25-2)

   1. In the lateral decubitus position, the patient lies with the operative side down when using hyperbaric solutions. The patient's shoulders and hips are positioned perpendicular to the bed (prevents rotation of the spine), the knees are drawn up to the chest, the neck is flexed, and the patient is asked to actively curve the back outward (spreads spinous processes apart).

TABLE 25-2

PATIENT POSITION FOR PERFORMANCE OF SPINAL ANESTHESIA

Lateral Decubitus Sitting
Easier to identify the midline in obese patients
Facilitates restriction of block to sacral segments

Prone (Jackknife)
Consider when surgery is to be performed in this position
Hypobaric solution produces sacral block for perirectal surgery

2. Using the iliac crests as landmarks, the L2–3, L3–4, and L4–5 interspaces are identified and the desired interspace chosen.

3. All antiseptic solutions are neurotoxic, and care must be taken not to contaminate spinal needles or local anesthetics.

B. **Midline Approach**

1. After infiltration of the selected needle insertion site with local anesthetic solution, the needle is advanced (subcutaneous tissue to supraspinous ligament to interspinous ligament to ligamentum flavum to epidural space to dura mater ["pop"] to arachnoid mater) until CSF is obtained (gentle aspiration may be helpful). The spinal meninges are typically at a depth of 4 to 6 cm.

2. If bone is encountered, the depth should be noted and the needle withdrawn to subcutaneous tissue and redirected more cephalad (Fig. 25-4).

3. If the patient experiences a paresthesia (differentiate from discomfort from contacting bone), it is important to immediately stop advancing the needle and to determine whether the needle tip has encountered a nerve root in the epidural space or in the subarachnoid space (presence of CSF confirms the needle has encountered a cauda equina nerve root).

4. After completing the injection of local anesthetic solution, a small volume of CSF is again aspirated to confirm the needle tip remained in the subarachnoid space.

5. Once the block is placed, strict attention must be directed to the patient's hemodynamic status with blood pressure and heart rate supported as necessary.

6. The level of anesthesia should be assessed by pin prick or temperature sensation. If the anesthesia is not rising high enough, the table may be tilted to influence spread of a hyperbaric or hypobaric local anesthetic.

C. **Paramedian approach** (patient cannot flex the spine or heavily calcified interspinous ligaments) is insertion of the needle 1 cm lateral to the desired interspace with advancement toward the midline (first significant resistance is ligamentum flavum as interspinous ligament is bypassed).

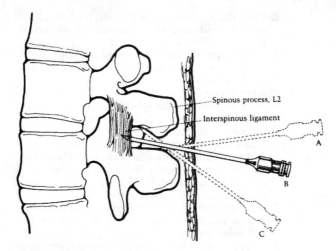

FIGURE 25-4. Midline approach to the subarachnoid space. The spinal needle is inserted with a slight cephalad angulation and advanced in the midline (**B**). If bone is contacted, it may be either the caudad (**A**) or cephalad (**C**) spinous process. The needle should be redirected slightly and if bone is encountered at a shallower depth, then the needle is likely walking up the cephalad spinous process. If bone is encountered at a deeper depth, then the needle is likely walking down the inferior spinous process. If bone is repeatedly contacted at the same depth, then the needle is likely off the midline and walking along the lamina.

    D. Lumbosacral approach is a paramedian approach directed at the L5 to S1 interspace.

IV. CONTINUOUS SPINAL ANESTHESIA

    A. The technique is similar to that used for a single-shot spinal anesthesia except that a needle large enough to accommodate the desired catheter must be inserted (catheter inserted 2 to 3 cm into the subarachnoid space).

    B. Although smaller catheters decrease the risk of postdural puncture headache, they have been associated with reports of neurologic injury (recommendation is not to use a catheter smaller than 24 gauge).

V. EPIDURAL ANESTHESIA

    A. Patient preparation, positioning, monitors, and needle approaches for epidural anesthesia are the same as for spinal anesthesia. Unlike spinal anesthesia, epidural anesthesia may be performed at any intervertebral space.

1. Using the midline approach, the epidural needle is inserted into the interspinous ligament ("gritty" feel) and then advanced slowly until the ligamentum flavum is contacted (increased resistance).

2. The epidural needle must traverse the ligamentum flavum and stop in the epidural space ("loss of resistance") before encountering the spinal meninges.

   a. A glass syringe containing 2 to 3 mL of saline and 0.1 to 0.3 mL of air is attached to the epidural needle and the plunger pressed. If the needle is properly placed in the ligamentum flavum, it should be possible to compress the air bubble without injecting the saline. If the air bubble cannot be compressed without injecting fluid, then the needle tip is most likely not in the ligamentum flavum but instead in the interspinous ligament or off midline in the paraspinous muscles.

   b. Once the ligamentum flavum is identified, the needle is slowly advanced with the nondominant hand while the dominant hand maintains constant pressure on the syringe plunger (Fig. 25-5).

   c. As the needle enters the epidural space, there will be a sudden and dramatic loss of resistance as the saline is rapidly injected (warn patient of possible pain). If the needle is advancing obliquely through the ligamentum flavum, it is possible to enter into the paraspinous muscles instead of the epidural space (loss of resistance less dramatic).

   d. When the syringe is disconnected from the needle, it is common to have a small amount of fluid flow from the needle hub (usually saline, which is at room temperature in contrast to CSF).

3. A test dose of local anesthetic solution is injected to help detect unrecognized intravenous or subarachnoid placement of the needle. After a negative test dose, the desired volume of local anesthetic solution should be administered in 5-mL increments (decreases risk of pain during injection and allows early detection of adverse reactions).

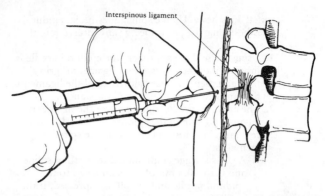

Interspinous ligament

FIGURE 25-5. Proper hand position when using the loss-of-resistance technique to locate the epidural space. After placing the tip of the needle in the ligamentum flavum, a syringe containing 2 to 3 mL of saline and an air bubble is attached. The dominant hand maintains constant pressure on the syringe plunger while the nondominant hand rests against the patient's back and is used to slowly advance the needle. If the needle is properly placed in the ligamentum flavum, it should be possible to compress the air bubble without injecting the saline. As the needle tip enters the epidural space, there will be a sudden loss of resistance and the saline will be easily ejected from the syringe.

VI. CONTINUOUS EPIDURAL ANESTHESIA

A. Use of a catheter for epidural anesthesia affords greater flexibility than the single-shot technique but introduces the risk of catheter migration (subarachnoid space, intervertebral foramen) and increases the likelihood of a unilateral epidural block.

B. Epidural catheters are usually inserted through a curved tip needle to help direct the catheter away from the dura mater. The catheter will typically encounter resistance as it reaches the curve of the needle, but steady pressure will usually result in its passage into the epidural space.

   1. The catheter should be advanced only 3 to 5 cm into the epidural space (minimizes risk of entering a vein, puncturing dura mater, exiting via an intervertebral foramen, wrapping around a nerve root).

   2. Once the catheter is appropriately positioned, the needle is slowly withdrawn with one hand as the catheter is stabilized with the other. The length of

the catheter in the epidural space is confirmed because this distance is important when trying to determine if a catheter used in the postoperative period has been dislodged.
3. A test dose of the local anesthetic solution is injected before the initial injection and any subsequent "top-up dose" (typically one-half the initial dose at an interval equal to two thirds the expected duration of the block).

VII. EPIDURAL TEST DOSE

A. The most common test dose is 3 mL of local anesthetic solution containing 5 μg/mL of epinephrine (1:200,000).
   1. This dose is sufficient to produce evidence of spinal anesthesia if accidental subarachnoid injection occurs.
   2. Intravenous injection of the epinephrine dose typically increases heart rate an average of 30 beats/min.
      a. Reflex bradycardia may occur in patients being treated with alpha-blockers (systolic blood pressure increase of $\geq$20 mm Hg may be a more reliable indicator of intravascular injection in these patients).
      b. The sensitivity of epinephrine as a test dose in parturients is questionable, because maternal heart rate increases during contractions are often as large as those produced by epinephrine.
B. Aspirating the catheter or needle to check for blood or CSF is helpful if positive, but the incidence of false-negative aspirations is too high to rely on this technique alone.

VIII. COMBINED SPINAL-EPIDURAL ANESTHESIA

A. This technique combines the rapid onset and dense block of spinal anesthesia with the flexibility afforded by an epidural catheter (see Fig. 25-3).
B. After the peak spinal block height is established, the injection of saline or a local anesthetic solution into the epidural space causes the block height to increase, presumably reflecting compression of the spinal

meninges forcing CSF cephalad as well as a local anesthetic effect.

C. A potential risk of this technique is that the meningeal hole made by the spinal needle may allow high concentrations of subsequently administered epidural drugs to reach the subarachnoid space.

IX. PHARMACOLOGY

A. Interindividual variability makes it difficult to reliably predict the height and duration of central neuraxial block that will result from a particular local anesthetic dose (Table 25-3).

B. Spinal Anesthesia

1. Block Height (Table 25-4)

a. Baricity and patient position. Of those factors that do exert significant influence on local anesthetic spread, the baricity of the local anesthetic solution relative to patient position is probably the most important.

b. Hyperbaric solutions (more dense than CSF) are typically prepared by mixing the local anesthetic solution with 5 to 8% dextrose. Gravity causes hyperbaric solutions to flow downward in the CSF to the most dependent regions of the spinal column. Spinal anesthesia can be restricted to the sacral and lower lumbar dermatomes ("saddle block") by administering a hyperbaric local anesthetic solution with the patient in the sitting position.

c. Hyperbaric solutions can be used to advantage for unilateral surgical procedures performed in the supine position if the operative site is dependent during drug injection and the patient is left in the lateral position for at least 6 minutes.

d. When the patient is turned supine following hyperbaric drug injection in the lateral position, the normal spinal curvature will influence subsequent movement of the injected solution. Hyperbaric solutions injected at the height of the lumbar lordosis will tend to flow cephalad to pool in the thoracic kyphosis and caudad to pool in the sacrum (Fig. 25-6).

e. Gravity influences the distribution of hyperbaric and hypobaric solutions only until they are

TABLE 25-3
REPRESENTATIVE SURGICAL PROCEDURES APPROPRIATE FOR SPINAL ANESTHESIA

Surgical Procedure	Suggested Block Height	Technique	Comments
Perianal Perirectal	L1–2	Hyperbaric solution/sitting position Hypobaric solution/jackknife position Isobaric solution/horizontal position	Patients must remain in relative head-up or head-down position when using hypobaric and hyperbaric solutions to maintain restricted spread during the procedure
Lower extremity	T10	Isobaric solution	Hypobaric and hyperbaric solutions are also suitable but may produce higher blocks than necessary
Hip Transurethral resection of the prostate Vaginal/cervical Herniorraphy	T6–8	Hyperbaric solution/horizontal position	Isobaric solutions injected at L2–3 interspace may also be suitable
Pelvic procedures Appendectomy Abdominal	T4–6	Hyperbaric solution/horizontal position	Upper abdominal procedures usually require concomitant general anesthesia to prevent vagal reflexes and pain from traction on the diaphragm and esophagus

TABLE 25-4

FACTORS THAT MAY INFLUENCE THE SPREAD OF LOCAL ANESTHETIC SOLUTIONS IN THE SUBARACHNOID SPACE

Characteristics of the Local Anesthetic Solution
Baricity relative to patient position (most important of all factors)
Local anesthetic dose (little effect with isobaric solutions)
Local anesthetic concentration
Volume injected

Patient Characteristics
Age, weight, height (poor predictors of extent of sensory blockade)
Gender
Pregnancy

Technique
Site of injection
Speed of injection
Barbotage
Direction of needle bevel
Addition of vasoconstrictors

Diffusion

sufficiently diluted in CSF so that they become isobaric (solution no longer moves in response to changes in position).

  f. **Dose, volume, and concentration.** Drug dose and volume appear to be relatively unimportant in predicting the spread of hyperbaric local anesthetic solutions injected in the horizontal plane (reflects predominate effect of baricity and patient position).

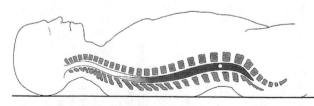

FIGURE 25-6. In the supine position, hyperbaric local anesthetic solutions injected at the height of the lumbar lordosis (*circle*) will flow down the lumbar lordosis to pool in the sacrum and in the thoracic kyphosis. Pooling in the thoracic kyphosis is thought to explain the fact that hyperbaric solutions produce blocks with an average sensory level of T4–6.

g. **Injection site** (same as for drug dose and volume).

h. **Patient characteristics.** The most important variable governing block height may be the patient's lumbosacral CSF volume. Patient age, weight, and height have not been proven to be important predictors of block height.

2. **Onset** of spinal anesthesia is within a few minutes regardless of the drug used, although time to reach peak block is different among drugs (lidocaine sooner than bupivacaine).

3. **Duration** of spinal anesthesia is characterized by gradual waning of the block beginning with the most cephalad dermatome.

   a. When speaking about duration of block, it is necessary to distinguish between duration at the surgical site and time required for anesthesia to completely resolve (influences discharge time) (Table 25-5).

   b. A thorough understanding of the factors that govern the duration of anesthesia is necessary for the anesthesiologist to choose techniques that result in an appropriate duration (Table 25-6).

C. **Epidural Anesthesia**

1. Any procedure that can be performed under spinal anesthesia can also be performed under epidural anesthesia and requires the same block height (see Table 25-3). As with spinal anesthesia, there is a great interindividual variability in the spread and duration of epidural anesthesia (Table 25-7).

2. **Block Spread.** To choose the most appropriate local anesthetic and dose for a particular clinical situation, the anesthesiologist must be familiar with the variables that affect spread and duration of epidural anesthesia (Table 25-8).

3. **Onset** of epidural anesthesia can usually be detected within 5 minutes in the dermatomes immediately surrounding the injection site.

   a. The time to peak effect is 15 to 20 minutes with shorter acting drugs and 20 to 25 minutes with longer acting drugs.

   b. Increasing the dose of local anesthetic speeds the onset of both motor and sensory block.

4. **Duration** (Table 25-9)

TABLE 25-5

DOSE AND DURATION OF LOCAL ANESTHETICS USED FOR SPINAL ANESTHESIA

Drug	Dose (mg)	Two-Dermatome Regression (min)	Complete Resolution (min)	Prolongation by Adrenergic Agonists (%)
Chloroprocaine	30–100	30–50	70–150	Not recommended
Lidocaine	25–100	40–100	140–240	20–50
Bupivacaine	5–20	90–140	240–380	20–50
Tetracaine	5–20	90–140	240–380	50–100

TABLE 25-6

FACTORS THAT MAY INFLUENCE THE DURATION OF SENSORY BLOCKADE PRODUCED BY SPINAL ANESTHESIA

Local anesthetic drug (principal determinant of duration)
Drug dose
Block height (higher blocks regress faster as cephalad spread results
   in relatively lower drug concentration in CBF)
Adrenergic agonists (effectiveness depends upon local anesthetic
   with which they are combined; tetracaine > bupivacaine)
      Epinephrine 0.2–0.3 mg
      Phenylephrine 2–5 mg
      Clonidine 75–150 μg

X. PHYSIOLOGY

A. Neurophysiology

1. **Site of action** of spinal and epidural anesthesia is not precisely known but can potentially occur at any or all points along the neural pathways extending from the site of drug administration to the interior of the spinal cord.
2. **Differential neural block** refers to the clinically important phenomenon in which nerve fibers subserving different functions display varying sensitivity to local anesthetic blockade.

TABLE 25-7

LOCAL ANESTHETICS USED FOR SURGICAL EPIDURAL ANESTHESIA

Drug	Two-Dermatome Regression (min)	Complete Resolution (min)	Prolongation by Epinephrine (%)
Chloroprocaine 3%	45–60	100–160	40–60
Lidocaine	60–100	160–200	40–80
Mepivacaine 2%	60–100	160–200	40–80
Ropivacaine 0.5–1%	90–180	240–420	None
Etidocaine 1–1.5%	120–240	300–460	None
Bupivacaine 0.5–0.75%	120–240	300–460	None

TABLE 25-8

FACTORS THAT MAY INFLUENCE THE SPREAD OF LOCAL ANESTHETIC SOLUTIONS IN THE EPIDURAL SPACE

Injection site (unlike spinal anesthesia, epidural anesthesia produces a segmental block that spreads both caudally and cranially from the site of injection)

Drug volume (increasing the volume will result in greater spread and density of block; increases cephalad distribution)

Drug dose (important with volume in determining spread and density of block)

Drug concentration (relatively unimportant in determining block spread)

Position (does not seem to have a clinically important effect on spread of the block from side to side)

Patient characteristics

Age (greater spread in elderly perhaps because of less compliant epidural space and decreased ability of local anesthetic solution to escape via intervertebral foramina)

Height and weight (weak correlation except at extremes)

Pregnancy (conflicting data)

Atherosclerosis (conflicting data)

   a. Sympathetic nervous system nerve fibers appear to be blocked by the lowest concentration of local anesthetic followed in order by fibers responsible for pain, touch, and motor function.

   b. Although the mechanism for differential block in spinal and epidural anesthesia is not known, it is

TABLE 25-9

FACTORS THAT INFLUENCE THE DURATION OF SENSORY BLOCKADE PRODUCED BY EPIDURAL ANESTHESIA

Local anesthetic drug (principal determinant of duration)

Dose (increasing dose results in increased duration and density)

Age (conflicting results)

Adrenergic agonists (epinephrine 1:200,000)

   Prolongs duration of lidocaine and mepivacaine > bupivacaine and etidocaine

   Mechanism may reflect decreased absorption from epidural space or direct inhibitory effect of epinephrine on sensory and motor neurons

clear that fiber diameter is not the only, nor perhaps even the most important, factor contributing to differential blockade.

c. During spinal and epidural anesthesia, differential block is manifest as a spatial separation in the modalities blocked (sympathetic block may extend 2 to 6 dermatomes higher than sensory block, which is 2 to 3 dermatomes higher than motor block). This spatial separation is believed to result from a gradual decrease in local anesthetic concentration within the CSF as a function of distance from the site of injection.

d. An occasional patient has intact touch and proprioception at the surgical site despite adequate blockade of pain sensation.

e. Central neuraxial block produces sedation, potentiates the effects of sedative drugs, and markedly decreases anesthetic requirements.

B. **Cardiovascular Physiology**

1. Understanding the homeostatic mechanisms responsible for control of blood pressure and heart rate is essential for understanding and treating the cardiovascular changes associated with spinal and epidural anesthesia (Fig. 25-7).

2. **Spinal Anesthesia.** Blockade of sympathetic nervous system efferent fibers is the principal mechanism by which spinal anesthesia produces cardiovascular derangements.

a. The incidence of significant hypotension or bradycardia is generally related to the extent of sympathetic nervous system blockade, which in turn parallels block height.

b. Hypotension during spinal anesthesia is the result of arterial (decreased systemic vascular resistance) and venous (decrease preload responsible for decreased cardiac output) dilation.

c. Heart rate slows significantly in 10 to 15% of patients (blockade of sympathetic cardioaccelerator fibers or diminished venous return and associated decreased stretch of intracardiac stretch receptors). Unexplained severe bradycardia and asystole during spinal and epidural anesthesia may require aggressive intervention with epinephrine.

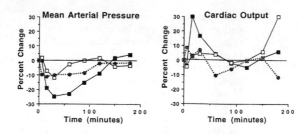

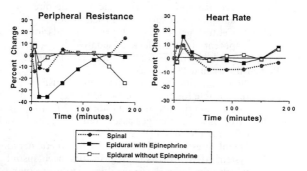

FIGURE 25-7. The cardiovascular effects of spinal and epidural anesthesia in volunteers with T5 sensory blocks. The effects of spinal anesthesia and epidural anesthesia without epinephrine were generally comparable and are both qualitatively and quantitatively different from the effects of epidural anesthesia with epinephrine added to the local anesthetic solution.

    d. Spinal anesthesia can also produce second and third-degree heart block. Preexisting first-degree heart block may be a risk factor for progression to higher grade heart block during spinal anesthesia.

  3. Epidural Anesthesia. The hemodynamic changes produced by epidural anesthesia are largely dependent on whether or not epinephrine is added to the local anesthetic solution (see Fig. 25-7).

    a. Hemodynamic changes of high epidural anesthesia without epinephrine in the local anesthetic solution resemble spinal anesthesia,

  although the magnitude is usually less than
  that seen with comparable levels of spinal
  block.
  b. When epinephrine is added to the local anesthetic
  solution the resulting beta-2-mediated
  vasodilation leads to a greater decrease in blood
  pressure than occurs in the absence of
  epinephrine.
  4. **Treating Hemodynamic Changes** (Table 25-10)
C. **Respiratory Physiology**
  1. Spinal and epidural anesthesia to midthoracic levels
  have little effect on pulmonary function in patients
  without preexisting disease (drugs used for sedation
  may have a greater effect).
  2. The adverse impact of high blocks on active
  exhalation suggests caution when using spinal or
  epidural anesthesia in patients with chronic
  obstructive pulmonary disease or those who rely on
  accessory muscles of respiration to maintain
  adequate ventilation.
  3. Patients with high spinal or epidural anesthesia may
  complain of dyspnea (loss of ability to feel chest
  move while breathing, which is usually adequately
  treated by reassurance). A normal speaking voice
  suggests ventilation is normal (faint gasping whisper
  with an excessively high block).

TABLE 25-10

**TREATING HEMODYNAMIC CHANGES SECONDARY TO
SPINAL AND EPIDURAL ANESTHESIA**

Vasopressors
Ephedrine (5–10 mg iv treats causes of hypotension by increasing
  cardiac output [venous return] and systemic vascular resistance)
Dopamine (long-term infusion because tachyphylaxis can develop
  to repeated doses of ephedrine)
Phenylephrine (increase blood pressure by increasing systemic
  vascular resistance, which may decrease cardiac output; may be
  specific treatment for hypotension during epidural anesthesia
  provided by epinephrine-containing local anesthetic solutions)

Fluid Administration
Prehydration with 500–1500 mL of crystalloid solution (cannot be
  relied on to prevent hypotension); 6% hetastarch 500 mL may be
  an alternative to crystalloids

D. **Gastrointestinal Physiology**
  1. Unopposed parasympathetic nervous system activity results in increased secretions, relaxation of sphincters, and constriction of the bowel.
  2. Nausea is a common complication of spinal and epidural anesthesia (cause unknown but often associated with blocks higher than T5, hypotension, and opioid administration).
E. **Endocrine-Metabolic Physiology.** Spinal anesthesia and epidural anesthesia inhibit many of the changes associated with the stress response to surgery (presumed to reflect blockade of afferent sensory information).

XI. COMPLICATIONS

A. **Backache**
  1. Postoperative backache occurs after general anesthesia but is more common following spinal (11%) or epidural anesthesia (30%).
  2. Possible explanations for backache include needle trauma, local anesthetic irritation, and ligamentous strain secondary to muscle relaxation.
B. **Postdural Puncture Headache**
  1. The headache is characteristically mild or absent when the patient is supine, but head elevation results in fronto-occipital headache. Occasionally, cranial nerve symptoms (diplopia, tinnitus) and nausea and vomiting are present.
     a. The headache is believed to result from the loss of CSF through the meningeal needle hole resulting in decreased buoyant support for the brain.
     b. In the upright position, the brain sags in the cranial vault, putting traction on pain-sensitive structures and possibly cranial nerves.
  2. The incidence of postdural puncture headache decreases with increasing age and with the use of small-diameter spinal needles with noncutting tips.
     a. Inserting cutting needles with the bevel aligned parallel to the long axis of the meninges results in a meningeal opening that is likely to be pulled closed by the longitudinal tension present on the dura mater.
     b. Up to 50% of young patients develop postdural puncture headache after accidental meningeal puncture with a large epidural needle.

   c. If age is considered, there does not seem to be a gender difference in the incidence of postdural puncture headache.
   d. Remaining supine does not decrease the incidence of postdural puncture headache.
   e. Use of fluid rather than air for determining loss of resistance during attempted location of the epidural space decreases the risk of developing postdural puncture headache in the event of an accidental meningeal puncture.
3. Postdural puncture headache usually resolves spontaneously in a few days with conservative therapy (bed rest, analgesics, and caffeine).
4. **Epidural blood patch** (10 to 20 mL of autologous blood is aseptically injected into the epidural space near the interspace where the meningeal puncture occurred) produces relief in 85 to 95% of patients within 1 to 24 hours (presumed to form a clot over the meningeal hole).
   a. The most common side effects of blood patch are backache and radicular pain.
   b. Prophylactic blood patch is effective in preventing postdural puncture headache in patients in whom the meninges are accidentally punctured during attempted epidural anesthesia.
   c. Epidural administered fibrin glue is an effective alternative to a blood patch for treatment of postdural puncture headache (meningeal patch rather than a blood patch).
C. **Hearing loss** (transient, lasting 1 to 3 days) is common after spinal anesthesia especially in female patients.
D. **Systemic toxicity** manifests as central nervous system and cardiovascular toxicity during epidural anesthesia (drug doses are too low during spinal anesthesia).
   1. Central nervous system toxicity may result from intravascular absorption from the epidural space but is more commonly due to accidental intravenous injection of the local anesthetic solution.
   2. Because plasma concentrations of local anesthetic required to produce cardiovascular toxicity are high, this complication likely results only from accidental intravenous injection of the local anesthetic solution.
   3. An adequate test dose and incremental injection of the local anesthetic solution are the most important methods to prevent systemic toxicity during epidural anesthesia.

E. **Total Spinal Anesthesia**
   1. Total spinal anesthesia occurs when the local anesthetic solution spreads high enough to block the entire spinal cord and occasionally the brainstem during either spinal or epidural anesthesia.
   2. Profound hypotension and bradycardia are secondary to sympathetic nervous system blockade. Apnea may occur as a result of respiratory muscle dysfunction or depression of brainstem control centers.
   3. Management includes administration of vasopressors, atropine, fluids, and oxygen, plus controlled ventilation of the lungs. If the cardiovascular and ventilatory consequences are managed appropriately, total spinal block will resolve without sequelae.

F. **Neurologic Injury**
   1. Neurologic injury occurs in approximately 0.03 to 0.1% of all spinal and epidural anesthesias (persistent paresthesias and limited motor weakness are the most common injuries).
   2. Hyperbaric 5% lidocaine has been implicated as a cause of cauda equina syndrome following subarachnoid injection through small-bore (high resistance) catheters during continuous spinal anesthesia (injection through these high-resistance catheters produces little turbulence and undiluted local anesthetic solution tends to pool around dependent cauda equina nerve roots).

G. **Transient Neurologic Symptoms (TNS)**
   1. TNS is defined as pain and/or dysesthesia in the buttocks or legs following spinal anesthesia (may follow use of all local anesthetics but the risk appears to be greater with lidocaine regardless of the dose).
   2. Surgery in the lithotomy position and obesity may increase the risk for developing transient radicular irritation.
   3. Pain usually resolves spontaneously in 72 hours.

H. **Chloroprocaine** (preservative free) is a short-acting spinal anesthetic and does not seem to be associated with TNS.

I. **Spinal hematoma** is a rare (estimated to be <1 in 150,000) complication of spinal or epidural anesthesia manifesting as lower extremity numbness or weakness (detection difficult in patients receiving perioperative spinal local anesthetic solutions pain control).

1. Early detection is critical as a delay of more than 8 hours in decompressing the spinal cord decreases the likelihood of neurologic recovery.
2. Coagulation defects are the principal risk factor for development of an epidural hematoma.
   a. Patients receiving nonsteroidal anti-inflammatory drugs with antiplatelet effects or subcutaneous unfractionated heparin for deep vein thrombosis prophylaxis are not considered to be at increased risk for development of a spinal hematoma.
   b. Patients taking antiplatelet drugs (thienoprydine derivatives such as ticlopidine and clopidogrel, GP IIb/IIIa antagonists such as abciximab) should generally not receive a neuraxial block.
   c. Patients receiving fractionated low-molecular weight heparin (enoxaparin, dalteparin, tinzaparin) are considered to be at increased risk for development of a spinal hematoma. Patients receiving these drugs preoperatively at thromboprophylactic doses should have the drug held for 10 to 12 hours before central neuraxial block.
   d. For patients in whom low-molecular weight heparin is begun after surgery, single-shot neuraxial blocks are not contraindicated provided the first doses of heparin is not administered until 24 hours postoperatively using twice-daily dosing regimens (6 to 8 hours if using once-daily dosing regimens).

TABLE 25-11

CONDITIONS THAT MAY INCREASE THE RISK OF SPINAL OR EPIDURAL ANESTHESIA

Hypovolemia
Increased intracranial pressure
Coagulopathy or thrombocytopenia (epidural hematoma)
Sepsis (increased risk of meningitis)
Infection at the puncture site
Preexisting neurologic disease (no evidence that epidural or spinal anesthesia alters the course)
Patient refusal (absolute contraindication)

TABLE 25-12

CHOICE OF SPINAL OR EPIDURAL ANESTHESIA

Spinal Anesthesia
Less time to perform
More rapid onset
Better quality sensory and motor block
Less pain during surgery

Epidural Anesthesia
Less risk of postdural puncture headache
Less hypotension if epinephrine is not added to local anesthetic solution
Ability to prolong or extend block via an indwelling catheter
Option of using an epidural catheter to provide postoperative analgesia

   e. If an indwelling central neuraxial catheter is in place, it should not be removed until 10 to 12 hours after the last dose of low-molecular weight heparin, and subsequent doses should not be begun until at least 2 hours after catheter removal.
   f. Patients who are fully anticoagulated (prolonged prothrombin time and plasma thromboplastin time) at the time of block placement or removal of the epidural catheter are considered to be at increased risk for the development of a spinal hematoma.
3. The risk of spinal hematoma during removal of an epidural catheter is nearly as great as with placement of the catheter. The timing for removal of the epidural catheter and the degree of anticoagulation need to be coordinated.
4. Drugs regimens not considered to increase the risk of neuraxial bleeding when used alone (minidose unfractionated heparin, nonsteroidal anti-inflammatory drugs) may increase the risk when combined.

XII. CONTRAINDICATIONS (Table 25-11)

XIII. SPINAL OR EPIDURAL ANESTHESIA? (Table 25-12)

CHAPTER 26 ■ PERIPHERAL NERVE BLOCKADE

Regional anesthesia of the extremities and of the trunk may be a useful alternative to general anesthesia in selected patients (Mulroy MF: Peripheral nerve blockade. In Barash PG, Cullen BF, Stoelting RK [eds]: *Clinical Anesthesia*, pp 718–745. Philadelphia, Lippincott Williams & Wilkins, 2006).

I. GENERAL PRINCIPLES

A. **Local Anesthetic Drug Selection and Doses** (see Table 17-1)
   1. Use of low concentrations of local anesthetics permits injection of large volumes of solution, which improves the reliability of peripheral nerve blocks.
   2. The addition of epinephrine (1:200,000) to the local anesthetic solution is recommended to prolong the duration of anesthesia (exceptions are blocks of end organs or intravenous regional blocks). The duration of blockade is also influenced by local blood flow.

B. **Nerve Localization**
   1. A known relationship of the nerve to be blocked to bones or arteries improves the likelihood of success when a peripheral nerve block is performed. Nerve block techniques associated with less reliable landmarks require either large volumes of local anesthetic solution or the establishment of paresthesia of the desired nerve.
      a. Paresthesias are considered the ultimate sign of nerve localization, but care must be taken to avoid intraneural injection (cramping or aching during injection).
      b. Even without intraneural injection, residual neuropathy of peripheral nerves appears more likely if paresthesias are elicited.
   2. **Nerve Stimulator.** A low-current electrical impulse (0.1 to 10.0 mA) delivered to the vicinity of a peripheral nerve through an insulated needle connected to a nerve stimulator produces

stimulation of motor fibers and thus identifies proximity to the nerve (an alternative to elicitation of a paresthesia). The accuracy of nerve localization can be improved by the use of insulated needles.

3. **Ultrasound guidance** may be used to localize nerves especially if located near an artery.

C. **Equipment**
   1. Use of disposable kits is a matter of personal preference based on cost, quality of contents, and assurance of sterility.
   2. **Needles** used for regional anesthesia have a shorter angulation to the bevel (to push the nerve away).
   3. **Syringes** (10 mL is the best compromise between bulk and the need to inject large volumes) may include **control rings** to facilitate control of the injection and allow the operator to refill the syringe with one hand (Fig. 26-1).
   4. **Continuous Catheters.** Continuous infusion catheters adapted for peripheral nerve blockade with an electrode in the tip permit localization of nerves for prolonged postoperative analgesia.
   5. Chlorhexadine, alcohol, and organic iodine preparations are useful for cleansing the skin.

D. **Common Complications** (Table 26-1)

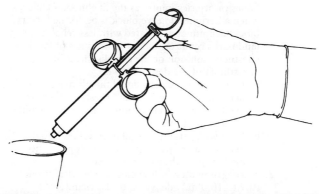

FIGURE 26-1. Three-ring syringe improves control of injection and ease of refilling.

TABLE 26-1

COMPLICATIONS OF PERIPHERAL NERVE BLOCK

Systemic toxicity
Peripheral nerve injury (intraneural injection versus position injury
  [take care in positioning "numb" extremities])
Pain at injection site
Local hematoma

II. PATIENT PREPARATION

A. **Patient Selection.** Most operations can be performed
   with a regional anesthetic technique, but the decision to
   select a peripheral nerve block may be influenced by
   several factors (Table 26-2).

B. **Premedication and Sedation**
   1. The best preparation for a regional technique is
      careful explanation of the planned procedure to the
      patient.
   2. Supplemental medication (titrate to effect) at the
      time of performance of the peripheral nerve block is
      commonly used. Sedation must be adjusted to the
      required level of patient cooperation (report
      paresthesias), need for analgesia (fentanyl, 50 to
      100 μg iv), and subsequent amnesia (midazolam,
      1 to 3 mg iv). Benzodiazepines increase the seizure
      threshold for local anesthetics.

C. **Monitoring** is the same as for patients undergoing
   general anesthesia although it is also important to
   maintain verbal contact as a means of assessing a
   patient's mental status and for detecting early signs of
   local anesthetic (systemic) toxicity.

D. **Discharge Criteria.** It is acceptable to discharge a
   patient from the postanesthesia care unit in the
   presence of residual numbness (analgesia) as long as

TABLE 26-2

CONTRAINDICATIONS TO PERIPHERAL NERVE BLOCKS

Patient refusal or objection to being "awake"
Local infection at block site
Coagulopathy
Preexisting neuropathy

blood pressure is stable (orthostatic hypotension absent) and mental status is acceptable.

III. SPECIFIC TECHNIQUES: HEAD AND NECK
(Table 26-3)

A. **Cervical plexus blockade** is useful for operations on the lateral (carotid endarterectomy) or anterior neck (thyroidectomy) (Table 26-4).

B. **Airway anesthesia** is useful to facilitate awake tracheal intubation or fiberoptic laryngoscopy, but caution must be exercised if loss of protective laryngeal reflexes could place a patient at increased risk for aspiration.

   1. Topical anesthesia is often provided with pledgets or an atomizer using a solution of 4% lidocaine. This higher concentration of lidocaine is required to penetrate mucosal membranes. Premedication with an anticholinergic to decrease secretions facilitates the onset of topical anesthesia.

      a. For effective anesthesia of the posterior pharyngeal wall, the tongue is first sprayed and the patient is encouraged to gargle and swallow the residual liquid in the mouth. The numb tongue is grasped with a gauze pad, and the patient is encouraged to take rapid deep breaths while the spray is delivered during inspiration.

      b. For nasal mucosal anesthesia, a mixture of 3 to 4% lidocaine with 0.25 to 0.5% phenylephrine on cotton pledgets is an alternative to 4% cocaine with its unique vasoconstrictive properties.

TABLE 26-3
REGIONAL ANESTHESIA OF THE HEAD AND NECK

Trigeminal nerve block (sensory and motor function of the face)
Gasserian ganglion block
Superficial trigeminal nerve branch block
Maxillary nerve block
Mandibular nerve block
Cervical plexus block (sensory and motor fibers of the neck and posterior scalp)
Occipital nerve block (sensory innervation to the posterior and lateral scalp)
Airway anesthesia

TABLE 26-4
COMPLICATIONS OF CERVICAL PLEXUS BLOCK

Phrenic nerve block (reason to avoid bilateral cervical plexus block)
Vertebral artery injection
Epidural injection
Subarachnoid injection
Recurrent laryngeal nerve block

2. Superior laryngeal nerve blockade (branch of the vagus) that provides anesthesia to the vocal cords, epiglottis, and arytenoids. The superior laryngeal nerve is blocked bilaterally as it penetrates the thyrohyoid membrane (Fig. 26-2).
3. Tracheal anesthesia is produced by rapid injection during inspiration of 4 mL of 4% lidocaine through a needle passed through the cricothyroid membrane into the trachea.

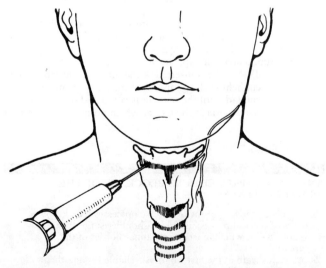

FIGURE 26-2. Superior laryngeal nerve block is performed through the thyrohyoid membrane.

IV. SPECIFIC TECHNIQUES: UPPER EXTREMITY

A. Innervation of the upper extremity is from nerve roots derived from C5 to T1. There are three anatomic locations where local anesthetic solutions are placed to block the brachial plexus (Table 26-5 and Fig. 26-3).

B. **Interscalene Approach**

1. The needle is inserted in the interscalene groove at the level of the cricoid cartilage and advanced perpendicular to the skin in all planes until the tubercle of C6 is contacted or a paresthesia is elicited, at which point 25 to 30 mL of 1% lidocaine or 0.25% bupivacaine is injected. Higher concentrations of local anesthetic are needed to produce a more profound motor blockade.

2. If arm surgery requiring the use of a tourniquet is planned, a subcutaneous ring of anesthetic across the axilla is often provided to block the superficial intercostobrachial fibers crossing the chest wall into the axilla.

3. Use of long-acting local anesthetics and insertion of a continuous catheter is effective for procedures such as rotator cuff repairs and provision of prolonged postoperative analgesia.

4. Complications of the interscalene approach are related to the structures located in the vicinity of the C6 tubercle (Table 26-6).

C. **Supraclavicular Approach**

1. The needle is inserted in the interscalene groove 1 cm behind the midpoint of the clavicle and advanced caudad until the first rib is contacted or a paresthesia is elicited, at which point 25 to 40 mL of

---

TABLE 26-5

ANATOMIC APPROACHES TO BLOCKADE OF THE BRACHIAL PLEXUS

Interscalene groove near the transverse processes (blocks lower fibers of cervical plexus; useful for shoulder surgery but may spare C8–T1, which innervate the ulnar border of the forearm)

Subclavian sheath at the first rib (most reliable for anesthesia of the forearm and hand)

Axillary sheath surrounding the artery in the axilla (technically easy but may not block the musculocutaneous nerve)

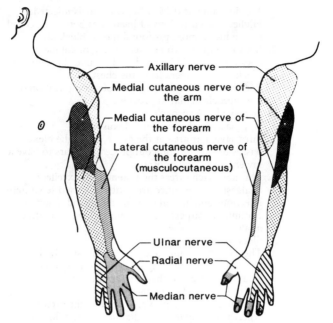

FIGURE 26-3. Sensory dermatomes of the arm.

TABLE 26-6

COMPLICATIONS OF THE INTERSCALENE APPROACH TO THE BRACHIAL PLEXUS

Pneumothorax (cough or chest pain while exploring for the nerve)
Spinal or epidural anesthesia
Vertebral artery injection
Diaphragm paralysis
Neuropathy of the C6 nerve root
Inadequate anesthesia in the ulnar distribution (use 30 to 40 mL of local anesthetic solution)

1% lidocaine or 0.25% bupivacaine is injected. Higher concentrations of local anesthetic are needed to produce a more profound motor blockade.

2. If a tourniquet is to be used, a ring of cutaneous anesthesia should be produced around the axilla to block sensory fibers from the chest wall.

3. Pneumothorax is the most serious complication of the supraclavicular approach.

D. Infraclavicular Approach

1. Approaching the brachial plexus in the infraclavicular area at the point where the plexus passes below the coracoid process appears to have a lower risk of pneumothorax.

2. This approach offers the potential of excellent analgesia of the entire area with only two separate injections and also allows for the introduction of continuous catheters for prolonged postoperative analgesia.

E. Axillary Technique

1. The axillary technique carries the least risk of pneumothorax, making it useful for outpatients.

2. The nerves are anesthetized around the axillary artery (Fig. 26-4). The median and musculocutaneous nerves are above the artery, whereas the ulnar and radial nerves lie below and behind the vessel.

a. Individual fascial septa may surround each nerve, necessitating separate injections into each compartment in contrast to other single-injection techniques possible with more peripheral procedures.

b. Another obstacle to the single-injection technique at this level is the early departure of the musculocutaneous branch from the sheath high in the axilla.

3. Basic Procedure

a. The axillary artery is located as high as practical in the axilla as it courses in the groove between the coracobrachialis and triceps muscles (Fig. 26-5). The needle is advanced alongside the artery, ideally seeking paresthesias of the nerves serving the area of the proposed surgery (see Fig. 26-4). Injection of 15 to 20 mL of 1% lidocaine or 0.25% bupivacaine with each paresthesia or a single injection of 25 to 40 mL is carried out.

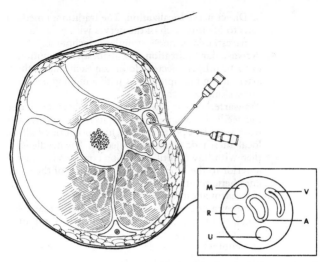

FIGURE 26-4. Needle location for block of the brachial plexus using the axillary technique.

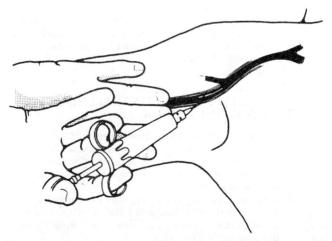

FIGURE 26-5. Hand position for block of the brachial plexus using the axillary technique.

b. **Direct nerve localization.** The traditional method is to identify each of the nerves with either a paresthesia or nerve stimulator technique.

4. **Perivascular Infiltration.** Local anesthetic solution (5 to 10 mL) is injected closely on each side of the artery using multiple passes with a moving needle not seeking paresthesias.

5. **Transarterial.** The artery is deliberately entered, and the needle is advanced until aspiration confirms it has passed just posterior, at which point one-half the local anesthetic solution is injected. The needle is then withdrawn until aspiration confirms it is just anterior to the artery and the other half of the local anesthetic solution is injected.

6. If forearm anesthesia is required, supplementary anesthesia of the musculocutaneous nerve may be obtained by injecting an additional 5 to 10 mL of anesthetic solution into the body of the coracobrachialis muscle (direct nerve response can be elicited with a stimulator).

7. If a continuous technique is desired, a catheter can be threaded centrally after nerve localization or by identifying the sheath by perceiving the characteristic fascial pop upon entry.

8. **Complications** of the axillary technique are rare and include neuropathy (the reason some routinely avoid paresthesias), hematoma (small-gauge needles decrease the risk), and accidental intravascular injection.

V. SPECIFIC TECHNIQUES: INTRAVENOUS REGIONAL ANESTHESIA

A. Intravenous regional anesthesia (Bier block) is produced by injection of local anesthetic solution without epinephrine (50 mL of 0.5% lidocaine) through a small-gauge intravenous catheter in the dorsum of the hand.

B. Injection is accomplished only after exsanguination of the extremity and subsequent inflation of a tourniquet around the upper arm to 2.5 times the systolic blood pressure (or 300 mm Hg).

1. For brief operations, the intravenous catheter may be removed at this point. If surgery may extend

beyond 1 hour, the catheter can be left in place and solution reinjected after 90 minutes.

2. Beyond 45 minutes of surgery, many patients experience discomfort at the level of the tourniquet (use "double-cuff" tourniquet and inflate the proximal cuff, first allowing production of anesthesia under the distal cuff).

C. Systemic toxicity may occur if the tourniquet fails or is released prematurely (within 40 minutes after intravenous injection of the local anesthetic solution). The duration of anesthesia is minimal beyond the time of tourniquet release.

VI. DISTAL UPPER EXTREMITY BLOCKADE

A. Nerves to the hand can be blocked at the elbow or wrist, where the muscles are thinned and prominent bony landmarks allow easier identification of the nerves. Blockade at the elbow does not produce greater anesthesia than blockade at the wrist, reflecting the extensive branching of the sensory nerves to the forearm, principally from the musculocutaneous nerve.

B. **Blockade at the Elbow** (Table 26-7)

C. **Blockade at the wrist** is often preferred to more proximal approaches, because the nerves are associated with easily identified landmarks, and anesthesia is produced with or without paresthesias using 3 mL of local anesthetic solution (Fig. 26-6).

D. **Suprascapular Block**

1. The suprascapular nerve is a terminal branch of the brachial plexus that can be anesthetized by a separate injection to provide pain relief following shoulder arthroscopy or reconstructive surgery.

TABLE 26-7

BLOCK OF PERIPHERAL NERVES AT THE ELBOW

Ulnar nerve (inject 1 to 4 mL of local anesthetic solution in the groove formed by the medial condyle of the humerus and the olecranon process of the ulna; seek paresthesias, but carefully avoid intraneural injection)

Median nerve (inject 5 mL of local anesthetic solution 1 cm medial to the brachial artery)

Radial nerve (inject local anesthetic solution in a fan-shaped pattern 2 cm lateral to the brachial artery)

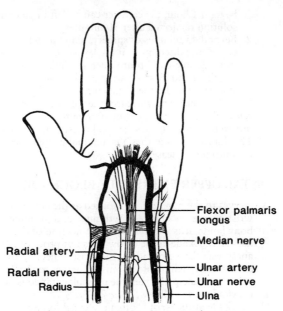

FIGURE 26-6. Terminal nerves at the wrist.

2. The spine of the scapula is identified with the patient sitting upright and leaning forward. The inferior tip of the scapula is identified and the original line of the spine is bisected at a point immediately superior to the inferior tip. The needle is inserted about 1 cm superior and 1 cm lateral from this midpoint until contact is made with the scapula. The needle is redirected until the edge of the suprascapular notch is identified (paresthesia to the shoulder joint may occur or the nerve stimulator may produce internal rotation of the arm).

VII. TRUNK

A. Intercostal Nerve Blockade
1. Anesthesia of the intercostal nerves provides both motor and sensory anesthesia of the entire abdominal wall from the xiphoid process to the

pubis without sympathetic nervous system blockade.

a. When the patient is in the prone, lateral, or sitting positions, the ribs are identified by palpation along the line of their most extreme posterior angulation (Fig. 26-7).

b. The needle is "walked off" the lower border of the rib and advanced 4 to 6 mm while

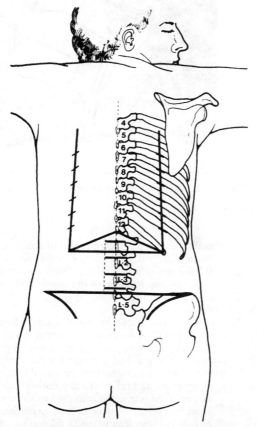

FIGURE 26-7. Landmarks for intercostal block.

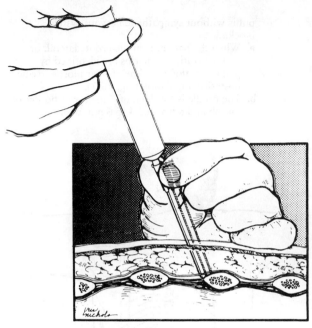

FIGURE 26-8. Hand and needle positions for intercostal block.

maintaining a 10-degree cephalad angle, at which point 3 to 5 mL of a solution containing 0.25 to 0.5% bupivacaine is injected after confirming an extravascular location of the needle (Fig. 26-8).

2. **Complications** (Table 26-8)

B. **Intrapleural Anesthesia**

1. This block is instituted by inserting an epidural catheter 5 to 6 cm into the intrapleural space (signaled by negative pressure that moves the plunger of the attached glass syringe forward) at the level of the seventh or eighth intercostal space.

   a. Bupivacaine (20 mL of 0.5% solution with epinephrine) is injected into the intrapleural space every 3 to 6 hours, or a constant infusion of 0.25% bupivacaine (0.125 mL/kg/hr) can be initiated.

TABLE 26-8

COMPLICATIONS OF INTERCOSTAL NERVE BLOCK

Pneumothorax
Intravascular injection
Systemic absorption (vascularity of the injection site is extensive)
Epidural or subarachnoid injection (most likely with an
  intrathoracic approach)

      b. The local anesthetic solution appears to diffuse
         through the parietal pleura onto the intercostal
         nerves.
   2. Risks of this technique include systemic toxicity
      from absorption of the local anesthetic and
      pneumothorax.
   3. The major limitation is unilateral analgesia, which
      limits this technique to procedures such as
      cholecystectomy or nephrectomy. Loss of local
      anesthetic solution to thoracotomy drainage
      makes this technique less reliable for thoracotomy
      pain.
 C. Ilioinguinal Blockade. The L1 nerve root (occasionally
   joined by a branch of the T12 root) provides sensory
   anesthesia in the area needed for hernia repair surgery
   (subcutaneous infiltration still necessary).
 D. Penile Blockade. Two skin wheals raised at the dorsal
   base of the penis just below and medial to the pubic
   spine followed by placement of 5 mL of local anesthetic
   solution bilaterally plus infiltration of 5 mL in the
   subcutaneous tissue around the underside of the shaft
   provides anesthesia for circumcision and urethral
   procedures. Epinephrine must not be added to the local
   anesthetic solution.
 E. Sympathetic Blockade
   1. Stellate Ganglion
      a. This block provides selective sympathetic nervous
         system blockade of the upper extremity and head,
         which is especially useful in the treatment of
         reflex sympathetic dystrophy.
      b. The needle is inserted at the medial border of the
         sternocleidomastoid muscle, 1.5 to 2 cm caudad
         to the level of the cricoid cartilage (about two
         fingerbreadths above the clavicle) and advanced
         until it contacts bone (C7), at which point a test

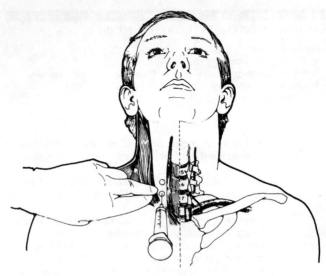

FIGURE 26-9. Landmarks for stellate ganglion block.

  dose (2 mL) is injected followed by up to 8 mL of
1% lidocaine or 0.25% bupivacaine (Fig. 26-9).
 c. The sternocleidomastoid muscle and carotid
sheath are retracted laterally. Paresthesia of the
brachial plexus implies that the needle is too far
lateral.
 d. Onset of ipsilateral sympathetic nervous system
blockade is usually evident within 10 minutes
after injection of the local anesthetic solution
(Table 26-9).

TABLE 26-9	
SIGNS OF SYMPATHETIC NERVOUS SYSTEM BLOCKADE FOLLOWING STELLATE GANGLION BLOCK (HORNER'S SYNDROME)	
Ptosis	Nasal congestion
Miosis	Vasodilation
Anhydrosis	Increased skin temperature

TABLE 26-10

COMPLICATIONS OF STELLATE GANGLION BLOCK

Pneumothorax
Intravascular injection (vertebral artery)
Block of cardioaccelerator fibers
Hoarseness from recurrent laryngeal nerve paralysis
Subarachnoid injection

    e. Potential complications of stellate ganglion block reflect the surrounding anatomy and detract from the use of neurolytic solutions (Table 26-10).

2. **Celiac Plexus**
    a. This block provides relief of pain from malignancy of upper abdominal organs, especially the pancreas.
    b. The celiac plexus is a sympathetic ganglion that results from the merger of the greater and lesser splanchnic nerves at the level of L1 in the retroperitoneal space along the aorta.
    c. The needle is advanced until it contacts the lateral border of L1 (T12 spinous process partially overlies L1), at which point it is withdrawn and the angle steepened so it may be walked off the anterior border of L1 (Fig. 26-10).
    d. **Radiographic verification** of needle location may be indicated, especially if neurolytic solutions are to be injected.
    e. A large volume of local anesthetic solution (20 to 25 mL of 0.75% lidocaine or 0.25% bupivacaine) is needed to diffuse in the retroperitoneal space to reach the ganglia.
    f. The most reliable sign of successful blockade is analgesia or hypotension (prehydration with 1000 mL of crystalloid solution blunts this response).
    g. Potential complications of celiac plexus block reflect the surrounding anatomy (Table 26-11).
    h. **Chronic pain relief** with a neurolytic block lasts 2 to 6 months and may be repeated as necessary, although a trial diagnostic block with local anesthetic is indicated before each use of neurolytic drugs.

3. **Hypogastric Plexus**

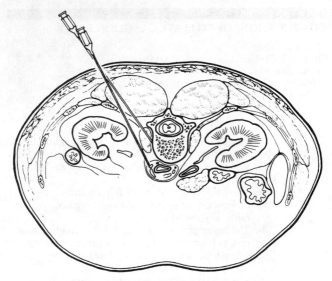

FIGURE 26-10. Landmarks for celiac plexus block.

    a. Fibers passing through this plexus provide visceral sensation to pelvic organs.
    b. Neurolytic block can produce significant pain relief for pelvic malignancies.

VIII. LOWER EXTREMITY

    A. Nerves to the lower extremities are most easily blocked by spinal or epidural anesthesia.

TABLE 26-11
COMPLICATIONS OF CELIAC PLEXUS BLOCK

Unrecognized subarachnoid injection (permanent paralysis if using a neurolytic solution)

Intravascular injection

Back pain if injecting neurolytic solution (treat with intravenous opioids)

Diaphragmatic irritation (shoulder pain)

Transiently increased peristalsis (reflects a shift in balance from sympathetic to parasympathetic nervous system innervation)

1. A peripheral nerve block may be indicated in the presence of sepsis, coagulopathy, or desire for selective anesthesia of the leg or foot.
2. The nerves of the leg arise from the spinal roots of L2-S3, which form the lumbar plexus (lateral femoral cutaneous, femoral, and obturator nerves produce sensory and motor innervation to the upper leg) and the sciatic nerve (divides into the tibial and common peroneal nerves to supply the lower leg).

B. **Sciatic Nerve Block: Classic Posterior Approach**
   1. This block provides adequate anesthesia for the sole of the foot and lower leg.
   2. The needle is inserted at a point 5 cm caudad along the perpendicular line that bisects the line joining the posterior superior iliac spine and greater trochanter; it is advanced perpendicular to the skin in all planes until a paresthesia is elicited, at which point 25 mL of 1.5% lidocaine or 0.5% bupivacaine is injected (Fig. 26-11).

C. **Ankle Blockade**
   1. At least five nerves must be blocked to produce adequate anesthesia (Fig. 26-12).

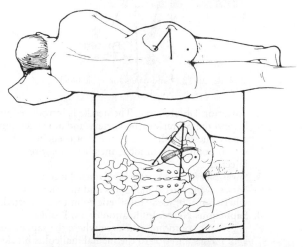

FIGURE 26-11. Landmarks for sciatic nerve block.

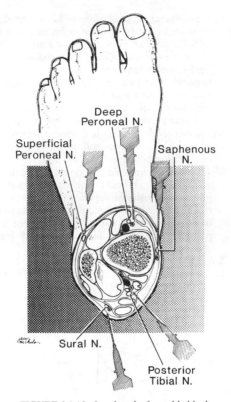

FIGURE 26-12. Landmarks for ankle block.

2. **Posterior Tibial Nerve.** The needle is introduced just behind the posterior tibial artery and advanced until a paresthesia to the sole of the foot is elicited, at which point 5 mL of local anesthetic solution is injected.
3. **Sural Nerve.** The needle is advanced into the groove between the lateral malleolus and the calcaneus, where 5 mL of local anesthetic solution is injected.
4. **Saphenous Nerve.** Infiltration of 5 mL of local anesthetic solution in the area where the saphenous vein passes anterior to the medial malleolus blocks this nerve.

5. **Deep Peroneal Nerve.** This is the major nerve to the dorsum of the foot, and it is blocked by placement of 5 mL of local anesthetic solution just lateral to the anterior tibial artery.
6. **Superficial Peroneal Branches.** A subcutaneous ridge of anesthetic solution (5 to 10 mL) is placed between the anterior tibial artery and the lateral malleolus.

CHAPTER 27 ■ ANESTHESIA FOR NEUROSURGERY

Knowledge of the neurobiology of the brain is necessary for the application of the principles of neuroanesthesia (Bendo AA, Kass IS, Hartung J, Cottrell JE: Anesthesia for neurosurgery. In Barash PG, Cullen BF, Stoelting RK [eds]: *Clinical Anesthesia*, pp 746–789. Philadelphia, Lippincott Williams & Wilkins, 2006).

I. NEUROPHYSIOLOGY

A. Membrane Potentials
1. Neurons have an electrical potential across their cell membranes (about -70 mV at rest) owing to different intracellular and extracellular ion concentrations.
2. The conductance of ions across the cell membranes is via ion-specific protein channels.
3. Neurons signal over long distances by propagating action potentials, which are brief and rapid depolarizations of the membrane.

B. Synaptic Transmission
1. Activation of $GABA_A$ receptors opens chloride channels (activity enhanced by benzodiazepines, barbiturates).
2. Activation of $GABA_B$ receptors by GABA opens potassium channels.
3. **Glutamate** is the principal excitatory neurotransmitter in the CNS. It acts to depolarize the postsynapitc neuron, causing it to be more likely to generate an action potential. The N-methyl-D-aspartate receptor is activated by glutamate.

C. Brain Metabolism
1. The principal substrate used for energy production (formation of adenosine triphosphate) in the brain is glucose. Entrance of glucose into the glycolytic pathway requires oxygen (3.5 mL/100 g/min in an adult and 5.2 mL/100 g/min in children).
2. Pumping ions (sodium, potassium, calcium) across cell membranes is the largest energy requirement of the brain.

D. Cerebral Blood Flow (CBF)
1. The brain receives about 15% of the cardiac output but represents only about 2% of total body weight reflecting its high metabolic rate. Regional CBF is coupled to metabolic rate, increasing dramatically when the local cerebral metabolic rate for oxygen $CMRO_2$ increases.
2. CBF parallels the $PaCO_2$ (increasing the $PaCO_2$ from 40 to 80 mm Hg doubles the CBF, whereas decreasing the $PaCO_2$ from 40 to 20 mm Hg halves the CBF) (Fig. 27-1).
   a. Decreasing the CBF by acute changes in the $PaCO_2$ or by the administration of drugs (thiopental) is an important principle of neuroanesthesia.
   b. The effects of increasing or decreasing the $PaCO_2$ are transient and the CBF returns to normal in 6 to 8 hours even if the altered $PaCO_2$ levels are maintained.
3. CBF is maintained at a constant rate (autoregulated) over a mean arterial pressure (MAP) of about 50 to

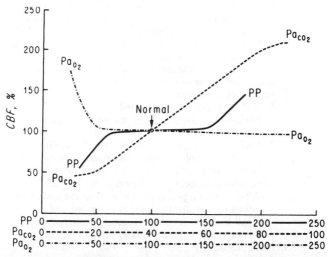

FIGURE 27-1. The effect of perfusion pressure (PP), $PaCO_2$, and PaO_2 on cerebral blood flow (CBF).

150 mm Hg in normotensive individuals reflecting appropriate adjustments of cerebral vascular resistance (see Fig. 27-1).

   a. This response takes 1 to 3 minutes to develop, such that an abrupt change in MAP is accompanied by a transient period of increased or decreased CBF.
   b. When MAP decreases below about 50 mm Hg, the CBF is decreased and mild symptoms of cerebral ischemia occur at a MAP of about 40 mm Hg.
   c. When MAP exceeds the autoregulated range, it may cause disruption of the blood-brain barrier and subsequent cerebral edema.
   d. Autoregulation can be abolished by trauma, hypoxia, and certain drugs used during anesthesia.
   e. Systemic hypertension that persists for 1 to 2 months (hypertrophy of vessel walls occurs in this time period) causes a shift of the autoregulation range to higher pressures such that cerebral ischemia may occur despite perfusion pressures >50 mm Hg.

E. **Cerebrospinal fluid (CSF)** is formed in the choroid plexus of the cerebral ventricles (0.3 to 0.4 mL/min) and reabsorbed into the venous system of the brain via the arachnoid villi (volume of CSF in the brain is 100 to 150 mL). Furosemide (inhibits transport of sodium and chloride ions) and acetazolamide (decreased bicarbonate ion transport) may be used clinically to decrease the rate of CSF formation.

F. **Intracranial Pressure (ICP)**
   1. ICP >15 mm Hg may impede CBF (cerebral perfusion pressure is MAP minus ICP) and introduces the risk of brain herniation.
   2. Under normal circumstances a small increase in intracranial volume does not greatly increase ICP because of the elasticity (compliance) of the components located in the cranium (Fig. 27-2). After a certain point, the capacity of the system to adjust to increased volume is exceeded and even a small increase in volume (vasodilation, hematoma, tumor, edema) increases ICP.

G. **Pathophysiology**
   1. The brain is the most sensitive of all organs to ischemic damage, which may be global (cardiac

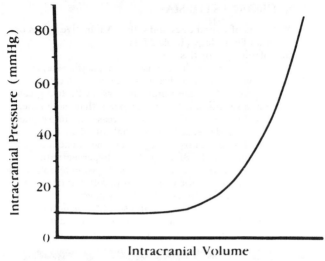

FIGURE 27-2. The effect of increasing intracranial volume on intracranial pressure.

arrest) or focal (localized stroke). Ischemic damage to neurons most likely reflects decreased energy production (blockage of oxidative phosphorylation), leading to decreased activity of adenosine triphosphate-dependent ion pumps and intracellular accumulation of sodium and calcium ions.

2. **Seizures** greatly increase CMR and must be suppressed in conditions in which CBF may be compromised.

3. **Brain trauma** may produce irreversible neuronal damage, although much of the injury may be secondary and follow the initial insult (calcium influx, release of vasoconstrictive substances).

4. **Brain tumors** may increase ICP (blood vessels supplying the tumor may have a leaky blood-brain barrier contributing to vasogenic brain edema).

5. Processes that lead to neuronal death are necrosis (disintegration of the cell and activation of microglia), the immune (inflammation) response, and apoptosis (reactivated when neurons are damaged as a result of ischemia)

II. NEUROANESTHESIA

A. **Effects of Anesthetics and Other Adjunctive Drugs on Brain Physiology** (Table 27-1)
B. **Volatile Anesthetics**
1. Halothane, enflurane, isoflurane, desflurane, and sevoflurane have direct vasodilatory effects that increase CBF. Desflurane increases CBF to a greater and sevoflurane to a lesser extent than isoflurane.
   a. Increases in CBF could increase ICP in patients with decreased intracranial compliance.
   b. It may be possible to negate the impact of increased CBF on ICP with hyperventilation. However, if ICP is increased it is preferable to use an intravenous agent (propofol) that does not have any direct vasodilatory effect.
2. Isoflurane, desflurane, and sevoflurane decrease $CMRO_2$ to a greater extent than halothane. It is

TABLE 27-1

EFFECTS OF DRUGS ON THE NEUROPHYSIOLOGY OF THE BRAIN

Drug	Cerebral blood flow	Cerebral metabolic oxygen requirements	Direct cerebral vasodilation
Halothane	+ + ++	−	yes
Enflurane	++	−	yes
Isoflurane	+	− −	yes
Desflurane	+	− −	yes
Sevoflurane	+	− −	yes
Nitrous oxide	+	+	
Nitrous oxide with a volatile anesthetic	++	+	
Nitrous oxide with an iv anesthetic	0	0	
Thiopental	− − −	− − −	no
Etomidate	− − −	− − − −	no
Propofol	− −	− −	no
Midazolam	− −	− −	no
Ketamine	++	+	yes
Fentanyl	−/0	−/0	no

+ = increase; − = decrease.

thought that isoflurane's metabolic effect serves to decrease CBF and impede this drug's direct vasodilatory effect, which serves to limit increases in CBF. Isoflurane is often recommended as the drug of choice for patients with cerebral ischemia or the potential to develop it.

3. Although nitrous oxide is commonly used in neuroanesthesia, its use should be carefully considered given its potential effects on CBF, $CMRO_2$, and ICP.

C. **Intravenous Anesthetics**

1. Barbiturates, etomidate, propofol, and benzodiazepines decrease CBF and $CMRO_2$. Opioids cause minimal effects on these parameters. Ketamine can increase CBF and $CMRO_2$ and is not commonly used in neuroanesthesia.

2. Thiopental in doses sufficient to produce a flat electroencephalogram (EEG) decreases $CMRO_2$ by 50%. The decrease in $CMRO_2$ results in constriction of the cerebral vasculature, leading to a decrease in CBF and ICP. An important problem with thiopental when used to lower ICP is decreased cerebral perfusion pressure.

3. Propofol decreases $CMRO_2$ similar to sevoflurane but does not increase CBF and is able to reduce ICP. Jugular bulb oxygen saturation may decrease during hyperventilation in patients receiving propofol.

4. Dexmedetomidine reduces arousal and decreases CBF.

III. BRAIN PROTECTION

A. **Cerebral preconditioning** in response to ischemia reflects an endogenous response to decreased blood flow and oxygen delivery (as during hibernation). Clinically acceptable means of accomplishing cerebral preconditioning are being evaluated (erythropoietin).

B. **Neurogenesis and Diaschisis.** It is possible that neural precursors in the brain initiate compensatory responses to stroke that results in productions of new neurons.

C. **Mild Hypothermia and Postoperative Fever.** Clinical evidence does not support induction of perioperative hypothermia for neurosurgical procedures (aneurysm

repair, head injury) that do not entail circulatory bypass.
  D. **Anesthetic and Adjuvant Drugs.** Clinically verified pharmacological brain protection is even more elusive than the benefits of mild hypothermia. Clinical decisions about which anesthetic is most appropriate should be based on considerations other than potential to provide cerebral protection.

IV. MONITORING

  A. **EEG** can be used to monitor cerebral function (early detection of cerebral ischemia) and localization of epileptic foci during general anesthesia (Table 27-2).
   1. Anesthetic drugs and physiologic changes may alter EEG waveforms and interpretation (Table 27-3).
   2. Efforts to use the EEG as a monitor of the depth of anesthesia have been unsuccessful because of the variety of drugs involved during an anesthetic and because some anesthetics do not follow a predictable pattern with respect to their effects on the EEG.
   3. Verification of electrical silence via EEG monitoring is useful when determining the dose of barbiturate needed to maintain "coma."
  B. **Computerized Electroencephalographic Processing**
   1. The most widely used technique is power-spectrum analysis (compressed spectral array format), which

TABLE 27-2
ELECTROENCEPHALOGRAM FREQUENCY CHANGES

delta-rhythm (0–3 Hz)	Deep sleep
	Deep anesthesia
	Pathologic states (brain tumors, arterial hypoxemia, metabolic encephalopathy)
theta-rhythm (4–7 Hz)	Physiologic sleep and general anesthesia in adults
	Hyperventilation in awake children
alpha-rhythm (8–13 Hz)	Resting awake adult with eyes closed
beta-rhythm (>13 Hz)	Mental activity
	Light anesthesia

TABLE 27-3

ELECTROENCEPHALOGRAPHIC CHANGES ASSOCIATED WITH DRUGS AND PHYSIOLOGIC CHANGES

Increased Frequency
Barbiturates (low dose)
Benzodiazepines (low dose)
Etomidate (low dose)
Propofol (low dose)
Ketamine
Nitrous oxide (30–70%)
Volatile anesthetics (<1 MAC)
Arterial hypoxemia (initially)
Hypercarbia (mild)
Seizures

Decreased Frequency and Increased Amplitude
Barbiturates (moderate dose)
Etomidate (moderate dose)
Propofol (moderate dose)
Opioids
Volatile anesthetics (>1 MAC)
Arterial hypoxemia
Hypocarbia (moderate to extreme)
Hypothermia

Decreased Frequency and Decreased Amplitude
Barbiturates (high dose)
Arterial hypoxemia (mild)
Hypercarbia (severe)
Hypothermia (<35°C)

Electrical Silence
Barbiturates (coma dose)
Etomidate (high dose)
Propofol (high dose)
Isoflurane (2 MAC)
Arterial hypoxemia (severe)
Hypothermia (<15°C–20°C)
Brain death

MAC = minimum alveolar concentration.

has value as a monitor of cerebral ischemia and possibly depth of anesthesia.

2. Control readings in awake patients should be obtained before induction of general anesthesia. Bilateral data must be obtained to distinguish between anesthetic and systemic effects (bilateral

changes) and surgical trauma or cerebral ischemia (ipsilateral changes).

C. **Evoked potentials** are used to monitor the functional integrity of ascending sensory pathways (sensory evoked potentials) and descending motor pathways (motor evoked potentials).

1. **Sensory evoked potentials** used clinically are somatosensory, auditory, and visual.

    a. Compromise or injury of a neurologic pathway (as during spinal column instrumentation for treatment of scoliosis) is manifested as an **increase** in the **latency** and/or a **decrease** in the **amplitude** of evoked potential waveforms.

    b. Anesthetics influence evoked potentials (Table 27-4). In general, volatile anesthetics cause a decrease in amplitude.

2. **Motor evoked potentials** (detect motor pathway compromise, which may occur independent of sensory pathway compromise) may obviate the need for an intraoperative wake-up test during scoliosis surgery and provide detection of intraoperative spinal cord dysfunction during aortic cross-clamping.

D. **Cranial nerve monitoring** during posterior fossa surgery and brainstem procedures can be accomplished with monitoring the electromyogram potential of cranial nerves with motor components (V, VII, IX, X, XI, XII).

1. Evoking the nerves with electrical stimulation facilitates identification and thus preservation of cranial nerves.

2. Neuromuscular blockade may interfere with monitoring electromyogram potentials.

E. **Intracranial Pressure Monitoring**

1. Techniques used to monitor ICP include ventricular catheters, subdural-subarachnoid bolts or catheters, epidural transducers, and intraparenchymal fiberoptic devices (Fig. 27-3).

2. The intraventricular catheter is the standard method for monitoring ICP. The intraparenchymal fiberoptic device is inserted through a 2-mm burr hole and in comparison to ventriculostomies is easier to place, is less disruptive to brain tissue, and because there is no fluid column, the risk of infection is probably smaller.

TABLE 27-4
EFFECTS OF INTRAVENOUS AND INHALED DRUGS ON SENSORY AND MOTOR EVOKED POTENTIALS

	Brainstem auditory potentials		Cortical somatosensory evoked potentials		Visual evoked potentials		Motor evoked potentials	
	Lat	Amp	Lat	Amp	Lat	Amp	Lat	Amp
Thiopental (4–6 mg/kg iv)	0	0	0	0	?	?	+	−\
Diazepam (0.1 mg/kg iv)	0	0	+	−	0	−	+	−
Midazolam	?	?	+/0	−	?	?	+/0	−
Fentanyl	0	0	+/0	−/0	0	−	0	0
Sufentanil	0	0	+/0	−/0	?	?		
Alfentanil	0	0	+/0	−/0	?	?		
Etomidate	+	0	+	+	+	0	0	0
Propofol (2–6 mg/kg iv)	0	0	+	0/−	?	?	0	−
Ketamine	+	0	+/0	+	+	+		
Nitrous oxide	0	−	0	−	+	−	+	−
Enflurane	+	0	+	+	+	−	+	−
Halothane	+	0	+	−	+	−	+	−
Isoflurane	+	0	+	−	+	−	+	−
Desflurane	+	0	+	−	?	?	+	−
Sevoflurane	+	0	+	−	?	?	+	−

+ = increased; − = decreased; 0 = no change; ? = no data; lat = latency; amp = amplitude.

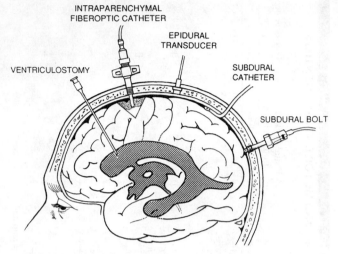

INTRAPARENCHYMAL
FIBEROPTIC CATHETER

EPIDURAL
TRANSDUCER

VENTRICULOSTOMY

SUBDURAL
CATHETER

SUBDURAL BOLT

FIGURE 27-3. Techniques used to measure intracranial pressure.

F. **Transcranial Doppler ultrasound** is used for clinical imaging of intracranial vasculature (does not measure CBF but rather direction and velocity of the moving column of blood in a major artery).
G. **Cerebral Oxygenation/Metabolism Monitors**
   1. **Brain tissue oxygenation** may be monitored by a sensor placed into the cerebral cortex.
   2. **Jugular venous bulb oximetry** provides an estimate of the global (not focal) balance between cerebral oxygen demand and supply (<50% indicates increased oxygen extraction and risk for ischemic injury).
   3. **Transcranial oximetry** is a noninvasive optical method for monitoring cerebral regional oxygenation (trend monitor with each patient acting as his or her control). In situations of potential regional ischemia (carotid endarterectomy, temporary clip application during intracranial aneurysm surgery) bilateral monitoring is recommended.

TABLE 27-5
METHODS USED FOR NEURORADIOLOGY

Computed tomography scan (contrast enhancement is provided by intravenous injection of dye)

Magnetic resonance imaging (provides excellent contrast between gray and white matter)

Positron emission tomography (detects positron energy emitted from the injected radionuclide as a reflection of processes involved in cerebral metabolism; can be overlaid on computed tomography or magnetic resonance imaging to improve anatomic location of detected activity [seizures])

Cerebral angiography (used to define the vasculature of the brain or spinal cord; hyperventilation of the patient's lungs slows cerebral blood flow and improves the clarity)

Myelography (avoid drugs that lower the seizure threshold in patients receiving the water-soluble contrast agent metrizamide)

Interventional neuroradiology (complications may be hemorrhagic [immediate heparin reversal] or occlusive)

V. **NEURORADIOLOGY** (Table 27-5). General anesthesia is required for very young or uncooperative patients because these procedures require a totally motionless patient.

VI. **ANESTHETIC MANAGEMENT OF NEUROSURGICAL PATIENTS**

   A. Neurosurgical procedures tend to be lengthy and require unusual positioning of the patient and the institution of special techniques such as hyperventilation of the patient's lungs, cerebral dehydration, and deliberate hypotension.

   B. Except for neurosurgical emergencies (head trauma, impending herniation), most neurosurgical procedures can be delayed until after the treatment of medically unstable conditions.

   C. **Preoperative evaluation** includes a complete neurologic evaluation with special attention to the patient's level of consciousness, the extent of focal neurologic deficits, and the presence or absence of signs and symptoms frequently associated with increased ICP (Table 27-6).

TABLE 27-6

SIGNS AND SYMPTOMS OF INCREASED
INTRACRANIAL PRESSURE

Headache
Nausea
Papilledema
Unilateral pupillary dilatation
Oculomotor or abducens palsy
Depressed level of consciousness
Irregular breathing
Midline shift (0.5 cm) or encroachment of expanding brain on
  cerebral ventricles (computed tomography or magnetic
  resonance imaging)

D. The location of the space-occupying lesion
   (supratentorial or infratentorial compartment)
   determines its clinical presentation and anesthetic
   management.
   1. **Supratentorial** lesions are usually associated with
      problems in the management of increased ICP.
   2. **Infratentorial** lesions cause problems related to
      pressure effects on vital brainstem structures and
      increased ICP produced by obstructive
      hydrocephalus.
E. Fluid and electrolyte abnormalities are common in
   patients with decreased levels of consciousness.

VII. SUPRATENTORIAL INTRACRANIAL TUMORS

A. Meningiomas, gliomas, and metastatic lesions
   eventually grow to the size at which compensatory
   mechanisms are exhausted, and additional increases in
   the size of the tumor (central area of hemorrhagic
   tissue, wider border of brain edema) manifest as
   progressive increases in ICP.
B. Anesthetic Techniques and Drugs
   1. The goal of neuroanesthetic care for patients with
      supratentorial tumors is to maximize therapeutic
      modalities that decrease ICP.
   2. ICP must be controlled before the cranium is opened
      and optimal operating conditions obtained by
      producing a slack brain.
C. Clinical Control of Intracranial Hypertension
   (Table 27-7)

TABLE 27-7
METHODS TO CONTROL INTRACRANIAL PRESSURE

Hyperventilation (PaCO$_2$ 25–30 mm Hg)
Diuresis (mannitol as an osmotic diuretic and furosemide as a loop diuretic)
Hypertonic saline (acts as osmotic diuretic but more data is needed to verify safety)
Drug-induced cerebral vasoconstriction (thiopental, etomidate, propofol, lidocaine)
Corticosteroids (dexamethasone effective for localized cerebral edema surrounding tumors; requires 12–36 hours)
Elevation of the head to 30° (encourages cerebral venous drainage)
Blood pressure control
CSF drainage
Fluid restriction
Hypothermia
Surgical decompression (epidural hematoma)

1. Rapid brain dehydration and decrease in ICP can be produced by administering an osmotic diuretic (mannitol 0.25 to 1 g/kg iv begins to work within 10 to 15 minutes and lasts about 2 hours) or a loop diuretic (furosemide 0.5 to 1 mg/kg iv alone or 0.15 to 0.3 mg/kg iv in combination with mannitol).

    a. Because mannitol may initially increase ICP (reflects mannitol-induced vasodilation), it should be administered slowly (10 minutes or longer) and in conjunction with maneuvers that decrease intracranial volume (steroids, hyperventilation). Furosemide may be a preferred choice to decrease ICP in patients with preexisting cardiovascular disease (mannitol produces a transient increase in intravascular fluid volume).

    b. Combined mannitol and furosemide diuresis is more effective than mannitol alone but produces more severe dehydration and electrolyte imbalance (monitor electrolytes intraoperatively and replace potassium as necessary).

2. **Corticosteroids** decrease edema around brain tumors but require several hours to days before a decrease in ICP occurs. Neurologic improvement that precedes a decrease in ICP may reflect a restoration of the previously abnormal blood-brain barrier.

3. **Hyperventilation** of the patient's lungs to maintain a $PaCO_2$ of 25 to 30 mm Hg (every mm Hg decrease below 40 mm Hg decreases CBF 1 to 2 mL/100 g/min, but the effect may be as brief as 4 to 6 hours) is the mainstay of acute and subacute management of increased ICP. Impaired responsiveness to changes in $PaCO_2$ occurs in areas of vasoparalysis (ischemia, trauma, tumor, infection) and interferes with effectiveness of hyperventilation.

4. **Restricted fluid intake** is rarely used to lower ICP because it can cause hypovolemia resulting in hypotension with induction of anesthesia.

   a. Fluid resuscitation and maintenance fluids (hourly maintenance fluids plus urine output) in the routine neurosurgical patient are provided with glucose-free isomolar crystalloid solutions to prevent increases in brain water content. Solutions containing glucose are avoided in neurosurgical patients with normal glucose metabolism, because these solutions may exacerbate ischemic damage and cerebral edema (hyperglycemia augments ischemic damage by promoting neuronal lactate production).

   b. Preoperative corticosteroids and general anesthesia-induced gluconeogenesis may elevate resting glucose levels. Blood glucose may be monitored during craniotomy and maintained at near low-normal values mainly by withholding exogenous glucose.

5. A **neutral** head position elevated 15 to 30 degrees is recommended to decrease ICP by improving venous drainage. Flexing or turning of the head, lowering the head, or application of positive end-expiratory pressure (>10 cm H_2O) acts to impair cerebral venous drainage with possible increases in ICP.

6. **Pharmacologic agents** (thiopental, propofol, etomidate) are potent cerebral vasoconstrictors that can acutely decrease ICP as may be associated with induction of anesthesia or painful stimulation.

7. Intraoperatively, a modest degree of **hypothermia** (34°C) is recommended as a way to confer neuronal protection during focal ischemia.

D. **Premedication** is not administered to lethargic patients.

E. **Monitoring** in addition to routine observations includes measurement of intra-arterial blood pressure, arterial blood gases, central venous pressure, and urine output. The need to measure ICP for supratentorial operations is controversial.

F. **Muscle Relaxants**

1. Succinylcholine and nondepolarizing muscle relaxants that evoke the release of histamine may accentuate coexisting intracranial hypertension or lower cerebral perfusion pressure.

2. To achieve muscle relaxation for intubation of the trachea, succinylcholine is not recommended for elective neurosurgical cases. The steroidal muscle relaxants may be better relaxants for neurosurgical patients because they do not affect ICP. When there is a risk of aspiration, succinylcholine should be used. Succinylcholine-induced hyperkalemia has been reported after closed head injury and ruptured cerebral aneurysms in patients who were not hemiplegic or paraplegic.

G. **Induction, Maintenance, and Emergence**

1. A common induction sequence is thiopental (3 to 5 mg/kg iv) or propofol (1.25 to 2.5 mg/kg) followed by fentanyl (3 to 5 μg/kg iv) and a nondepolarizing muscle relaxant.

2. Before direct laryngoscopy for tracheal intubation is initiated, an additional dose of thiopental (2 to 3 mg/kg iv) is administered and endotracheal intubation is performed as rapidly and smoothly as possible.

3. After induction of anesthesia, ventilation of the patient's lungs is controlled mechanically (routine institution of hyperventilation is not recommended because of the risk of cerebral ischemia).

4. The most commonly administered maintenance anesthetics are either propofol-opioid (remifentanil or fentanyl) or isoflurane-opioid. There is a question of cerebral hypoperfusion in the presence of propofol especially in the presence of hyperventilation.

5. Intracranial hematoma and cerebral edema are the most feared complications after intracranial surgery. Emergence should be smooth to avoid arterial hypertension (causes hematomas and edema). Muscle relaxants are not reversed until the head dressing is applied and lidocaine (1.5

mg/kg iv) can be administered 90 seconds before
extubation.

6. A brief neurologic examination is performed after
extubation of the trachea and the patient is
transported with the head elevated at about
30 degrees to the postanesthesia care unit.

H. **Awake craniotomy** with functional mapping is
recommended for removal of tumors involving the
eloquent cortex.

VIII. INFRATENTORIAL INTRACRANIAL TUMORS

A. Patients with infratentorial tumors (posterior fossa
contains the medulla, pons, cerebellum, and lower
cranial nerve nuclei) may exhibit depressed levels of
consciousness secondary to increased ICP from
obstructive hydrocephalus and/or exhibit signs of
brainstem compression, with depressed ventilation and
cranial nerve palsies.

B. **Special Anesthetic Considerations**

1. **Surgical Position**

a. Exploration of the posterior fossa has been
traditionally performed with the patient in the
sitting position because it provides excellent
surgical exposure and facilitates venous and CSF
drainage. Other positions (lateral and prone)
have been advocated because of the lower
incidence of venous air embolism and greater
cardiovascular stability.

b. Pneumocephalus occurs frequently in patients
who have surgery performed in the sitting
position (nitrous oxide may contribute to the
development of tension pneumocephalus in the
postoperative period resulting in neurologic
dysfunction).

2. **Monitoring**

a. The electrocardiogram is monitored for changes
in heart rate and cardiac rhythm during
posterior fossa exploration because surgical
retraction or manipulation around the
brainstem or cranial nerves can cause significant
cardiac dysrhythmias or alterations in blood
pressure.

b. Alternatively, sensory evoked potentials
(brainstem auditory evoked potentials during

TABLE 27-8
DIAGNOSIS OF VENOUS AIR EMBOLISM

Precordial Doppler ultrasonic transducer (placed over right sternal border between third and sixth intercostal spaces; verify correct positioning by central venous injection of 10 mL of saline; most sensitive noninvasive monitor detecting amounts of air as small as 0.25 mL)

Transesophageal echocardiography (slightly more sensitive than the Doppler but invasive and cumbersome; advantages of monitoring air in the right and left heart so can detect both venous and arterial air embolism)

Capnography (air embolism is reflected as decreased end-tidal CO_2; Doppler changes without evidence of changes in end-tidal CO_2 are not hemodynamically significant)

Mass spectrometry (end-expired nitrogen reflects the volume of the entrained air)

Pulmonary artery catheter (increase in pressure correlates with the hemodynamic significance of the embolus)

acoustic neuroma surgery; somatosensory evoked potentials to monitor brainstem ischemia) have been used to monitor compromise of the brainstem or cranial nerves.
   c. Electromyography is used to test seventh nerve function when the face is not accessible to palpation or visual assessment.
3. **Venous air embolism** may occur whenever the operative field is elevated above the right atrial level (Tables 27-8 and 27-9).
4. **Anesthetic Management**
   a. Postural hypotension (minimized by adequate preoperative hydration, wrapping the legs, and

TABLE 27-9
TREATMENT OF VENOUS AIR EMBOLISM

Flood surgical field with saline and wax bone edges
Discontinue nitrous oxide
Compress neck veins
Aspirate air (maximum retrieval of air can be obtained from a multiorificed tip that is positioned at the junction of the superior vena cava and the right atrium)
Give vasopressors and volume infusion (treat hypotension)
Administer positive end-expiratory pressure to the airways (avoid in patients with a probe patent foramen ovale)

TABLE 27-10

POSTOPERATIVE CONCERNS FOLLOWING POSTERIOR
FOSSA SURGERY

Central apnea
Impaired swallowing and pharyngeal sensation (at risk for
  aspiration)
Hypertension (requires prompt treatment to prevent brain edema
  and hematoma formation)
Cardiac dysrhythmias
Delayed awakening (brainstem compression)

flexing the patient's hips and knees at heart level)
and the risk of venous air embolism (physiologic
effect may be increased in the presence of nitrous
oxide) are considerations when selecting an
anesthetic technique for patients in the sitting
position.

b. A nitrous oxide-oxygen-opioid-muscle relaxant
anesthetic combined with controlled
hyperventilation of the patient's lungs may be
recommended for maximal cardiovascular
stability and control of ICP.

5. **Postoperative Concerns** (Table 27-10)

IX. PITUITARY TUMORS

A. Pituitary tumors can be categorized as
nonfunctioning (chromophobe adenomas that enlarge
and compress the normal gland) and **hypersecreting**
(most often adenomas secreting prolactin or growth
hormone).

B. **Special Anesthetic Considerations**

1. **Preoperative evaluation** of patients with pituitary
tumors requires an assessment of endocrine function
and associated medical disorders (systemic effects of
excess cortisol; airway changes associated with
acromegaly).

a. **Panhypopituitarism** replacement therapy includes
oral administration of corticosteroids and
thyroxine and possibly intranasal instillation of
synthetic vasopressin.

b. All patients scheduled for pituitary surgery are
given supplemental short-acting corticosteroid
therapy preoperatively.

  c. The computed tomographic scan or magnetic resonance imaging scan and the neurologic examination are evaluated for signs of increased ICP.

  2. **Surgical Considerations.** Transsphenoidal excision has been recommended for all pituitary tumors that do not have marked suprasellar extension. The incidence of permanent diabetes insipidus and anterior pituitary insufficiency is increased when a transcranial approach is needed.

  3. **Anesthetic considerations** for patients undergoing pituitary surgery include measures to control ICP if a transcranial approach is used and right atrial catheterization for treatment of potential venous air embolism if a transsphenoidal procedure is planned.

     a. Visual evoked potential monitoring may be used to monitor compromise of blood supply to the optic nerves and chiasm.

     b. Cocaine-soaked pledgets (4%) and epinephrine (1:200,000) used to prepare the nasal approach for transsphenoidal surgery may initially cause hypertension, tachycardia, cardiac dysrhythmias, and myocardial ischemia that necessitate treatment.

     c. Following transsphenoidal surgery, the patient awakens with nasal packing in place emphasizing the need for full return of consciousness before extubation of the trachea is performed.

  4. **Postoperative concerns** include the need for continued corticosteroid supplementation and strict attention to fluid balance (diabetes insipidus may manifest in the first 12 hours postoperatively).

X. CEREBROSPINAL MALFORMATIONS

A. **Intracranial Aneurysms**
   1. Diagnosis of subarachnoid hemorrhage (SAH) is by clinical findings (severe headache associated with stiff neck, photophobia, nausea and vomiting, transient loss of consciousness) and computed tomography.

   2. **Complications** of SAH and surgical treatment include rebleeding, cerebral vascular vasospasm, intracranial hypertension, and hydrocephalus.

       a. Rebleeding occurs most commonly during the
          first 24 hours following SAH.
       b. Cerebral vascular vasospasm occurs most often 4
          to 12 days following SAH and is heralded by
          worsening ache and hypertension. The diagnosis
          of cerebral vascular vasospasm is confirmed by
          angiography, whereas the transcranial Doppler is
          a noninvasive method to evaluate the
          effectiveness of various therapies (efficacy of
          nimodipine is questionable).
       c. **Triple H therapy** (hypervolemia, hypertension,
          and hemodilution) has become the mainstay
          for treatment (efficacy unproven) of neurologic
          deficits caused by cerebral vascular vasospasm.
       d. Cerebral angioplasty may be a method to treat
          symptomatic cerebral vascular vasospasm.
  B. Endovascular Treatment of Cerebral Aneurysms
     1. Endovascular embolization is a therapeutic
       alternative to surgical clipping of some cerebral
       aneurysm (insertion of Guglielmi detachable
       coils).
  C. Special Anesthetic Considerations
     1. Preoperative Evaluation (Table 27-11)
     2. Anesthetic management is designed to avoid
       aneurysm rupture (occurs intraoperatively in 20%
       of patients), maintain cerebral perfusion pressure,
       and provide optimal surgical access ("slack brain")
       (Table 27-12).
       a. The potential benefits of deliberate hypotension
          for cerebral aneurysm clip ligation must be
          weighed against the risk of causing cerebral
          ischemia or ischemia to other organs.

TABLE 27-11

PREOPERATIVE EVALUATION OF THE PATIENT WITH A SUBARACHNOID HEMORRHAGE

Increased ICP
Hyponatremia (diabetes insipidus; syndrome of inappropriate
   antidiuretic hormone secretion)
Hypernatremia and hyperosmolarity
Hypertension
Cardiac dysrhythmias
ST segment depression or elevation on the electrocardiogram
   (subendocardial infarction is a possibility)

TABLE 27-12

MANAGEMENT OF ANESTHESIA FOR TREATMENT OF SUBARACHNOID HEMORRHAGE AS A RESULT OF AN INTRACRANIAL ANEURYSM

Minimize hypertension associated with tracheal intubation (establish a surgical level of anesthesia, give a short-acting opioid just before initiating direct laryngoscopy, and assure a brief duration of laryngoscopy)

Mechanical control of ventilation to maintain the $PaCO_2$ at 25–30 mm Hg

Thiopental and fentanyl frequently used in conjunction with isoflurane to maintain anesthesia

CSF drainage and osmotic diuretics

Consider monitoring evoked potentials to reflect adequacy of cerebral perfusion during deliberate hypotension or aneurysm clip application

Be prepared to treat sudden hemorrhage

Avoid reaction to tracheal tube at conclusion of surgery (patient remains intubated and mechanically ventilated if neurologic status is depressed)

      b. Low-grade hypothermia (32°C to 34°C) is recommended during aneurysm surgery to enhance the brain's ability to tolerate ischemia.

    3. Intraoperative cerebral protection is most often provided with thiopental (only drug shown to be useful in humans for protection against local [not global] ischemia). Mild intraoperative hypothermia (32°C to 34°C) is of unproven value.

  D. Postoperative concerns include hypertension leading to cerebral edema or hematoma (requires pharmacologic treatment) and vasospasm (maintain higher than normal intravascular fluid volume).

  E. Arteriovenous Malformations (AVMs)

    1. Clinical features of AVMs include signs and symptoms of SAH, development of focal epilepsy, and progressive focal neurologic sensory motor deficits occurring in a child or young adult.

    2. Special Anesthetic Considerations

      a. Closed embolization of cerebral AVMs may be performed with sedation (fentanyl-midazolam), which allows neurologic examinations during the procedure and permits immediate diagnosis of complications (stroke, hemorrhage).

      b. The anesthetic management of a patient with an
AVM is similar to management of patients
for intracranial aneurysm surgery. When the
AVM is large, hypothermia and high-dose
barbiturates may be recommended for brain
protection.

      c. Deliberate hypotension may be instituted to
decrease the size of the AVM.

      d. After removal of the AVM, breakthrough
cerebral edema (blood flow diverted to vessels
not accustomed to high blood flows),
hemorrhage, or hypertension (beta antagonists
may be useful) may occur.

XI. HEAD INJURY

    A. Motor vehicle accidents are responsible for the
majority of head injuries, and >50% of these patients
have multiple injuries resulting in significant blood loss,
hypotension, and arterial hypoxemia.

    B. **Classification** of severe head injury is based on the
Glasgow Coma Scale (score <7 persisting for longer
than 6 hours is severe head injury) (Table 27-13).

TABLE 27-13
GLASGOW COMA SCALE

Parameter	Response	Score
Eye opening	Spontaneously	4
	To command	3
	To pain	2
	No response	1
Motor response	Obeys verbal commands	6
	Localizes pain	5
	Flexion withdrawal	4
	Decorticate rigidity	3
	Decerebrate rigidity	2
	No response	1
Verbal response	Oriented and converses	5
	Disoriented and converses	4
	Inappropriate words	3
	Incomprehensible words	2
	No response	1

C. Following head trauma, the primary injury resulting from the biomechanical effect of forces applied to the skull and brain (concussion, contusion, laceration, hematoma) is irreversible. Secondary injury caused by arterial hypoxemia, anemia, hypotension, hypercarbia, or increased ICP is treatable.

1. Nonoperative treatment of diffuse cerebral edema includes hyperventilation of the patient's lung, diuresis produced with mannitol and furosemide, depression of the CMR with barbiturates, and ICP monitoring.

2. Depressed skull fractures and acute epidural, subdural, and intercerebral hematomas usually require craniotomy.

D. **Emergency Therapy** (Table 27-14)

1. Before securing the airway in a head-injured patient, a quick assessment of the patient's neurologic status and concomitant injuries should be made (incidence of cervical spinal injuries in victims of head-first falls or motor vehicle accidents is >10%).

2. When multiple trauma complicates head injury, there is no ideal crystalloid resuscitation fluid. A major concern during resuscitation is the development of cerebral edema (crystalloid solutions

---

TABLE 27-14

EMERGENCY TREATMENT OF SEVERE HEAD INJURY AND INTRACRANIAL HYPERTENSION

Insert ICP monitor
Maintain cerebral perfusion pressure >70 mm Hg
Treat increased ICP
  First-tier therapy
    Ventricular drainage
    Mannitol 0.25–1.0 g/kg iv (may repeat if serum osmolarity
      <320 mOsmol/L and patient euvolemic)
    Hyperventilation to $PaCO_2$ 30–35 mm Hg
  Second-tier therapy
    Hyperventilation to $PaCO_2$ <30 mm Hg (Sjo_2, $AVDO_2$
      and/or cerebral blood flow recommended)
    High-dose barbiturate therapy
    Consider hypothermia
    Consider hypertensive therapy
    Consider decompressive craniectomy

containing sodium in concentrations lower than in the plasma [0.45% NaCl and lactated Ringer's solution] are more likely than isoosmolar fluids [0.9% saline] to increase brain water content). Glucose-containing solutions are not recommended because of a significant association between plasma glucose levels and poor neurologic outcome in head-injured patients.
3. Hypertension, tachycardia, and increased cardiac output may result from a surge of epinephrine (labetalol or esmolol effective treatment).
4. Hyperventilation of the patient's lungs to lower the $PaCO_2$ to 25 to 30 mm Hg is indicated when control of increased ICP is the primary concern. When the clinical situation no longer requires hyperventilation or there is evidence of cerebral ischemia, normocapnic ventilation is indicated.
5. All head-injured patients are assumed to have full stomachs.
E. **Anesthetic Management**
   1. The patient is evaluated by computed tomography and taken directly to the operating room (Table 27-15).
   2. Major goals of anesthetic management are to optimize cerebral perfusion and oxygenation. Cerebral perfusion pressure should be maintained between 60 and 110 mm Hg
   3. A period of postoperative ventilation is often recommended because brain swelling is maximal 12 to 72 hours after injury.
   4. Hypertension and reacting to the tracheal tube should be avoided because these responses can lead

TABLE 27-15

PREANESTHETIC ASSESSMENT OF THE HEAD-INJURED PATIENT

Airway (cervical spine)
Breathing (ventilation and oxygenation)
Circulatory status
Associated injuries
Neurologic status (Glasgow Coma Score)
Preexisting chronic illness
Circumstances of the injury (time of the injury, duration of unconsciousness, associated alcohol or other drug use)

TABLE 27-16
SYSTEMIC SEQUELAE OF HEAD INJURY

Cardiopulmonary Problems
Airway obstruction
Arterial hypoxemia
Shock
Adult respiratory distress syndrome
Neurogenic pulmonary edema
Aspiration

Hemorrhagic Problems
Disseminated intravascular coagulation

Endocrine Problems
Diabetes insipidus
Syndrome of inappropriate antidiuretic hormone secretion

Gastrointestinal Problems
Stress ulcers
Hemorrhage

to intracranial bleeding. Labetalol or esmolol can be used to treat hypertension and supplemental barbiturates are given to sedate the patient.
F. **Systemic sequelae** of head injury are diverse and can complicate its management (Table 27-16).

CHAPTER 28 ■ RESPIRATORY FUNCTION IN ANESTHESIA

Anesthesiologists manipulate pulmonary function greatly, emphasizing the importance of a thorough knowledge of pulmonary physiology for the safe conduct of anesthesia (Stock MC: Respiratory function in anesthesia. In Barash PG, Cullen BF, Stoelting RK [eds]: *Clinical Anesthesia*, pp 790–812. Philadelphia, Lippincott Williams & Wilkins, 2006).

I. FUNCTIONAL ANATOMY OF THE LUNGS

A. **Muscles of Ventilation**
   1. The muscles of ventilation are endurance muscles that are adversely affected by poor nutrition, chronic obstructive pulmonary disease, and increased airway resistance.
   2. The primary ventilatory muscle is the diaphragm with minor contributions from the intercostal muscles. The muscles of the abdominal wall are important for expulsive efforts such as coughing.
B. **Lung Structures**
   1. The visceral and parietal pleura are constantly in contact, creating a potential intrapleural space in which pressure decreases when the diaphragm descends and the rib cage expands.
   2. The lung parenchyma is subdivided into three airway categories based on functional lung anatomy (Table 28-1).
      a. Airways with diameters of >2 mm create 90% of total airway resistance.
      b. The number of alveoli increases progressively with age, starting at about 24 million at birth and reaching the final adult count of 300 million by the age of 8 to 9 years. There is an estimated 70 m^2 of surface area for gas exchange.
      c. The adult trachea is 10 to 12 cm long with an outside diameter of about 20 mm. The cricoid cartilage corresponds to the level of the sixth cervical vertebral body. Both ends of the trachea

TABLE 28-1

FUNCTIONAL AIRWAY DIVISIONS

Type	Function	Structure
Conductive	Bulk gas movement	Trachea to terminal bronchioles
Transitional	Bulk gas movement	Respiratory bronchioles
	Limited gas exchange	Alveolar ducts
Respiratory	Gas exchange	Alveoli
		Alveolar sacs

are attached to mobile structures, and in an adult the carina can move an average of 3.8 cm with flexion and extension of the neck (important in intubated patient). In a child tracheal tube movement is even more critical because displacement of even 1 cm can move the tube out of the trachea or below the carina.

d. In the adult the right mainstem bronchus leaves the trachea at approximately 25 degrees from the vertical tracheal axis, whereas the angle of the left mainstem bronchus is approximately 45 degrees (accidental endobronchial intubation or aspiration most likely to occur on the right). In children younger than 3 years, the angles created by the right and left mainstem bronchi are approximately equal.

e. The right mainstem bronchus is approximately 2.5 cm long prior to its initial branching (left is about 4.5 cm) and in 2 to 3% of adults the right upper lobe bronchus opens into the trachea above the carina (important for placement of a double-lumen tube).

3. **Respiratory Airways and the Alveolar–Capillary Membrane**

a. The alveolar–capillary membrane is important for transport of alveolar gases (oxygen, carbon dioxide) and metabolism of circulating substances.

b. Type I alveolar cells provide the extensive surface for gas exchange and these cells are susceptible to injury (adult respiratory distress syndrome).

   c. Type III alveolar cells are macrophages and
      provide protection against infection and
      participate in the lung inflammatory
      response.
4. **Pulmonary Vascular Systems**
   a. Two major circulatory systems supply blood to
      the lungs: the pulmonary (gas exchange and
      metabolic needs of the alveolar parenchyma) and
      bronchial (oxygen to the conductive airways and
      pulmonary vessels) vascular networks.
   b. Anatomic connections between the bronchial and
      pulmonary venous circulations create an absolute
      shunt of about 2% of the cardiac output
      ("normal or physiologic shunt").

II. LUNG MECHANICS

A. Lung movement is entirely passive and responds to
   forces external to the lungs (during spontaneous
   ventilation the external forces are produced by ventilatory muscles).
B. **Elastic Work**
   1. The lung's natural tendency is to collapse (elastic
      recoil) such that normal expiration at rest is passive.
   2. Surface tension at an air-fluid interface is responsible
      for keeping alveoli open (during inspiration surface
      tension increases ensuring that gas tends to flow
      from larger to smaller alveoli and thereby
      preventing collapse).
   3. **Esophageal pressure** is a reflection of the intrapleural
      pressure and allows an estimation of the patient's
      work of breathing (elastic work and resistive work
      to overcome resistance to gas flow in the airway).
   4. Patients with low lung compliance typically breathe
      with smaller tidal volumes at more rapid rates.
      Patients with diseases that increase lung compliance
      (gas trapping because of asthma or chronic
      obstructive pulmonary disease) must use ventilatory
      muscles to actively exhale.
C. **Resistance to Gas Flow.** Both laminar and turbulent
   flow exist within the respiratory tract.
   1. **Laminar flow** is not audible and is influenced only
      by viscosity (helium has a low density, but its
      viscosity is close to air).

TABLE 28-2
PHYSIOLOGIC CHANGES IN RESPIRATORY FUNCTION ASSOCIATED WITH AGING
Dilation of alveoli
Enlargement of airspaces
Decrease in exchange surface area
Loss of supporting tissue
Decreased lung recoil
Increased functional residual capacity
Decreased chest compliance (increased work of breathing)
Decreased respiratory muscle strength (nutrition, cardiac index)
Decreased expiratory flow rates
Blunted respiratory response to hypoxemia and hypercapnia (manifests during heart failure, airway obstruction, pneumonia)

    2. Turbulent flow is audible and is almost invariably present when high resistance to gas flow is problematic (helium will improve flow).

  D. Increased Airway Resistance
    1. The normal response to increased inspiratory resistance is increased inspiratory muscle effort.
    2. The normal response to increased expiratory resistance is use of accessory muscles to force gas from the lungs. Patients who chronically use accessory muscles to exhale are at risk for ventilatory muscle fatigue if they experience an acute increase in ventilatory work, most commonly precipitated by pneumonia or heart failure.
    3. An increased $PaCO_2$ in the setting of increased airway resistance may signal that the patient's compensatory mechanisms are nearly exhausted.

  E. Physiologic Changes in Respiratory Function Associated with Aging (Table 28-2). Despite changes, the respiratory system is able to maintain adequate gas exchange at rest and during exertion throughout life with only modest decrements in PaO_2 and no change in $PaCO_2$.

III. CONTROL OF VENTILATION

  A. Mechanisms that control ventilation are complex, requiring integration with many parts of the central and peripheral nervous systems (Fig. 28-1).

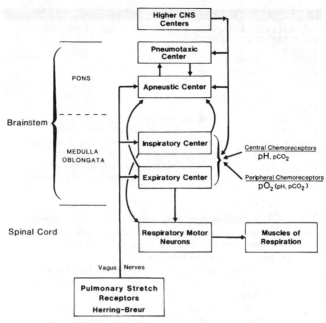

FIGURE 28-1. Diagram of central nervous system respiratory centers, neurofeedback circuits, primary neurohumoral sensory inputs, and mechanical outputs.

B. Generation of a Ventilatory Pattern (Table 28-3)
1. The medulla oblongata contains the most basic ventilatory control centers in the brain.
2. The pontine centers process information that originates in the medulla.
3. The reticular activating system in the midbrain increases the rate and amplitude of ventilation.
4. The cerebral cortex can affect the breathing pattern.

C. Reflex Control of Ventilation
1. Reflexes that directly influence the ventilatory pattern (swallowing, coughing, vomiting) usually do so to prevent airway obstruction.

TABLE 28-3
DEFINITION OF RESPIRATORY

Term	Definition
Eupnea	Continuous inspiratory and expiratory movement without interruption
Apnea	Cessation of ventilatory effort at passive end-expiration
Apneusis	Cessation of ventilatory effort at end-inspiration
Apneustic ventilation	Apneusis with periodic expiratory spasms
Biot's ventilation	Ventilatory gasps interposed between periods of apnea (agonal ventilation)

2. The Herring-Breur reflex (apnea during sustained lung distention) is only weakly present in humans.

D. Chemical Control of Ventilation

1. Peripheral chemoreceptors include the carotid bodies (ventilatory effects characterized by increased breathing rate and tidal volume) and aortic bodies (circulatory effects characterized by bradycardia and hypertension).

a. Both carotid and aortic bodies are stimulated by decreased PaO_2 (below about 60 mm Hg) but not by arterial hemoglobin saturation with oxygen, arterial oxygen concentration (anemia), or $PaCO_2$.

b. Patients who depend on hypoxic ventilatory drive have PaO_2 values around 60 mm Hg.

c. Potent inhaled anesthetics depress hypoxic ventilatory responses by depressing the carotid body response to hypoxemia.

2. Central Chemoreceptors

a. Approximately 80% of the ventilatory response to inhaled carbon dioxide originates in the central medullary centers.

b. The chemosensitive areas of the medullary ventilatory centers are exquisitely sensitive to the extracellular fluid hydrogen ion concentration (carbon dioxide indirectly determines this concentration by reacting with water to form carbonic acid).

       c. Increased $PaCO_2$ is a more potent stimulus (increased breathing rate and tidal volume within 60 to 120 seconds) to ventilation than is metabolic acidosis (carbon dioxide but not hydrogen ions can easily cross the blood-brain barrier).

       d. Normalization of the cerebrospinal fluid pH (active transport of bicarbonate ions) over time results in a decline in ventilation despite persistent increases in the $PaCO_2$. The reverse sequence occurs when acute ascent to altitude initially stimulates ventilation leading to an abrupt decrease in $PaCO_2$.

E. Breath Holding

  1. The rate of increase in $PaCO_2$ in awake, preoxygenated adults with normal lungs who hold their breaths without previous hyperventilation is 7 mm Hg in the first 10 seconds.

  2. The rate of increase in $PaCO_2$ in apneic anesthetized patients is 12 mm Hg during the first minute and 3.5 mm Hg for every subsequent minute (reflects decreased metabolic rate and carbon dioxide production in the anesthetized compared with awake patients).

  3. Hyperventilation is rarely followed by an apneic period in awake humans despite a decreased $PaCO_2$. In contrast, even mild hyperventilation during general anesthesia will produce apnea.

F. Quantitative Aspects of Chemical Control of Breathing (Fig. 28-2)

  1. The carbon dioxide response curve approaches linearity at $PaCO_2$ values between 20 and 80 mm Hg (above 100 mm Hg carbon dioxide acts as a ventilatory depressant).

  2. The slope of the carbon dioxide response curve is considered to represent carbon dioxide sensitivity (normally 0.5 to 0.7 l/min/mm Hg CO_2).

  3. The apneic threshold occurs at a $PaCO_2$ of about 32 mm Hg.

  4. Various events cause a shift in the position and/or change in the slope of the carbon dioxide response curve (Table 28-4).

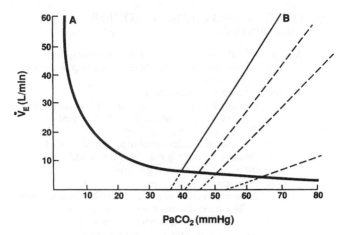

FIGURE 28-2. Carbon dioxide–ventilatory response curves. Curve A is generated by varying minute ventilation (VE) and measuring changes in the $PaCO_2$. Curve B is the classic carbon dioxide–ventilatory response curve that is generated by varying the $PaCO_2$ and measuring the resultant VE. The slope of the curve defines sensitivity to the ventilatory stimulating effects of carbon dioxide. Volatile anesthetics and opioids shift the curve to the right and eventually depress the slope (*dashed lines*).

TABLE 28-4

CLINICAL STATES ASSOCIATED WITH CHANGES IN THE VENTILATORY RESPONSE TO CARBON DIOXIDE

Left Shift and/or Increased Slope
Hyperventilation (increased minute ventilation resulting in decreased $PaCO_2$ and respiratory alkalosis)
Arterial hypoxemia
Metabolic acidosis
Central etiologies (drugs [salicylates], intracranial hypertension, cirrhosis, anxiety)

Right Shift and/or Decreased Slope
Physiologic sleep ($PaCO_2$ increases up to 10 mm Hg)
Metabolic alkalosis
Denervation of peripheral chemoreceptors
Opioids (decreased breathing rate and increased tidal volume)
Volatile anesthetics

IV. OXYGEN AND CARBON DIOXIDE TRANSPORT

A. The movement of gas across the alveolar-capillary membrane depends on the integrity of the pulmonary and cardiac systems.

B. **Bulk Flow of Gas (Convection)**
1. The greatest part of airway resistance occurs in the larger airways (>2 mm in diameter), where gas molecules travel more quickly.
2. During normal quiet ventilation, gas flow within convective airways is mainly laminar, thus decreasing resistance to gas flow.

C. **Gas Diffusion**
1. Diffusion defects that create arterial hypoxemia are rare. The most common reason for a measured decrease in diffusing capacity is mismatching of ventilation-to-perfusion that functionally results in a decreased surface area available for diffusion.
2. Hypercarbia is never the result of diffusion defects (carbon dioxide is 20 times more diffusible than oxygen).

D. **Distribution of Ventilation and Perfusion**
1. The efficiency with which oxygen and carbon dioxide exchange at the alveolar-capillary membrane depends on the matching of capillary perfusion and alveolar ventilation.
2. **Distribution of blood flow** within the lung is mainly gravity dependent, depending on the relationship between pulmonary artery pressure, alveolar pressure, and pulmonary venous pressure (Fig. 28-3).
3. **Distribution of ventilation** is preferentially directed to more dependent areas of the lung.
4. The ideal matching of ventilation-to-perfusion (V/Q = 1) is believed to occur at approximately the level of the third rib. Above this level, ventilation occurs slightly in excess of perfusion, whereas below this level the ratio becomes <1 (Fig. 28-4).
   a. **Hypoxic pulmonary vasoconstriction** decreases blood flow to unventilated (hypoxic) alveoli in an attempt to maintain a desirable V/Q ratio.
   b. Increases in dead space ventilation primarily affect carbon dioxide elimination and have little

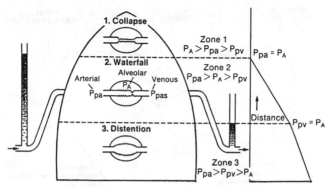

FIGURE 28-3. Distribution of blood flow in the isolated lung. PA = alveolar pressure; Ppa = pulmonary artery pressure; Ppv = pulmonary venous pressure.

effect on arterial oxygenation, whereas physiologic shunt primarily affects arterial oxygenation with little effect on carbon dioxide elimination.

E. **Physiologic Dead Space**

1. **Anatomic dead space** (2 mL/kg) accounts for the majority of dead space ventilation and is a result of ventilation of structures that do not participate in oxygenation (oronasopharynx to the terminal and respiratory bronchioles). Clinical conditions that modify anatomic dead space include tracheal intubation, tracheostomy, and large lengths of ventilatory tubing between the tracheal tube and the ventilator Y-piece.

2. **Alveolar dead space** arises from ventilation of alveoli where there is little or no perfusion.

3. Increases in physiologic dead space are most often because of increases in alveolar dead space (decreased cardiac output as may occur with decreased venous return following institution of positive-pressure ventilation of the lungs, pulmonary embolism, and chronic obstructive pulmonary disease).

   a. Decrease in pulmonary blood flow associated with pulmonary embolism is more a result of

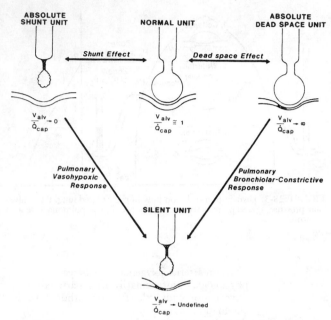

FIGURE 28-4. Continuation of ventilation-to-perfusion relationships. Gas exchange is maximally effective in normal lung units and only partially effective in shunt and dead space units. It is totally absent in silent units, absolute shunt, and dead space units.

reflex bronchoconstriction than mechanical obstruction to blood flow.

    4. **Assessment of physiologic dead space**

        a. A comparison of the minute ventilation and $PaCO_2$ allows a gross qualitative assessment of physiologic dead space ventilation.

        b. The difference between $PETCO_2$ and $PaCO_2$ is because of dead space ventilation.

F. Physiologic Shunt

    1. The physiologic shunt is that portion of the cardiac output that returns to the left heart without being exposed to ventilated alveoli (absolute shunt and oxygenation will not be improved by administration of supplemental oxygen).

a. An anatomic shunt arises from the venous return from the pleural, bronchiolar, and thebesian veins (2 to 5% of the cardiac output).

b. Anatomic shunts of the greatest magnitude usually are associated with congenital heart disease.

2. **Shunt effect (venous admixture)** occurs in areas where alveolar ventilation is deficient compared with perfusion (oxygenation will be improved by administration of supplemental oxygen). Disease entities that tend to produce venous admixture include mild pulmonary edema, postoperative atelectasis, and chronic obstructive pulmonary disease.

3. **Assessment of arterial oxygenation and physiologic shunt.** The simplest assessment of oxygenation is qualitative comparison of the patient's inspired oxygen concentration and resulting PaO_2 (venous admixture will magnify the effect of a small shunt).

4. **Physiologic shunt calculation** includes the contribution of mixed venous blood (may be extremely desaturated in critically ill patients owing to low cardiac output, anemia, arterial hypoxemia, and increased metabolic oxygen requirements) and is the best estimate of how well the lungs can oxygenate the arterial blood.

V. PULMONARY FUNCTION TESTING

A. Screening spirometry permits classification of pulmonary dysfunction as an obstructive defect or restrictive defect (Table 28-5).

1. An obstructive defect is suggested by a decreased forced exhaled volume in 1 second/forced vital capacity (FEV1/FVC) or forced expiratory flow between 25 and 75% of total exhaled volume (FEF 25 to 75%). A decision to institute bronchodilator therapy may be based on these measurements (Fig. 28-5).

2. A restrictive defect is suggested by a proportional decrease in all lung volumes (vital capacity [VC], FVC, FEV1), but the FEV1/FVC remains normal.

TABLE 28-5

PULMONARY FUNCTION TESTS IN RESTRICTIVE AND OBSTRUCTIVE LUNG DISEASE

Measurement	Restrictive disease	Obstructive disease
FVC	Decreased	Normal to slightly decreased
FEV1	Decreased	Normal to slightly decreased
FEV1/FVC	Normal	Decreased
FEF 25–75%	Normal	Decreased
FRC	Decreased	Normal to slightly increased
TLC	Decreased	Normal to slightly increased

FVC = forced vital capacity; FEV1 = forced exhaled volume in 1 second; FEF 25–75% = forced expiratory flow between 25 and 75% of total exhaled volume; FRC = functional residual capacity; TLC = total lung capacity.

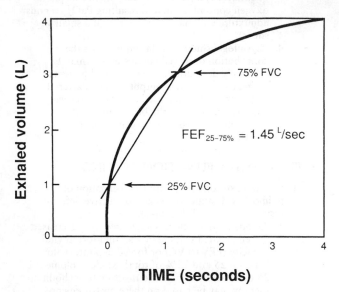

FIGURE 28-5. The spirogram depicts a 4-liter forced vital capacity (FVC) on which the points representing 25 and 75% FVC are marked. The slope of the line connecting the points is the forced expiratory flow (FEF 25 to 75%).

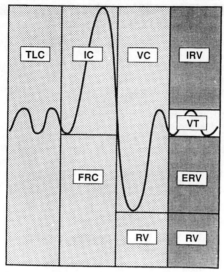

FIGURE 28-6. Lung volumes and capacities. The darkest bar depicts the four basic lung volumes that sum to create total lung capacity (TLC). ERV = expiratory reserve volume; FRC = functional residual capacity; IC = inspiratory capacity; IRV = inspiratory reserve volume; RV = residual volume; VT = tidal volume; VC = vital capacity.

B. **Lung Volumes and Capacities** (Fig. 28-6)
C. **Flow-Volume Loops.** Imaging techniques (MRI) provide more precise and useful information in the diagnosis of upper airway and extrathoracic obstruction and have replaced use of flow-volume loops.
D. **Carbon Monoxide Diffusing Capacity (D_{LCO})**
   1. Decreased hemoglobin concentration decreases the D_{LCO} whereas an increased $PaCO_2$ increases the D_{LCO}.
   2. D_{LCO} is deceased by alveolar fibrosis associated with oxygen toxicity and pulmonary edema.
E. **Preoperative Pulmonary Assessment** (Table 28-6)
   1. Specific measurements of lung function do not predict postoperative complications.
   2. History of smoking >40 pack years, COPD, asthma, cough, exercise intolerance <1 flight of

TABLE 28-6

PREOPERATIVE PULMONARY ASSESSMENT

Anticipate impaired pulmonary function in specific patients/
situations
  Chronic lung disease
  Smoking history
  Persistent cough or wheezing
  Morbid obesity
  Requirement for one lung anesthesia or lung resection
  Neuromuscular disease
History determines need for testing (exercise tolerance)
  Chest X ray
  Arterial blood gases
  Screening spirometry (identify patients who will benefit from
    preoperative therapy, provide baseline prior to lung resection)

stairs is more predictive of postoperative
complications.

3. Baseline pulmonary function data is reserved for
   patients with severely impaired preoperative
   pulmonary function (quadriplegics, myasthenics) so
   assessment for weaning from mechanical ventilation
   and/or tracheal extubation may be guided by
   preoperative values.

4. Arterial blood gases are not indicated unless the
   patient's history suggests hypoxemia or carbon
   dioxide retention (identify reversible disease or to
   define severity as a baseline).

5. Defining baseline PaO_2 and $PaCO_2$ are important
   if it is anticipated that patients with severe COPD
   will require postoperative mechanical ventilation
   (Table 28-7).

VI. ANESTHESIA AND OBSTRUCTIVE PULMONARY DISEASE

A. Patients with marked obstructive pulmonary disease
   are at increased risk for intraoperative (reflex
   bronchoconstriction during direct laryngoscopy and
   tracheal intubation) and postoperative complications.

1. Patients with asthma and chronic obstructive
   pulmonary disease may benefit from preoperative
   bronchodilator therapy.

TABLE 28-7

**RESPIRATORY VALUES FOR GUIDING WEANING FROM
MECHANICAL VENTILATION AND/OR TRACHEAL
EXTUBATION**

	Normal values (70 kg)
Alveolar oxygen tension	110 mm Hg (FIO2 0.21)
Alveolar-arterial oxygen gradient	<10 mm Hg (FIO2)
Arterial-to-alveolar oxygen ratio	>0.75
Arterial oxygen content	20 mL/100 mL blood
Mixed venous oxygen content	15 mL/100 mL blood
Arterial–venous oxygen content	4–6 mL/100 mL blood
Intrapulmonary shunt	<5%
Physiologic dead space	0.33
Oxygen consumption	250 mL/min
Oxygen transport	1000 mL/min
Respiratory quotient	0.8

2. Controlled ventilation of the lungs at <10 breaths/
minute should prevent hypercarbia, minimize V/Q
mismatch, and allow time for exhalation.
3. Tidal volume and inspiratory flow rates are adjusted
to keep peak airway pressure <40 cm H_2O.
B. Tracheal extubation as soon as possible after the end of
the operation is desirable in an attempt to decrease the
risk of iatrogenic infection.

VII. ANESTHESIA AND RESTRICTIVE DISEASE

A. These patients typically breathe rapidly and shallowly
because more pressure is required to expand stiff lungs.
B. Positive end-expiratory pressure will increase the
functional residual capacity and reverse arterial
hypoxemia.
1. High peak airway pressures may be required to
expand stiffened lungs yet large tidal volumes are
avoided because of the risk of barotrauma and
volutrauma.
2. Arterial hypoxemia can develop rapidly (as during
apnea for tracheal intubation, transportation from
the operating room), reflecting the limited oxygen
stores in the lungs because of the decreased
functional residual capacity.

3. General anesthesia further decreases the functional residual capacity that persists into the postoperative period (offset with positive airway pressure).
C. The single most important aspect of postoperative pulmonary care is getting the patient out of bed, preferably walking.

VIII. THE EFFECT OF CIGARETTE SMOKING ON PULMONARY FUNCTION (Table 28-8)

A. Cessation of smoking for 12 to 24 hours is sufficient to decrease carboxyhemoglobin levels to near normal but does not predictably influence the incidence of postoperative pulmonary complications.
   1. Normalization of mucociliary function requires 2 to 3 weeks of abstinence from smoking, during which time sputum increases.
   2. Smokers who decrease but do not stop cigarette consumption continue to acquire the same amount of nicotine (change in smoking technique) and it is unlikely that postoperative pulmonary complications will be altered.
B. Smoking patients should be advised to stop smoking 2 months prior to elective operations to maximize the effect of smoking cessation, or for at least 4 weeks to gain some benefit from mucociliary function.

TABLE 28-8

EFFECT OF SMOKING

Decreased ciliary motility
Increased sputum production
Increased airway reactivity
Development of obstructive pulmonary disease
Ventilation-to-perfusion mismatch (venous admixture and arterial hypoxemia)
Gas trapping
Increased minute ventilation
Barrel chest deformity
Decreased lung compliance (exhale forcibly to prevent gas trapping)
Increased carboxyhemoglobin concentration (normal <1%, may be 8–10% in smokers)

C. Smoking is one of the main risk factors associated with postoperative morbidity (pneumonia).

IX. PULMONARY FUNCTION POSTOPERATIVELY

A. **Postoperative Pulmonary Function**
   1. Changes in pulmonary function that occur postoperatively are primarily restrictive (gauged by the decrease in functional residual capacity).
   2. The operative site is the single most important determinant of postoperative pulmonary restriction and pulmonary complications (Table 28-9).
B. **Postoperative Pulmonary Complications**
   1. Atelectasis and pneumonia, as reflected by changes in the color and quantity of sputum, oral temperature >38°C, and a new infiltrate on the chest X ray, are the two most common postoperative complications.
   2. The risk of postoperative pulmonary complications can be minimized by ensuring the absence of active pulmonary infection and use of therapeutic bronchodilation if reactive airway disease is associated with increased airway resistance.
   3. Strategies to decrease the risk of postoperative pulmonary complications include the use of lung-expanding therapies, choice of analgesia, and cessation of smoking.
      a. Stir-up regimens (walking) are as effective as incentive spirometry.
      b. After median sternotomy, functional residual capacity does not return to normal for several

TABLE 28-9

RELATION OF OPERATIVE SITE TO POSTOPERATIVE DECREASES IN FUNCTIONAL RESIDUAL CAPACITY (FRC)

Operative site	Decrease in FRC (%)
Nonlaparoscopic upper abdominal surgery	40–50[a]
Lower abdominal and thoracic surgery	30
Intracranial	15–20
Peripheral vascular	15–20

[a]In presence of conventional postoperative analgesic techniques.

weeks regardless of postoperative pulmonary therapy.

c. Postoperative analgesia influences the risk of postoperative pulmonary complications (epidural analgesia especially for abdominal and thoracic operations decreases the risk).

CHAPTER 29 ■ ANESTHESIA FOR THORACIC SURGERY

The number of noncardiac thoracic surgical operations has increased, reflecting the fact that lung cancer is the most common cause of cancer mortality in the world (Cohen E, Neustein SM, Eisenkraft JB: Anesthesia for thoracic surgery. In Barash PG, Cullen BF, Stoelting RK [eds]: *Clinical Anesthesia*, pp 813–855. Philadelphia, Lippincott Williams & Wilkins, 2006).

I. PREOPERATIVE EVALUATION

A. Preoperative evaluation should focus on the extent and severity of pulmonary disease and cardiovascular involvement.

B. **History** (Table 29-1)

C. **Physical Examination** (Table 29-2)

D. **Laboratory Studies** (Table 29-3)

1. A vital capacity at least three times the tidal volume is necessary for an effective cough. A vital capacity <50% of predicted or <2 liters is an indicator of increased risk.

2. Thoracoscopic surgery and improved postoperative pain management have made it possible for patients with even smaller lung volumes to successfully undergo surgery.

3. The ratio of forced exhaled volume to forced vital capacity (FEV1/FVC) is useful in differentiating restrictive (normal ratio as both are decreased) from obstructive (low ratio as FEV1 is decreased) disease.

4. A 15% improvement in pulmonary function tests following bronchodilator therapy is an indication for continued preoperative therapy.

5. A mass that is seen on computed tomography is more likely to be malignant if it also demonstrates enhanced glucose uptake on the positron emission tomography scan.

TABLE 29-1
HISTORY PRIOR TO THORACIC SURGERY

Dyspnea (quantitate as to activity required to produce it; may warn of need for postoperative ventilation)

Cough (characteristics of sputum)

Cigarette smoking

Exercise tolerance (increased risk when unable to climb two flights of stairs)

Risk factors for acute lung injury (alcohol abuse, high ventilatory pressures, excessive fluid administration)

II. PREOPERATIVE PREPARATION

A. Several conditions predispose to postoperative complications, and their treatment preoperatively is associated with decreases in morbidity and mortality (Table 29-4).

B. Patients scheduled for lung resection may benefit from tests to determine the extent of resection that will be tolerated as well as cardiopulmonary function in the presence of unilateral pulmonary artery occlusion (Fig. 29-1).

III. INTRAOPERATIVE MONITORING

A. Invasive monitoring and pulse oximetry have improved patient care (Table 29-5).

B. An arterial catheter is essential to provide continuous recordings of blood pressure because surgical manipulations or intravascular volume shifts can cause sudden changes in blood pressure.

TABLE 29-2
PHYSICAL EXAMINATION PRIOR TO THORACIC SURGERY

Respiratory system

    Cyanosis

    Clubbing

    Breathing rate and pattern (distinguish between obstructive and restrictive disease)

    Breath sounds (wet sounds versus wheezing)

Cardiovascular system (presence of pulmonary hypertension)

TABLE 29-3
LABORATORY STUDIES PRIOR TO THORACIC SURGERY

Electrocardiogram (evidence of right ventricular hypertrophy)
Chest X ray
Arterial blood gas analysis (blue bloaters versus pink puffers)
Pulmonary function tests (evaluation of lung resectability)
Computed tomography and positron emission tomography scan
Diffusing capacity for carbon monoxide
Maximal oxygen consumption

    C. Serial arterial blood gas determinations are necessary to confirm the adequacy of ventilation and oxygenation as suggested by capnography and pulse oximetry.

    D. During thoracotomy, the radial artery catheter is often placed in the dependent arm to aid in stabilizing the catheter. This catheter can also be used to monitor for possible axillary artery compression (avoid compression of artery and brachial plexus with placement of "axillary roll" under dependent hemithorax).

IV. PHYSIOLOGY OF ONE LUNG VENTILATION

    A. Physiology of the Lateral Decubitus Position

       1. In an open-chested, anesthetized, and paralyzed patient, the dependent lung is overperfused (gravity-dependent blood flow) and underventilated.

       2. Underventilation reflects minimal pressure of abdominal contents pressing against the upper

TABLE 29-4
FACTORS THAT PREDISPOSE TO COMPLICATIONS FOLLOWING THORACIC SURGERY

Smoking (carboxyhemoglobin decreases in 48 hr; improvement of ciliary function and decrease in sputum production require 8–12 weeks)
Infection
Hypovolemia and electrolyte balance (facilitate removal of bronchial secretions)
Wheezing (sympathomimetic drugs, steroids, cromolyn, parasympatholytic drugs)

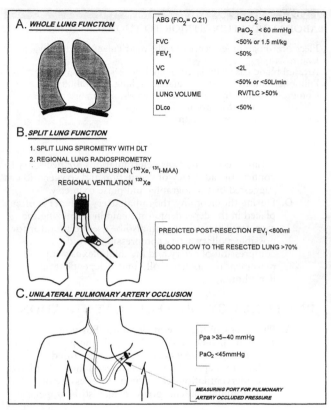

FIGURE 29-1. The order of tests to determine the cardiopulmonary function status of the patient and the extent of resection that will be tolerated by the patient.

diaphragm, making it easier for positive-pressure ventilation to distend the nondependent lung.

V. ONE-LUNG VENTILATION

A. Indications for one-lung ventilation may be categorized as absolute and relative (Table 29-6).
B. Methods of Lung Separation
   1. Bronchial Blockers

TABLE 29-5

INVASIVE MONITORING FOR THORACIC SURGERY

Direct arterial catheterization (place in dependent arm for thoracotomy; right radial warns of innominate artery compression during mediastinoscopy)

Central venous pressure (acceptable in patients with good ventricular function undergoing pneumonectomy)

Pulmonary artery catheter (during one-lung ventilation the accuracy of measurements may depend on position of the catheter)

Transesophageal echocardiography (reflects ventricular and valvular function; wall motion abnormalities may be because of myocardial ischemia)

Noninvasive digital sensor placed on ear lobe (continuous monitoring of $PaCO_2$, SpO_2, and heart rate)

    a. Selective airway occlusion can be achieved by the use of an arterial embolectomy (Fogarty) catheter. The catheter is placed with the aid of a fiberoptic bronchoscope and a conventional endotracheal tube is then placed alongside the catheter.

    b. Univent tube is a single-lumen endotracheal tube with a built-in movable endobronchial blocker, which is manipulated into the desired mainstem bronchus with the aid of a fiberoptic bronchoscope. Since it is a single lumen tube it does not need to be replaced at the conclusion of the surgical procedure.

TABLE 29-6

INDICATIONS FOR ONE-LUNG VENTILATION

Absolute Indications
Prevent contamination of healthy lung (abscess, hemorrhage)
Control distribution of ventilation (bronchopleural fistula)
Minimally invasive cardiac procedures

Relative Indications
Surgical exposure, high priority
Thoracic aneurysm
Pneumonectomy
Upper lobe lobectomy
Surgical exposure, low priority
Esophageal resection
Middle and lower lobe lobectomy

2. **Double-Lumen Endobronchial Tubes**
   a. These tubes are the most widely used means of achieving lung separation and one-lung ventilation. The design of double-lumen tubes (many different types but the design is similar for all) is characterized by two catheters bonded together with one lumen long enough to reach a mainstem bronchus while the other shorter catheter portion remains in the trachea above the carina. Lung separation is achieved by inflation of the tracheal and bronchial cuffs. The bronchial cuff on a right-sided tube is slotted to allow ventilation of the right upper lobe because the right mainstem bronchus is too short to accommodate both the right lumen tip and cuff.
   b. **Robershaw tube** is available as a left- or right-sided clear plastic disposable tube without a carinal hook. Lumina are of sufficient size to facilitate suctioning and offer low resistance to gas flow. The blue endobronchial cuff is easily recognized when fiberoptic bronchoscopy is used to confirm its position.
3. **Positioning double-lumen tubes (Robershaw)**
   a. Initial insertion of the tube is performed with the distal concave curvature facing anteriorly. After the tip of the tube is past the vocal cords, the stylet is removed and the tube is rotated 90 degrees to direct the bronchial lumen appropriately toward the desired mainstem bronchus. Advancement of the tube is ended when moderate resistance to further passage is encountered (about 29 cm in most adults), indicating that the tube tip has been firmly seated in the mainstem bronchus (Fig. 29-2).
   b. Once the tube is judged to be in the proper position, a sequence of steps is performed to check its location (Table 29-7).
   c. Confirmation of placement using a fiberoptic bronchoscope is recommended (Table 29-8 and Figs. 29-3 and 29-4).
4. **Lung separation in the patient with a difficult airway** may include use of a flexible fiberoptic endoscope, a double-lumen or a Univent tube using a tube exchanger plus laryngoscopy, or a tube exchanger and bronchial blocker.

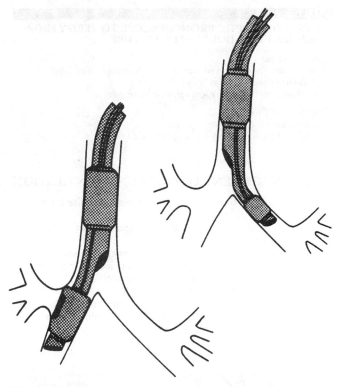

FIGURE 29-2. Schematic depiction of the proper placement of a right or left endobronchial tube.

TABLE 29-7

STEPS TO VERIFY PROPER POSITION OF A DOUBLE-LUMEN TUBE

Inflate tracheal cuff and confirm bilateral and equal breath sounds
Inflate bronchial cuff (rarely >2 mL of air) and confirm bilateral and equal breath sounds (ensures that bronchial cuff is not obstructing the contralateral hemithorax)
Selectively clamp each lumen and confirm one-lung ventilation
Perform bronchoscopy using a fiberoptic bronchoscope (nearly one-half of tubes thought to be properly positioned by auscultation and examination were not confirmed by bronchoscopy; see Table 29-8)

TABLE 29-8

USE OF A FIBEROPTIC BRONCHOSCOPE TO VERIFY PROPER PLACEMENT OF A DOUBLE-LUMEN TUBE

Left-Sided Tube
Tracheal lumen (carina visualized and upper surface of blue endobronchial cuff just below the carina)
Bronchial lumen (identify left upper lobe orifice)

Right-Sided Tube
Tracheal lumen (carina visualized)
Bronchial lumen (identify right upper lobe orifice)

VI. MANAGEMENT OF ONE-LUNG VENTILATION

A. A goal of one-lung ventilation is to optimize arterial oxygenation (Table 29-9).

B. Clinical Approach to the Management of One-Lung Ventilation

1. The position of the double-lumen tube should be rechecked after the patient is placed in the lateral decubitus position. Two-lung ventilation is maintained as long as possible.

2. After initiation of one-lung ventilation, PaO_2 can continue to decrease for up to 45 minutes (pulse oximetry a vital monitor).

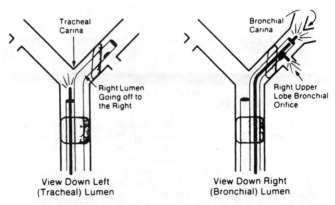

FIGURE 29-3. Use of a fiberscope to verify position of a double-lumen tube.

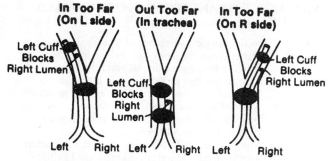

FIGURE 29-4. Examples of double-lumen tube malpositions.

      a. If arterial hypoxemia occurs during one-lung
        ventilation, it is important to verify proper tube
        position using a fiberscope.
      b. If arterial hypoxemia persists after verification of
        tube position, consider addition of continuous
        positive airway pressure or positive
        end-expiratory pressure.
      c. Monitor airway pressure because a sudden
        increase may reflect tube displacement.
    3. Never hesitate to reinstitute two-lung ventilation
      until a patient can be stabilized or the cause of a
      patient's instability (arterial hypoxemia,
      hypotension, cardiac dysrhythmias) is corrected.

TABLE 29-9

**METHODS TO OPTIMIZE OXYGENATION DURING
ONE-LUNG VENTILATION**

Maximize delivered oxygen concentration
Tidal volume to dependent lung is 10–12 mL/kg, and the rate is
    adjusted to maintain the $PaCO_2$ near 35 mm Hg (consider
    decreasing the tidal volume as necessary to avoid increase in
    airway pressure thereby making acute lung injury less likely)
Positive end-expiratory pressure to the dependent lung (10 cm
    H_2O increases functional residual capacity; consider when
    PaO_2 is low)
Continuous positive airway pressure to the nondependent lung
    (5–10 cm H_2O improves the $PaCO_2$ most reliably, distends
    alveoli, and diverts blood flow to the dependent lung)

VII. CHOICE OF ANESTHESIA FOR THORACIC SURGERY

A. Consider the likely presence of increased airway reactivity (cigarette smoking, chronic bronchitis, obstructive pulmonary disease) and the effect of volatile anesthetics or ketamine on bronchomotor tone.

   1. Propofol infusion in combination with remifentanil is useful for producing anesthesia associated with one lung anesthesia and no effect on hypoxic pulmonary vasoconstriction.

   2. Lidocaine (1 to 2 mg/kg iv) has been used before airway manipulations to decrease the likelihood of reflex bronchospasm.

B. An adequate depth of anesthesia before airway manipulation is the most important goal for managing patients with increased airway reactivity.

VIII. HYPOXIC PULMONARY VASOCONSTRICTION

A. Hypoxic pulmonary vasoconstriction is a homeostatic mechanism that normally diverts blood flow away from hypoxic (atelectatic) regions of the lungs (local increases in pulmonary vascular resistance) and thereby optimizes oxygenation.

B. Inhibition of hypoxic pulmonary vasoconstriction during one-lung ventilation could accentuate arterial hypoxemia. Nevertheless, inhaled anesthetics do not seem to interfere with hypoxic pulmonary vasoconstriction.

IX. ANESTHESIA FOR DIAGNOSTIC PROCEDURES

A. **Bronchoscopy** is most often performed with a fiberoptic bronchoscope that easily passes through a tracheal tube of 8.0 to 8.5-mm internal diameter.

B. **Mediastinoscopy** (Table 29-10)

C. **Thoracoscopy**

   1. Insertion of an endoscope into the thoracic cavity and pleural space is used for the diagnosis of pleural disease, effusions, and infectious diseases (especially acquired immunodeficiency syndrome) and for staging procedures and lung biopsy.

   2. Anesthesia can be provided using local, regional, or general anesthesia, depending on the expected

TABLE 29-10

ANESTHETIC CONSIDERATIONS DURING MEDIASTINOSCOPY

Signs of Eaton-Lambert syndrome
Hemorrhage
Pneumothorax
Venous air embolism
Recurrent laryngeal nerve injury
Pressure on the innominate artery (manifests as a decreased right radial pulse and necessitates repositioning of the mediastinoscope, especially in the presence of cerebrovascular disease)

duration of the procedure and the physical status of the patient.

   a. If general anesthesia is required, either a single- or a double-lumen tube may be used. Positive-pressure ventilation interferes with visualization via the endoscope and, therefore, a double-lumen tube is preferred.

   b. The spontaneous partial pneumothorax that occurs when the endoscope is inserted results in improved surgical visualization. The spontaneous pneumothorax is usually well tolerated even in awake patients because the skin and chest wall form a seal around the thoracoscope and limit the degree of lung collapse.

D. **Video-assisted thoracoscopic surgery (VATS)** entails making small incisions in the chest wall, which allows the introduction of a video camera and surgical instruments into the thoracic cavity.

   1. **Anesthesia Considerations**

      a. As with traditional thoracotomy, for VATS the patient needs to be positioned in the lateral decubitus position and lung collapse is needed for adequate surgical exposure.

      b. The need for one-lung ventilation is greater with VATS than with open thoracotomy because it is not possible to retract the lung during a VATS as it is during an open thoracotomy.

      c. The operated lung should be deflated as soon as possible following tracheal intubation because it may take as long as 30 minutes for complete lung collapse to occur.

      d. Carbon dioxide insufflation into the pleural cavity to facilitate visualization. Insufflation pressures should be kept low (<15 mm Hg) because high pressures can cause mediastinal shift and hemodynamic compromise.

      e. Continuous positive airway pressure as commonly used to treat arterial hypoxemia during one-lung ventilation for an open thoracotomy will be unacceptable during VAT (interfere with surgical procedure). During VATS positive end-expiratory pressure to the nonoperated (dependent) lung should be used.

2. Postoperative Concerns

      a. Pain following VATS is less than after an open thoracotomy.

      b. Respiratory function is better preserved following VATS.

X. ANESTHESIA FOR SPECIAL SITUATIONS

A. High-frequency jet ventilation techniques are often appropriate.

B. Bronchopleural fistula and empyema are more likely to occur after a pneumonectomy than after other types of lung resection. Management of anesthesia in such patients includes several considerations (Table 29-11).

    1. An alternative to tracheal intubation in awake patients is placement of a double-lumen tube under general anesthesia with the patient breathing spontaneously.

TABLE 29-11

ANESTHETIC CONSIDERATIONS IN MANAGEMENT OF A PATIENT WITH A BRONCHOPLEURAL FISTULA

Drain empyema before induction of anesthesia

Awake tracheal intubation with a double-lumen tube (bronchial lumen directed to the side opposite the fistula; anticipate outpouring of pus from the tracheal lumen if an empyema is present)

Instituting controlled ventilation before placement of a double-lumen tube may result in hypoventilation because of a large air leak

Leave the chest drainage tube open to prevent tension pneumothorax

2. Rapid sequence induction of anesthesia plus a muscle relaxant, followed by placement of a single-lumen tracheal tube, may be acceptable if the air leak is small and an empyema is not present.

3. For a large bronchopleural fistula, high-frequency jet ventilation may be the nonsurgical treatment of choice.

C. **Lung Cysts and Bullae**

1. These disorders usually represent end-stage emphysematous destruction of the lungs associated with severe obstructive pulmonary disease and carbon dioxide retention.

2. Positive-pressure ventilation or nitrous oxide may cause bullae to expand or rupture (tension pneumothorax).

3. Ideally, a double-lumen tube is inserted with a patient breathing spontaneously while awake or during general anesthesia.

4. Gentle positive-pressure ventilation with rapid, small tidal volumes and pressures not to exceed 10 cm H_2O may be used during the induction and maintenance of anesthesia, especially if the bullae have been shown to have no or only poor bronchial communication.

D. **Lung Volume Reduction Surgery**

1. This surgery is intended to relieve dyspnea and improve airflow in patients with severe emphysema.

2. In contrast to lung volume reduction surgery the excision of giant bullae is presumed to improve lung function, exercise tolerance, and oxygenation secondary to reexpansion of more normal, underlying compressed lung.

3. The role of lung volume reduction surgery in the treatment of emphysema remains controversial.

4. **Anesthetic Management**

   a. The presence of polycythemia may erroneously suggest that intravascular fluid volume and hydration are adequate.

   b. Adequate postoperative pain relief is essential to permit early tracheal extubation (thoracic epidural catheter).

   c. One-lung ventilation is required.

   d. In the early recovery period, it is important to recognize signs of tension pneumothorax.

TABLE 29-12

ANESTHETIC CONSIDERATIONS FOR TRACHEAL RESECTION

Left radial artery cannulation (permits continuous monitoring of blood pressure during periods of innominate artery compression)

Corticosteroids to decrease tracheal edema

Deliver 100% oxygen to facilitate periods of apneic oxygenation

Consider placing a small anode (wire reinforced) tracheal tube above the stenosis, followed by distal placement of a sterile tracheal or bronchial tube after the trachea is exposed (other options include high-frequency jet ventilation or cardiopulmonary bypass)

Postoperatively, keep the head flexed and strive for early tracheal extubation

    E. **Anesthesia for resection of the trachea** may be necessary to relieve stenosis that may follow prolonged tracheal intubation or tracheotomy (Table 29-12).

    F. **Bronchopulmonary lavage** is performed under general anesthesia using a double-lumen tube, most often for the treatment of cystic fibrosis.

XI. MYASTHENIA GRAVIS

    A. Myasthenia gravis is caused by a decrease in the number of postsynaptic acetylcholine receptors (circulating antibodies to the receptors), resulting in a decrease in the margin of safety of neuromuscular transmission (exercise-induced weakness).

    B. **Medical Therapy**
        1. Anticholinesterase drugs are administered in an attempt to prolong the duration of action of acetylcholine. Anticholinesterase overdose causes a cholinergic crisis (treat with intravenous atropine), whereas underdose causes a myasthenic crisis (improves with edrophonium, 2 to 10 mg iv).
        2. Plasmapheresis decreases antibody titers, resulting in transient improvement (also causes a decrease in plasma cholinesterase).

    C. **Thymectomy**
        1. This surgery is considered the treatment of choice in most patients with myasthenia gravis.

TABLE 29-13

ANESTHETIC CONSIDERATIONS IN MANAGEMENT OF THYMECTOMY FOR TREATMENT OF MYASTHENIA GRAVIS

Evaluate the adequacy of drug therapy (corticosteroids, anticholinesterases)

Pulmonary function tests

Continue anticholinesterase drugs preoperatively (controversial)

Modest preoperative medication (benzodiazepines, avoid opioids)

Induction of anesthesia with an intravenous drug followed by a volatile anesthetic to facilitate tracheal intubation

Anticipate the need for postoperative support of ventilation of the patient's lungs

Avoid drugs with skeletal muscle relaxing properties (antiarrhythmics, diuretics, aminoglycosides)

Sensitivity to nondepolarizing muscle relaxants

Nonrelaxant techniques (avoids risks of muscle relaxants by utilizing combinations of propofol, opioids, and short-acting inhaled anesthetics)

    2. The gland is removed by a median sternotomy or transcervically using a technique similar to mediastinoscopy (lower incidence of postoperative ventilatory failure).

  D. **Management of General Anesthesia** (Table 29-13)

  E. **Nondepolarizing Muscle Relaxants**

    1. It is prudent to assume that even treated patients are sensitive to the effects of muscle relaxants and the initial dose should be decreased. One approach is to titrate to effect using a peripheral nerve stimulator, beginning with doses of muscle relaxant that are one-tenth to one-twentieth the usual dose.

    2. Muscle relaxants that undergo rapid clearance from the plasma (atracurium, mivacurium) are useful.

    3. Antagonism with anticholinesterases has been safely accomplished but introduces the risk of a cholinergic crisis (titrate the anticholinesterase dose against the responses to peripheral nerve stimulation). Spontaneous recovery from rapidly cleared muscle relaxants is an advantage if pharmacologic antagonism is deemed undesirable.

  F. **Depolarizing Relaxants.** Patients treated with anticholinesterases may be sensitive to succinylcholine, reflecting slowed metabolism of the muscle relaxant.

TABLE 29-14

POSTOPERATIVE CONSIDERATIONS FOLLOWING
THORACIC SURGERY

Postoperative pain control (optimizes ventilation)
Patient-controlled analgesia
Intercostal nerve blocks (2–3 mL of 0.5% bupivacaine)
Cryoanalgesia
Neuraxial opioids (epidural or intrathecal morphine diluted in
  saline; intrathecal dose about one-tenth the epidural dose;
  administer opioid before surgical incision as "preemptive
  analgesia")
Atelectasis (rapid shallow breathing in response to pain;
  treatment is any maneuver that increases functional residual
  capacity)
Low cardiac output syndrome (replace intravascular fluid
  volume; consider inotropes and/or vasodilators)
Cardiac dysrhythmias (supraventricular tachycardias; consider
  prophylactic digitalis if normokalemic)
Hemorrhage (reexplore if blood loss >200 mL/hr)
Tension pneumothorax
Peripheral nerve injury (intercostal, brachial plexus, recurrent
  laryngeal)

G. **Postoperative Care.** Decrease the opioid dose by
   one-third, as anticholinesterases may increase the
   analgesic effect of these drugs.

XII. POSTOPERATIVE MANAGEMENT AND
COMPLICATIONS (Table 29-14)

CHAPTER 30 ■
CARDIOVASCULAR ANATOMY
AND PHYSIOLOGY

Perioperative management of patients during either cardiac or non-cardiac surgery requires a knowledge of cardiovascular anatomy and physiology (Lake CL: Cardiovascular anatomy and physiology. In Barash PG, Cullen BF, Stoelting RK [eds]: *Clinical Anesthesia*, pp 856–885. Philadelphia, Lippincott Williams & Wilkins, 2006). In the future, an understanding of genomics (sequencing, modification, and functioning of deoxyribonucleic acid and messenger ribonucleic acid) and proteomics (sequencing, modification, and functioning of the proteins of a biological system) will be important.

I. ANATOMY

A. **Heart.** The functional anatomy of the four cardiac chambers, four valves, and great vessels is easily visualized using transesophageal echocardiography (Fig. 30-1).

1. **Right Atrium.** Systemic veins drain into the right atrium via the superior vena cava, inferior vena cava, and the coronary sinus. Connecting the papillary muscles to the valve leaflets are strong, fibrous structures known as the chordae tendineae.

2. **Right Ventricle.** Anatomically, the right ventricle is a pocket wrapped around one-third of the left ventricle, and its fibers are continuous with those of the left ventricle.

3. **Pulmonary Artery and Peripheral Pulmonary Circulation**
   a. The pulmonic valve is a trileaflet valve that is normally about 4 cm² in area.
   b. The pulmonary artery originates from the superior portion of the right ventricle and then passes under the aorta before it bifurcates.
   c. The pulmonary circulation is innervated by the sympathetic nervous system and alpha-2 and probably alpha-1 receptors are present.

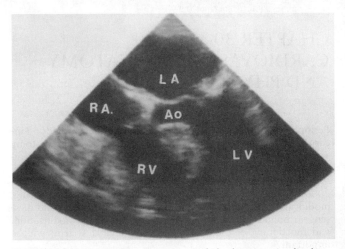

FIGURE 30-1. The functional anatomy of the heart is visualized using transthoracic or transesophageal echocardiography. All four cardiac chambers, atrioventricular valves, aortic outflow tract, and interatrial and interventricular septa are visible on the transesophageal view. When viewed in real time, the function of both valves and ventricles can be assessed.

4. **Left Atrium**
   a. The left atrium is slightly larger than the right and receives one or two pulmonary veins on its left and two or three on its right side.
   b. The major functions of the left atrium are a reservoir for pulmonary venous blood, conduit to empty its contents into the left ventricle, and an active contractile chamber.
   c. The normal adult mitral valve in area is about 6 to 8 cm^2 (valves <1 cm^2 are severely stenotic). The blood supply to the mitral chordae and papillary muscles is often tenuous.
5. **Left Ventricle**
   a. The left ventricle is thicker (8 to 15 mm) than the right ventricle. Both ventricles consist of an inner layer (endocardium covered with endothelium), which is important for its probable release of a contracting factor (endocardin) and myocardium relaxing factor.

6. **Aorta and Its Branches**
   a. A normal aortic valve is about 3 to 4 cm^2 in area.
   b. The aorta at the level of the aortic valve dilates to form the sinuses of Valsalva in which the coronary ostia are located.
   c. Major branches of the aorta are the innominate (divides into the right subclavian and right carotid arteries), left carotid artery, and left subclavian artery.

B. **Coronary Circulation**
   1. The right and left coronary arteries originate from the sinuses of Valsalva to supply blood to the myocardium (Fig. 30-2). Ischemic changes on the electrocardiogram (ECG) are reflected in leads that monitor the diseased coronary artery (Table 30-1).
   2. **Coronary dominance** is determined by which artery crosses the junction between atria and ventricles to supply the posterior descending coronary branch (right coronary in 50%, left in 20%, balance between the two arteries remainder).

C. **Cardiac Conduction System.** The system for electrical activation of the heart consists of the sinoatrial (SA) node (located in the right atrial wall at the junction of

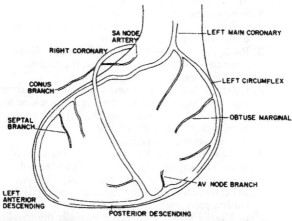

FIGURE 30-2. In this lateral view, the normal left coronary artery divides into the left anterior descending and circumflex coronary arteries. The right coronary artery usually gives off the arteries to the sinus and atrioventricular nodes before terminating on the inferior surface of the heart as the posterior descending artery.

TABLE 30-1
DISTRIBUTION OF CORONARY ARTERY CIRCULATION

Left Coronary Artery
Anterior descending artery (ischemic changes in leads V3 to V5 of the ECG)
Right bundle branch
Left bundle branch
Anterior and posterior papillary muscles (mitral valve)
Anterolateral left ventricle
Circumflex artery (ischemic changes in leads I and aVL of the ECG)

Right Coronary Artery (ischemic changes in leads II, III, and aVF as well as conduction abnormalities on the ECG)
SA and AV nodes
Right atrium and ventricle
Posterior interventricular septum
Posterior fascicle of left bundle branch
Interatrial septum

the right atrium with the superior vena cava), the bundle of His, right and left bundle (anterior and posterior fascicles) branches, and the Purkinje system.

D. Cardiac and Vascular Nerves
  1. **Sympathetic System.** Sympathetic fibers from the stellate ganglion form a nerve that follows the course of the left main coronary artery.
  2. **Parasympathetic System.** Parasympathetic fibers enter the thorax as branches from the recurrent laryngeal and thoracic vagus nerve.
  3. **Cerebral Vasomotor Center.** The vasomotor center independently regulates arterial pressure, blood flow distribution, and cardiac contractility with influences from higher centers such as the cerebral cortex, hypothalamus, and pons.
  4. **Cardiac Receptors.** Vagal receptors in cardiac chambers may be important in maintenance of cardiac volume, coronary vasospasm, ischemia-induced dysrhythmias, and perception of cardiac pain.
      a. Vagal innervation affects principally the atrial musculature and SA node. Sympathetic nerve fibers extend to all portions of the atria, ventricles, and conduction system (beta-1 receptors more dominant than beta-2 receptors).

> b. Stimulation of cardiac parasympathetic nerves causes negative chronotropic and dromotropic effects.

5. **Neural Supply of the Peripheral Vasculature.** Innervation of the peripheral circulation, with the exception of the cerebral and coronary vasculature, originates from the thoracolumbar sympathetic fibers. Vasodilation results from decreased sympathetic nervous system tone or activation of vasodilatory receptors.

II. CARDIOVASCULAR DIAGNOSTIC PROCEDURES

A. **Cardiac Magnetic Resonance Imaging (CMRI)**
  1. CMRI is a comprehensive technique for evaluation and quantification of global and regional wall motion, contractility, ejection fraction, and shunts (complementary to echocardiography for diagnosis of congenital cardiac defects).
  2. The combination of CMRI and pharmacologic stress with dobutamine or adenosine assesses contractile reserve (alternative to resting/stress echocardiography, thallium scintigraphy, positive emission tomography).
  3. CMRI cannot substitute for coronary angiography in the evaluation of small branching arteries.

B. **Catheterization** is usually performed via the femoral vessels with the passage of catheters under fluoroscopic control and subsequent measurement of pressures and oxygen saturations (Table 30-2).
  1. Oxygen saturation is greater in the inferior vena cava than in the superior vena cava owing to the contribution of blood from the renal veins.
  2. Measurements commonly made or calculated include cardiac output and index, stroke volume and index, systemic and pulmonary vascular resistance, valve area, and shunt flows.

C. **Angiography** is performed to quantitate ventricular contractility, shunting between cardiac chambers, and cardiac valvular regurgitation.
  1. Iodinated dyes that are injected are hyperosmolar substances that depress the myocardium, dilate the coronary arteries, decrease blood pH, increase serum osmolarity, and cause allergic reactions.

TABLE 30-2
NORMAL CARDIAC CATHETERIZATION DATA

Site	Pressure (mm Hg)	Oxygen saturation (%)
Inferior vena cava	0–8	75–85
Superior vena cava	0–8	65–75
Right atrium	0–8	70–80
Right ventricle	15–30/0–8	70–80
Pulmonary artery	15–30/4–12	70–80
Pulmonary wedge	5–12 (mean)	70–80
Left atrium	12 (mean)	94–96
Left ventricle	100–140/4–12	94–96
Aorta	100–140/60–90	94–96

2. Adequate fluid replacement must be given after contrast angiography to prevent hypovolemia from the induced osmotic diuresis.

D. **Coronary arteriography** may cause cardiac dysrhythmias, bradycardia, hypotension, and T wave changes on the ECG (changes revert to normal when the catheter is removed from the coronary ostia or the blood pressure is increased by having the patient cough).

E. **Determination of Shunts**
   1. A 10% step-up in oxygen saturation at the atrial level indicates left-to-right shunting into the right atrium.
   2. A 5% step-up at the ventricular or aorticopulmonary level indicates shunting at that site.

III. PHYSIOLOGY

A. **Cardiac Cycle** (Fig. 30-3)
   1. Effective atrial systole at resting heart rates contributes 5 to 20% of the stroke volume. Acute atrial fibrillation increases atrial pressures and eliminates the contribution of the atria to ventricular filling.
   2. Atrial systole (A wave on the venous pressure waveform and P wave on the ECG) concludes ventricular filling.
   3. Time available for ventricular filling decreases from 400 to 500 msec at a heart rate of 60 beats/min to <10 msec at a heart rate of 160 beats/min. Mitral

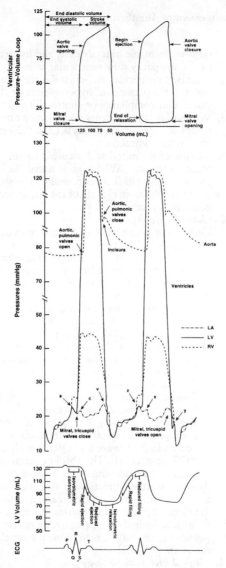

FIGURE 30-3. The events of the cardiac cycle from filling of the atria to ventricular emptying are demonstrated using waveforms from the aorta, pulmonary artery, right and left ventricles, and central veins. The relationship between the ECG and the phases of the cardiac cycle shows that ventricular systole occurs immediately following the QRS complex. The changes in ventricular pressure–volume waveform coincide with ventricular ejection and filling.

stenosis, ischemic heart disease, and hypertrophic cardiomyopathy slow ventricular filling.

4. Increased ventricular end-diastolic pressure may occur in the presence of hypervolemia or changes in ventricular compliance or contractility.

5. Ventricular systole occurs immediately after the QRS complex on the ECG, about 0.12 to 0.20 second after atrial contraction.

6. Closure of the mitral and tricuspid valves (atrioventricular [AV] valves) is noted clinically by the normally split first heart sound. The second heart sound results from closure of the aortic and pulmonic valves.

B. Cardiac Electrophysiology

1. **Cellular Electrophysiology.** Cardiac pacemaker cells contain channels named for the ion most rapidly transferred (calcium, sodium, potassium) and receptors (beta). Beta-adrenergic receptor stimulation augments subsarcolemmal calcium release via ryanodine receptors.

   a. Automaticity (rate of spontaneous phase IV depolarization) decreases in order from the SA node, AV node, His bundle, proximal Purkinje fibers, and distal Purkinje fibers. Interactions between sympathetic and parasympathetic innervations also affect the intrinsic depolarization rate.

   b. The compound action potential in cells results from local ionic transmembrane fluxes through the channels (Fig. 30-4). The spread of depolarization throughout the atrial and ventricular muscle results in the P wave and QRS complex of the ECG, respectively. The absolute refractory period ends at the beginning of the T wave on the ECG.

2. **Action Potential Alterations.** Events that determine the rate of firing of automatic cardiac cells include the slope of phase IV depolarization and are influenced by body temperature, oxygenation, serum potassium, the resting membrane potential, and threshold potential.

3. **Clinical Electrophysiology**

   a. An electrical impulse travels from the SA node to the AV node in 0.04 second at which point transmission is further delayed. The P-R interval on the ECG (normally <0.2 msec) is nearly

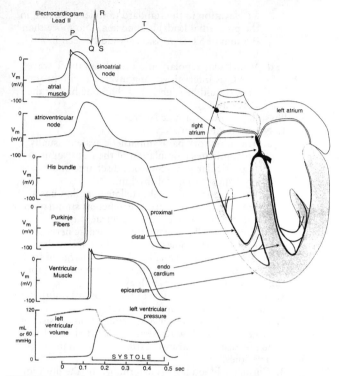

FIGURE 30-4. The action potential of an automatic cell as present in the sinoatrial node differs from that of the ventricular muscle cell in that the pacemaker cell depolarizes spontaneously during phase IV. An action potential occurs due to rapid influx of sodium ions into the cell (phase 0). Phase II is the plateau of the action potential resulting principally from calcium entry through slow channels of the cell membrane. During phase III repolarization of the cell occurs.

  isoelectric because atrial repolarization is not recordable.
  b. Ventricular repolarization begins about 0.12 to 0.20 second after depolarization of the SA node to produce the QRS complex. The entire QRS complex should be <10 msec.
  c. On the ECG, the time from the end of ventricular depolarization to the beginning of repolarization, the ST segment, is isoelectric. More than 1 mm of

ST elevation in the standard limb leads (2 mm in the precordial leads) is abnormal. No more than 0.5 mm of ST depression should be seen in any lead.

    d. Ventricular repolarization results in the T wave. The Q-R interval, varying inversely with heart rate, should be slightly less than one half of the R-R interval.

C. **Physiology of the Cardiac Nerves**
1. **Neural Regulation**
    a. The inhibitory parasympathetic system usually predominates (stimulation of the right vagus nerve in particular slows SA node discharge and predisposes to nodal rhythm).
    b. Stimulation of the right stellate ganglion has a greater effect on heart rate, whereas stimulation of the left has more effect on contractility. Abnormalities of sympathetic cardiac nerve tone occur in syndromes with long Q-T intervals.
    c. Myocardial ischemia increases discharge of both vagal and sympathetic nervous system receptors.

D. **Coronary Circulatory Physiology**
1. About 5% of the cardiac output (250 mL/min) of an adult perfuses the coronary arteries.
2. Physiologically, the coronary circulation consists of large-diameter, low-resistance epicardial vessels and high-resistance intramyocardial arteries and arterioles.
3. Coronary blood flow is determined by the duration of diastole and the difference between diastolic aortic pressure and left ventricular end-diastolic pressure.
    a. The majority of left coronary artery blood flow occurs in diastole because intramyocardial pressure is lowest at this time (Fig. 30-5).
    b. Right coronary artery blood flow occurs in both systole and diastole because intramyocardial pressure is lower in the thinner right ventricle.
4. Myocardial oxygen consumption is high as reflected by a PO_2 of 18 to 20 mm Hg (saturation 30%) in coronary venous blood. Because oxygen extraction cannot be further increased, coronary blood flow must increase if the heart requires additional oxygen.

E. **Coronary Autoregulation**
1. Coronary perfusion is autoregulated to maintain a constant flow between perfusion pressures of

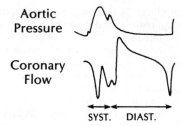

FIGURE 30-5. This diagrammatic relationship between aortic pressure and coronary flow demonstrates that little coronary flow occurs during systole while the majority occurs during diastole. This relationship is particularly true for the left coronary artery, which supplies the left ventricle. The right ventricle, being thinner and developing less pressure, produces less impediment to coronary flow during systole.

approximately 50 to 120 mm Hg (coronary blood flow becomes pressure dependent at perfusion pressures outside the range of autoregulation).

    a. The principal site of coronary autoregulation is the coronary arteriole (<150 mm diameter).

    b. The PO_2 of coronary arterial blood flow influences autoregulation (local hypoxemia results in adenosine-induced vasodilation).

2. Reactive hyperemia is increased coronary blood flow that occurs immediately after occlusion of a coronary artery.

3. Delivery of a vasodilator to a vascular bed served by a normal and a stenotic coronary artery connected by collaterals will dilate the normal arterioles (increased flow) but produce little change in the arterioles served by the stenotic artery because they are maximally dilated. The increased flow via normal arterioles is termed coronary steal.

4. Endocardial/Epicardial Flow Ratio. The distribution of coronary blood flow is as important as total flow. Severe anemia decreases the endocardial/epicardial ratio (subendocardial ischemia), whereas hypoxemia increases both coronary blood flow and the endocardial/epicardial ratio.

5. Neural Influences

    a. Parasympathetic stimulation activates coronary muscarinic receptors inducing vasodilation.

    b. Sympathetic stimulation causes coronary vasodilation as a result of the metabolic factors produced by increased myocardial oxygen requirements and direct beta-receptor stimulation.

c. Coronary artery spasm may result from unopposed alpha-1 stimulation in the presence of beta-adrenergic blockade or when a pure alpha agonist is administered.

F. **Cardiac Output** (Table 30-3)

1. **Determinants** of cardiac output include preload (blood volume), afterload (systemic vascular resistance is an estimate of the wall stress faced by the myocardium during ventricular ejection), heart rate (automaticity of the sinus node; when heart rate is >160 beats/min the cardiac output decreases because filling time is inadequate), myocardial contractility, and ventricular compliance.

2. The **ejection fraction** is the ratio of the stroke volume to the end-diastolic volume. Normally, the ratio is 0.6 to 0.7 and severe impairment of ventricular function is present when the ejection fraction is <0.4.

TABLE 30-3
HEMODYNAMIC VARIABLES: CALCULATIONS AND NORMAL VALUES

Variable	Calculation	Normal values
Cardiac index (CI)	CO/BSA	2.5–4.0 l/min/m^2
Stroke volume (SV)	CO/HR	60–90 mL/beat
Stroke index (SI)	SV/BSA	40–60 mL/beat/m^2
Mean arterial pressure (MAP)	Diastolic blood pressure plus one-third pulse pressure	80–120 mm Hg
Systemic vascular resistance (SVR)	MAP-CVP/COX80	1200–1500 dynes/cm/sec^{-5}
Pulmonary vascular resistance (PVR)	PAP-PWP/COX80	100–300 dynes/cm/sec^{-5}
Right ventricular stroke work index (RVSWI)	0.0136 (PAP-CVP)/SI	5–9 g-m/beat/m^2
Left ventricular stroke work index (LVSWI)	0.136 (MAP-PWP)/SI	45–60 g-m/beat/m^2

CVP = central venous pressure; BSA = body surface area; CO = cardiac output; PAP = mean pulmonary artery pressure; PWP = pulmonary wedge pressure; MAP = mean arterial pressure; g-m = gram meter.

G. **Myocardial Mechanics**
   1. **Ventricular (Starling) Function Curve.** If cardiac muscle is stretched, it develops greater contractile tension because of changes in myofibril calcium sensitivity and alterations in the amount of activator calcium.
      a. An increase in venous return stretches the muscle fibers to increase contractility and improve cardiac output.
      b. Ventricular function curves are influenced by afterload.
      c. Ventricular function curves are used clinically when weaning patients from cardiopulmonary bypass, to assess the effects of anesthetic drugs on the heart, and to guide fluid and pharmacologic therapy in the perioperative period.
   2. **Pressure-volume loops** are an index of ventricular function (myocardial contractility and compliance) that is less affected by preload and afterload than ventricular function curves (Fig. 30-6).
   3. **Cardiac work** describes myocardial function in terms of load carried and distance moved. Advantages of using cardiac work rather than cardiac output to describe cardiac function include the use of heart rate, preload, and afterload (the major variables affecting cardiac function) in the calculation.

H. **Myocardial Metabolism**
   1. Knowledge of myocardial metabolism (substrate utilization and oxygen consumption) is important for preservation of the heart during conditions of stress, cardiac arrest, or cardiac asystole during cardiac surgery.
   2. **Sources of energy** for the heart are derived primarily from lactate and fatty acids delivered by the coronary blood. Glucose is the only substrate used by the heart anaerobically.
   3. **Myocardial oxygen consumption** (8 to 10 mL/100 g/min, making it one of the highest of all organs) is determined by heart rate, wall tension, and myocardial contractility.
   4. **Myocardial Supply/Demand Ratio**
      a. A balance must always exist between oxygen consumption (demand) and myocardial oxygen supply if ischemia is to be avoided (Table 30-4).

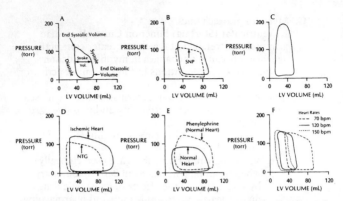

FIGURE 30-6. The relationship of ventricular pressure and volume over the entire cardiac cycle is the pressure-volume loop shown in *A*. The loop begins on the bottom left with opening of the mitral valve and filling of the left ventricle to end-diastolic volume. Isovolumetric contraction begins at the lower right portion of the curve with closure of the mitral valve. The aortic valve opens at the upper right portion of the loop and ventricular ejections begins. At the upper left of the loop, the aortic valve closes (end-systolic volume) and isovolumetric relaxation returns the loop to the starting point. Stroke volume is the difference between the volume at the end of diastole and the end of systole. The area of the loop is stroke work. The effects of afterload reduction on the pressure-volume loop are depicted in loop *B*, while loop *E* shows the changes that occur with increased afterload. Loop *C* shows changes in a patient with aortic stenosis.

TABLE 30-4

FACTORS INVOLVED IN MYOCARDIAL OXYGEN SUPPLY AND DEMAND

Myocardial Oxygen Consumption
Heart rate
Contractile state
Myocardial wall tension
Arterial oxygen consumption
Basal oxygen requirements
Oxygen cost of muscle fiber shortening
Oxygen cost of electrical activation

Myocardial Oxygen Supply
Aortic diastolic pressure
Left ventricular end-diastolic pressure
Coronary artery diameter
Arterial oxygen content

TABLE 30-5

DISTRIBUTION OF CARDIAC OUTPUT

	Amount of total cardiac output (%)
Brain	12
Heart	4
Liver	24
Kidneys	20
Skeletal muscle	23
Skin	6
Intestines	8

   b. Heart rate and diastolic ventricular volume are the two factors most likely to produce ischemia if either or both are increased.
 I. Distribution of Cardiac Output (Table 30-5)
 J. Peripheral Circulatory Physiology. The peripheral circulation consists of resistance (>60% of peripheral resistance is in the arterioles and precapillary vessels) and capacitance (venous) vessels.
 K. Arterial Pulses and Blood Pressure
   1. The arterial pulse is a wave of vascular distention (forward-propagating pressure wave and its reflectance back toward the heart) resulting from the impact of the stroke volume being ejected into a closed system.
   2. The velocity of the pulse wave depends on the elasticity of the vessel (velocity is most rapid in the least distensible vessels).
     a. In the aortic arch the pulse wave travels 3 to 5 m/sec and the aortic pulse wave precedes the brachial waveform by about 0.05 second.
     b. In large distensible arteries (subclavian) the pulse wave travels 7 to 10 m/sec, whereas in small nondistensible peripheral arteries it travels 15 to 30 m/sec. Such differences become important when timing the counterpulsation of an intra-aortic balloon.
   3. The arterial pressure waveform changes as it moves peripherally (Fig. 30-7).
     a. These changes are best explained by a tubular model of the vascular system in which the contour of the pulse wave depends on the velocity of the

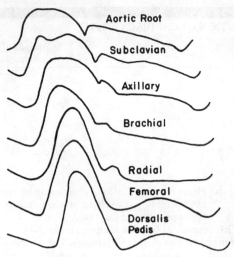

FIGURE 30-7. The changes in pulse waveform as it moves from the aortic root to the dorsalis pedis artery.

pressure wave, the duration of the pulse, and length of the tube (vessel).

   b. In central aortic waveforms, the closure of the aortic valve is indicated by a notch (incisura) on the descending limb. By contrast, peripheral pulse waveforms have a greater amplitude.

4. **Blood pressure** is the lateral pressure exerted by the contained blood on the walls of the vessels.

   a. Mean arterial pressure (product of the cardiac output and systemic vascular resistance) remains constant, whereas pulse pressure and systolic blood pressure increase as blood moves peripherally in the circulation.

   b. Blood pressure normally decreases <6 mm Hg during inspiration (exaggerated in the presence of cardiac tamponade) because pulmonary venous capacitance increases during inspiration to a greater extent than the increase in right-sided venous return and output, thus causing a decrease in left ventricular stroke volume.

5. **Factors Controlling Peripheral Vascular Tone** (Table 30-6)

TABLE 30-6

FACTORS CONTROLLING BLOOD PRESSURE

Central and peripheral autonomic nervous system function (sympathetic tone maintains blood vessels in a partially constricted state [vasomotor tone])

Cardiac output

Systemic vascular resistance

Nitric oxide (endothelium-derived relaxing factor) causes relaxation of vascular smooth muscle

  Basal release of nitric oxide occurs in all but cerebral and coronary vasculature (atherosclerosis impairs relaxation)

  Decreased production of nitric oxide may contribute to systemic and pulmonary hypertension

  Hypoxia impairs nitric oxide production and inhibits platelet aggregation and adhesion

Antidiuretic hormone

Catecholamines

  Norepinephrine is the most important agonist at alpha-1 receptors mediating smooth muscle vasoconstriction in arteries and veins independent of neural supply

  Epinephrine is more potent as a beta-2 agonist than norepinephrine resulting in vasodilation

Renin-angiotensin system

  Renin release from the kidneys is inversely related to renal perfusion

  Renin initiates the formation of angiotensin I (inactive), which is converted to angiotensin II in the lungs (angiotensin-converting enzyme), which stimulates the secretion of aldosterone and inhibits renin release

Atrial natriuretic peptide

  Stored principally in atrial myocytes and released in response to increased vascular volume (atrial distention)

  Decreases blood pressure by direct peripheral vasodilation, natriuresis, and diuresis

IV. SPECIFIC PERIPHERAL CIRCULATIONS

A. Pulmonary Circulation

1. The pulmonary circulation is a low-pressure, high-flow system and has five principal functions (Table 30-7).

2. **Measurement of pulmonary tone** is most often via a flow-directed catheter that measures the pulmonary artery wedge pressure or occluded pressure (as blood runs away from the tip of the catheter beyond the

TABLE 30-7

FUNCTION OF THE PULMONARY CIRCULATION

Metabolic Transport of Humoral Substances and Drugs
Norepinephrine and prostaglandings (E and F series) are removed
   in the lungs by a carrier-mediated process
Acetylcholine and bradykinin are inactivated in the lungs
Drugs (propranolol, lidocaine, bupivacaine, captopril, fentanyl)
   are removed during passage across the lungs
Epinephrine, histamine, and dopamine are not altered by the lungs

Transport of Blood Through the Lungs

Reservoir for the Left Ventricle

Filtration of Venous Drainage

*Transport of Gas, Fluid, and Solutes Across the Walls of
   Exchanging Vessels*

point of occlusion, the pressure in the pulmonary
artery equilibrates with the left atrial pressure).
   a. Left atrial pressure is similar to left ventricular
      end-diastolic pressure in the absence of mitral
      stenosis or increased airway pressure.
   b. Normally, the pulmonary artery wedge pressure is
      1 to 4 mm Hg lower than the pulmonary artery
      end-diastolic pressure.
3. **Effects of Drugs and Maneuvers on Pulmonary Tone**
   a. A hypoxic gas mixture in alveoli causes the
      precapillary arterial vessels supplying that area to
      constrict to divert blood flow away from that area
      (hypoxic pulmonary vasoconstriction).
      Nitroprusside, nitroglycerin, and inhaled
      anesthetics inhibit this protective response and
      may result in a decreased PaO_2.
   b. Pulmonary hypertension occurs if alveolar
      hypoxia is generalized.
B. **Renal Circulation.** The main purpose of excessive renal
   blood flow is to provide energy for active renal tubular
   resorption of sodium.
C. **Physiology of the Venous System**
   1. Systemic veins have a conduit and reservoir function.
      About 60% of the systemic blood volume is in small
      veins and venules. Venodilation to accommodate as
      much as 70 to 75% of the systemic blood volume

buffers sudden increases in arterial blood pressure by allowing sequestration of blood in systemic veins.

2. The compliance of the venous system is regulated by venomotor tone, which is controlled by cerebral autonomic impulses (sympathetically mediated venoconstriction adds about 1 liter of blood to the circulation).

3. **Venous return** is a major determinant of cardiac preload. An increase in right atrial pressure decreases the pressure gradient and venous return. Loss of venous tone, as in autonomic neuropathy or during anesthesia, limits the normal compensatory increases in venous tone in response to changes in posture, positive airway pressure, or hypovolemia.

CHAPTER 31 ■ ANESTHESIA FOR CARDIAC SURGERY

Management of anesthesia for cardiac surgery requires a thorough understanding of normal and altered cardiac physiology; knowledge of the pharmacology of anesthetic, vasoactive, and cardioactive drugs; and familiarity with the physiologic derangements associated with cardiopulmonary bypass (CPB) and the specific surgical procedures (Skubas N, Lichtman AD, Sharma A, Thomas SJ: Anesthesia for cardiac surgery. In Barash PG, Cullen BF, Stoelting RK [eds]: *Clinical Anesthesia*, pp 886–932. Philadelphia, Lippincott Williams & Wilkins, 2006).

I. CORONARY ARTERY DISEASE (CAD)

A. Prevention or treatment of myocardial ischemia during coronary artery bypass graft (CABG) surgery decreases the incidence of perioperative myocardial infarction. Optimizing oxygen delivery to the myocardium is equally important to hemodynamic management.

B. **Myocardial Oxygen Demand.** The principal determinants of myocardial oxygen demand are wall tension and contractility. Interventions that prevent or promptly treat ventricular distention and decrease myocardial oxygen consumption will decrease myocardial oxygen demand.

C. **Myocardial Oxygen Supply.** Increases in myocardial oxygen requirements can only be met by raising coronary blood flow.

   1. **Coronary Blood Flow** (Table 31-1)

      a. The left ventricular subendocardium is most vulnerable to ischemia because myocardial oxygen requirements are high and predictable perfusion can occur only during diastole. The time available for diastole decreases with an increasing heart rate.

      b. A low ventricular filling pressure is desirable for improving perfusion (higher pressure gradient) and decreasing myocardial oxygen requirements (decreased ventricular volume and wall tension).

TABLE 31-1
DETERMINANTS OF CORONARY BLOOD FLOW

Perfusion pressure
Vascular tone
Time available for perfusion (heart rate)
Severity of intraluminal obstructions
Presence of collateral circulation

        c. It is not uncommon during an anesthetic for a patient to exhibit signs of myocardial ischemia without any change in blood pressure, heart rate, or ventricular filling pressure.

  D. Hemodynamic Goals
    1. Although the precise relationship between intraoperative myocardial ischemia and postoperative myocardial infarction remains controversial, there is consensus that a primary goal of a successful anesthetic is the prevention of myocardial ischemia.
    2. Combinations of anesthetics, sedatives, muscle relaxants, and vasoactive drugs are selected to decrease myocardial oxygen requirements and thus prevent or decrease the likelihood of myocardial ischemia.

  E. Monitoring for Ischemia (Table 31-2)
  F. Intraoperative Transesophageal Echocardiography (TEE) (Table 31-3)
  G. Selection of Anesthesia
    1. There is no one ideal anesthetic for patients with CAD. The choice of anesthetic depends primarily on

TABLE 31-2
MONITORING FOR MYOCARDIAL ISCHEMIA

Electrocardiogram (ST segment analysis of leads V5 and II)
Heart rate and blood pressure (rate-pressure product not a sensitive predictor of myocardial ischemia)
Pulmonary artery catheter (V waves reflect ischemia-induced papillary muscle dysfunction but probably not a sensitive indicator of myocardial ischemia)
TEE (regional wall motion abnormalities most sensitive indicator of myocardial ischemia)

TABLE 31-3

USES OF INTRAOPERATIVE TRANSESOPHAGEAL ECHOCARDIOGRAPHY

Evaluation of ventricular volume

Assessment of segmental wall motion abnormalities (myocardial ischemia)

Quantification of ventricular function (diastolic function and filling pressures)

Detect aortic atherosclerotic disease (aorta)

Visualization of the thoracic aorta and intracardiac air

Measurement of valve gradients and quantitation of valvular regurgitation

---

the extent of preexisting myocardial dysfunction and the pharmacologic properties of the specific drugs. Myocardial depression and associated decreases in myocardial oxygen requirements are only harmful in a patient whose heart cannot be further depressed without precipitating congestive heart failure.

2. Early tracheal extubation is popular for both on as well as off-pump cardiac procedures.

   a. Volatile anesthetics in combination with low-dose opioids or total intravenous anesthesia with short-acting drugs (midazolam, alfentanil, propofol) have been used to facilitate the likelihood of early tracheal extubation.

   b. Neuraxial opioids placed before induction of anesthesia decrease postoperative pain and facilitate early tracheal extubation.

3. **Opioids** lack myocardial depressant effects and are useful in patients with severe myocardial dysfunction.

   a. In critically ill patients, opioids such as fentanyl (50 to 100 g/kg iv) can be administered as the sole anesthetic.

   b. In patients with good left ventricular function, opioids may be inadequate to depress sympathetic nervous system activity, requiring the addition of a volatile anesthetic or vasoactive drug.

4. **Inhalation anesthetics** have the advantages of dose dependency, easy reversibility, titratable myocardial depression, amnesia, and reliable suppression of sympathetic nervous system responses to surgical

stress and CPB. Disadvantages include myocardial depression, systemic hypotension, and lack of postoperative analgesia.
  a. **Combinations of opioids and volatile anesthetics** may produce the advantages of each with minimal undesirable side effects. It is likely that any volatile anesthetic could be used as an adjuvant anesthetic if appropriate doses are used.
  b. **Isoflurane** is a coronary vasodilator (more so than other volatile anesthetics), but this effect is clinically insignificant in doses <1 minimum alveolar concentration (MAC) (no evidence of an increased incidence of myocardial ischemia or worsened outcome).
  c. **Desflurane** and **sevoflurane** possess hemodynamic profiles similar to isoflurane but have the advantage of faster recovery. A sudden increase in the inspired concentration of desflurane can result in increased heart rate, systemic blood pressure, and plasma epinephrine concentrations.
  5. **Intravenous Sedative Hypnotics.** An alternative adjuvant anesthetic to the low-dose opioid technique is a titratable infusion of a short-acting sedative (propofol, midazolam, dexmedetomidine) that can be continued postoperatively and after discontinuation afford a predictable and fairly rapid awakening.
H. **Treatment of Ischemia** (Table 31-4)
  1. **Nitroglycerin** is the drug of choice for the treatment of coronary vasospasm. As a venodilator, this drug decreases venous return and decreases ventricular filling pressures and thus wall tension.
  2. **Phenylephrine** increases myocardial oxygen requirements, but this increase is offset by improvements in oxygen delivery produced by the increased coronary perfusion pressure.
  3. **Calcium channel blockers**
    a. **Verapamil** is useful in the treatment of supraventricular tachycardia and slowing the ventricular response in atrial fibrillation and/or flutter. Myocardial depressant effects may limit its usefulness in some patients.
    b. **Nifedipine** and **diltiazem** are coronary vasodilators and are used as antianginal drugs and in the prevention of coronary vasospasm.

TABLE 31-4	
TREATMENT OF INTRAOPERATIVE MYOCARDIAL ISCHEMIA	
Event associated with ischemia	Treatment[a]
Increased blood pressure and pulmonary capillary wedge pressure	Increase anesthetic depth Nitroglycerin (0.5–3 μg/kg/min iv) Sodium nitroprusside (0.5–3 μg/kg/min iv)
Increased heart rate	Beta-antagonist Calcium channel blockers
Decreased blood pressure	Decrease anesthetic depth Phenylephrine
Decreased blood pressure and increased pulmonary capillary wedge pressure	Phenylephrine Nitroglycerin Inotrope
Normal hemodynamics	Nitroglycerin Calcium entry blocker

[a] Goal is to return heart to a slow, small, perfused state.

II. **VALVULAR HEART DISEASE** is characterized by pressure or volume overload of the atria or ventricles. TEE has become a commonly used monitor in the perioperative management of patients undergoing cardiac surgery.

A. **Aortic Stenosis**
   1. The normal aortic valve is composed of three semilunar cusps attached to the wall of the aorta. The normal annular diameter is 1.9 to 2.3 cm with an aortic valve area of 2 to 4 cm^2. The normal diameter of the left ventricular outflow tract is 2.2 cm.
   2. **Pathophysiology** (Fig. 31-1). Chronic obstruction to left ventricular ejection results in concentric ventricular hypertrophy, which makes the heart susceptible to myocardial ischemia even in the absence of CAD. Because the ventricle is stiff, atrial contraction is critical for ventricular filling and stroke volume.
   3. **Anesthetic Considerations.** Maintenance of adequate ventricular volume and sinus rhythm is crucial. Hypotension must be prevented and treated early if it

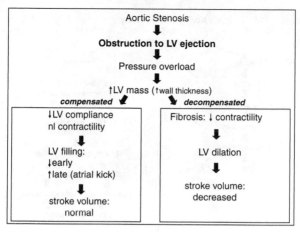

FIGURE 31-1. The physiological consequences of aortic stenosis.

develops to prevent the catastrophic cycle of hypotension-induced ischemia, subsequent ventricular dysfunction, and worsening hypotension. Bradycardia is a common cause of hypotension in patients with aortic stenosis.

4. **TEE in Aortic Stenosis.** A systolic leaflet separation ≥1.3 cm reliably excludes severe aortic stenosis.

B. **Hypertrophic cardiomyopathy** is a genetically determined disease characterized by development of a hypertrophic intraventricular septum, resulting in left ventricular outflow obstruction (resembles aortic stenosis). Outflow obstruction is increased by increases in myocardial contractility or heart rate or decreases in preload or afterload. Anesthetic management is based on maintenance of left ventricular filling and controlled myocardial depression as produced by volatile anesthetics, especially halothane.

C. **Aortic Insufficiency**

1. **Pathophysiology** (Fig. 31-2). Chronic volume overload of the left ventricle evokes eccentric hypertrophy but only minimal changes in filling pressures.

2. **Anesthetic Considerations.** Maintenance of adequate ventricular volume in the presence of mild vasodilation and increases in heart rate is most likely

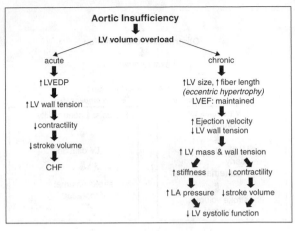

FIGURE 31-2. The physiological consequences of aortic insufficiency.

to optimize forward left ventricular stroke volume. An incompetent aortic valve may prevent the delivery of cardioplegia to the coronary system to produce diastolic arrest of the heart (alternative is injecting cardioplegia directly into the coronary ostia or into the coronary sinus).

3. **TEE in Aortic Insufficiency.** Echocardiographic examination demonstrates structural findings of aortic regurgitation and the effects of volume overload on the left ventricle.

D. **Mitral Stenosis**

1. **Pathophysiology** (Fig. 31-3). Increased left atrial pressure and volume overload are inevitable consequences of the narrowed mitral orifice. Persistent increases in left atrial pressure are reflected back through the pulmonary circulation, leading to right ventricular hypertrophy and perivascular edema in the lungs.

2. **Anesthetic Considerations.** Avoiding tachycardia is crucial for preventing inadequate left ventricular filling with concomitant hypotension. Continued preoperative administration of digitalis and antagonists, selection of anesthetics with minimal

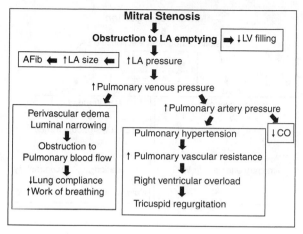

FIGURE 31-3. The physiological consequences of mitral stenosis.

propensity to increase heart rate, and achievement of an anesthetic depth sufficient to suppress sympathetic nervous system responses are recommended.

3. **TEE in Mitral Stenosis.** The mitral annulus is D shaped, and the posterior leaflet is continuous with the atrial and the ventricular myocardium, making this leaflet more prone to being displaced when either chamber enlarges. During diastole, the leaflet opens and drops inside the left ventricle, forming a funnel-shaped orifice, 4 to 6 cm^2 in diameter.

E. **Mitral Regurgitation**
1. **Pathophysiology** (Fig. 31-4). Chronic volume overload of the left atrium is the cardinal feature of mitral regurgitation.
2. **Anesthetic Considerations.** Selection of anesthetics that promote vasodilation and increase the heart rate is useful.
3. **TEE in Mitral Regurgitation.** Valve disease localized to the posterior leaflet or to a focal portion of the anterior leaflet and in the absence of calcification is most amenable to surgical repair.

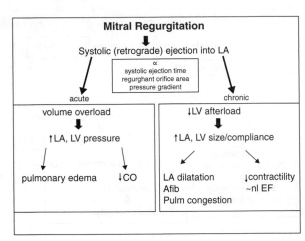

FIGURE 31-4. The physiological consequences of mitral regurgitation.

III. CARDIOPULMONARY BYPASS

A. CPB incorporates a circuit to oxygenate venous blood and return it to the patient's arterial circulation (Table 31-5 and Fig. 31-5).

B. **Blood Conservation in Cardiac Surgery**

1. Intraoperative autologous hemodilution involves the removal of whole blood before bypass (spared damaging effects [coagulopathy] of the bypass circuit) for reinfusion after bypass. Red blood cells may also be salvaged from the surgical field and bypass tubing, washed, and retransfused (Cellsaver). Cellsaver blood may worsen coagulopathy as factors causing coagulopathy are not removed by the filtering process.

2. Pharmacologic measures include antifibrinolytics (epsilon-aminocaproic acid and aprotinin) to decrease bleeding after bypass and reduce the risk of blood transfusion.

    a. Aprotinin introduces platelet protective effects and is effective in decreasing blood loss in high-risk patients (reoperation, known coagulopathy, sepsis, Jehovah's Witness). Disadvantages of aprotinin

---

TABLE 31-5

COMPONENTS OF CARDIOPULMONARY BYPASS

Circuit (blood is drained from the right atrium and returned to the ascending aorta)
Oxygenator
  Bubble (time-dependent trauma to the blood)
  Membrane (less damage to the blood)
Pump (generate pressure required to return perfusate to the patient)
  Roller (nonpulsatile)
  Centrifugal
  Pulsatile (controversy exists whether better than standard flow)
Heat exchanger (allows production of systemic hypothermia)
Prime (decreased hematocrit offset changes in blood viscosity because of hypothermia)
Anticoagulants (activated coagulation time >480 sec; resistance to heparin occurs in patients with antithrombin III deficiency and is treated with fresh frozen plasma or antithrombin III concentrate)
Myocardial protection (hypothermia to $10°C–15°C$ and potassium to ensure diastolic arrest)
  Aortic root (not feasible in patients with aortic insufficiency, must cannulate coronary ostia)
  Retrograde via coronary sinus
  Newly created bypass grafts

---

include a risk of anaphylaxis on reexposure (an animal-derived protein) and its high cost (offset by cost savings because of a decrease in transfusion requirements, operating room time, or need for reoperation).

  b. DDAVP may benefit a subgroup of cardiac surgical patients who have abnormal platelet function.

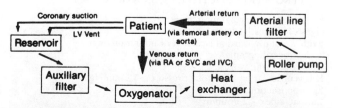

FIGURE 31-5. Diagram of a cardiopulmonary bypass circuit.

C. **Myocardial Protection.** The most common method of myocardial protection used today is that of intermittent hyperkalemic cold cardioplegia (diastolic electrical arrest) and moderate systemic hypothermia.
   1. During CPB the onset of left ventricular distention and lack of rapid electrical arrest may be evidence of poor myocardial protection and the possibility of difficulty in separation from bypass.
   2. TEE is helpful in diagnosing ventricular distention and its relief by venting or manual decompression.

IV. PREOPERATIVE EVALUATION

A. Data from the history, physical examination, and laboratory investigation are used to delineate the degree of left ventricular or right ventricular dysfunction (Table 31-6).
B. **Current drug therapy** is usually continued until the time of surgery, including beta-adrenergic antagonists, calcium channel blockers, ACE inhibitors, and digitalis preparations (heart rate or rhythm control).
C. **Premedication** for cardiac surgery often combines an opioid (morphine 0.1 to 0.2 mg/kg im) with scopolamine (0.006 mg/kg im) and/or a benzodiazepine (diazepam 0.05 to 0.1 mg/kg or lorazepam 0.05 to 0.07 mg/kg orally). Patients with valvular heart disease may be more susceptible to the ventilatory depressant effects of premedication than those with CAD scheduled for CABG operations.

TABLE 31-6

DATA FROM PREOPERATIVE EVALUATION

History of myocardial infarction
Signs of congestive heart failure
Evidence of myocardial ischemia or infarction on electrocardiogram
Chest radiograph
Left ventricular end-diastolic pressure >18 mm Hg
Ejection fraction <0.4
Cardiac index <2 l/min/m^2
TEE (wall motion abnormalities)

TABLE 31-7

MONITORS FOR CARDIAC SURGERY REQUIRING CARDIOPULMONARY BYPASS

Pulse oximeter (place as first monitor to detect unsuspected episodes of hypoxemia during catheter placement)

Electrocardiogram

Temperature (observe gradients during cooling and rewarming)

Intra-arterial blood pressure (radial artery blood pressure may be lower than central aortic pressure early after CPB)

Central venous pressure catheter (infusion of cardioselective drugs; assumed to reflect left-sided filling pressures in the absence of left ventricular dysfunction)

Pulmonary artery catheter (awake versus asleep placement; distal migration occurs during CPB and some recommend withdrawing catheter a few centimeters before initiation of CPB)

TEE (provides information about cardiac structure and function that exceeds any other monitor [valve function, ventricular filling, myocardial contractility, myocardial ischemia, presence of intracardiac air, assess aorta for plaques, congenital heart lesion repairs])

Central nervous system function (electroencephalogram, somatosensory evoked potentials)

   D. **Monitoring** should emphasize those areas particularly relevant to cardiac surgery (Table 31-7) (see Chapter 24).

   E. **Selection of Anesthetic Drugs.** There is no single-best drug with the most critical factor governing anesthetic selection being the degree of left ventricular dysfunction. The anticipated time to tracheal extubation may influence the choice of anesthetic ("fast track"). It is useful to be able to alter anesthetic depth to accommodate the varying intensity of the surgical stimulus (intense with tracheal intubation, sternotomy, and manipulation of the aorta and minimal during hypothermic CPB).

     1. **Potent inhalation anesthetics** are useful as the primary anesthetic and as adjuvants to treat or prevent hypertension associated with high-dose opioid techniques. Volatile anesthetics can be administered during CPB through a vaporizer incorporated into the CPB circuit.

     2. **Opioids** lack negative inotropic effects and in high doses (fentanyl, 50 to 100 μg/kg iv; sufentanil, 10 to 20 μg/kg iv) may be used as the sole anesthetic.

   a. In patients with good left ventricular function, it is
      often necessary to include adjuvant drugs to
      provide amnesia (benzodiazepines) and
      control hypertension (volatile anesthetics,
      vasodilators).
   b. Excessive bradycardia may accompany the use of
      opioids, especially if nondepolarizing muscle
      relaxants without heart rate effects are
      administered.
3. **Nitrous oxide** has limited usefulness because of its
   myocardial depressant effects in the presence of
   opioids and the ability to enhance the size of air
   emboli, which may be present in coronary arteries
   after CABG operations.
F. **Neuromuscular Blocking Drugs.** Selection of muscle
   relaxants is influenced by the hemodynamic and
   pharmacokinetic properties associated with each drug,
   the patient's myocardial function, and the anesthetic
   technique.

V. INTRAOPERATIVE MANAGEMENT (Table 31-8)

A. **Preinduction Period**
   1. Supplemental oxygen is administered via nasal
      cannula once the patient is transferred to the
      operating table. Angina is promptly treated with
      oxygen and nitroglycerin (sublingual or iv).
   2. Placing a pulse oximeter with the pulse tone audible
      should precede line placement.
B. **Induction and Intubation**
   1. The dose, speed of administration, and specific drugs
      selected depend primarily on a patient's
      cardiovascular reserve and desired cardiovascular
      profile.
   2. A brief duration of laryngoscopy is desirable,
      although intubation of the trachea may be associated
      with myocardial ischemia even in the absence of
      blood pressure and/or heart rate changes.
C. **The preincision period** between tracheal intubation and
   skin incision is one of minimal stimulation (blood
   pressure may need to be supported).
D. **Incision to bypass** is characterized by periods of intense
   surgical stimulation, which often require alteration in the
   depth of anesthesia or administration of a vasodilator to
   blunt responses (hypertension, tachycardia) that may

TABLE 31-8

CHECKLIST FOR MANAGEMENT OF PATIENT UNDERGOING CARDIOPULMONARY BYPASS

Before Cardiopulmonary Bypass
  Laboratory values
    Heparinization adequate (activated coagulation time or other method)
    Hematocrit
  Anesthetic
    Adequate depth utilizing amnestics, opioids
    Nitrous oxide off
    Muscle relaxants supplemented
  Monitors
    Arterial pressure (initial hypotension and then return)
    Central venous pressure (indicates adequate venous drainage)
    Pulmonary capillary wedge pressure (elevated with left ventricular distention reflecting inadequate drainage, aortic insufficiency)
  Patient/Field
    Cannulas in place (no clamps or air locks)
    Face (suffusion reflects inadequate superior vena cava drainage, unilateral blanching reflects innominate artery cannulation)
    Heart (signs of distention reflect ischemia, aortic insufficiency)
  Support
    Usually not necessary

During Cardiopulmonary Bypass
  Laboratory values
    Heparinization adequate
    Arterial blood gases (evidence of acidosis)
    Hematocrit, electrolytes, ionized calcium, glucose
  Anesthetic
    Discontinue ventilation
  Monitors
    Arterial hypotension (inadequate venous return, low pump flow, aortic dissection, decreased vascular tone, dampened waveform)
    Arterial hypertension (high pump flow, vasoconstriction)
    Venous pressure (transducer higher than atrial level, obstruction to chamber drainage)
    EEG
    Adequate body perfusion (acidosis, mixed venous oxygen saturation)
    Temperature
    Urine output
  Patient/Field
    Conduct of operation (heart distention, fibrillation)

(continued)

TABLE 31-8
CONTINUED

Venous engorgement
Signs of light anesthesia (movement, breathing)
Support
  Assist adequacy of pump flow (anesthetics/vasodilators for
  hypertension, constrictors for hypotension)

Before Separation from Cardiopulmonary Bypass
Laboratory values
  Hematocrit and arterial blood gases
  Potassium (may be elevated from cardioplegia)
  Ionized calcium
Anesthetic/Machine
  Initiate ventilation (evaluate lung compliance)
  Vaporizers off
  Alarms on
Monitors
  Normothermia (37°C nasopharyngeal, 35.5°C bladder)
  Electrocardiogram (rate, rhythm, ST wave)
  Transducers zeroed and calibrated
  Arterial and filling pressures
  Activate recorder
Patient/Field
  Look at heart (contractility, rhythm, size)
  De-aired (TEE)
  Bleeding
  Vascular resistance
Support
  As necessary (inotrope, vasodilator)

predispose to myocardial ischemia. Any evidence of new myocardial ischemia (ST segment changes on the electrocardiogram) should be treated appropriately and the surgeon notified.

E. **Cardiopulmonary Bypass**
  1. CPB is initiated after confirmation of adequate anticoagulation with heparin.
  2. There is no consensus about the optimal mean arterial pressure during CPB, although pump flows of 50 to 60 mL/kg usually produce perfusion pressures of 50 to 60 mm Hg.
    a. The effect of decreased viscosity (acute hemodilution) and loss of pulsatile flow may initially cause the perfusion pressure to decrease below 40 mm Hg.

   b. Phenylephrine may be administered to increase
      perfusion pressure if it is deemed necessary for
      maintenance of organ blood flow.
   3. Once full CPB is established, there is no need to
      continue ventilation of the patient's lungs. There is no
      consensus about management of the lungs (positive
      end-expiratory pressure versus zero airway pressure,
      oxygen versus room air) during CPB.
   4. Anesthetic requirements are decreased during
      hypothermic CPB, an effect that may offset the
      dilutional effect of CPB on plasma concentrations of
      injected drugs.
   5. Continued skeletal muscle paralysis is desirable to
      prevent increases in oxygen requirements owing to
      skeletal muscle activity.
F. Monitoring and Management During Bypass
   1. It is important to continuously observe the surgical
      field and cannulae to permit early detection of
      mechanical causes of hypotension or hypertension
      during CPB.
   2. Maintenance of adequate depths of anesthesia is
      important during bypass although clinical signs are
      few. Use of brain wave monitoring (BIS) may aid
      in determining the approximate depth of
      anesthesia.
   3. Maintenance of urine output with diuretics is a
      common practice during CPB. Nevertheless,
      postoperative renal failure is most likely because of
      aggravation of preexisting renal dysfunction
      or persistent low cardiac output following CPB.
G. Rewarming is begun when the surgical repair is nearly
   complete, remembering that patients may regain
   awareness as the anesthetic effects of hypothermia
   dissipate (consider administration of a volatile anesthetic
   if a smooth postbypass course is anticipated and early
   weaning from mechanical ventilation and extubation are
   planned). TEE is useful in assessing the effectiveness of
   the de-airing process.
H. Discontinuation of CPB is considered when rewarming is
   adequate. A low cardiac output must prompt a search
   for explanations (kinked grafts, air in coronary grafts,
   coronary artery spasm, global ischemia from inadequate
   myocardial protection) and consideration of
   pharmacologic support (inotropes, vasodilators)
   (Tables 31-9 and 31-10).

TABLE 31-9

ETIOLOGY OF RIGHT OR LEFT VENTRICULAR
DYSFUNCTION AFTER CARDIOPULMONARY BYPASS

Ischemia
  Inadequate myocardial protection
  Intraoperative infarction
  Reperfusion injury
  Coronary spasm
  Coronary embolism (air, thrombus)
  Technical difficulties (kinked or clotted grafts)

Uncorrected Structural Defects
  Nongraftable vessels
  Diffuse coronary artery disease
  Residual or new valve pathology
  Shunts
  Preexisting cardiac dysfunction

Cardiopulmonary Bypass–Related Factors
  Excessive cardioplegia
  Unrecognized cardiac distention

I. **Intra-Aortic Balloon Pump** (Table 31-11)
   1. The balloon pump functions as a mechanical assist
      device in the thoracic aorta (25-cm balloon on a
      90-cm vascular catheter) that uses the principle of
      synchronized counterpulsation to enhance left
      ventricular stroke volume.
      a. The balloon deflates immediately before systole to
         decrease afterload and myocardial oxygen
         requirements. Subsequently, the balloon inflates
         during diastole to provide diastolic
         augmentation that increases coronary blood flow.
      b. It is crucial to control heart rate and to suppress
         cardiac dysrhythmias to ensure proper balloon
         timing.
   2. As cardiac function improves, the assist ratio is
      gradually weaned from every beat to every other beat
      and then removed.
J. **Ventricular Assist Device.** When the heart is unable to
   meet systemic metabolic demands despite maximal
   pharmacologic therapy and insertion of the intra-aortic
   balloon pump, a device that pumps blood and
   bypasses the left or right ventricle may be
   useful.

TABLE 31-10

DIAGNOSIS AND THERAPY OF CARDIOVASCULAR DYSFUNCTION FOLLOWING CARDIOPULMONARY BYPASS

Blood pressure	Filling pressures	Cardiac output	Diagnosis	Treatment
Increased	Increased	Increased	Hypervolemia	Remove volume, vasodilation
Increased	Increased	Decreased	Vasoconstriction	Vasodilation
			Poor contractility	Inotrope
Increased	Decreased	Increased	Hyperdynamic	Anesthetic, beta-antagonist
Increased	Decreased	Decreased	Vasoconstriction	Vasodilation, give volume
Decreased	Increased	Increased	Hypervolemia	Wait
Decreased	Increased	Decreased	Poor contractility	Inotrope, vasodilation, mechanical assist
Decreased	Decreased	Increased	Vasodilation	Vasoconstriction
Decreased	Decreased	Decreased	Hypovolemia	Give volume

TABLE 31-11

INDICATIONS AND CONTRAINDICATIONS FOR
INTRA-AORTIC BALLOON PUMP

Indications
  Complications of myocardial ischemia
    Hemodynamic (cardiogenic shock)
    Mechanical (mitral regurgitation, ventricular septal defect)
    Intractable dysrhythmias
    Extension of infarct
  Acute cardiac instability
    Unstable angina
    Failed PTCA
    Cardiac contusion
    ? septic shock
  Open heart surgery
    Separation from cardiopulmonary bypass
    Ventricular failure
    Increasing inotropic requirements
    Progressive hemodynamic deterioration
    Refractory ischemia

Contraindications
  Severe aortic insufficiency
  Technical difficulties with insertion
  Irreversible cardiac disease
  Irreversible brain damage

K. Postcardiopulmonary Bypass
  1. **Reversal of Anticoagulation.** Heparin is partially
     reversed with protamine administered intravenously
     while the arterial cannula remains in place for
     continued transfusion of pump contents. Adequate
     reversal of anticoagulation with protamine is verified
     by measurement of the activated coagulation time.
     Protamine administration may be accompanied by
     side effects (Table 31-12). Whether protamine should
     be administered through the right atrium, left atrium,
     aorta, or a peripheral vein remains controversial.
  2. **Postbypass Bleeding**
    a. Persistent oozing following heparin reversal is not
      uncommon and usually reflects inadequate surgical
      hemostasis or platelet dysfunction.
    b. Closure of the chest is occasionally associated with
      transient decreases in blood pressure. If
      hypotension persists despite volume replacement,

TABLE 31-12
SIDE EFFECTS OF PROTAMINE

Hypotension (less likely when administered over 5 min)
Allergic reaction (more likely in patients receiving protamine-containing insulin preparations [NPH, PZI])
Pulmonary hypertension (mediated by release of thromboxane and C5a anaphylatoxin)

the chest must be reopened to rule out cardiac tamponade or kinking of a venous graft.

L. **Minimally Invasive Cardiac Surgery.** The desire to avoid the complications of CPB (stroke, neurocognitive defects, renal failure, pulmonary insufficiency, coagulopathy, activation of the systemic inflammatory response) as well as complications of sternotomy led to the development of techniques not requiring CPB (minimally invasive direct coronary artery bypass [MIDCAB], off-pump coronary bypass [OPCAB], robotic surgery).

M. **Postoperative Considerations**
1. **Bring-backs** of the patient for postoperative reexploration are necessary in 4 to 10% of cases, usually in the first 24 hours (Table 31-13).
2. **Tamponade** must always be included in the differential diagnosis of unexplained low cardiac output (Table 31-14). Ketamine is useful for induction and maintenance of anesthesia in patients with cardiac tamponade, because the goal is to avoid vasodilation or cardiac depression.
3. **Postoperative Pain Management**
   a. The emerging emphasis on early awakening and tracheal extubation after cardiac surgery has resulted in a deemphasis of high-dose opioid

TABLE 31-13
REASONS FOR POSTOPERATIVE REEXPLORATION

Persistent bleeding
Excessive blood loss
Cardiac tamponade
Unexplained low cardiac output

TABLE 31-14

MANIFESTATIONS OF CARDIAC TAMPONADE

Hypotension
Equalization of diastolic filling pressures (when the pericardium is no longer intact, loculated areas of clot may compress only one chamber, causing isolated increases in filling pressures)
Fixed stroke volume (cardiac output and blood pressure become dependent on heart rate)
Peripheral vasoconstriction
Tachycardia
Potential for concurrent myocardial ischemia

---

anesthetic techniques but the continued need for analgesia postoperatively.
  b. Intrathecal or epidural administration of opioids may be alternatives to intravenous opioids. Use of nonsteroidal anti-inflammatory drugs may play an

---

TABLE 31-15

CLASSIFICATION OF CONGENITAL HEART DEFECTS

Volume Overload of the Ventricle or Atrium Resulting in Increased Pulmonary Blood Flow
Atrial septal defect (high flow, low pressure)
Ventricular septal defect (high flow, high pressure)
Patent ductus arteriosus (high flow, high pressure)
Endocardial cushion defect (high flow, high pressure)

Cyanosis Resulting from Obstruction to Pulmonary Blood Flow
Tetralogy of Fallot
Tricuspid atresia
Pulmonary atresia

Pressure Overload on the Ventricle
Aortic stenosis
Coarctation of the aorta
Pulmonary stenosis

Cyanosis Because of a Common Mixing Chamber
Total anomalous venous return
Truncus arteriosus
Double outlet right ventricle
Single ventricle

Cyanosis as a Result of Separation of the Systemic and Pulmonary Circulations
Transposition of the great vessels

increasing role in management of postoperative
pain after cardiac surgery.

VI. ANESTHESIA FOR CHILDREN WITH CONGENITAL HEART DISEASE

A. Congenital heart defects cause either too much blood
flow to a cardiac chamber or obstruction of flow to a
chamber (Table 31-15). Since "anatomy dictates
physiology" the anesthetic management of children with
congenital heart disease requires knowledge of
anatomical defects and planned surgical procedures and
comprehensive understanding of the altered physiology.
B. **Preoperative Evaluation** (Table 31-16)

TABLE 31-16
PREOPERATIVE EVALUATION OF CHILDREN WITH CONGENITAL HEART DISEASE

History
Symptoms (poor weight gain, respiratory distress, easily
exhausted, cyanosis, upper respiratory infections)
Medications (potential interactions with anesthetics)
Previous surgical procedures

Physical Examination
Evidence of cardiac failure (irritability, diaphoresis, rales,
jugular venous distention, hepatomegaly)
Failure to thrive (pulmonary hypertension, poor peripheral
oxygenation)
Blood pressure in arms and legs
Auscultation of the heart (murmur reflects lesion)
Airway evaluation

Laboratory Evaluation
Hemoglobin (anemia versus polycythemia)
Coagulation profile (platelet count, prothrombin time, partial
thromboplastin time)
Potassium (diuretic therapy), glucose, calcium
Arterial blood gases
Chest radiography (cardiac size, abnormal vessels, pneumonia)
Electrocardiogram (rate and rhythm)

Echocardiography and Cardiac Catheterization
TEE delineates cardiac anatomy and permits noninvasive
measurement of ventricular size, function and cardiac output

C. **Premedication**
  1. Choice of premedication is based on the child's physiology with the goal being to produce a calm child without hemodynamic compromise (midazolam, fentanyl, ketamine, atropine).
  2. Small infants should not be kept without fluids while awaiting surgery
D. **Monitoring.** TEE is useful as a diagnostic and monitoring tool.
E. **Induction**
  1. Inhalation agents are useful for induction and may be continued for maintenance. Nitrous oxide is acceptable and does not increase pulmonary vascular resistance except in the presence of preexisting pulmonary hypertension. Nitrous oxide is limited to induction because of the risk of enlarging bubbles of air.
  2. Ketamine is a useful induction drug in children with cyanotic lesions.
F. **Maintenance.** The choice of anesthetic drugs following induction of anesthesia is influenced by ventricular function, the use of CPB, and anticipation of controlled mechanical ventilation or tracheal extubation at the end of the operation (Table 31-17).
G. **Cardiopulmonary Bypass**
  1. An aprotinin infusion may be initiated prior to beginning CPB and continued until the end of surgery in hopes of decreasing bleeding. Aprotinin may evoke an antibody response and children undergoing repeat procedures are at risk for anaphylaxis.
  2. During the course of CPB, vasodilating drugs (nitroprusside) are often administered to promote uniform cooling and rewarming.
  3. Separation from CPB may require pharmacologic intervention (Table 31-18).
H. **Tracheal Extubation and Postoperative Ventilation**
  1. Children undergoing correction of congenital cardiac defects that do not require ventricular incisions (atrial septal defect, ventricular septal defect repaired across the tricuspid valve) can often have their tracheas extubated at the conclusion of surgery.
  2. Those with risk factors for ventilatory failure must fulfill tracheal extubation criteria (risk factors include complex surgery, circulatory arrest, pulmonary hypertension, preexisting pulmonary disease) (Table 31-19).

TABLE 31-17

CHOICE OF DRUGS DURING MAINTENANCE OF ANESTHESIA FOR CORRECTION OF CONGENITAL CARDIAC DEFECTS

Intravenous Agents (fentanyl 50–100 μg/kg, remifentanil 1 μg/kg/min, bradycardia a risk)

Inhalational Agents
  Isoflurane (myocardial contractility may be better preserved than with halothane; propensity for laryngospasm if used for induction of anesthesia)
  Sevoflurane (ability to use for inhalation induction and lacks significant myocardial depression as decreases in systemic blood pressure are principally because of decreases in systemic vascular resistance)

Neuromuscular Blocking Drugs
  Succinylcholine (bradycardia limits usefulness)
  Nondepolarizing relaxants (facilitate tracheal intubation and provide paralysis during surgery; pancuronium is useful when increased heart rate is desirable)

TABLE 31-18

MEDICATIONS ADMINISTERED BY CONTINUOUS INTRAVENOUS INFUSION

Drug	Usual initial dose (μg/kg/min)	Usual dose range (μg/kg/min)
Amrinone[a]	2–5	2–20
Dopamine	2–5	2–20
Dobutamine	2–5	2–20
Epinephrine	0.1	0.1–1
Isoproterenol	0.05–1[b]	0.1–1
Lidocaine	20	20–50
Nitroglycerin	0.5	0.5–5
Norepinephrine	0.1	0.1–1
Phentolamine	0.1–1	0.5–5
Phenylephrine	1	1–3
Prostaglandin E1	0.05–1	0.05–0.2
Vasopressin	1μg–4u	0.0004

[a]Requires initial bolus of 750 μg/kg over 3 minutes before start of infusion.
[b]For chronotropic effect following cardiac transplantation, doses of 0.005 to 0.01 μg/kg/min are used.

TABLE 31-19

CRITERIA FOR TRACHEAL EXTUBATION FOLLOWING COMPLEX PROCEDURES

Ability to maintain oxygenation during spontaneous respiration

Coordination of thoracic and abdominal components of respiration

Acceptable chest X ray (absence of significant atelectasis, effusions, infiltrates)

Short period of time without caloric support

Stable inotropic support

CHAPTER 32 ■ ANESTHESIA FOR VASCULAR SURGERY

The heart is the principal focus for the anesthesiologist in the management of patients undergoing peripheral vascular surgery, emphasizing the fact that myocardial dysfunction is the single most important cause of morbidity following vascular surgery (Ellis JE, Roizen MF, Mantha S, Schwarze ML, McKinsey J, Lubarsky D, Kenaan C: Anesthesia for vascular surgery. In Barash PG, Cullen BF, Stoelting RK [eds]: *Clinical Anesthesia*, pp 933–973. Philadelphia, Lippincott Williams & Wilkins, 2006). Preservation of other organ systems (particularly the kidneys and brain) is also crucial. Low serum albumin values and high American Society of Anesthesiologists (ASA) physical classification are predictors of morbidity and mortality after vascular surgery.

I. VASCULAR DISEASE: EPIDEMIOLOGIC, MEDICAL, AND SURGICAL ASPECTS

A. Pathophysiology of Atherosclerosis
1. Atherosclerosis is a generalized inflammatory disorder of the arterial tree with associated endothelial dysfunction.
   a. Markers of inflammation (C-reactive protein) may be useful in predicting an increased risk of coronary artery disease.
   b. Risk factors for atherosclerosis include many aspects of the metabolic syndrome (Table 32-1).
2. Recommendations for more aggressive treatment of hypertension are based on studies that suggest this will delay progression of atherosclerotic disease (cardiovascular disease doubles for each increment increase of 20/10 mm Hg beginning at 115/75 mm Hg).
3. Morbidity associated with atherosclerosis arises from plaque enlargement and lumen obstruction (coronary arteries, carotid bifurcation, infrarenal abdominal aorta, iliofemoral vessels), plaque ulceration, embolization, thrombus formation, and aneurysmal dilatation owing to weakening of the artery wall.

TABLE 32-1

RISK FACTORS FOR ATHEROSCLEROSIS

Predisposing Risk Factors (Aspects of the Metabolic Syndrome)
Abdominal obesity
Atherogenic dyslipidemia
Raised blood pressure
Insulin resistance
Proinflammatory state
Prothrombotic state

Major Risk Factors
Cigarette smoking
Elevated low density lipoprotein cholesterol (LDL-C)
Low high density lipoprotein (HDL-C)
Family history of premature coronary artery disease
Aging

Emerging Risk Factors
Elevated triglycerides
Small LDL particles

B. **Natural History of Patients with Peripheral Vascular Disease**
1. Elderly patients with peripheral vascular disease have increased mortality rates (6- to 15-fold increases), particularly from cardiovascular causes.
   a. Carotid atherosclerosis increases the risk for ischemic stroke and identifies patients that are at risk for myocardial infarction.
   b. Renal artery atherosclerosis increases the risk of severe and refractory hypertension as well as renal failure.
2. The presence of disease in one vascular territory (peripheral arterial disease and claudication) is associated with increased risk of myocardial infarction and stroke.
3. Abdominal aortic aneurysms (AAAs) occur in up to 5% of males >65 years of age. AAAs between 4 and 5 cm in diameter are followed every 6 to 12 months to determine whether they are increasing in size.

C. **Medical Therapy for Atherosclerosis**
1. Medical therapy including use of antihypertensives (beta-blockers, ACE inhibitors), statin drugs, aspirin, and control of hyperglycemia (hypoglycemics and/or insulin) may reduce perioperative morbidity

and mortality in vascular surgery
(Table 32-2).
2. Cessation of smoking may be the most effective
medical therapy.
3. Antiplatelet therapy is a mainstay of medical therapy
for peripheral vascular disease and many patients
presenting for vascular surgery will be taking aspirin,
clopidogrel, ticlopidine, or COX-2 inhibitors
(Table 32-3).
   a. Adverse effects of aspirin (bleeding tendency,
   gastritis, renal vasoconstriction) must be weighed
   against the benefits (reduce risk of myocardial
   infarction and stroke after vascular
   surgery).
   b. COX-2 inhibitors are useful in providing
   perioperative analgesia but negative effects include
   inhibition of prostacyclin production, increased
   blood pressure, and thrombotic potential.
D. **Chronic Medical Problems and Risk Prediction in
Peripheral Vascular Disease Patients**
   1. Disorders associated with peripheral vascular disease
   most often include diabetes mellitus and cigarette
   smoking with its associated sequelae (chronic
   obstructive pulmonary disease, hypertension,
   coronary artery disease). Understanding the end-organ
   effects of these diseases can influence perioperative
   therapy.
   2. The dramatic decrease in the incidence of renal failure
   after abdominal aortic reconstruction has been
   attributed to better perioperative fluid management.
   3. Perioperative mortality and factors limiting patient
   progress after vascular surgery are primarily related to
   the heart.

II. CORONARY ARTERY DISEASE IN PATIENTS WITH PERIPHERAL VASCULAR DISEASE

A. Patients with peripheral vascular disease have a high
incidence of severe and correctable coronary artery
disease as documented by coronary angiography. The
presence of uncorrected coronary artery disease increases
mortality after vascular surgery.
B. Noncardiac surgery is associated with considerable risk
in the first 6 weeks following coronary stent placement
(clopidogrel and surgical bleeding versus risk of acute

TABLE 32-2
MANAGEMENT OF PREOPERATIVE DRUG THERAPY

Medication	Side effect or potential concern in the perioperative period	Recommendation for perioperative use
Aspirin	Platelet inhibition may increase bleeding Decreased GFR	Continue until day of surgery, especially for carotid and peripheral cases Monitor fluid and urine status
Clopidogrel	Platelet inhibition may increase bleeding Rare thrombotic thrombocytopenic purpura	Hold for 7 days before surgery except for CEA and severe CAD Consider additional crossmatch of blood Avoid neuraxial anesthesia if not held for at least 7 days
HMG COA reductase inhibitors (statins)	Liver function test abnormalities Rhabdomyolysis	Assess liver function tests and continue through morning of surgery Check CPK if myalgias

Beta-blockers	Bronchospasm Hypotension Bradycardia Heart block	Continue through perioperative period
ACE inhibitors	Induction hypotension Cough	Continue through perioperative period Consider 1/2 dose on day of surgery
Diuretics	Hypovolemia Electrolyte abnormalities	Continue through morning of surgery Monitor fluid and urine status
Calcium channel blockers	Perioperative hypotension especially with amlodipine	Continue through perioperative period (consider withholding amlodipine on the morning of surgery)
Oral hypoglycemics	Hypoglycemia preoperatively and intraoperatively Lactic acidosis with metformin	When feasible switch over to insulin preoperatively Monitor glucose status perioperatively

GRF, glomerular filtration rate; HMG, 3-hydroxy-3-methylglutaryl-coenzyme A reductase; ACE, angiotensin-converting enzyme.

TABLE 32-3

NEURAXIAL ANESTHESIA IN THE PATIENT RECEIVING THROMBOPROPHYLAXIS (AMERICAN SOCIETY OF REGIONAL ANESTHESIA AND PAIN MEDICINE)

Antiplatelet medications	No contraindication with NSAIDs Discontinue ticlopidine 14 days Discontinue clopidogrel 7 days Discontinue GP IIb/IIIa inhibitors 8–48 hr in advance
Unfractionated heparin Subcutaneous	No contraindication (consider delaying heparin until after block if technical difficulty anticipated)
Intravenous	Heparinize 1 hour after neuraxial technique Remove catheter 2–4 hr after last heparin dose No mandatory delay if traumatic
Low-molecular weight heparin Twice daily dosing	Initiate 24 hr after surgery regardless of technique Remove neuraxial catheter 2 hr before first dose
Once daily dosing	Neuraxial technique 10–12 hr after heparin dose Next dose of heparin 4–12 hr after needle or catheter placement Catheter removal 10–12 hr after heparin and 4 hr prior to next dose Postpone heparin 24 hr if traumatic
Warfarin	Document normal INR after discontinuation (prior to neuraxial technique) Remove catheter when INR ≤ 1.5 (initiation of therapy)
Thrombolytics	No data on safety interval for performance of neuraxial technique or catheter removal Follow fibrinogen level
Herbal therapy	No evidence for mandatory discontinuation prior to neuraxial technique Be aware of potential drug interactions

NSAIDs, nonsteroidal anti-inflammatory drugs; GP IIb/IIIa, platelet glycoprotein receptor IIb/IIIa inhibitors; INR, international normalized ratio.

TABLE 32-4
VALUE OF PREOPERATIVE CARDIAC RISK STRATIFICATION

Forego surgery or perform a more conservative surgical procedure in those at high risk

Determine those patients who should undergo myocardial revascularization (left main coronary artery disease, triple-vessel disease, poor left ventricular function)

Identify those who might benefit from aggressive therapy in the first 24–72 hr postoperatively

perioperative coronary stent thrombosis). After 6 weeks the stent is generally endothelialized.

  C. Perioperative myocardial infarction is more often non–Q wave, occurring on the operative day or first postoperative day.

   1. Myocardial infarction occurring in the perioperative period is associated with sustained elevation of heart rate, absence of chest pain, and prolonged premonitory episodes of ST segment depression.

   2. Elevations of cardiac troponin levels are associated with adverse perioperative outcomes.

   3. Three purposes are served by preoperative cardiac risk stratification (Table 32-4).

   4. The patient's preoperative history and physical examination can provide important prognostic information (Table 32-5).

     a. A waiting period of 6 months after a myocardial infarction before surgery may no longer apply to most patients (acute thrombolysis, angioplasty,

TABLE 32-5
PROGNOSTIC INFORMATION FROM HISTORY AND PHYSICAL EXAMINATION

Congestive heart failure
Coronary artery disease
Advanced age
Limited exercise tolerance
Renal insufficiency
Uncontrolled hypertension with left ventricular hypertrophy

control of hyperglycemia during acute care decrease infarct size).

   b. If coronary stenting has been performed, waiting 6 weeks before elective surgery is a consideration.
5. Exercise tolerance (may be limited by claudication or orthopedic problems) may be a useful prognostic indicator.
   a. When a patient can walk briskly for two blocks without angina or dyspnea, it is unlikely that left main disease, triple-vessel disease, or left ventricular dysfunction is present. These patients can probably undergo surgery without noninvasive testing as they are unlikely to experience adverse postoperative cardiac events or have severe coronary artery disease.
   b. Patients with stable symptoms who cannot walk two blocks briskly are at intermediate risk and may benefit from noninvasive testing (value of screening tests remains controversial) (Table 32-6).
   c. Dipyridamole-thallium scintigraphy may be utilized to establish risk stratification (Table 32-7).
6. Congestive heart failure is a strong predictor of morbid postoperative events.

TABLE 32-6

CLINICAL PREDICTORS OF INCREASED PERIOPERATIVE CARDIOVASCULAR RISK

Major Risk Factors (when present mandates intensive management including delay of surgery)
Acute myocardial infarction (<7 days)
Recent myocardial infarction (7–30 days)
Unstable angina
Decompensated congestive heart failure
Significant cardiac arrhythmias

Intermediate Risk Factors
Current or prior angina pectoris
Prior myocardial infarction
Congestive heart failure
Advanced age (70 years or older)
Limited exercise tolerance
Chronic renal insufficiency (serum creatinine >2 mg/100 mL)
Cerebrovascular accident
Diabetes mellitus

TABLE 32-7

SPECIALIZED TESTING OF CARDIAC FUNCTION IN THE
PREOPERATIVE PERIOD

Dipyridamole-thallium scintigraphy
Radionuclide ventriculography
Dobutamine stress echocardiography
Ultrasound assessment of brachial artery flow (endothelial
  dysfunction)
Coronary angiography

D. **Preoperative Coronary Revascularization**
   1. Myocardial revascularization prior to peripheral
      vascular surgery may be indicated in patients with
      triple-vessel coronary artery disease, poor left
      ventricular function (ejection fraction <0.35), or left
      main coronary artery disease.
   2. Stent thrombosis and increased surgical bleeding from
      clopidogrel are concerns in the patient with a recent
      coronary stent.
   3. Whether preoperative coronary revascularization
      protects against perioperative cardiac events is
      controversial.
      a. Once the patient has recovered from successful
         coronary artery revascularization (1 week after
         angioplasty and 6 to 8 weeks after coronary
         stenting or coronary artery bypass graft [CABG]
         surgery), peripheral vascular surgery is usually
         performed.
      b. In some cases, CABG surgery can be combined
         with peripheral vascular surgery (most commonly
         carotid endarterectomy).
      c. Elective abdominal aortic aneurysm repair should
         probably be performed before, simultaneously, or
         within 2 weeks of CABG surgery because of
         increased risk of aneurysm rupture seen after this
         period.
E. **Perioperative Cardiac Monitoring** (Table 32-8)
F. **Management of Perioperative Myocardial Ischemia and
   Infarction in Vascular Patients**
   1. Myocardial infarctions are more likely to occur in the
      first 24 hours following surgery.
   2. Stable coronary ischemic syndromes likely occur in
      response to increased oxygen demand by the

TABLE 32-8

PERIOPERATIVE MONITORING FOR DETECTION OF MYOCARDIAL ISCHEMIA

Electrocardiogram (lead V5 most sensitive for intraoperative detection of ST segment depression or elevation; automated ST segment monitors may facilitate clinician's ability to detect signs of ischemia)

Holter monitoring (demonstrates that immediate postoperative period is the time when myocardial ischemia is most likely [pain, adrenergic stress, hypothermia, shivering, hypercoagulability])

Pulmonary capillary wedge pressure (low sensitivity)

Transesophageal echocardiography (wall motion abnormalities)

CK-MB isoenzymes (false-positive results because of skeletal muscle damage)

Cardiac troponins (increased specificity in patients with skeletal muscle damage)

---

myocardium in a setting of fixed coronary plaques. Unstable coronary ischemic syndromes may reflect plaque rupture with local thrombus and vasoreactivity that produces intermittent critical decreases in coronary oxygen supply.

3. Patients undergoing vascular surgery are most likely to manifest myocardial ischemia in the immediate postoperative period with its associated pain, adrenergic stimulation, hypothermia, hypercoagulability, anemia, shivering, and sleep deprivation.

   a. Factors increasing the likelihood of postoperative myocardial ischemia that the anesthesiologist can control include tachycardia, hypertension, hypotension, anemia, shivering, endotracheal tube suctioning, and suboptimal analgesia.

   b. Continual myocardial ischemia lasting >2 hours is associated with a marked increase in the likelihood of adverse postoperative cardiac events.

G. **Perioperative Cardiac Risk Reducing Strategies** (Table 32-9)

   1. Of the various risk-reducing strategies, growing evidence suggests that perioperative beta-blockade provides benefit in preventing cardiac morbidity and mortality. Asthma, chronic obstructive airway disease, and cardiac conduction disease in the absence of a

pacemaker are contraindications to beta-blocker therapy.

2. High-dose opioid anesthetics reduce the stress response and may improve overall outcome after major surgery.

3. Epidural anesthesia may improve outcome in other organ systems, but its ability to decrease the incidence of myocardial infarction is speculative.

4. Anemia (hematocrit <28%) may increase the incidence of postoperative myocardial ischemia in high-risk patients undergoing noncardiac surgery (more likely to transfuse high-risk patients or those who demonstrate myocardial ischemia with packed red blood cells to augment the hematocrit to 30%).

5. Hypothermia is associated with increased adrenergic tone and postoperative myocardial ischemia in vascular surgery patients (aggressively warm patients and conserve heat during and after surgery).

6. Suctioning, tracheal extubation, and weaning from mechanical ventilation may produce myocardial ischemia (early tracheal extubation versus sedation and analgesia to permit tolerance of tracheal tube).

H. **Other Medical Problems in Vascular Surgery Patients** (Table 32-10)

III. CAROTID ENDARTERECTOMY

A. Anesthetic management of carotid endarterectomy (CEA) involves attempts to optimize cerebral perfusion in patients with a high prevalence of coronary artery disease (Table 32-11).

1. Alternatives to traditional CEA include carotid angioplasty (stroke from distal embolization of plaque) and stenting. Placement of an umbrella device to retrieve atheromatous debris may be useful.

2. The ischemic time for angioplasty and stenting is shorter than for CEA.

B. Risk factors for carotid occlusive disease (atherosclerosis) include advanced age, hypertension, and tobacco use (elevated serum lipids and a history of diabetes mellitus are less powerful indicators). Patients with left main coronary artery disease and other peripheral vascular disease are more likely to have carotid disease.

1. Embolism or hypoperfusion is presumed to result in development of neurologic symptoms (transient

TABLE 32-9

PHARMACOLOGIC PROPHYLAXIS AGAINST ACUTE VASCULAR EVENTS IN PATIENTS UNDERGOING VASCULAR SURGERY

Intervention	Regimen and comments	Recommendation
Perioperative beta-blockade	Preoperative oral beta-1 selective beta-blocker (bisoprolol, metoprolol, atenolol) initiated at least 30 days before surgery and intravenous therapy during intraoperative and postoperative period (metoprolol, atenolol, esmolol) Titrate heart rate to ≤65 beats/min	Class I
Alpha-2 blockers	Pretreatment with oral clonidine 300 μg at least 90 min before surgery and therapy continued for 72 hr (oral or transdermal 0.2 mg/day) Intravenous clonidine 300 μg/day can also be administered for 72 hr	Class IIa
Statin therapy	Typical dose of atorvastatin is 20 mg/day initiated at least 45 days prior to surgery. Continued use after surgery for at least 2 weeks. Statin use is also associated with improved graft patency, limb salvage, and decreased amputation rate in patients undergoing infrainguinal bypass	Class I

ACE inhibitors	Potential benefits include decreased stroke rate, limitation of ventricular remodeling that follows acute myocardial infarction, and decreased long-term mortality following infrainguinal bypass surgery	Class IIb
Calcium channel blockers	Reduced perioperative adverse cardiac events including supraventricular tachycardia in patients undergoing noncardiac vascular surgery	Class IIb
Nitroglycerin	Not indicated for myocardial ischemia prophylaxis or initial treatment	Class III
	May be used to treat arterial hypertension or elevated filling pressure	

Class I recommendations—evidence or general agreement that useful or protective.
Class II recommendations—conflicting evidence or a divergence of opinion regarding usefulness.
Class IIa—weight of evidence in favor of usefulness.
Class IIb—usefulness is less well established by evidence or opinion.
Class III—evidence that not useful.

TABLE 32-10

COEXISTING MEDICAL PROBLEMS IN PATIENTS WITH PERIPHERAL VASCULAR DISEASE

Hypertension (treat with oral doses of atenolol or metoprolol if poorly controlled)
Diabetes mellitus (increased incidence of postoperative death when autonomic neuropathy is present; intraoperative euglycemia may be particularly important during thoracic and carotid surgery)
Hypercoagulability
Chronic obstructive pulmonary disease (tobacco abuse)
Renal insufficiency

    ischemic attack resolves in 24 hours, reversible ische-mic neurologic deficit lasts longer than 24 hours, stroke).

2. The presence of a cervical bruit may reflect the need for further testing (duplex scan, magnetic resonance imaging).

3. Most patients presenting for carotid endarterectomy will be taking aspirin and/or clopidogrel (continue throughout the perioperative period).

4. Comparisons of angioplasty plus stenting to traditional CEA suggest superiority for stenting.
   a. These patients will generally receive clopidogrel and aspirin before stenting plus periprocedural heparin to maintain the activated clotting time twice normal.
   b. Bradycardia and hypotension is a risk during balloon inflation and stent deployment (consider prophylactic atropine).

TABLE 32-11

APPROACHES TO OPTIMIZE CEREBRAL PERFUSION DURING VASCULAR REPAIR

Preoperative testing to predict cerebral ischemic potential
Routine shunting
Neurologic monitoring of the awake patient
    EEG, SSEP, auditory evoked potentials
    Transcranial Doppler
    Jugular vein oxygenation
    Stump pressure
    Cerebral oximetry

5. Factors that consistently predict neurologic and cardiac morbidity and mortality after carotid endarterectomy include age >75 years, history of angina, preexisting neurologic symptoms, and diastolic blood pressure >110 mm Hg.

C. **Preoperative Evaluation and Preparation**
1. Coronary artery disease is common in patients presenting for carotid endarterectomy.
2. CEA is acceptable in the presence of stable coronary artery disease.

D. **Monitoring and Preserving Neurologic Integrity**
1. The two main goals of intraoperative management are to protect the brain and to protect the heart.
2. Blood pressure is maintained in a high-normal range assuming that blood vessels in ischemic or hypoperfused areas of brain have lost normal autoregulation (disadvantage is increased oxygen demands to the heart).
   a. Judicious use of phenylephrine to increase blood pressure only in specific instances of electroencephalographically detected reversible cerebral ischemia seems to be without detriment to the heart. Indiscriminate use of phenylephrine to increase blood pressure during deep general anesthesia with a volatile anesthetic increases the incidence of intraoperative segmental wall motion abnormalities.
   b. Embolic events may be as important as hypotension and hypoperfusion as the precipitating or sole cause of stroke after carotid endarterectomy.
3. Maintenance of normocarbia or moderate hypocarbia is recommended (hypercapnia may dilate vessels in normal areas of brain, while vessels in ischemic areas are already maximally dilated resulting in a "steal" phenomenon).
4. Moderate hyperglycemia may worsen ischemic brain injury (cerebral lactic acidosis resulting from the anaerobic glycolysis of increased brain glucose stores).
   a. Administration of dextrose-containing solutions may exacerbate hyperglycemia (similar effect from lactate-containing solutions because lactate is metabolized to glucose).
   b. Normal saline may be a recommended intraoperative fluid.

    c. Isovolemic hemodilution with Dextran or Hetastarch may be beneficial in cases of cerebral ischemia because blood viscosity is decreased and attendant microcirculatory disturbances are thus ameliorated.

5. Isoflurane is viewed as the volatile anesthetic with the most potential protective effect against cerebral ischemia (notion that decreased cerebral metabolism is associated with cerebral protection has been questioned).

6. Barbiturates may offer a degree of brain protection during periods of regional ischemia (maximal 50% decrease in cerebral metabolic oxygen requirements corresponds to a silent electroencephalogram and beyond this point additional doses are not helpful).

    a. In cases of massive global ischemia in which basal cellular metabolism has already deteriorated, even high doses of barbiturates will not improve neurologic outcome.

    b. Some clinicians use thiopental not only for induction of anesthesia but also for continuous intravenous infusion and/or as a 4- to 6-mg/kg iv bolus just before carotid occlusion.

    c. The cardiac depressant effects of barbiturates may require inotropic support.

7. Hypothermia can decrease neuronal activity sufficiently to decrease cellular oxygen requirements below the minimum levels normally required for continued cell viability (allow patients to cool passively in the operating room to about 35°C).

8. Temporary occlusion ("cross-clamping") of the carotid artery acutely disrupts blood flow and in the absence of a surgically placed shunt continued blood supply to the brain will depend entirely on adequate collateral blood flow through the circle of Willis.

    a. Routine use of shunts is not risk free (dislodgment of atheromatous material, air embolism, impaired surgical access).

    b. The use of a shunt is beneficial only if the cause of neurologic dysfunction is inadequate blood flow. Most studies suggest that as many as 65 to 95% of all neurologic deficits during and following carotid endarterectomy are caused by thromboembolic events that may occur when the carotid artery is dissected.

9. Surgeons who use shunts selectively need a monitoring device of cerebral perfusion to help decide when to place the shunt (transcranial Doppler, SSEP, EEG, cerebral oximetry, xenon cerebral blood flow).

10. Because embolism and not hypoperfusion is probably the most common cause of perioperative stroke, the real value of cerebral monitoring may lie in the avoidance of interventions such as the placement of shunts (can cause stroke) and blood pressure augmentation (detrimental effects on the heart).

E. **Anesthetic and Monitoring Choices for Elective Surgery** (Table 32-12)

1. The decision to select general or regional anesthesia is based on the experience and expertise of the anesthesiologist and preference of the surgeon (most studies show no difference between techniques for neurologic or cardiac complications or hospital stay).

   a. Possible advantages cited for regional anesthetic techniques include ease of cerebral monitoring, greater stability of blood pressure (absence of negative inotropic effects of volatile anesthetics), and avoidance of tracheal intubation.

TABLE 32-12

ANESTHETIC AND MONITORING CHOICES FOR PATIENTS UNDERGOING ELECTIVE CAROTID ENDARTERECTOMY

Intra-arterial catheter (before surgery compare blood pressure in each arm)

Electrocardiogram (leads II and V5 for ST segment changes)

Transesophageal echocardiography (selectively in patients at high risk for intraoperative myocardial ischemia)

Preoperatively establish range of patient's blood pressure and heart rate

Continue chronic medications to day of surgery

Avoid intraoperative fluid overload (may contribute to postoperative hypertension)

Restrict use of opioids (sedation may confound results of early neurologic assessment)

Avoid use of continuous infusions of phenylephrine (rely on patient's endogenous pressure sustaining responses)

Ask surgeon to infiltrate carotid bifurcation with 1% lidocaine

Confirm neurologic integrity before leave the operating room

     b. Possible disadvantages cited for regional anesthetic techniques include need for patient cooperation, difficult airway management should seizures or loss of consciousness occur, and absence of potential pharmacologic brain protection.

  2. Heparin is typically given in a dose of 50 to 100 units/kg prior to cross-clamping.

  3. Time is of the essence to help prevent neurologic deficits (shunt placement and removal requires 1 to 4 minutes and total occlusion time rarely exceeds 40 minutes).

  4. Carotid angioplasty and stenting includes heparinization and may include sedation.

  5. Decreases in blood pressure may occur with reperfusion following open CEA and stenting because of alterations in baroreceptor function.

F. Postoperative Management (Table 32-13)

  1. Severe hypertension (systolic blood pressure >200 mm Hg) seems to occur more often in patients with poorly controlled preoperative hypertension.

     a. Hypertension may precipitate acute myocardial ischemia (incidence is increased in first few hours after surgery) and congestive heart failure and may lead to cerebral edema and/or hemorrhage (postoperative hypertension is associated with an increased incidence of neurologic deficits).

     b. Causes of postoperative hypertension (rule out pain, arterial hypoxemia, hypercarbia, bladder

---

TABLE 32-13

POSTOPERATIVE COMPLICATIONS FOLLOWING CAROTID ENDARTERECTOMY

New neurologic dysfunction (ability to move extremities excludes possibility of acute thrombosis of the endarterectomy site)

Hemodynamic instability (hypertension more common than hypotension)

Hyperperfusion syndrome (manifests several days postoperatively as ipsilateral headache that may progress to seizures; transcranial Doppler may predict susceptible patients; steroids may be used in treatment)

Respiratory insufficiency (recurrent laryngeal nerve palsy, carotid body denervation)

Wound hematomas (airway compression)

distention) are unclear but may include denervation of the carotid sinus and overzealous administration of intravenous fluids.

    c. Hypertension usually peaks 2 to 3 hours after surgery but in some individuals may persist for 24 hours.

    d. Treatment of hypertension is with titration of short-acting drugs (nitroglycerin, labetalol, esmolol, tracheal lidocaine spray).

2. Hypotension and bradycardia after carotid endarterectomy are less frequent than hypertension (surgical removal of the atheroma again exposes the carotid sinus baroreceptors to higher levels of transmural pressure leading to brain stem–mediated vagal responses).

    a. Chemical denervation of the carotid sinus with local anesthetic by the surgeon results in fewer hypotensive patients but increases the incidence of postoperative hypertension.

    b. The baroreceptors seem to adjust over time and the hypotensive phase resolves in 12 to 24 hours.

    c. Treatment may not be necessary in the absence of myocardial ischemia or changes in neurologic status. Nevertheless, blood pressure is often restored to a low-normal range with intravenous infusion of fluids or administration of drugs (ephedrine, phenylephrine, dopamine).

G. **Management of Emergent Carotid Surgery**

1. The patient who awakens with a major new neurologic deficit or who develops a suspected stroke in the immediate postoperative period represents a surgical emergency (prompt removal of a carotid thrombosis can produce significant neurologic improvement).

2. Neck exploration for a wound hematoma following carotid endarterectomy may be associated with airway obstruction (acceptable to drain wound externally before induction of anesthesia).

IV. AORTIC RECONSTRUCTION

A. **Aneurysmal Disease.** Aneurysms pose a threat to life because of their unpredictable tendency to rupture or embolize (aggressive surgical management is warranted even in the absence of symptoms).

1. Epidemiology and Pathophysiology of Abdominal Aortic Aneurysm
    a. Risk factors for atherosclerosis are associated with an increased risk for abdominal aortic aneurysm.
    b. The risk of rupture of the abdominal aortic aneurysm is directly related to the luminal diameter of the aortic aneurysm (risk increases when aneurysm is >4.5 to 5 cm and surgical treatment is generally recommended).
B. Pathophysiology of Aortic Occlusion and Reperfusion. Prolonged cross-clamp time associated with treatment of supraceliac aortic occlusion is associated with visceral (kidneys, liver, gastrointestinal tract) and spinal cord ischemia.
    1. Cardiovascular Changes (Table 32-14)
    2. Renal Hemodynamics and Renal Protection
        a. The level of aortic clamping is the most important factor as it impacts renal blood flow.
        b. Hydration is the most important factor for maintaining renal blood flow during and after clamp release.

TABLE 32-14

HEMODYNAMIC CHANGES DURING AORTIC CROSS-CLAMPING AND UNCLAMPING

Unclamping

Increased mean arterial pressure and systemic vascular resistance (reflects increased afterload, activation of renin, and release of catecholamines and prostaglandins)

Decreased cardiac output in presence of increased systemic vascular resistance (may be accompanied by increased cardiac filling pressures if underlying coronary artery disease)

Administration of a vasodilator (nitroprusside) concomitant or immediately before placement of cross-clamp allows body to adapt

Level of clamping affects hemodynamic response (infrarenal better tolerated than suprarenal)

Hypotension may accompany unclamping (pretreat with fluid loading with or without vasoconstrictors [phenylephrine] or calcium [high potassium and acid load])

Gradual unclamping is preferable

    c. Dopamine and diuretics have not been shown to improve outcome.

    d. Intraoperative urinary output is not predictive of postoperative renal function.

3. **Humoral and Coagulation Profiles**

    a. In addition to volume redistribution following removal of the clamp, humoral mediators from underperfused areas also contribute to hemodynamic changes.

    b. Administration of bicarbonate does not prevent immediate postunclamping hypotension.

    c. Mannitol administration before and after unclamping may be beneficial because of its hydroxyl free radical scavenger properties.

    d. Sequestration of microaggregates and neutrophils contribute to postoperative pulmonary dysfunction.

4. **Visceral and Mesenteric Ischemia.** Bowel ischemia during cross-clamping is associated with increased mortality and leads to gut permeability and bacterial translocation.

5. **CNS and Spinal Cord Ischemia and Protection**

    a. The definitive preventive measures to spinal cord ischemia are short cross-clamping time, fast surgery, maintenance of normal cardiac function, and higher perfusion pressures.

    b. Cerebrospinal fluid (CSF) drainage, distal perfusion, and hypothermia may be beneficial in high aortic clamping.

C. **Surgical Procedures for Aortic Reconstruction**

1. **Approach.** Abdominal aortic reconstruction can be performed through a transperitoneal or retroperitoneal exposure.

2. **Clamp Level.** Infrarenal aortic clamping carries the lowest risk while supraceliac clamping carries the highest risk.

3. **Thoracic Aneurysm Repair**

    a. Lung separation is required to facilitate surgical access and to avoid intraogenic pulmonary contusion in the left lung.

    b. Edema of the head and neck after high cross-clamping may be present at the conclusion of the procedure.

4. **Aortic-Mesenteric Revascularization.** Partial cross-clamping of the aorta is preferred if possible and may mitigate hemodynamic changes.

5. **Aortorenal revascularization** can be performed by several surgical techniques (endarterectomy, reimplantation, bypass, ex-vivo renal artery reconstruction).
6. **Infrarenal Operations**
   a. Distal ischemic complications are likely a result of dislodgment of atheromatous material off the diseased aorta.
   b. Systemic use of heparin in the absence of distal occlusive disease is unnecessary.
7. **Thoracic Aortic Surgery**
   a. Endovascular thoracoabdominal aortic aneurysm repair is an alternative to open surgery (frequent complications).
   b. Paraplegia may occur with both approaches but seems to be less with the endovascular technique (consider SSEP monitoring whereas motor evoked potentials are more appropriate for monitoring anterior spinal column).
D. **Endovascular surgery for aortic aneurysms** generally requires bilateral common femoral artery or iliac artery access, and arterial sheaths are then advanced into the abdominal aortic aneurysm sac.
   1. Preimplantation calibrated angiography is required to identify the renal vessels (dye loads considerable and risk of renal insufficiency especially in diabetics).
   2. Endoleak is persistent perfusion of the aneurysm sac through attachment site leakage points.
   3. **Goals of Anesthesia for Endovascular Aneurysm Repair** (Table 32-15)
   4. **Managing Intraoperative Complications During Endovascular Aneurysm Repair.** Visceral ischemia may accompany misdeployment.

TABLE 32-15

GOALS OF ANESTHESIA FOR ENDOVASCULAR ANEURYSM REPAIR

Preserve organ function (as with open repair)
Anticipate significant blood loss and fluid requirements (invasive monitors)
Provide mild hypotension (nitroglycerin) and motionless patient at time of deployment

5. **Complications of Anesthesia**
   a. Endovascular aneurysm repair is often advocated for patients with chronic obstructive pulmonary disease (COPD) but the value of regional anesthesia, in contrast to open repair, is probably less.
   b. Anticoagulation can complicate management of regional anesthesia.
E. **Protecting the Spinal Cord and Visceral Organs** (Table 32-16)
F. **Monitoring and Anesthetic Choices for Aortic Reconstruction**
   1. Placement of arterial catheters above and below the level of the aortic cross-clamp is a consideration in patients undergoing aortic reconstruction.
   2. Placement of a pulmonary artery catheter is a consideration when a suprarenal aortic cross-clamp (rarely if infrarenal) will be needed or in patients with a history of congestive heart failure, poor left ventricular function by echocardiography (ejection fraction <0.35), diabetes with end-organ damage, cor pulmonale, or renal insufficiency.

TABLE 32-16
STRATEGIES TO PROTECT SPINAL CORD DURING DESCENDING THORACIC AORTIC SURGERY

Limitation of cross-clamp duration
Distal circulatory support (Gott shunt)
Reattachment of critical intercostal arteries
Cerebrospinal fluid drainage
Hypothermia
Maintenance of proximal blood pressure
  Pharmacotherapy
    Systemic (corticosteroids, barbiturates, calcium channel antagonists, oxygen free radical scavengers, NMDA antagonists, mannitol, magnesium, vasodilators)
    Intrathecal (papaverine, magnesium, tetracaine)
Avoidance of postoperative hypotension
Sequential aortic clamping
Enhanced monitoring for spinal cord ischemia
  Somatosensory evoked potentials
  Motor evoked potentials

3. Cerebrospinal fluid drainage is a consideration for patients undergoing thoracic aneurysm resection.

4. Ability to maintain hemodynamic equilibrium is more important than the anesthetic drug or technique that is selected.

   a. Volatile anesthetics (typically isoflurane) permit titration and manipulation of hemodynamic variables including treatment of stress-induced increases in left-ventricular filling pressures.

   b. An important reason to include volatile anesthetics is their ability to improve preconditioning mechanisms and reduce the size of myocardial infarction should it occur.

   c. If opioids are selected, it may be necessary to add other drugs (volatile anesthetics, nitroglycerin, nitroprusside) during cross-clamping of the aorta. Postoperative analgesia is an advantage of opioids, whereas lingering effects may jeopardize maintenance of adequate spontaneous ventilation.

   d. Combined general-epidural or spinal anesthesia has been advocated for aortic reconstruction (postoperative pain management and early assessment of neurologic function are considered important features of this approach).

G. **Management of Elective Aortic Surgery**

1. Prehydration is recommended to reduce variations in blood pressure that may accompany the induction of anesthesia (goal is to keep hemodynamic variables within 20% of each patient's preoperative "normal" values as long as pulmonary capillary wedge pressure does not exceed 15 mm Hg, heart rate does not exceed 80 to 90 beats/min, and signs of organ ischemia are absent).

2. Antihypertensive medications including diuretics are administered before arriving in the operating room. It is common to provide a continuous infusion of insulin throughout the operative period insulin-dependent diabetics.

3. For the half hour preceding placement of the aortic cross-clamp the patient is maintained slightly hypovolemic (examine ventricular volume by echocardiography or maintain pulmonary capillary wedge pressure 5 to 15 mm Hg).

      a. Alternatively, the concentration of volatile anesthetic or injection of local anesthetic into the epidural catheter may be utilized to facilitate volume loading so as to reduce hypotension after unclamping.

      b. Acceptance of proximal hypertension when the aorta is occluded may be a consideration in hopes of obtaining higher distal perfusion pressures and preventing distal ischemia.

   4. At the time of placement of the aortic cross-clamp a vasodilating drug (nitroprusside, nitroglycerin) is available for rapid iv administration through a central venous catheter should hypertension occur.

   5. Administration of exogenous vasopressors is avoided if possible (phyenylephrine increases the incidence of wall motion abnormalities observed by echocardiography). Rather than relying on vasopressors, adequate volume at the time of cross-clamp removal is obtained by replacing blood loss (including autotransfusion devices) during occlusion to keep the hematocrit slightly above 30%.

   6. Evisceration of bowel that is often necessary for optimal surgical exposure of the thoracoabdominal aorta further depletes intravascular fluid volume.

   7. Pathophysiologic events that accompany removal of the aortic cross-clamp are associated with inadequate preload (infuse fluids or blood at moment of removal of the cross-clamp and open the aorta gradually).

   8. During emergence from anesthesia, it may be necessary to treat hemodynamic variations (esmolol nitroglycerin). If a predominantly inhalational anesthetic technique has been used, it is common to place an epidural catheter and to administer epidural opioids and local anesthetics for postoperative analgesia.

   9. Prophylactic beta-blockade is provided in the postoperative period (metoprolol 5 to 10 mg iv every 6 hours as long as heart rate is >55 beats/min and systolic blood pressure >110 mm Hg).

H. Anesthesia for Emergency Aortic Surgery

   1. The most common cause of emergency aortic reconstruction is a leaking or ruptured aortic aneurysm (symptoms include back pain, syncope, vomiting). Rupture occurs most often into the retroperitoneum, resulting in a life-saving tamponade effect.

2. Patients with dissection may have severe hypertension, which must be controlled immediately if rupture is to be prevented.

   a. When rupture is suspected, rapid control of the proximal portion of the aorta (consider passage of a balloon from the femoral artery to occlude the aorta above the rupture) is more important than volume replacement.

   b. Vasopressin may be effective in restoring blood pressure with hemorrhagic shock resistant to catecholamines.

3. Because of hypothermia from massive fluid resuscitation and placement of the aortic cross-clamp above the hepatic artery, replacement blood may not pass through the liver in amounts adequate to allow for metabolism of citrate.

4. As opposed to elective aortic reconstruction, during which preserving myocardial function is the primary goal, in emergency resection the crucial factor for patient survival is (1) rapid control of blood loss and reversal of hypotension and then (2) preservation of myocardial function.

V. LOWER EXTREMITY REVASCULARIZATION

A. These patients are often elderly with complex medical histories and diseases of multiple organ systems.

   1. Endovascular repair may involve angioplasty and/or stenting of smaller vessels, including femoral arteries (restenosis may require repeated percutaneous or surgical revascularization procedures).

   2. In addition to maintaining adequate cardiac function (high risk for myocardial ischemia and infarction, low cardiac output syndrome, pulmonary edema), another goal of anesthetic management is to ensure adequate perfusion and prevent hypercoagulable responses to surgery so as to maintain graft patency.

B. The most common inflow peripheral vascular procedure is aortofemoral bypass, whereas the most common outflow procedure below the inguinal ligament is placement of a bypass graft (saphenous vein associated with highest patency rates) from the femoral artery to the popliteal or tibial artery.

1. The quality of the repair is determined from the pulse quality, Doppler ultrasound studies, or completion angiography.
2. Heparin is not likely to be reversed at the end of the operation as bleeding is not a problem and graft patency may be improved by anticoagulation.
3. If graft thrombosis develops early in the postoperative period, the patient is promptly returned to the operating room for graft thrombectomy (significant blood loss can be anticipated during flushing of the graft).

C. **Anesthetic Management of Elective Lower Extremity Revascularization**
1. Most cardiac problems occur in the postoperative period and it is during this time that analgesia and correction of hemodynamic and fluid imbalances are likely to be needed.
2. Care must be taken not to allow overhydration to occur intraoperatively in support of blood pressure only to result in congestive heart failure when epidural sympathectomy wanes.
3. Continuous monitoring of blood pressure with an arterial catheter is often recommended as is placement of a central venous pressure catheter (most helpful in recognizing and treating postoperative hypovolemia).
4. The choice of anesthetic for lower extremity revascularization is individualized for each patient (Table 32-17).
   a. Formation of an epidural hematoma (severe back pain or pressure earliest symptom) can be diagnosed with computed tomography or magnetic resonance imaging. Time is of the essence for if the spinal cord compression persists longer than 6 to 12 hours catastrophic paralysis may result.
   b. Anticoagulation represents a relative contraindication to regional anesthesia (use of nonsteroidal anti-inflammatory drugs, aspirin, or subcutaneous heparin does not seem to be problematic).
   c. Placement of an epidural catheter with subsequent heparinization appears to be safe.

TABLE 32-17

CHOICE OF ANESTHESIA FOR LOWER EXTREMITY
REVASCULARIZATION

Anesthetic technique	Advantages	Disadvantages
Regional	Effective blockade of stress response	Time consuming, especially for postoperative management
	Postoperative analgesia	Sympathectomy requires volume loading
	Patient serves as monitor for myocardial ischemia (angina, dyspnea)	Respiratory depression if level of blockade becomes high or patient becomes overly sedated
	Possible prevention of postoperative hypercoagulability	Patient discomfort lying during long procedure
	Improved graft blood flow	Rare neurologic sequelae
		Precludes thrombolytic therapy
		Technically difficult in patients with obesity, kyphoscoliosis, previous laminectomy
General	Hemodynamics easily controlled during surgery	Hyperdynamic state after surgery must usually be treated
	No patient discomfort during long procedures	Postoperative hypercoagulability not inhibited
	Reliable	

    d. Despite the absence of supporting data, it may be
recommended to wait until cessation of
heparinization to remove an epidural
catheter.

  **D. Anesthesia for Emergency Surgery for Peripheral
Vascular Insufficiency**

    1. Emergency surgery for peripheral vascular
insufficiency is required when acute arterial occlusion
results in severe ischemia and threatens viability of a
limb (occluding material may originate from heart or
other major arteries).

2. The anesthesiologists must be prepared for either a simple procedure (Fogarty embolectomy) or complex and prolonged procedure (bypass reconstruction).
3. Free radical scavengers such as mannitol and N-acetyl cysteine may be administered to mitigate reperfusion responses.

CHAPTER 33 ■ ANESTHESIA AND THE EYE

Anesthesia for ophthalmic surgery presents unique anesthetic challenges and requirements (Table 33-1) (McGoldrick KE, Gayer SI: Anesthesia and the eye. In Barash PG, Cullen BF, Stoelting RK [eds]: *Clinical Anesthesia*, pp 974–996. Philadelphia, Lippincott Williams & Wilkins, 2006). Patients undergoing ophthalmic surgery may represent extremes of age (macular degeneration is the leading cause of blindness in individuals >65 years of age) and coexisting medical diseases.

I. OCULAR ANATOMY

A. The supraorbital notch, infraorbital foramen, and lacrimal fossa are clinically palpable and function as important landmarks for performance of regional anesthesia (Fig. 33-1).

B. The coat of the eye is composed of three layers: sclera, uveal tract, and retina.
  1. The fibrous outer layer of the sclera is protective, providing sufficient rigidity to maintain the shape of the eye, whereas the anterior portion of the sclera, the **cornea**, is transparent, permitting light to enter the internal ocular structures.
  2. The uveal tract consists of the iris, ciliary body, and choroid.
    a. The pupil is part of the iris that controls the amount of light that enters by dilation (sympathetic innervation) or constriction (parasympathetic innervation).
    b. The ciliary body produces aqueous humor.
  3. The retina is a neurosensory membrane that converts light impulses to neural impulses that travel via the optic nerve to the brain.

C. Six intraocular muscles move the eye within the orbit.

D. The **conjunctiva** is a mucous membrane (topical administration of ophthalmic drugs) that

TABLE 33-1

REQUIREMENTS FOR OPHTHALMIC SURGERY

Akinesia
Profound analgesia
Minimal bleeding
Avoidance of the oculocardiac reflex
Control of IOP
Awareness of possible drug interactions
Awakening without coughing, straining, or vomiting

covers the globe and serves as a lining of the eyelids.

E. Blood supply to the eye is from branches of the internal and external carotid arteries.

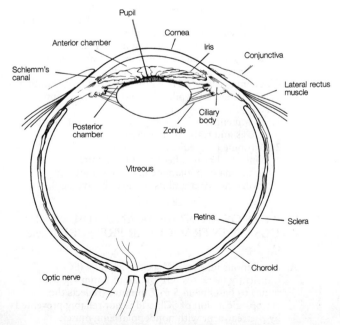

FIGURE 33-1. Diagram of ocular anatomy.

II. OCULAR PHYSIOLOGY

A. **Formation and Drainage of Aqueous Humor**
  1. Aqueous humor is formed in the posterior chamber by the ciliary body in an active secretory process involving carbonic anhydrase as well as by passive filtration from the vessels on the anterior surface of the iris.
  2. Drainage of aqueous humor is via a network of connecting venous channels (includes Schlemm's canal) that empty into the superior vena cava (any obstruction between the eye and right atrium impedes aqueous drainage and increases intraocular pressure [IOP]).

B. **Maintenance of Intraocular Pressure**
  1. IOP normally varies between 10 and 21.7 mm Hg but becomes atmospheric when the globe is opened. The major determinant of IOP is the volume of aqueous humor.
  2. Any sudden increase in IOP when the globe is open may lead to prolapse of the iris and lens, extrusion of the vitreous, and blindness.
  3. Straining, vomiting, or coughing (as during laryngoscopy and tracheal intubation) greatly increases venous pressure and IOP.

C. **Glaucoma** is characterized by increased IOP, resulting in impairment of capillary blood flow to the optic nerve.
  1. Treatment consists of topical medication to produce miosis and trabecular stretching.
  2. Atropine premedication in the dose range used clinically has no effect on IOP in patients with glaucoma (scopolamine may have a greater mydriatic effect and its use may be avoided).

III. EFFECTS OF ANESTHESIA AND ADJUVANT DRUGS ON INTRAOCULAR PRESSURE (Table 33-2)

A. Intravenous injection of succinylcholine (SCh) transiently increases IOP by about 8 mm Hg with return to baseline in 5 to 7 minutes (reflects the cycloplegic action of SCh and is not reliably prevented by pretreatment with nondepolarizing muscle relaxants or intravenous administration of lidocaine).

TABLE 33-2
EVENTS THAT ALTER INTRAOCULAR PRESSURE

Decreased	Increased
Volatile anesthetics	Increased venous pressure owing to coughing or vomiting
Injected anesthetics (?ketamine)	Direct laryngoscopy
Hyperventilation	Hypoventilation
Hypothermia	Arterial hypoxemia
Mannitol	Succinylcholine
Glycerin	
Nondepolarizing muscle relaxants	
Timolol	
Bextaxolol	

    B. Etomidate-induced myoclonus may be hazardous in the setting of an open globe.

IV. OCULOCARDIAC REFLEX

    A. This reflex manifests as bradycardia (and occasionally cardiac dysrhythmias) that is elicited by pressure on the globe and by traction on the extraocular muscles (strabismus surgery), especially the medial rectus.

    B. Monitoring of the electrocardiogram is useful for early recognition of this reflex.

    C. Atropine given iv within 30 minutes of surgery is thought to effect a reduced incidence of the reflex (controversial). Atropine as administered intramuscularly for preoperative medication is not effective for preventing this reflex.

V. ANESTHETIC RAMIFICATIONS OF OPHTHALMIC DRUGS

    A. **Echothiophate** is a long-acting anticholinesterase miotic that decreases IOP and prolongs the duration of action of SCh.

    B. **Cyclopentolate** is a mydriatic and may produce central nervous system toxicity.

    C. **Phenylephrine** is a mydriatic that may produce cardiovascular effects.

D. **Acetazolamide** when administered chronically to lower IOP may be associated with renal loss of bicarbonate and potassium ions.

E. **Timolol** lowers IOP, but systemic absorption may result in cardiac depression and increased airway resistance.

F. **Sulfur hexafluoride (SF6)** is injected into the vitreous to mechanically facilitate retinal reattachment. Nitrous oxide (N_2O) (blood/gas solubility 0.47) should be avoided for 10 days following intravitreous injection of SF6 (blood/gas solubility 0.004). A Medic-Alert bracelet might be helpful to identify patients at risk.

VI. PREOPERATIVE EVALUATION

A. **Establishing Rapport and Assessing Medical Conditions.** Preoperative testing should be based on the history and physical examination.

B. Many elderly adult candidates for ophthalmic surgery are on antiplatelet or anticoagulant therapy owing to a history of coronary or vascular pathology.

VII. ANESTHESIA TECHNIQUES

A. Most ophthalmic procedures in adults can be performed with either local or general anesthesia. Data have failed to demonstrate a difference in complications between local and general anesthesia for cataract surgery (Table 33-3).

B. **Retrobulbar and Peribulbar Blocks.** Retrobulbar block may be associated with significant complications, emphasizing that local anesthesia does not necessarily involve less physiologic trespass than general

---

TABLE 33-3
FACTORS THAT INFLUENCE CHOICE OF ANESTHESIA

Nature and duration of procedure
Coagulation status
Patient's ability to communicate and cooperate
Personal preference of the anesthesiologist

TABLE 33-4

COMPLICATIONS OF NEEDLE-BASED OPHTHALMIC ANESTHESIA

Stimulation of the oculocardiac reflex arc
Superficial hemorrhage–circumorbital hematoma
Retrobulbar hemorrhage
Retinal perfusion compromise (loss of vision)
Globe penetration and intraocular injection (retinal detachment, loss of vision)
Trauma to optic nerve or orbital cranial nerves (loss of vision)
Optic nerve sheath injection (orbital epidural anesthesia)
Extraocular muscle injury (postoperative strabismus, diplopia)
Intra-arterial injection (immediate convulsions)
Central retinal artery occlusion
Accidental brainstem anesthesia (apnea, hypotension, coma)

anesthesia (Table 33-4). Akinesia of the eyelids is obtained by blocking the branches of the facial nerve supplying the orbicularis muscle.

C. **Topical analgesia** can be achieved with local anesthetic drops or gels.

1. **Choice of Local Anesthetics, Block Adjuvants, and Adjuncts.** Anesthetics for ocular surgery are selected based upon onset and duration needed (mix local anesthetics to obtain desired onset and duration). Osmotic agents (mannitol, glycerin, carbonic anhydrase) may be administered iv to reduce vitreous volume and IOP.

D. **General Principles of Monitored Anesthesia Care (MAC)** (Table 33-5). Cataract surgery (number one Medicare expenditure) is most commonly performed with the patient under some form of regional anesthesia (retrobulbar block, topical anesthesia) plus monitoring equipment and often the presence of an anesthesiologist (MAC).

VIII. ANESTHETIC MANAGEMENT OF SPECIFIC SITUATIONS

A. **Open Eye–Full Stomach.** Anesthesiologists must balance the risk of aspiration against the risk of blindness in an injured eye that could result from an acute increase in IOP and extrusion of ocular contents.

TABLE 33-5

GENERAL PRINCIPLES OF MONITORED ANESTHESIA CARE (MAC)

Avoid combinations of local anesthetics with heavy sedation (opioids, benzodiazepines, hypnotics)

After placement of block patient should be relaxed but awake to avoid head movement

Able to maintain airway patency

Avoid undersedation and associated hypertension and tachycardia (especially in patients with coronary artery disease)

Provide adequate ventilation about the face to avoid carbon dioxide accumulation

Continuous monitoring of the electrocardiogram (oculocardiac reflex) and oxygen saturation

1. Consider preoperative administration of H2 antagonists and/or metoclopramide.
2. **Induction of anesthesia** is often with propofol or thiopental plus a high dose ($3 \times ED95$) of an intermediate- or short-acting nondepolarizing muscle relaxant (avoids any drug-induced increase in IOP as occurs with SCh).
   a. The advantage of a nondepolarizing muscle relaxant may be offset by a delayed onset and prolonged duration of action for what otherwise may be a short operation.
   b. Although controversial, there is no published report of loss of intraocular contents when using a nondepolarizing muscle relaxant for pretreatment followed by a barbiturate-SCh induction sequence when used in this setting.
3. Regardless of the muscle relaxant selected, any premature attempt at tracheal intubation may produce coughing, straining, and an abrupt increase in IOP, emphasizing the potential value of confirming the onset of drug effect with a peripheral nerve stimulator.
4. Awake intubation of the trachea is not a likely approach because any reaction by the patient could adversely increase IOP.

B. **Strabismus surgery** is the most common pediatric ocular operation and may introduce unique concerns (Table 33-6).

TABLE 33-6
CONSIDERATIONS FOR STRABISMUS SURGERY

Oculocardiac reflex
Increased incidence of malignant hyperthermia
Interference by succinylcholine in interpretation of forced duction test
Increased incidence of postoperative nausea and vomiting

1. The laryngeal mask airway has the potential advantage of not requiring the use of muscle relaxants and being associated with less straining or coughing with its removal.
2. The incidence of postoperative nausea and vomiting may be decreased by use of an intravenous anesthetic technique with propofol, avoidance of opioids (ketorolac 750 μg/kg iv as an alternative), and prophylactic administration of an antiemetic (droperidol 20 μg/kg iv, metoclopramide 250 μg/kg iv, or ondansetron 150 μg/kg iv) immediately after induction of anesthesia.
C. **Intraocular surgery** (glaucoma drainage surgery, open eye vitrectomy, corneal transplants, cataract extraction) introduces unique concerns and requirements (Table 33-7).
   1. Epinephrine 1:200,000 may be infused into the anterior chamber of the eye to produce mydriasis. Systemic absorption and resulting cardiac dysrhythmias in the presence of volatile anesthetics have not been recognized as a problem.
   2. Nondepolarizing muscle relaxants administered to provide akinesia and to facilitate performance and interpretation of the forced duction test (differentiate between a paretic muscle and a

TABLE 33-7
CONSIDERATIONS FOR INTRAOCULAR SURGERY

Control of IOP
Continue miotics in glaucoma patients
Need for complete akinesia
Provide an antiemetic effect

restrictive force preventing ocular motion) can be safely antagonized even in patients with glaucoma because the combination of anticholinesterase and anticholinergic drugs, in conventional doses, has minimal effects on pupil size and IOP.

D. Retinal Detachment Surgery

1. Internal tamponade of the retinal break may be accomplished by injecting the expandable gas SF6 into the vitreous. Owing to the blood/gas partition coefficient differences, the concomitant administration of N_2O may enhance the internal tamponade effect of SF6 intraoperatively, resulting in increases in IOP and interference with retinal circulation. For this reason, N_2O probably should be discontinued for at least 15 minutes before injection of SF6, and likewise N_2O probably should not be administered for 10 days after the injection.

2. Decrease in IOP is often provided by intravenous administration of acetazolamide or mannitol.

3. Akinesia is not critical, and inhalation anesthetics need not be accompanied intraoperatively by nondepolarizing muscle relaxants.

IX. POSTOPERATIVE OCULAR COMPLICATIONS
(Table 33-8)

A. The incidence of eye injuries associated with nonocular surgery is very low (0.056%). Certain types of surgery, including complex spinal surgery in the prone position, operations involving extracorporeal circulation, and nasal or sinus surgery, may increase the risk of serious postoperative visual complications. Injuries associated with regional anesthesia for ophthalmic surgery are typically permanent and related to the block technique.

B. Corneal abrasion is the most common ocular complication after general anesthesia. Patients complain of pain and a foreign body sensation that is exacerbated by blinking.

1. An ophthalmology consultation is appropriate and treatment is prophylactic topical application of antibiotic ointment and patching of the injured eye.

2. Healing usually occurs within 24 to 48 hours.

C. Ischemia optic neuropathy is the most common cause of visual loss in patients older than 50 years of age. The incidence of postoperative vision loss after spine

TABLE 33-8

POSTOPERATIVE OCULAR COMPLICATIONS

Corneal abrasion
Chemical injury (Hibiclens)
Photic injury (laser beams, protect eyes with moist gauze pads and
  metal shields)
Mild visual symptoms
  Photophobia
  Diplopia
  Blurred vision (residual effects of petroleum-based ophthalmic
    ointment, or ocular effects of anticholinergic drugs)
Hemorrhagic retinopathy
Retinal ischemia (external pressure on globe, increased ocular
  venous pressure associated with a steep head-down position
  combined with the prone position, deliberate hypotension and
  infusion of large amounts of crystalloid solution)
Central retinal arterial occlusion
Branch retinal arterial occlusion
Ischemic optic neuropathy (anterior ischemic optic neuropathy or
  posterior ischemic optic neuropathy)
Cortical blindness (reflects brain injury rostral to the optic nerve,
  emboli or profound hypotension are common causes,
  differential diagnosis includes normal optic disc on fundoscopy
  and normal pupillary responses)
Visual symptoms after transurethral resection of the prostate
  (glycine toxicity)
Acute glaucoma
Postcataract ptosis

surgery performed in the prone position may be as
high as 1%.

1. **Anterior ischemic optic neuropathy** is thought to
   reflect temporary hypoperfusion or nonperfusion of
   the vessels supplying the anterior portion of the
   optic nerve.
   a. Male patients undergoing prolonged spine
      surgery in the prone position and operations
      requiring cardiopulmonary bypass may be at
      increased risk for development of anterior
      ischemic optic neuropathy.
   b. The etiology is very likely multifactorial
      although intraoperative anemia, controlled
      hypotension, and increased IOP or orbital
      venous pressure (prone and head down) may
      contribute to the ischemia of the optic nerve.

    c. Patients typically experience painless visual loss in the early postoperative period that is associated with an afferent pupillary defect and optic disc edema or pallor. Magnetic resonance imaging initially shows enlargement of the optic nerve followed by optic atrophy. Visual loss is usually permanent.

2. **Posterior ischemic optic neuropathy** is produced by decreased oxygen delivery to the retrolaminar part of the optic nerve.

    a. Male patients undergoing surgery involving the neck, nose, or spine may be at increased risk for development of posterior ischemic optic neuropathy.

    b. The etiology is unclear but systemic hypotension, anemia, and venous stasis are often associated. Facial edema may be present.

    c. Patients typically experience a symptom-free period that often precedes the loss of vision associated with a nonreactive pupil. Bilateral blindness is more common than following anterior ischemic optic neuropathy. Disc edema is not a feature of posterior ischemic optic neuropathy owing to its retrobulbar location.

CHAPTER 34 ■ ANESTHESIA FOR OTOLARYNGOLOGIC SURGERY

Anesthetic management of the patient undergoing head and neck surgery often challenges the anesthesiologist to devise an anesthetic plan that includes unique considerations (Table 34-1) (Ferrari LR, Gotta AW, Joseph R: Anesthesia for otolaryngologic surgery. In Barash PG, Cullen BF, Stoelting RK [eds]: *Clinical Anesthesia*, pp 997–1012. Philadelphia, Lippincott Williams & Wilkins, 2006).

I. EVALUATING THE AIRWAY

A. Significant upper airway obstruction because of tumor, infection, or trauma may be present despite the absence of clinical symptoms.

B. In the presence of tumor or infection in the airway, a radiologic evaluation may be useful.

II. ANESTHESIA FOR PEDIATRIC EAR, NOSE, AND THROAT SURGERY

A. **Tonsillectomy and Adenoidectomy**

1. Patients with cardiac valvular disease are at risk for endocarditis from recurrent streptococcal bacteremia secondary to infected tonsils.

2. Tonsillar hyperplasia may lead to chronic airway obstruction, resulting in obstructive sleep apnea syndrome, carbon dioxide retention, and cor pulmonale.

3. **Preoperative evaluation** includes a thorough history (antibiotics, aspirin-containing medications, sleep apnea) and physical examination (wheezing, stridor, mouth breathing, tonsillar size). In those children with a history of cardiac abnormalities, an echocardiogram may be indicated.

4. **Anesthetic Management**

   a. **Premedication** often includes an antisialagogue.

   b. **Induction** of anesthesia is usually with a volatile anesthetic and nitrous oxide (parental presence is a consideration especially with an anxious child)

TABLE 34-1

UNIQUE CONSIDERATIONS IN ANESTHETIC MANAGEMENT
OF PATIENTS UNDERGOING HEAD AND NECK SURGERY

Diagnose alterations in anatomy of upper airway because of
 tumor, infection, trauma, congenital defect
Create a shared operative field
Select anesthetic drugs compatible with the surgical procedure
Define the appropriate time for tracheal extubation

followed by administration of a nondepolarizing
muscle relaxant to facilitate tracheal intubation.

c. A specially designated laryngeal mask airway
(LMA) that easily fits under the mouth gag
permits surgical access while the lower airway is
protected from exposure to blood during the
procedure. Positive pressure ventilation should be
avoided, although gentle assisted ventilation is
both safe and effective if peak inspiratory
pressure is kept below 20 cm H_2O.

d. **Emergence** should be rapid and the child should
be able to clear blood or secretions from the
oropharynx (maintenance of a patent upper
airway and pharyngeal reflexes is important in
the prevention of aspiration, laryngospasm, and
airway obstruction).

e. It is recommended that patients be observed for
early hemorrhage (first 6 hours) and be free from
significant nausea, vomiting, and pain prior to
discharge.

5. **Complications** (Table 34-2)

a. Preoperative preparation of the patient who
requires return to the operating room for surgical
hemostasis includes hydration (check for
orthostatic changes).

b. A rapid sequence induction of anesthesia with a
styletted endotracheal tube is often
recommended.

c. Dependable suction is mandatory because blood
in the pharynx may impair visualization.

d. Acute postoperative pulmonary edema
(negative-pressure pulmonary edema) is an
infrequent but potentially life-threatening
complication encountered when airway

TABLE 34-2

POSTOPERATIVE COMPLICATIONS OF TONSILLECTOMY

Emesis (occurs in 30–65% of patients, mechanism unknown but may include presence of irritant blood in the stomach)

Dehydration

Hemorrhage (75% occurs in first 6 hours after surgery; if requires surgical hemostasis, consider a full stomach and hypovolemia)

Pain (minimal after adrenoidectomy and severe after tonsillectomy)

Postobstructive pulmonary edema (rare but possible if prior acute upper airway obstruction, treatment may include supplemental oxygen and administration of diuretics)

obstruction is suddenly relieved. Treatment is supportive and maintenance of a patent airway, oxygen administration, and diuretic therapy in some cases are required.

e. Examples of patients in whom early discharge is not advised after tonsillectomy include those younger than 3 years of age, those with abnormal coagulation values, those with evidence of obstructive sleep disorder or apnea, presence of a peritonsillar abscess, and those with conditions (distance, weather, social conditions) that would prevent close observation and/or prompt return to the hospital.

B. **Peritonsillar abscess** (Quinsy tonsil) may interfere with swallowing and breathing (fever, pain, trismus).

1. Treatment consists of surgical drainage and intravenous antibiotic therapy.

2. Although the upper airway seems compromised, the abscess is usually in a fixed location in the lateral pharynx (visualization of the vocal cords should not be impaired because the pathology is supraglottic and well above the laryngeal inlet) and does not interfere with ventilation of the patient's lungs by mask after induction of general anesthesia.

3. Direct laryngoscopy must be carefully performed to minimize the risk of rupture of the abscess and spillage of purulent material into the patient's trachea.

III. EAR SURGERY

    A. Myringotomy and Tube Insertion
        1. Anesthesia may be provided with a volatile anesthetic and nitrous oxide.
        2. Recurrent upper respiratory infections may not resolve until there is eradication of middle ear fluid. Because tracheal intubation is not required, the presence of symptoms of an upper respiratory infection may not mandate delay of surgery.
    B. Middle Ear and Mastoid
        1. Tympanoplasty and mastoidectomy are two of the most common procedures performed on the middle ear.
        2. **Anesthetic Considerations** (Table 34-3)

IV. AIRWAY SURGERY

    A. Stridor is noisy breathing as a result of airway obstruction (Table 34-4).
        1. Inspiratory stridor results from upper airway obstruction, expiratory stridor results from lower airway obstruction, and biphasic stridor is present with midtracheal lesions.
            a. Information indicating positions that make the stridor better or worse are helpful for positioning the patient to take advantage of gravity in decreasing airway obstruction during induction of anesthesia.

TABLE 34-3

ANESTHETIC CONSIDERATIONS FOR TYMPANOPLASTY AND MASTOIDECTOMY

Head placed in head rest and laterally rotated (avoid tension of heads of the sternocleidomastoid muscles)

Preservation of facial nerve (preserve a 30% response on twitch monitor if muscle relaxants are administered)

Minimize bleeding (relative hypotension [mean arterial pressure 25% below baseline] and local injection of epinephrine [1:1000])

Discontinue nitrous oxide during placement of tympanic membrane graft

TABLE 34-4
CAUSES OF STRIDOR

Supraglottic airway	Larynx	Subglottic airway
Laryngomalacia	Laryngocele	Tracheomalacia
Vocal cord paralysis	Infection (tonsillitis, peritonsillar abscess)	Vascular ring
Subglottic stenosis	Foreign body	Foreign body
Hemangiomas	Choanal atresia	Infection (croup, epiglottis)
Cysts	Cysts	
	Mass	
	Large tonsils	
	Large adenoids	
	Craniofacial abnormalities	

    b. Laryngomalacia as a result of a long epiglottis that prolapses posteriorly is the most common cause of stridor in infants.
  2. Signs and Symptoms (Table 34-5)
B. Bronchoscopy
  1. Goals of anesthesia include a quiet surgical field (coughing or straining during instrumentation with a rigid bronchoscope may result in damage to the patient's airway), use of an antisialagogue to decrease secretions that may obscure the view through the bronchoscope, and rapid return to consciousness with intact upper airway reflexes.

TABLE 34-5
SIGNS AND SYMPTOMS SPECIFICALLY EXAMINED IN PATIENTS WITH STRIDOR

Breathing rate
Heart rate
Wheezing
Cyanosis
Chest retractions
Nasal flaring
Level of consciousness

2. In children an inhalation induction of anesthesia is common, whereas intravenous drugs are usually administered to adults. Maintenance of anesthesia often includes a volatile anesthetic and muscle relaxant.

   a. Because ventilation of the lungs may be intermittent, it is recommended that 100% oxygen be used as the carrier gas during bronchoscopic examination.

   b. If a rigid bronchoscope is used, ventilation of the lungs is accomplished through a side port (manual versus Sander's jet ventilation).

   c. At the conclusion of rigid bronchoscopy, an endotracheal tube is usually placed to control the patient's airway during recovery of anesthesia.

V. PEDIATRIC AIRWAY EMERGENCIES

A. **Epiglottitis** is an infectious disease (*Haemophilus influenzae*) of children (usually 2 to 7 years of age) and adults that can progress rapidly from sore throat to total upper airway obstruction.

   1. Characteristic signs and symptoms include sudden onset of fever, dysphagia, and preference for the sitting position.

   2. Direct visualization of the epiglottis and sedation outside the operating room should not be attempted because total upper airway obstruction may result.

   3. If the clinical situation allows, oxygen should be administered by mask and lateral radiographs of the soft tissues in the neck may be obtained.

   4. The child with severe airway compromise should proceed from the emergency room to the operating room accompanied by the anesthesiologist and surgeon.

   5. In all cases of epiglottitis, an artificial airway is established by means of tracheal intubation (Table 34-6).

B. **Laryngotracheobronchitis (LTB, croup)**

   1. LTB is usually a viral illness that occurs most often in children 6 months to 6 years of age.

TABLE 34-6

ESTABLISHMENT OF AN ARTIFICIAL AIRWAY IN THE PRESENCE OF EPIGLOTTITIS

Bring patient to operating room (child may be accompanied by a parent)

Place monitors (child may remain sitting)

Induce anesthesia by mask (halothane [sevoflurane] in oxygen)

Intravenous access may be accomplished after loss of consciousness

Place an orotracheal tube with use of muscle relaxants (select a tube size at least one size smaller than normal)

Replace orotracheal tube with a nasotracheal tube after the surgeon has examined the larynx

Extubation of the trachea is usually possible after 48–72 hr (leak develops around tracheal tube)

      2. Onset is more insidious than epiglottitis, with the child presenting with a low-grade fever, inspiratory stridor, and a barking cough.

      3. Treatment includes cool humid mist and oxygen and in severe cases nebulized racemic epinephrine and a short course of steroids.

  C. Foreign Body Aspiration

      1. This diagnosis should be suspected in any patient who presents with wheezing and a prior history of coughing or choking while eating.

      2. Most foreign bodies are radiolucent and the only findings on X ray are air trapping, infiltrate, and atelectasis.

      3. Aspirated foreign bodies are considered an emergency requiring removal in the operating room.

         a. Inhalation induction of anesthesia with halothane (sevoflurane an alternative) in oxygen may be prolonged secondary to obstruction of the airway.

         b. Nitrous oxide may be avoided to decrease the likelihood of air trapping distal to the obstruction.

         c. Spontaneous ventilation may be preserved until the location and nature of the foreign body have been determined.

d. Respiratory compromise secondary to airway edema or infection is a possible complication in the postoperative period.

VI. ANESTHESIA FOR PEDIATRIC AND ADULT SURGERY

A. Laser Surgery of the Airway

1. The laser (light amplification by stimulated emission of radiation) provides precision in targeting lesions, minimal bleeding, and edema as well as preservation of surrounding structures and rapid healing.

   a. The CO_2 laser has particular application in the treatment of laryngeal or vocal cord papillomas and coagulation of hemangiomas.

   b. Misdirected laser beams may cause injury to the patient or to unprotected operating room personnel (eye goggles with side protectors).

   c. Laser smoke plumes may cause damage to the lungs or serve as a vehicle for spread of viral particles (?human immunodeficiency virus).

2. **Anesthetic Management** (Table 34-7) (Fig. 34-1)

B. Nasal Surgery

1. Regardless of the anesthetic technique selected (general anesthesia or conscious sedation), it is likely that local vasoconstriction (topical local anesthetics, cocaine, and epinephrine) will be used.

2. A moderate degree of controlled hypotension combined with head elevation serves to decrease bleeding at the surgical site.

TABLE 34-7

ANESTHESIA FOR LASER SURGERY

Primary gas for anesthetic maintenance should be delivered with lowest safe concentration of oxygen (nitrous oxide and oxygen support combustion)

Recognize that polyvinylchloride tracheal tubes can ignite and vaporize when in contact with laser beam (use reflective tape or specially designed tubes)

Inflate tracheal tube cuff with saline to which methylene blue has been added (detect cuff rupture from a misdirected laser beam)

Apneic oxygenation techniques or jet ventilation are alternatives to tracheal intubation

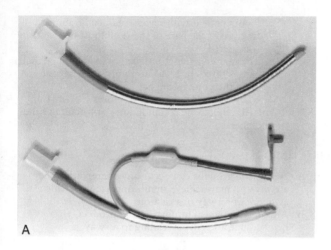

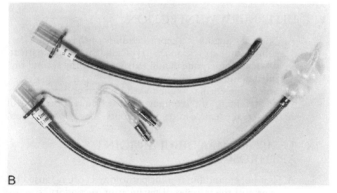

FIGURE 34-1. **A.** Cuffed and uncuffed rubber endotracheal tubes wrapped with reflective metallic tape. **B.** Cuffed and uncuffed flexible metal endotracheal tubes for use during laser surgery of the airway.

C. Maxillofacial Trauma

1. Challenges to the anesthesiologist in caring for patients with maxillofacial trauma include securing the upper airway in the presence of unknown anatomic alterations, sharing the airway with the surgeon, and determining when it is safe to extubate the patient's trachea.

   a. In any patient with severe midfacial trauma, a fracture of the base of the skull must be considered.
   b. The mandible has a unique horseshoe shape that causes forces to occur at points often distant from the point of impact.
2. **The LeFort classification of fractures** (LeFort I, II, and III) depicts the common lines of fracture of the midface.

VII. TUMORS

A. Neoplastic growths can occur anywhere within the airway and may achieve significant size with little evidence of airway obstruction.
B. Attempted tracheal intubation can produce hemorrhage and edema leading to airway obstruction.

VIII. UPPER AIRWAY INFECTION

A. Ludwig's angina is a septic cellulitis of the submandibular region that typically occurs in a patient who has undergone dental extraction of the second or third mandibular molars.
B. Soft tissue edema coupled with upward and posterior displacement of the tongue and the frequent presence of laryngeal edema can result in upper airway obstruction.

IX. TEMPOROMANDIBULAR JOINT ARTHROSCOPY

A. Temporomandibular joint pathology is often caused by spasm of the muscles of mastication secondary to chronic tension of these muscles (as an involuntary mental tension relieving mechanism).
B. Many patients with chronic temporomandibular joint dysfunction have significant psychopathology (depression, preoccupation with facial pain) and use mood-altering or tension-abating drugs.
C. Nasotracheal intubation is usually chosen.
D. Extracapsular extravasation of fluid used to irrigate the joint during arthroscopy can compromise the patency of the airway that manifests on tracheal extubation.

X. PATIENT EVALUATION

A. Patients who have sustained facial trauma should be evaluated for other injuries (cervical spine fractures, cranial fractures, intracranial injury).

B. The patient with Ludwig's angina is often septic and poorly hydrated.

C. Tumors of the head and neck are usually associated with cigarette and alcohol abuse with associated abnormalities of pulmonary and hepatic function.

XI. SECURING THE AIRWAY

A. Awake tracheal intubation or tracheostomy may be indicated in patients with upper airway tumor, infection, or trauma.

B. The technique of an "awake look" prior to a decision to induce anesthesia and administer a muscle relaxant may be misleading as skeletal muscle tone in the awake state that helps identify anatomic structures is absent once anesthesia and skeletal muscle paralysis are produced.

C. After maxillofacial trauma the ability to open the mouth may be limited because of pain, trismus, edema, or mechanical dysfunction of the temporomandibular joint.

1. Pain will not influence mouth opening in an anesthetized and paralyzed patient.

2. Trismus will succumb to an anesthetic and muscle relaxant unless there is fibrosis of the masseter muscles (possible if trismus presents for 2 weeks or longer).

XII. AWAKE INTUBATION

A. The airway must be anesthetized using a combination of topical anesthesia and superior laryngeal nerve block.

B. **Superior Laryngeal Nerve Block**

1. The external branch of the superior laryngeal nerve innervates the cricothyroid muscle (tensor of the vocal cords) and the internal branch provides sensory innervation from the base of the tongue to the vocal cords.

2. With the patient lying supine, a 22-gauge needle attached to a syringe containing 2 mL of 2% lidocaine is introduced until it contacts the hyoid bone.

   a. When the needle contacts the hyoid bone, it is redirected caudad until it just steps off the bone penetrating the thyrohyoid membrane.

   b. Following negative aspiration, the local anesthetic is injected and the block repeated on the opposite side.

   c. Complications of superior laryngeal nerve block include intravascular injection of local anesthetic solution (carotid artery lies just posterior to the site of needle placement for performance of the block).

C. Topical anesthesia includes local anesthetic instilled into the nose (add a vasoconstrictor such as 0.5% phenylephrine to shrink the nasal mucosa) and/or mouth (nebulized in a hand-held nebulizer and inhaled by the patient).

   1. Topical anesthesia may be applied below the level of the vocal cords by introducing a 22-gauge needle through the cricothyroid membrane and rapidly injecting 4 mL of 2% lidocaine.

   2. The resulting cough reflex will distribute the local anesthetic along the tracheal mucosa and inferior surface of the vocal cords.

D. The LMA may be useful in temporarily securing a compromised airway whereas a tracheal tube is necessary to protect the airway from aspiration of blood. The LMA-Fastrach is a modification of the intubating LMA, designed specifically for the anatomically difficult airway.

XIII. LEFORT III FRACTURES

A. This type of fracture may involve the cribiform plate of the ethmoid bone and cause the separation of the nasopharynx and base of the skull.

B. Nasotracheal intubation introduces the risk of delivering foreign material from the nasopharynx into the subarachnoid space.

   1. Even positive-pressure ventilation of the patient's lungs can increase pressure in the nasopharynx and force foreign material or air into the skull.

2. The problems of securing the airway in a patient with a LeFort III fracture are usually obviated by performing a preliminary tracheostomy.

XIV. ANESTHETIC MANAGEMENT FOR THE TRAUMATIZED UPPER AIRWAY

A. After tracheal intubation or tracheostomy has been performed, general or intravenous drugs may be administered.
B. Because there is a significant incidence of intracranial injury associated with maxillofacial trauma, the brain must be protected from increases in intracranial pressure.

XV. EXTUBATION

A. When a tracheostomy has been performed, the decision at the conclusion of surgery is whether to allow spontaneous breathing or to create suitable conditions (opioids, muscle relaxants) for continued mechanical ventilation of the patient's lungs.
B. After trauma, infection, or extensive oral resection for tumor, the endotracheal tube must not be removed until there is subsidence of edema (especially submandibular edema) or infection that might compromise the unprotected airway.
C. An orotracheal tube may be removed over a tube changer.

CHAPTER 35 ▪ THE RENAL SYSTEM AND ANESTHESIA FOR UROLOGIC SURGERY

The kidney plays a central role in implementing and controlling a variety of homeostatic functions, including excreting metabolic waste products in the form of urine while keeping extracellular fluid volume and composition constant (O'Hara JF, Cywinski JB, Monk TG: The renal system and anesthesia for urologic surgery. In Barash PG, Cullen BF, Stoelting RK [eds]: *Clinical Anesthesia*, pp 1013–1039. Philadelphia, Lippincott Williams & Wilkins, 2006). Renal dysfunction may occur perioperatively as a direct result of surgical or medical disease, prolonged decreases in oxygen delivery, nephrotoxin insult, or, frequently, a combination of the three.

I. RENAL ANATOMY AND PHYSIOLOGY

A. Anatomy and Innervation of the Genitourinary System

1. Nociceptive projection to the spinal cord for the kidneys and ureters is via sympathetic nerves (T10–L1) (Fig. 35-1). Parasympathetic fibers from S2–4 spinal segments supply the ureters (see Fig. 35-1). These spinal segments also provide somatic innervation to the lumbar area, flank, ilioinguinal area, scrotum, or labia. Accordingly, pain from the kidney and ureter is referred to those areas.

2. The bladder receives its innervation from sympathetic nerves originating from T11–L2, which conduct pain while bladder stretch sensation is transmitted via parasympathetic fibers from S2–4. Parasympathetics also provide the bladder with the majority of its motor innervation.

   a. The prostate, penile urethra, and penis also receive sympathetic and parasympathetic fibers from T11–L2 and S2–4 segments.

   b. The pudendal nerve provides pain sensation to the penis via the dorsal nerve of the penis.

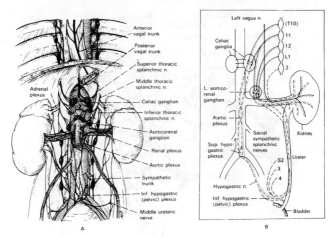

FIGURE 35-1. **A.** Anatomy of the kidney and ureters. **B.** Schematic illustration of the autonomic and sensory nerve pathways supplying the kidney and ureters.

  B. Anatomy of the Nephron (Fig. 35-2)
    1. The glomerulus is a capillary network receiving blood from the afferent arteriole, thus serving as the filtering unit of the nephron.
      a. The glomerulus is enveloped by the initial segment of the renal tubular system called Bowman's capsule from which the glomerular filtrate passes into the proximal tubule.
  C. Renal Physiology
    1. The kidney fulfills its dual roles of waste excretion and body fluid management by filtration of large amounts of fluid and solutes from the blood, resorption of needed components of this filtrate, and secretion of waste products into the tubular fluid.
    2. **Glomerular Filtration**
      a. Urine production begins with the filtration of water and solutes from blood flowing through the afferent arteriole. The glomerular membrane serves as the filter while Bowman's capsule acts as the initial receptacle for the filtrate. More than 99% of the filtered fluid is reabsorbed and returned to the circulation, resulting in 1 to 2 liters of urine output per day in the adult.

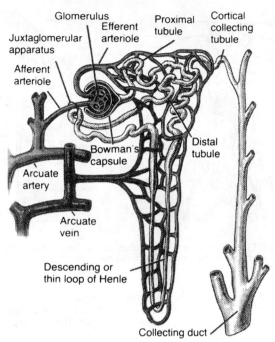

FIGURE 35-2. Anatomy of the nephron.

    b. Glomerular filtration rate (GFR) is a measure of glomerular function expressed as milliliters of filtrate produced per minute. The two major determinants of glomerular filtration pressure are glomerular capillary pressure (directly related to renal artery pressure and influenced by afferent and efferent arteriolar tone [sympathetic nervous system stimulation, angiotensin]) and glomerular oncotic pressure (directly dependent on plasma oncotic pressure and related to rate of blood flow through the glomerulus).

3. Autoregulation of Renal Blood Flow (RBF) and Glomerular Filtration Rate

    a. Autoregulation of RBF over a wide range of arterial blood pressures is necessary for the

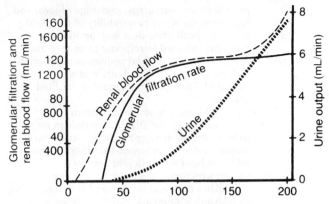

FIGURE 35-3. Autoregulation of glomerular filtration rate and renal blood flow over a wide range of mean arterial pressures. Note that urine output is not subject to autoregulation.

kidney to maintain relatively constant rates of glomerular filtration (Fig. 35-3). Renal autoregulation of blood flow and filtration is accomplished by local feedback signals that modulate glomerular arteriolar tone.

b. Autoregulation of urine flow does not occur, and there is a linear relationship between mean arterial pressure above 50 mm Hg and urine output.

4. **Tubular Resorption of Sodium and Water**
   a. Sodium (energy dependent) and water (passive osmotically driven and antidiuretic hormone) resorption are closely related to the homeostatic mechanisms involved in the response to physiologic stress.
   b. The neurohumoral response to surgical stress and critical illness is primarily directed at maintaining blood pressure, circulating blood volume, and essential organ blood flow.
   c. Conservation of water and excretion of excess solute by the kidneys are accomplished by establishing a hyperosmotic medullary interstitium (dependent on the vasa recta, which

provides a countercurrent exchange of ions) and regulating the water permeability of the distal tubule and collecting duct with antidiuretic hormone (released in response to an increase in either the extracellular sodium concentration or the extracellular osmolarity and a perceived decrease in the intravascular fluid volume).

5. **Renin–Angiotensin Aldosterone System**
   a. Renin release by the afferent arteriole in response to hypotension or sympathetic nervous system stimulation leads to angiotensin II production, which induces renal efferent arteriolar vasoconstriction and aldosterone release (stimulates the distal tubules and collecting ducts to reabsorb sodium and water, resulting in an expansion of the intravascular fluid volume).
   b. The body's response to surgical stress (decrease in GFR and salt and water retention) manifests as oliguria and edema formation that may persist for several days into the postoperative period because of ongoing stress (pain, sepsis, hypovolemia).

6. **Renal Vasodilator Mechanisms**
   a. Opposing the salt and water retention and vasoconstriction observed in stress states are the actions of atrial natriuretic peptide (released by cardiac atria in response to conditions of increased stretch as produced by relative hypervolemia, nitric oxide, and prostaglandins).
   b. Nitric oxide and prostaglandins are produced by the kidneys to increase sodium and water excretion.

II. RENAL DYSFUNCTION AND ANESTHESIA

A. Although direct anesthetic effects on the kidneys are generally not harmful, indirect effects of regional or general anesthesia (protracted decrease in cardiac output or hypotension that coincides with a period of intense renal vasoconstriction) may combine with hypovolemia, shock, nephrotoxin exposure, or other vasoconstrictive states to produce renal dysfunction. There are no comparative studies demonstrating superior renal protection or improved renal outcome with general versus regional anesthesia.

TABLE 35-1
CHARACTERISTICS OF ACUTE RENAL FAILURE
Accumulation of creatinine and urea in blood (reflects loss of ability to excrete waste products)
Decreased urine production (nonoliguric forms of acute renal failure are common in the postoperative period)
Multiple organ system failure
Sepsis
High mortality (50–70%)

B. **Acute Renal Failure (ARF)** (Table 35-1 and Fig. 35-4)
1. **Prerenal azotemia** is defined as the increase in blood urea nitrogen (BUN) associated with renal hypoperfusion or ischemia that has not caused renal parenchymal damage.
2. **Intrinsic ARF** implies a primary renal etiology of ARF but also includes ischemia (acute tubular necrosis), toxins (drugs, contrast media), and parenchymal diseases.
3. **Intraoperative Oliguria**
   a. Oliguria (urine output <0.5 mL/kg/hr) may be a useful sign of renal hypoperfusion when other

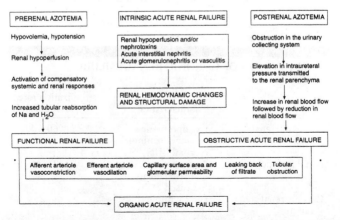

FIGURE 35-4. Mechanisms of acute renal failure.

objective signs of decreased systemic blood flow are present. If a fluid bolus does not improve urine flow rate, or heart rate and blood pressure indicate hypovolemia, further fluid administration is indicated.

   b. If oliguria persists and signs of congestive heart failure or volume overload appear, the patient's hemodynamic profile should be further assessed with a pulmonary artery catheter.

   c. When sepsis is responsible for oliguria, hypotension is a common finding and is usually secondary to systemic vasodilation, hypovolemia, and decreased myocardial contractility.

C. **Chronic Renal Failure** (Table 35-2)
   1. Uremia is associated with electrolyte and acid-base disorders and multiple organ system dysfunction (Table 35-3).
   2. Renal failure patients are predisposed to develop hyperkalemia (Table 35-4).

D. **Anesthetic Agents in Renal Failure**
   1. **Induction Agents and Sedatives**
      a. Thiopental induction dose requirements are decreased in uremic patients as a result of decreased protein binding.
      b. The pharmacokinetics of ketamine are not altered by renal failure (redistribution and hepatic

TABLE 35-2

CLASSIFICATION OF CHRONIC RENAL FAILURE

	Characteristics	Glomerular filtration rate (% of normal)
Decreased renal reserve	Asymptomatic Normal creatinine Normal BUN	60–75
Renal insufficiency	Nocturia Increased creatinine Increased BUN	25–40
Chronic renal failure	Fatal without dialysis	<25
Uremia	Frequent dialysis	<10

TABLE 35-3

CHARACTERISTICS OF UREMIA

Water Homeostasis
Extracellular fluid expansion

Electrolyte and Acid-Base
Hyponatremia
Hyperkalemia
Hypercalcemia
Hypocalcemia
Hyperphosphatemia
Hypermagnesemia
Metabolic acidosis

Cardiovascular
Congestive heart failure
Hypertension
Pericarditis
Myocardial dysfunction
Dysrhythmias

Respiratory
Pulmonary edema
Central hyperventilation

Gastrointestinal
Delayed gastric emptying
Nausea and vomiting
Hemorrhage

Neuromuscular
Encephalopathy
Seizures
Sensory and motor polyneuropathy
Autonomic nervous system dysfunction

Hematologic
Anemia
Platelet hemostatic defect

Immunologic
Cell-mediated and humoral immunity defects

Endocrine Metabolism
Renal osteodystrophy
Decreased glucose intolerance
Hypertriglyceridemia
Atherosclerosis

TABLE 35-4

FACTORS CONTRIBUTING TO HYPERKALEMIA IN CHRONIC RENAL FAILURE PATIENTS

Potassium Intake
Increased dietary intake
Exogenous intravenous supplementation
Potassium salts of drugs
Blood transfusions
Gastrointestinal hemorrhage

Potassium Release from Intracellular Stores
Increased catabolism
Sepsis
Metabolic acidosis
Beta-adrenergic-blocking drugs
Digitalis intoxication
Insulin deficiency
Succinylcholine

Potassium Excretion
Acute decrease in glomerular filtration rate
Potassium-sparing diuretics
ACE inhibitors (decreased aldosterone secretion)
Heparin (decreased aldosterone effect)

ACE = angiotensin-converting enzyme.

metabolism responsible for termination of effects
with <3% of the drug excreted unchanged in the
urine).

c. Etomidate has a larger free fraction in the
presence of uremia, but clinical effects seem
unchanged.

d. Propofol undergoes extensive hepatic metabolism
to inactive metabolites that are renally excreted.
Pharmacokinetics of propofol appear to be
unchanged in patients with renal failure.

e. Benzodiazepines are extensively protein bound,
and in the presence of renal failure their clinical
effect may be prolonged (decrease initial dose).
Certain benzodiazepine metabolites are
pharmacologically active and have the potential
to accumulate with repeated administration of
the parent drug to anephric patients. ARF may
slow the plasma clearance of midazolam.

f. Dexmedetomidine produces prolonged sedative
effects in patients with renal dysfunction.

TABLE 35-5

OPIOIDS IN CHRONIC RENAL FAILURE PATIENTS

Morphine (chronic administration results in accumulation of morphine-6-glucuronide, which is a more potent analgesic than its parent compound)

Meperidine (normeperidine is neurotoxic and depends on renal excretion)

Codeine (potential for producing prolonged effects)

Fentanyl (absence of active metabolites; small doses are tolerated by uremic patients whereas large doses [25 μg/kg] may result in a prolonged effect)

Alfentanil (extensively metabolized to inactive compounds)

Sufentanil (an active metabolite is dependent on renal excretion)

Remifentanil (rapidly metabolized to weakly active metabolites that depend on renal clearance)

---

   2. **Opioids** (Table 35-5)
   E. **Muscle Relaxants**
      1. Only succinylcholine, atracurium, mivacurium, and cisatracurium appear to have minimal renal excretion of the unchanged parent compound.
         a. The clearance and duration of action of atracurium and cisatracurium are not altered by renal failure. Consistent with its greater potency, cisatracurium metabolism results in lower blood levels than atracurium.
         b. The duration of action of vecuronium may be prolonged because of its decreased clearance and accumulation of an active metabolite.
      2. Anticholinesterase and anticholinergic drugs are highly dependent on renal excretion such that a change in dose in patients with decreased renal function is not necessary.

III. PRESERVATION OF RENAL FUNCTION

   A. To prevent ARF, one must first identify those patients who are at risk for perioperative renal damage and then focus on preserving renal function in that group.
   B. **Patient-Based Risk Factors for ARF** (Table 35-6)
   C. **Perioperative Assessment of Renal Function** (Table 35-7)
   D. **Nephrotoxins and Perioperative ARF** (Table 35-8)

TABLE 35-6
RISK FACTORS FOR POSTOPERATIVE RENAL FAILURE
Patient-Based Indicators
Preoperative renal dysfunction
Perioperative cardiac dysfunction
Hepatic failure (obstructive jaundice, ascites)
Hypovolemia
Advanced age?
Nephrotoxic Exposure
High-Risk Surgical Procedures
Cardiopulmonary bypass
Aortic cross-clamping
Trauma
Burns
Emergency surgery
Hepatic transplantation
Renal transplantation

IV. HIGH-RISK SURGICAL PROCEDURES

A. Emergency surgery owing to trauma is a risk factor for ARF. Acute tubular necrosis is the preeminent renal lesion associated with trauma and may be produced by any number of ischemic mechanisms (hypovolemic shock, multiple organ failure, pigmenturia, exogenous nephrotoxins).

1. ARF that develops in the trauma patient may be characterized by an early oliguric picture related to hypovolemia (up to 90% mortality) or a late-onset nonoliguric syndrome associated with multiple organ failure, nephrotoxin exposure, or sepsis (mortality 20 to 30%).

2. Prevention of ARF in the trauma patient presenting for emergency surgery includes restoration of euvolemia, maintenance of cardiac output (renal blood flow), and systemic oxygen delivery.

   a. Invasive hemodynamic monitoring may be required to guide the intraoperative management of ongoing cardiovascular instability as a result of surgical manipulation, blood loss, fluid shift, and anesthetic effects.

TABLE 35-7

CLINICAL USEFULNESS OF RENAL FUNCTION TESTS

Test	Distinguish ATN from PRA	Predict early ATN	Comments
Urine flow rate	Poor	Poor	
Urine specific gravity	Poor	Poor	Many nonrenal factors
Urine osmolarity	Poor	Poor	Many nonrenal factors
Serum creatinine, BUN	Poor	Late findings	Rapid preoperative screen
U/P creatinine, BUN	Poor	Poor	
Urine sodium	Poor	Poor	
Fraction excretion sodium	Good in late ATN	Poor	
Free water		Good with creatinine	Less sensitive than creatanine
Creatinine clearance	Good	Good	2-hour versus 24-hour collection

PRA = prerenal azotemia; ATN = acute tubular necrosis.

TABLE 35-8

NEPHROTOXINS ENCOUNTERED IN THE PERIOPERATIVE PERIOD

Antibiotics
Volatile anesthetics (enflurane, sevoflurane)
Nonsteroidal anti-inflammatory drugs (ketorolac)
Chemotherapeutic/immunosuppressive drugs (cyclosporin A)
Contrast media
Myoglobin (rhabdomyolysis because of acute skeletal muscle injury or ischemia; compartment syndrome; extreme lithotomy position)
Hemoglobin (hemolysis)

   b. Nephrotoxin exposure (radiocontrast media, nonsteroidal anti-inflammatory drugs, myoglobin) should be minimized.

   c. Furosemide or mannitol therapy is not recommended in the early resuscitative phase of trauma management except when massive rhabdomyolysis is suspected.

   d. Postoperatively, creatinine clearance determinations (1 or 2 hours) can help identify those patients with impending ARF.

B. Vascular surgery requiring cross-clamping of the aorta (regardless of the level of the clamp) has deleterious effects on renal function.

  1. Two major predictors of ARF following aortic surgery are preexisting renal dysfunction and perioperative hemodynamic instability.

  2. Attempts to improve renal outcome in aortic surgery begin with meticulous, rapid surgical technique to lessen ischemia time and prevent atheromatous renal artery emboli. There are few data to support the use of mannitol or "renal dose dopamine" to prevent the renal injury associated with aortic surgery.

C. Cardiac surgery requiring cardiopulmonary bypass can be expected to result in renal dysfunction or failure in up to 5% of patients. Preoperative renal dysfunction is a major risk factor for postoperative ARF in this population.

  1. The type of cardiopulmonary bypass (pulsatile versus nonpulsatile) and perfusion pressure on bypass are less important factors in the pathogenesis of ARF than is protracted hemodynamic instability (renal hypoperfusion).

  2. Careful hemodynamic management is the basis of any strategy designed to avoid renal hypoperfusion in cardiac surgery.

   a. Mannitol can be used to protect against hemoglobin-induced ARF, promote urine flow, and decrease renal cell swelling that can occur on cardiopulmonary bypass.

   b. Renal dose dopamine has been used as a renal vasodilator in cardiac surgery with mixed success. An increased incidence of postoperative cardiac dysrhythmias may accompany the use of dopamine.

D. **Hepatic failure** and **cholestatic jaundice** are risk factors for the development of postoperative ARF. When such patients are exposed to intraoperative hemodynamic instability, massive transfusions, and nephrotoxins, ARF frequently follows. Renal dose dopamine has been shown to be no better than preoperative hydration for preserving renal function in patients with obstructive jaundice.

E. Perioperative sepsis is a common cause of renal dysfunction (renal autoregulation is impaired, RBF and GFR are decreased).

V. ANESTHESIA FOR ENDOUROLOGIC PROCEDURES

A. Incisional surgery in urology is being replaced by endoscopic procedures (Table 35-9).

B. **Cystourethroscopy and Ureteral Procedures**
   1. Local anesthesia with or without conscious sedation techniques is often sufficient for patients to tolerate cystoscopic procedures. If general anesthesia is required for cystoscopy or urethral procedures, laryngeal mask airways are useful alternatives to a traditional face mask.
   2. Ureteroscopy usually requires dilation of the ureteral orifice and intramural ureter, often necessitating regional or general anesthesia.

TABLE 35-9

COMMON ENDOUROLOGIC PROCEDURES

Cystourethroscopy
Internal optical urethrotomy
Ureteroscopy
Placement of ureteral stent
Distal stone manipulation/laser lithotripsy
Transurethral resection of the prostate
Transurethral incision of the prostate
Balloon dilation of the prostate
Transurethral resection of bladder tumors
Extracorporeal shock wave lithotripsy
Percutaneous nephrostomy, nephroscopy, and nephrolithotomy

C. Transuretheral Resection of the Prostate (TURP)
   1. The prostate gland contains a rich plexus of veins
      that can be opened during the surgical resection,
      which may result in intravascular absorption of the
      irrigating fluid leading to unique perioperative
      complications.
   2. **Irrigating Solutions for TURP** (Table 35-10)
   3. **Transurethral resection (TURP) syndrome** (water
      intoxication syndrome) is a general term used to
      describe a wide range of neurologic and
      cardiopulmonary symptoms that occur when
      irrigating fluid is absorbed (20 mL for every minute
      of resection time). In an attempt to prevent excessive
      fluid absorption, it is recommended that resection
      time be limited to <1 hour and the bag of irrigating
      fluid be suspended no more than 60 cm above the
      operating table. Ethanol-labeled irrigating fluid can
      be used to assess the degree of fluid absorption
      (measure ethanol concentration in the patient's
      exhaled gases).
      a. Hypertension and bradycardia are the result of
         acute hypervolemia, which may lead to
         pulmonary edema.
      b. Prompt intervention is necessary when the
         neurologic or cardiovascular complications of

TABLE 35-10
IRRIGATING SOLUTIONS FOR TRANSURETHRAL RESECTION OF THE PROSTATE

Solution	Osmolarity (mOsm/l)	Advantages	Disadvantages
Glycine (1.5%)	200	Less likelihood of TURP syndrome	Transient postoperative visual impairment Hyperammonemia Hyperoxaluria
Sorbitol (3.3%)	165	Same as glycine	Hyperglycemia Possible lactic acidosis Osmotic diuresis
Mannitol (5%)	275	Isoosmolar Nonmetabolized	Osmotic diuresis Hypervolemia

TURP = transurethral resection of the prostate.

TABLE 35-11
TREATMENT OF TRANSURETHRAL RESECTION SYNDROME

Ensure oxygenation and circulatory support
Notify surgeon and terminate procedure as soon as possible
Consider insertion of invasive monitors if cardiovascular instability is present
Send blood to laboratory for measurement of electrolytes, creatinine, glucose, and arterial blood gases
Obtain 12-lead electrocardiogram
Treat mild symptoms in presence of serum sodium concentration >120 mEq/l with fluid restriction and loop diuretic (fur-furosemide)
Treat severe symptoms in presence of serum sodium concentration <120 mEq/l with 3% sodium chloride at a rate <100 mL/hr iv
Discontinue 3% sodium chloride when serum sodium concentration >120 mEq/l

TURP procedures are recognized (Table 35-11).

4. **Other Complications of TURP**
    a. Bleeding associated with TURP is difficult to quantitate (estimated to be 2 to 4 mL per minute of resection). Serial hematocrits and the patient's vital signs are used to determine the need for transfusion.
    b. Disseminated intravascular coagulation (<1% of resections) may be caused by the release of thromboplastin, especially in the patient with prostate cancer. Treatment is supportive including the administration of plasma, platelets, and deficient factors (use of heparin is controversial).
    c. Perforation of the prostatic capsule (occurs in 1 to 2% of resections) usually results in extraperitoneal extravasation of fluid.
    d. Fever suggests bacteremia secondary to spread of bacteria via open prostatic channels that is enhanced by the presence of an indwelling catheter (most patients receive prophylactic antibiotics). The risk of sepsis is increased when irrigation pressure during the procedure exceeds 30 cm H_2O.

e. Hypothermia (body temperature decreases 1°C for every hour of surgery) is a particular risk in elderly patients with decreased thermoregulatory capacity (warming irrigation fluids may be recommended).

5. **Anesthetic Techniques for TURP**
   a. General or regional anesthesia is acceptable with the choice being influenced by the unique needs of each individual patient. Regional anesthesia allows the patient to remain awake, which should facilitate early diagnosis of the TURP syndrome or the extravasation of irrigation fluid. Perioperative morbidity and postoperative cognitive function is not dependent on the type of anesthesia administered. Patients receiving a regional anesthesia may have less postoperative pain than those receiving a general anesthetic.
   b. The incidence of myocardial ischemia is increased following TURP surgery but there is no difference between patients receiving regional versus general anesthesia.
   c. Spinal anesthesia (T10 sensory level) is generally preferred over lumbar epidural anesthesia because sacral segments are more reliably blocked.

6. **Morbidity and Mortality Following TURP** (Table 35-12)

7. **The Future of TURP**
   a. Less invasive surgical treatments include balloon dilatation, prostate stents, transurethral incision of the prostate, and laser prostatectomy.
   b. These procedures can usually be preformed on an outpatient basis and decrease the risk of TURP syndrome.

D. **Transurethral Resection of Bladder Tumors (TURB)**

1. Endoscopic resection of superficial transitional cell cancer of the bladder (accounts for 90% of bladder cancers) requires either general anesthesia (bladder tumor near the obturator nerve) or regional anesthesia (T10 sensory level to block pain associated with distension of the bladder).

2. **Complications During TURB**
   a. Bladder perforation is suggested by an abnormal irrigation pattern in which fluid is instilled into the bladder but not recovered and, in an awake

TABLE 35-12

COMPLICATIONS ACCOMPANYING TRANSURETHRAL
RESECTION OF THE PROSTATE

Intraoperative
Bleeding requiring transfusion
Transurethral resection of the prostate syndrome
Cardiac dysrhythmias
Extravasation of irrigating fluid

Immediate Postoperative Problems
Inability to void
Bleeding
Clot retention
Infection

Characteristics of Patients at Risk for Perioperative Morbidity
Large prostate gland (>45 g)
Long resection time (>90 minutes)
Acute urinary retention
Advanced age (>80 yr)

patient, sudden abdominal pain often associated
with referred pain to the shoulder.
   b. The intraperitoneal accumulation of irrigating
      fluid (especially sterile water) can be life
      threatening (open laparotomy for drainage and
      bladder perforation is recommended).
E. Extracorporeal Shock Wave Lithotripsy (SWL)
   1. Technical Aspects of SWL
      a. All lithotriptors have four main components: an
         energy source, a focusing device, a coupling
         medium, and a stone localization system. The
         water bath transmits the shock wave to the
         patient and serves as the coupling medium,
         allowing the shock wave to pass into the body
         without dissipation because the acoustic
         impedance of body tissue is close to that
         of water.
      b. Shock waves are triggered off the
         electrocardiogram to occur 20 msec after the R
         wave during the refractory period of the
         heart.
   2. Physiologic Effects of Immersion Lithotripsy
      (Table 35-13)

TABLE 35-13
PHYSIOLOGIC EFFECTS OF IMMERSION LITHOTRIPSY

Cardiovascular System
Peripheral venous compression
Increased central blood volume
Increased central venous pressure
Increased pulmonary capillary wedge pressure
Increased venous return

Respiratory System
Increased work of breathing
Decreased vital capacity and functional residual capacity

Temperature Regulation

3. Patient Selection and Complications of SWL
   a. The only absolute contraindications to SWL are pregnancy (pregnancy test in women of child-bearing potential because fetal damage is possible from shock waves and/or radiation), abnormal coagulation parameters (risk of perinephric hematoma; preoperative prothrombin time, partial thromboplastin time, and platelets), and active urinary tract infection (all patients are treated with antibiotics).
   b. Patients with artificial cardiac pacemakers are acceptable candidates for SWL if an alternative pacing device is available and the patient is positioned so the pacemaker is not in the shock wave path.
   c. Relative contraindications to SWL include the presence of an orthopedic prosthesis, renal insufficiency (serum creatinine >3 mg/dL) and the presence of an abdominal aneurysm that is >6 cm in diameter.
4. Complications of SWL (Table 35-14)
5. Anesthetic Techniques for SWL
   a. The impact of shock waves in the skin and viscera is responsible for the pain experienced during the procedure.
   b. Conscious sedation (propofol and fentanyl and midazolam) combined with local anesthetic infiltration of the flank (alternatively combined

TABLE 35-14
COMPLICATIONS OF SHOCK WAVE LITHOTRIPSY

Hematuria (renal parenchymal damage)
Transient renal failure (avoid bilateral lithotripsy at same
   treatment)
Postoperative flank pain
Petechiae and soft tissue swelling at entry site
Urinary tract colic ("steinstrasse" reflects broken stone
   fragments in the ureter)
Damage to adjacent organs by the shock wave (lungs, pancreas,
   gastrointestinal tract)
Sepsis
Brachial plexus injuries

with intercostal blocks and topical application of
local anesthetic cream) is the preferred anesthetic
technique for procedures performed using the
newer generation lithotriptors.
   c. General anesthesia offers the advantages of
      control of patient ventilation and movement, but
      the need to position an unconscious patient is a
      major disadvantage. Regional anesthesia (T6
      sensory level necessary) simplifies patient
      positioning, but sympathetic nervous system
      blockade is associated with a higher incidence of
      intraoperative hypotension.
F. **Percutaneous Renal Procedures**
   1. Dilation of the nephrostomy tract (most often for
      removal of renal calculi too large to be treated with
      lithotripsy) is associated with considerable
      discomfort and requires either general or regional
      anesthesia.
   2. Complications of percutaneous surgical techniques
      include trauma to the spleen, liver, or kidney,
      resulting in acute blood loss and the need for open
      surgical exploration, colon injury, and pleural
      injury.
   3. Extravasation of irrigation fluid into the
      retroperitoneal, intraperitoneal, intravascular, or
      pleural space can create a situation similar to that
      seen with TUR syndrome. For this reason, it is
      common to compare the quantity of irrigation fluid
      used with output from the patient. Because

electrocautery is rarely used, the preferred irrigating solution is 0.9% sodium chloride (change to sorbitol if electrocautery is needed).

VI. LASER SURGERY IN UROLOGY

A. Advantages of laser for urologic surgery over traditional surgical approaches are minimal blood loss, decreased postoperative pain, and tissue denaturation, which decreases the risk of tumor implantation.

B. Damage to the eye is the potential injury that requires the greatest attention.

C. During carbon dioxide laser therapy for condyloma acuminatum, the plume (smoke) from the vaporization of tissue contains active human papilloma virus particles (operating room personnel should wear protective laser masks that prevent small particles from being inhaled).

VII. UROLOGIC LAPAROSCOPY

A. Laparoscopic urologic procedures differ from conventional laparoscopy in that many structures in the genitourinary system are extraperitoneal (carbon dioxide absorption may be greater compared with intraperitoneal insufflation). The increased absorption of carbon dioxide during extraperitoneal laparoscopic techniques mandates that the anesthesiologist carefully monitor and adjust the patient's ventilation as needed to maintain normocarbia.

B. Laparoscopic procedures in urology may be lengthy (general anesthesia needed to ensure patient comfort with prolonged pneumoperitoneum) and associated with oliguria (prolonged increases in intra-abdominal pressure of >15 mm Hg results in decreased urine output despite adequate circulating blood volume and cardiac output). Administration of large volumes of iv fluids to treat this oliguria may lead to hypervolemia and congestive heart failure.

VIII. RADICAL CANCER SURGERY

A. These procedures are often lengthy, require intraoperative patient positions that may be associated with significant impact on cardiorespiratory function, and have the potential for hemorrhage and large intraoperative blood and fluid requirements. In addition, patients undergoing these procedures are often elderly with preexisting medical conditions.

B. **Radical Prostatectomy**

1. General anesthesia or regional anesthesia (sensory level to T6–8) with sedation may be used for this procedure. Epidural patient-controlled analgesia to maintain postoperative analgesia is used regardless of the technique selected.

2. The surgical approach is either retropubic (operating room table is broken in the midline or the kidney rest is elevated with the patient in a head-down position) or perineal (exaggerated lithotomy position with the patient in a head-down position). Because of the positioning during radical perineal prostatectomy, most anesthesiologists prefer either general or a combined epidural-general anesthetic during the procedure.

   a. The head-down position required by either surgical approach produces physiologic changes in respiration (abdominal contents compress the diaphragm), circulation, and cerebrovascular systems (increased intracranial pressure). Jugular venous distention can lead to edema of the airway, tongue, and face.

   b. Rhabdomyolysis with associated ARF may follow perineal prostatectomy performed in the exaggerated lithotomy position.

   c. Venous air embolism may occur if the prostatic venous network is opened while the patient is in the head-down position (some recommend monitoring with a precordial Doppler and placement of a multiorificed central venous pressure catheter).

3. The most common intraoperative problem is hemorrhage. The potential for rapid blood loss is the reason to recommend direct arterial blood pressure monitoring, especially in elderly or high-risk patients. Hemodynamic monitoring of volume status with a central venous pressure catheter may be necessary because the bladder is opened during the procedure, making it impossible to monitor fluid status with urinary output.

TABLE 35-15

CHARACTERISTICS OF BLEOMYCIN PULMONARY
TOXICITY

Onset of respiratory failure 3–10 days postoperatively
Risk factors include preoperative evidence of pulmonary injury,
  total bleomycin dose >50 mg, creatinine clearance <5 mL/min
Role of intraoperative hyperoxia (inspired oxygen concentration
  >30%) is controversial
Limit intravenous fluid replacement (colloid preferred) to amount
  necessary to maintain hemodynamic stability and adequate
  urine output

   C. **Radical Cystectomy**
      1. Patient positioning and monitoring requirements are
        as described for a radical prostatectomy performed
        using the retropubic approach. The need for urinary
        diversion prolongs the procedure such that general
        anesthesia or a combined general-epidural anesthetic
        is used.
      2. Previous treatment with chemotherapeutic drugs
        may result in adverse effects (doxorubicin [cardiac
        toxicity], methotrexate [hepatic toxicity, renal
        toxicity, neurotoxicity]).
   D. **Radical Nephrectomy**
      1. General anesthesia or combined epidural-general
        anesthesia is used for patients placed in the "kidney
        position."
      2. Acute blood loss is a possibility. The patient needs to
        be adequately hydrated to optimize blood flow to
        the remaining kidney and to prevent hypotension
        from positioning. Pneumothorax may occur during
        surgery if the chest is accidentally entered (chest
        X ray in the postanesthesia care unit if suspected).
   E. **Radical Surgery for Testicular Cancer**
      1. Testicular cancer is the most common malignancy in
        young men between 15 and 34 years of age.
      2. Following an orchiectomy the subsequent treatment
        may include radiation, chemotherapy, and/or
        retroperitoneal lymph node dissection.
      3. Bleomycin, used as an antitumor antibiotic against
        germ cell tumors of the testis, is associated with
        pulmonary toxicity and postoperative respiratory
        failure following retroperitoneal lymph node
        dissection (Table 35-15).

CHAPTER 36 ■ ANESTHESIA AND OBESITY

Obesity is a condition of excessive body fat with adverse health implications including increased risk for hypertension, coronary artery disease, hyperlipidemia, diabetes mellitus, gallbladder disease, degenerative joint disease, obstructive sleep apnea (OSA), and psychological and socioeconomic impairment (Ogunnaike BO, Whitten CW: Anesthesia and obesity. In Barash PG, Cullen BF, Stoelting RK [eds]: *Clinical Anesthesia*, pp 1038–1052. Philadelphia, Lippincott Williams & Wilkins, 2006). In *android* (central) obesity, adipose tissue is located predominantly in the upper body (truncal distribution) and is associated with increased oxygen consumption and increased incidence of cardiovascular disease. In *gynecoid* (peripheral) obesity, adipose tissue is located predominantly in the hips, buttocks, and thighs. This fat is less metabolically active so it is less closely associated with cardiovascular disease. *Ideal body weight* (IBW) is the weight associated with the lowest mortality rate for a given height and gender. In clinical practice, *body mass index* (BMI = weight in kg/height^2 in meters) is used to estimate the degree of obesity (*morbid obesity* is BMI >30 kg/m^2). Waist circumference (>102 in men and >89 in women) strongly correlates with abdominal fat and is an independent risk predictor of disease distribution of body fat.

I. PATHOPHYSIOLOGY OF OBESITY

A. **Respiratory System.** Fat accumulation on the thorax and abdomen decreases chest wall and lung compliance. Polycythemia from chronic hypoxemia contributes to increased total blood volume and may lead to pulmonary hypertension and cor pulmonale. Increased elastic resistance and decreased compliance of the chest wall further reduces total respiratory compliance while supine, leading to shallow and rapid breathing. Decreased pulmonary compliance leads to decreased functional residual capacity (FRC), vital capacity (VC), and total lung capacity (TLC). Reduced FRC can result in lung volumes below CC in the course of normal tidal ventilation, leading to small airway closure, ventilation–perfusion mismatch, right-to-left shunting, and arterial hypoxemia (anesthesia worsens this situation such that up to a 50% reduction in FRC occurs in the obese anesthetized patient compared with 20% in the nonobese). Obesity increases oxygen consumption and carbon dioxide production because of the metabolic activity of excess fat and the increased workload on supportive tissues. Arterial oxygen tension in morbidly obese patients' breathing room air is lower than that predicted for similarly aged nonobese subjects in both sitting and supine positions.

1. **Obstructive Sleep Apnea (OSA).** OSA (present in up to 50% of obese patients) is characterized by frequent episodes of apnea or hypopnea during sleep, snoring, and daytime symptoms, which include sleepiness, impaired concentration, memory problems, and morning headaches. OSA is defined as 10 seconds or more of total cessation of airflow despite continuous respiratory effort against a closed glottis. Long-term OSA can lead to the *obesity hypoventilation (Pickwickian) syndrome*, which is seen in 5 to 10% of morbidly obese patients. These patients also have an increased sensitivity to respiratory depressant effects of general anesthetics.

B. **Cardiovascular System.** Total blood volume is increased in the obese, but on a volume-to-weight basis, it is less than in nonobese individuals (50 mL/kg compared with 70 mL/kg). Cardiac output increases with increasing weight with resulting left ventricular hypertrophy, reduced compliance, and impairment of left ventricular filling (diastolic dysfunction and eventual biventricular failure). Obesity accelerates atherosclerosis but symptoms such as angina or exertional dyspnea occur only occasionally because morbidly obese patients often have very limited mobility and may appear asymptomatic even when they have significant cardiovascular disease. Intraoperative ventricular failure may occur from rapid intravenous fluid administration. Many obese patients have mild to moderate hypertension with a 3- to 4-mmHg increase in systolic and a 2-mmHg increase in diastolic arterial pressure for every 10 kg of weight gained.

C. **Gastrointestinal System.** Gastric volume and acidity may be increased, hepatic function altered (fatty liver infiltration, abnormal liver function tests), and drug metabolism adversely affected by obesity. Delayed gastric emptying may occur because of increased abdominal mass that causes antral distention, gastrin release, and a decrease in pH with parietal cell secretion. An increased incidence of hiatal hernia and gastroesophageal reflux may also increase aspiration risk. Gastric emptying has been said to be actually faster in the obese, especially with high energy content intake such as fat emulsions, but because of their larger gastric volume (up to 75% larger), the residual volume is larger. Nonpremedicated, nondiabetic fasting obese surgical patients who are free from significant gastroesophageal pathology should follow the same fasting guidelines as nonobese patients and be allowed to drink clear liquids (up to 300 mL does not adversely affect pH and volume of gastric contents at induction of anesthesia) until up to 2 hours before elective surgery. Morbidly obese patients who have undergone intestinal bypass surgery have a particularly high prevalence of hepatic dysfunction and cholelithiasis.

D. **Renal and Endocrine Systems.** Impaired glucose tolerance in the morbidly obese is reflected by a high prevalence of type II diabetes mellitus because of resistance of peripheral fatty tissues to insulin. Exogenous insulin may be required perioperatively even in obese patients with type II diabetes mellitus to oppose the catabolic response to surgery. With prolonged obesity there may be a loss of nephron function, with further impairment of natriuresis and further increases in arterial pressure.

E. **Airway.** Anatomic changes of obesity that affect the airway include limitation of movement of the atlantoaxial joint and cervical spine by upper thoracic and low cervical fat pads; excessive tissue folds in the mouth and pharynx; short thick neck; suprasternal, presternal, and posterior cervical fat; and a very thick submental fat pad. OSA predisposes to airway difficulties during anesthesia.

II. **PHARMACOLOGY.** The volume of the central compartment in which drugs are first distributed remains unchanged in obese patients, but absolute body water content and lean body and adipose tissue mass are increased, affecting lipophilic and polar drug distribution. Plasma albumin concentrations and plasma protein binding are not significantly changed by obesity. There is no significant difference in absorption and bioavailability of orally administered medication when comparing obese and normal weight subjects. Histologic abnormalities of the liver are common in the obese, with concomitant deranged liver function tests, but drug clearance is not usually affected. Renal clearance of drugs is increased in obesity as a result of increased renal blood flow and glomerular filtration rate (GFR). Highly lipophilic substances such as barbiturates and benzodiazepines show significant increases in volume of distribution (VD) for obese individuals. Less lipophilic compounds have little or no change in VD with obesity. Drugs with weak or moderate lipophilicity can be dosed on the basis of IBW or lean body mass (LBM). About 20 to 40% of an obese patient's increase in total body weight can be attributed to an increase in LBM. Adding 20% to the estimated IBW dose of hydrophilic medications (nondepolarizing muscle relaxants) is sufficient to include the extra lean mass.

III. SPECIFIC INTRAVENOUS AGENTS (Table 36-1)

IV. MEDICAL THERAPY FOR OBESITY. Medications used to treat obesity are formulated to reduce energy intake, increase energy utilization, or decrease absorption of nutrients.

A. **Sibutramine** inhibits the reuptake of norepinephrine to increase satiety after the onset of eating rather than reduce appetite. It does not promote the release of serotonin, unlike fenfluramine and dexfenfluramine, which may explain the absence of reports of sibutramine causing cardiac valvular lesions. Sibutramine also results in transient dose-related increases in systolic and diastolic blood (2 to 4 mmHg) and a slight increase in heart rate (3 to 5 bpm)

B. **Orlistat** blocks the absorption and digestion of dietary fat by binding lipases in the GI tract. Chronic dosing of

TABLE 36-1
DETERMINANTS OF DOSING FOR INTRAVENOUS DRUGS IN THE OBESE PATIENT

Drug	Dosing	Comments
Propofol	Induction: IBW	Systemic clearance and V_D at steady state correlates
	Maintenance: TBW	High affinity for excess fat and other well-perfused organs. High hepatic extraction and conjugation
Thiopental	TBW	Increased V_D
		Increased blood volume, cardiac output, and muscle mass
		Increased absolute dose
		Prolonged duration of action
Midazolam	TBW	Central V_D increases in line with body weight
		Increased absolute dose
		Prolonged sedation because higher loading doses needed to achieve adequate serum concentrations
Succinylcholine	TBW	Plasma cholinesterase activity increases in proportion to body weight
		Increased absolute dose
Vecuronium	IBW	Recovery may be delayed if given according to
		TBW because of increased V_D and impaired hepatic clearance
Rocuronium	IBW	Faster onset and longer duration of action
Atracurium and Cisatracurium	TBW	Pharmacokinetics and pharmacodynamics not altered in obese subjects
		Absolute clearance, V_D, and elimination half-time do not change.
		Unchanged dose per unit body weight without prolongation of recovery because of organ independent elimination
Fentanyl and Sufentanil	TBW	Increased V_D and elimination half-time, which correlates positively with degree of obesity
	Induction: TBW	Distributes as extensively in excess body mass as in lean tissues
	Maintenance: IBW	Dose should account for total body mass
		Fentanyl dosing based on a derived pharmacokinetic mass correlates better with clearance
Remifentanil	IBW	Systemic clearance and V_D corrected per kg ot TBW—significantly smaller in the obese
		Pharmacokinetics is similar in obese and non-obese patients
		Age and lean body mass should be considered for dosing

IBW = ideal body weight; TBW = total body weight; VD = volume of distribution.

orlistat results in an increase in warfarin's anticoagulant effect because of decreased absorption of vitamin K. This leads to an abnormal prothrombin time (PT) with a normal partial thromboplastin time (PTT), because of deficiency of clotting factors II, VII, IX, and X. The resulting coagulopathy should be corrected 6 to 24 hours before elective surgery with a vitamin K analogue such as phytonadione and fresh frozen plasma for emergency surgery or active bleeding.

V. BARIATRIC SURGERY.

Bariatric surgery encompasses a variety of surgical procedures (classified as malabsorptive, restrictive, or combined) used to treat morbid obesity. Gastric restriction (gastroplasty) creates a small upper pouch (15 to 30 mL) in the stomach and is the most commonly performed bariatric procedure in the United States. Adjustable gastric banding (AGB) is a restrictive gastric operation usually done by minimally invasive laparoscopic approach. Laparoscopic bariatric surgery is minimally invasive with less postoperative pain, lower morbidity, and faster recovery. Profound muscle relaxation is important during laparoscopic bariatric procedures to facilitate ventilation and to maintain an adequate working space for visualization, safe manipulation of laparoscopic instruments, and extraction of excised tissues. Laparoscopic bariatric surgery requires maneuvering the operating table into various surgically favorable positions (a malleable "bean-bag" in addition to belts and straps, may help to keep the patient secured). Anesthesia personnel may be asked to facilitate the proper placement of an intragastric balloon to help the surgeon size the gastric pouch and also facilitate performance of leak tests with saline or methylene blue through a nasogastric (NG) tube. After the gastric pouch is created, insertion of an NG tube should be aided by viewing the lasparoscope monitor and carefully watching to avoid disruption of the anastomosis. Cephalad displacement of the diaphragm and carina from a pneumoperitoneum during laparoscopy can cause a firmly secured endotracheal tube to displace into a mainstem bronchus.

A. **Rhabdomyolysis** is more common in morbidly obese patients undergoing laparoscopic procedures when compared to the open procedure. Unexplained elevations in serum creatinine and creatine phosphokinase (CPK) levels or complaints of buttock, hip, or shoulder pain in the postoperative period should raise suspicion of rhabdomyolysis and should be investigated.

B. **Gastric electrical stimulation** by means of an implantable gastric stimulator (IGS) causes smooth muscles of the stomach to stop peristalsis so that the patient feels full. Possible lead dislodgment from violent stomach contractions during postoperative nausea and vomiting is a consideration for the anesthesiologist. The stimulating pulses emitted by the IGS can be picked up on the ECG, which may lead to false readings.

VI. PREOPERATIVE CONSIDERATIONS

A. **Preoperative Evaluation** (Table 36-2)

B. **Concurrent, Preoperative, and Prophylactic Medications.** The patient's usual medications should be continued until the time of surgery with the possible exception of insulin and oral hypoglycemics. Antibiotic prophylaxis is important because of an increased incidence of wound infections in the obese. Anxiolysis and prophylaxis against both aspiration pneumonitis and deep vein thrombosis (DVT) should be addressed at premedication. Morbid obesity is a major independent risk factor for sudden death from acute postoperative pulmonary embolism (PE). Subcutaneous heparin 5,000 IU administered before surgery and repeated every 8 to 12 hours until the patient is fully mobile reduces the risk of DVT. Other risk factors include venous stasis disease, BMI ≥ 60, truncal obesity, and obesity hypoventilation syndrome (OHS)/sleep apnea syndrome (SAS). It is suggested that enoxaparin dosing in the obese be varied with age and lean body mass.

C. **Airway.** Neck circumference has been identified as the single biggest predictor of problematic intubation in morbidly obese patients (probability of a problematic intubation is approximately 5% with a 40-cm neck circumference compared with a 35% probability at 60-cm neck circumference.

TABLE 36-2

PREOPERATIVE CONSIDERATIONS IN OBESE PATIENTS

Evaluation of cardiorespiratory systems and airway (previous
anesthetic experiences)

Evaluate for systemic hypertension, pulmonary hypertension,
signs of ventricular failure and ischemic heart disease

Examine for signs of cardiac failure (elevated jugular venous
pressure, added heart sounds, pulmonary crackles,
hepatomegaly and peripheral edema activity)

Chest radiographs (evidence of underlying lung disease and
prominent pulmonary arteries)

Metabolic and nutritional abnormalities (scheduled for repeat
bariatric surgery)

Postoperative polyneuropathy (vitamin and nutritional
deficiency, known as acute postgastric reduction surgery
[APGARS]) neuropathy

Protracted postoperative vomiting, hyporeflexia, and muscular
weakness (implications for neuromuscular blocking drugs)

Electrolyte and coagulation indices should be checked before
surgery (vitamin K analog or fresh frozen plasma may be
needed)

Evidence of OSA and OHS should be sought preoperatively
(OSA patients on a continuous positive airway pressure
[CPAP] device at home should be instructed to bring it with
them to the hospital as it may be needed postoperatively)

Possibility of invasive monitoring, prolonged intubation, and
postoperative mechanical ventilation should be discussed
with the patient

Arterial blood gas measurement (routine pulmonary function
tests and liver function tests are not cost-effective in
asymptomatic obese patients)

VII. INTRAOPERATIVE CONSIDERATIONS

A. **Positioning.** Specially designed tables or two regular
operating tables may be required for safe anesthesia
and surgery in obese patients (regular operating tables
have a maximum weight limit of approximately 205
kg). Brachial plexus injury, ulnar neuropathy, and
lower extremity nerve injuries are frequent. Supine
positioning causes ventilatory impairment and inferior
vena cava and aortic compression in obese patients.
FRC and oxygenation are decreased further with
supine positioning. Trendelenburg positioning (avoid if

possible), as may be required during bariatric procedures, further worsens FRC. The head-up reverse Trendelenburg position provides the longest safe apnea period (SAP) during induction of anesthesia. Lateral decubitus positioning allows for better diaphragmatic excursion and should be favored over prone positioning whenever the surgical procedure permits.

B. **Monitoring.** Invasive arterial pressure monitoring may be indicated for the morbidly obese patient, those patients with cardiopulmonary disease, and for those patients where the noninvasive blood pressure cuff may not fit properly. Blood pressure measurements can be falsely elevated if a cuff is too small.

C. **Induction, Intubation, and Maintenance.** Adequate preoxygenation is vital in obese patients because of rapid desaturation after loss of consciousness as a result of increased oxygen consumption and decreased FRC. Larger doses of induction agents may be required by obese patients because blood volume, muscle mass and cardiac output increase linearly with the degree of obesity. If a difficult intubation is anticipated, awake intubation utilizing topical or regional anesthesia is a prudent approach. Towels or folded blankets under the shoulders and head can compensate for the exaggerated flexed position of posterior cervical fat. Continuous infusion of a short-acting intravenous agent, such as propofol, or any of the inhalational agents or a combination may be used to maintain anesthesia. Evidence does not support the suggestion that significant delayed recovery and awakening from volatile anesthetic agents occurs in obese patients when compared to the non-obese. Rapid elimination and analgesic properties make nitrous oxide an attractive choice for anesthesia in obese patients, but high oxygen demand in this patient population limits its use. Positive end-expiratory pressure (PEEP) is the only ventilatory parameter that has consistently been shown to improve respiratory function in obese subjects. PEEP may, however, decrease venous return and cardiac output.

D. **Regional anesthesia** is a useful alternative to general anesthesia in the morbidly obese patient as it may help avoid potential intubation difficulties. It can, however, be technically difficult because of inability to identify usual bony landmarks. Epidural vascular engorgement and fatty infiltration reduce the volume of the space, making dose requirements of local anesthetics for epidural anesthesia 20 to 25% less in obese patients. Subarachnoid blocks are not technically as difficult as epidural blocks but the height of a subarachnoid block in obese patients can be unpredictable.

VIII. POSTOPERATIVE CONSIDERATIONS

A. **Emergence.** Prompt extubation reduces the likelihood that the morbidly obese patient, who may have underlying cardiopulmonary disease, will become ventilator dependent. Supplemental oxygen should be administrated after extubation. There is an increased incidence of atelectasis in morbidly obese patients after general anesthesia, which persists into the postoperative period.

B. **Postoperative Analgesia.** Perioperative use of regional anesthesia and analgesia reduces the incidence of postoperative respiratory complications. Potential advantages of epidural analgesia in obese patients include prevention of DVT, improved analgesia, and earlier recovery of intestinal motility. Delayed respiratory depression is one of the known complications of central neuraxial opioids.

IX. RESUSCITATION. The possible need for cardiopulmonary resuscitation should be entertained during anesthesia for the morbidly obese. Chest compressions may not be effective and mechanical compression devices may be required. The maximum 400 joules of energy on regular defibrillators is sufficient for the morbidly obese because their chest wall is usually not much thicker, but the higher transthoracic impedance from the fat may obligate several attempts. The laryngeal mask airway (LMA) and the esophageal tracheal Combitube® are temporary supraglottic airway devices that are useful during resuscitation of the obese.

CHAPTER 37 ■ ANESTHESIA AND GASTROINTESTINAL DISORDERS

I. ESOPHAGUS

A. **Upper Esophageal Sphincter.** The cricopharyngeus muscle, one of the two inferior muscles of the pharynx, together with the circular fibers of the upper esophagus, acts as the functional *upper esophageal sphincter* (UES) at the pharyngoesophageal junction (Ogunnaike BO, Whitten CW: Anesthesia and gastrointestinal disorders. In Barash PG, Cullen BF, Stoelting RK [eds]: *Clinical Anesthesia*, pp 1052–1060. Philadelphia, Lippincott Williams & Wilkins, 2006). The UES helps prevent aspiration by sealing off the upper esophagus from the hypopharynx in conscious healthy patients. UES function is impaired during both normal sleep and anesthesia. Most anesthetic agents, except ketamine, will reduce UES tone and increase the likelihood of regurgitation of material from the esophagus into the hypopharynx.

B. The border between the stomach and esophagus is formed by the *lower esophageal sphincter* (LES) (Table 37-1). The LES is the major barrier to gastroesophageal reflux. The major physiological derangement in gastroesophageal reflux is a reduction in LES pressure. The difference between the LES pressure and gastric pressure is "barrier pressure" and is more important than the LES tone in the production of gastroesophageal reflux. Anesthetic agents that may reduce the barrier pressure, thereby reducing LES pressure, include thiopental, propofol, opioids, anticholinergics, and inhaled anesthetics, while antiemetics, cholinergics, antacids, and succinylcholine increase LES pressure. Nondepolarizing muscle relaxants and H2-receptor antagonists have no effect on LES pressure. Cricoid pressure in both conscious and unconscious patients decreases LES tone because of a significant reduction in esophageal barrier pressure while gastric pressure remains normal. The evidence that succinylcholine increases LES tone, while cricoid pressures decreases

TABLE 37-1

FACTORS AFFECTING LOWER ESOPHAGEAL SPHINCTER TONE

Decrease tone	Increase tone	No change in tone
Inhaled anesthetics	Anticholinesterases—	H2-receptor
Opioids	neostigmine,	antagonists—
	edrophonium	cimetidine,
		ranitidine
Anticholinergics—	Cholinergics	Nondepolarizing
atropine,	Acetylcholine	muscle
glycopyrrolate		relaxants—
		atracurium
		vecuronium
Thiopental	Alpha adrenergic	
	stimulants	
Propofol		Propranolol
Beta-blockers	Antacids	
Ganglion blockers	Metoclopramide	
Tricyclic	Gastrin	
antidepressants		
Secretin	Serotonin	
Glucagon	Histamine	
Cricoid pressure	Pancreatic	
	polypeptide	
Obesity	Metoprolol	
Hiatal hernia		
Pregnancy		

LES tone, makes the necessity for application of cricoid pressure during a rapid sequence induction questionable.

II. **STOMACH.** The stomach is very distensible with the capacity to store large amounts of material (up to 1.5 L of fluid) without a significant increase in intragastric pressure. There is a dose-response relationship in the severity of aspiration pneumonitis for both gastric volume and acidity that directly reaches the lung. Human breast milk predisposes to an increased severity of aspiration pneumonitis when compared to other types of milk.

III. **PROTECTIVE AIRWAY REFLEXES** include apnea with laryngospasm, which causes closure of both the false and true vocal cords and coughing. Premedicated and anesthetized patients and the elderly have reduced airway reflexes, putting them at an increased risk for perioperative aspiration pneumonitis.

IV. REDUCING PERIOPERATIVE ASPIRATION RISK
(Table 37-2)

A. **Control of gastric contents** involves minimizing intake, increasing gastric emptying with prokinetics, and reducing gastric volume and acidity with a nasogastric tube, antacids, H2-receptor antagonists, and proton pump inhibitors (PPIs). Clear liquids can be administered to children and adults up to 2 and 3 hours, respectively, prior to anesthesia without increased risk for regurgitation and aspiration. Altered physiological states (pregnancy and diabetes mellitus) and GI pathology (bowel obstruction and peritonitis) may adversely affect the rate of gastric emptying, thereby increasing aspiration risk. The extent of delayed gastric emptying with diabetes mellitus correlates well with the presence of autonomic neuropathy. The American Society of Anesthesiologists (ASA) recommends a fasting period of 4 hours for breast milk, 6 hours for both nonhuman milk and

---

TABLE 37-2
METHODS TO REDUCE THE RISK OF REGURGITATION AND PULMONARY ASPIRATION

Minimize intake
  Adequate preoperative fasting
  Clear liquids only if necessary
Increase gastric emptying
  Prokinetics (metoclopramide)
Reduce gastric volume and acidity
  Nasogastric tube
  Nonparticulate antacid (sodium citrate)
  H2-receptor antagonists (famotidine)
  Proton pump inhibitors (lansoprazole)
Airway management and protection
  Cricoid pressure
  Cuffed endotracheal intubation
  Esophageal-tracheal combitube
  Proseal LMA

LMA = laryngeal mask airway.

infant formula, and also 6 hours for a light solid meal. Presence of a nasogastric (NG) tube does not guarantee an empty stomach and may impair the function of the LES and UES, but it does not diminish the effectiveness of cricoid pressure. The NG tube also provides a direct connection to the outside for passive drainage of gastric contents and is best left in place and open to freely drain during induction of anesthesia.

B. **Prevention of Pulmonary Aspiration**

1. **Cricoid pressure** may be used to occlude the upper end of the esophagus to prevent passive regurgitation of gastric contents and decrease the risk of pulmonary aspiration during rapid sequence induction, intubation technique. The technique has not been subjected to outcome analysis as to its effectiveness in patients. Also, application of cricoid pressure reduces LES tone and may cause the esophagus to be displaced to the side rather than to be compressed. The force applied to the cricoid cartilage should be sufficient to prevent aspiration but not so great as to cause airway obstruction or allow the possibility of esophageal rupture if vomiting occurs. The recommended force is estimated to range between 20N and 44N. Awake patients experience pain, coughing, and retching with pressures greater than 20N, so this amount of force should be applied only after loss of consciousness. A reasonable approach is to apply 10N force to the cricoid in the awake state and increase to 30N after loss of consciousness. Cricoid pressure by itself, before laryngoscopy and intubation, increases the incidence of hypertension and tachycardia during induction of anesthesia.

C. **Airway Protection.** A cuffed endotracheal tube is the mainstay of prevention of regurgitated material from reaching the trachea and lungs. Of the other airway devices used, the laryngeal mask airway (LMA) reduces barrier pressure at the LES with an increased incidence of reflux in comparison with the cuffed endotracheal tube.

V. **THE INTESTINES.** The small intestine (SI) is the site of most of the absorption of fluids and nutrients from the GI tract. Parasympathetic stimulation and antagonism increases and decreases the activity of the SI respectively. Suppression of sympathetic activity increases SI activity while stimulation results in a decrease. Hypokalemia, peritonitis, and laparotomy all suppress intestinal activity for up to 48 hours. Neostigmine increases colonic activity while morphine and other opioids decrease both activity and tone.

A. **Splanchnic Blood Flow.** Splanchnic blood flow is influenced predominantly by the autonomic nervous system. Alpha-adrenergic stimulation leads to vasoconstriction and beta-2 adrenergic stimulation causes vasodilation. Splanchnic vascular resistance increases with severe hemorrhage, which helps divert blood flow to other vital organs. Hypocapnia significantly reduces splanchnic blood flow while hypercapnia does the opposite. Neostigmine reduces mesenteric blood flow because of induced exaggerated contraction. Atropine partially offsets the blood flow reduction.

B. **Postoperative Anastomotic Leakage.** Anastomotic leakage after colon surgery can be related to patient factors (anemia, comorbidity), surgical factors (bowel preparation, operative expertise), and anesthesia and pain management–related factors (morphine, epidural analgesia, neostigmine). Anesthesia-related factors increase the incidence of anastomotic dehiscence by increasing intestinal motility and intraluminar pressure. Prokinetics like metoclopramide have been associated with colonic anastomotic dehiscence during the early postoperative period; however, clinical observations and animal studies have largely discounted the suggestions that neostigmine has a deleterious effect on bowel anastomosis.

C. **Postoperative Ileus.** Multiple mechanisms contribute to ileus after intestinal surgery (Table 37-3). Epidural analgesia that includes local anesthetics has been most effective in minimizing postoperative ileus. Minimally invasive surgery (including laparoscopy) reduces inflammatory responses, thereby reducing ileus; so also does early enteral nutrition and early mobilization.

D. **Mesenteric traction syndrome** consists of sudden tachycardia, hypotension, and decreases in PaO_2. Nonsteroidal anti-inflammatory drugs and aspirin, which inhibit cyclooxygenase, significantly ameliorate

TABLE 37-3
MECHANISMS OF ILEUS AFTER ABDOMINAL SURGERY

Abdominal pain (activates a spinal reflex that inhibits motility)
Sympathetic hyperactivity
Opioids
Electrolyte imbalance
Immobility
Intestinal wall swelling from fluid administration

these clinical features, suggesting a prostacyclin mediated etiology. Prophylactic administration of H1 and H2 antihistamines also reduces the incidence of dysrhythmias as a result of the mesenteric traction syndrome.

E. **Nitrous Oxide and the Bowel.** Because nitrous oxide is 30 times more soluble than nitrogen in blood, nitrous oxide diffuses into gas-containing body cavities from the blood stream faster than the nitrogen in those cavities can diffuse out into circulation. This can contribute to excessive distension of gas-containing bowels, possible bowel ischemia, and increased difficulty with surgical exposure. Factors that determine the extent of distension include the amount of gas within the bowel, the duration of nitrous oxide administration, and the concentration of nitrous oxide used. Use of 80% nitrous oxide can potentially result in a 5-fold increase in bowel gas, whereas use of a 50% concentration can result in no more than a doubling of bowel gas. Nitrous oxide is best avoided in situations when the bowels are distended. On the other hand, use of low concentrations of nitrous oxide during elective abdominal operations where no significant amount of gas is present in the bowels is reasonable.

VI. **CARCINOID TUMORS** are usually asymptomatic although nonspecific symptoms such as abdominal pain, diarrhea, intermittent intestinal obstruction, and GI bleeding are occasionally seen. Nonmetastatic carcinoid tumors secrete hormones that are usually transported to the liver through the portal vein where they are subsequently inactivated. Carcinoid tumors, especially those arising in the midgut, secrete a variety of hormones, mediators, and biogenic amines including large quantities of serotonin that produce increased platelet serotonin levels and increased urinary levels of 5-hydroxy-indole-acetic-acid (5-HIAA), a metabolite of serotonin. Other secreted substances include histamine, substance P, catecholamines (including dopamine), bradykinin, tachykinin, motilin, corticotrophin, prostaglandins, kallikrein, and neurotensin. Bradykinin produces cutaneous flushing, bronchospasm and hypotension while serotonin causes hypertension or hypotension.

A. **Carcinoid Syndrome.** Metastatic carcinoid tumor releases vasoactive peptides into the systemic circulation, which leads to signs and symptoms (bronchoconstriction, hypotension, hypertension, diarrhea, carcinoid heart disease). There is no correlation between the blood level of serotonin and the severity of symptoms.

B. **Carcinoid heart disease** is seen in up to 60% of patients with carcinoid syndrome. Cardiac involvement is usually right sided affecting tricuspid (tricuspid regurgitation) and pulmonary valves. The predominance of right-sided cardiac lesions suggests that the substances secreted from liver metastasis into the hepatic vein never reach the left side of the heart because of pulmonary metabolism.

C. **Perioperative Management of the Carcinoid Patient.** Complete surgical excision is the most effective treatment for carcinoid tumors. Management should focus on blocking histamine and serotonin receptors and avoidance of drugs that facilitate mediator release from tumor cells. Mediator release can be triggered by opioids and muscle relaxants that release histamine. Patients with carcinoid may have diarrhea and high gastric output. Therefore fluid resuscitation may be required, and serum electrolytes and glucose should be measured at regular intervals.

1. **Somatostatin** is a GI regulatory peptide that reduces the amount of serotonin released from carcinoid tumors. Somatostatin has a very short half-life of about 3 minutes and must therefore be given as an infusion.

2. **Octreotide** is a synthetic somatostatin analogue with a half-life of approximately 2.5 hours. Preoperative preparation should include 100 mg octreotide

subcutaneously three times daily in the preceding 2 weeks. Preoperative anxiolytics should be administered to prevent stress-triggered release of serotonin, and patients receiving octreotide preoperatively should continue with their normal dose on the morning of surgery. Octreotide effectively treats intraoperative carcinoid crises.

D. **Anesthetic Management.** Any of the currently available induction agents and muscle relaxants including propofol, etomidate, synthetic opioids, vecuronium, cisatracurium, and rocuronium can be used successfully. Caution should be exercised with drugs such as thiopental and succinylcholine that can release histamine. All current inhalation agents can be used successfully; however, desflurane may be the better choice in patients with liver metastasis because of its low rate of metabolism. Administration of octreotide prior to manipulation of the tumor will attenuate adverse hemodynamic responses. The sympathetic blockade produced by epidural or spinal anesthesia may worsen hypotension, which can be minimized by dosing the epidural catheter with opioids or dilute local anesthetic solutions. Intraoperative hypotension from sympathetic blockade should be treated with volume expansion and intravenous infusion of octreotide rather than with sympathomimetics like ephedrine, which can trigger release of vasoactive substances from carcinoid tumors. Intense hemodynamic monitoring and octreotide administration should continue into the postoperative period as secretion of vasoactive substances can still occur from residual tumor or metastasis.

CHAPTER 38 ■ ANESTHESIA FOR MINIMALLY INVASIVE PROCEDURES

I. **MINIMAL ACCESS INTRA-ABDOMINAL GYNECOLOGIC PROCEDURES.** Minimal access surgical procedures produce significantly less trauma than conventional open procedures, with the potential advantages of reduced postoperative pain, shorter hospital stays, more rapid return to normal activities, and significant cost savings (Cunningham AJ, Nolan C: Anesthesia for minimally invasive procedures. In Barash PG, Cullen BF, Stoelting RK [eds]: *Clinical Anesthesia*, pp 1061–1071. Philadelphia, Lippincott Williams & Wilkins, 2006).

A. Laparoscopic cholecystectomy is a routinely performed procedure and has replaced conventional open cholecystectomy as the procedure of choice for symptomatic cholelithiasis.

B. Laparoscopy produces significant physiological changes associated with peritoneal insufflation and alteration in patient position, which can have a major impact on cardiopulmonary function.

1. Specific intraoperative complications as a result of traumatic injuries and gas embolism may occur and present significant challenges in anesthetic management.

2. The duration of some procedures, the risk of vascular or visceral injury, and difficulty in evaluating blood loss add to the anesthetic challenge.

3. The physiologic effects of intraperitoneal carbon dioxide insufflation combined with variations in patient positioning can have a major impact on cardiorespiratory function particularly in elderly patients with comorbidities.

4. Intraoperative complications may include traumatic injuries associated with blind trocar insertion, gas embolism, pneumothorax, and surgical emphysema associated with extraperitoneal insufflation.

II. SURGICAL TECHNIQUE

A. Laparoscopic operative techniques involve intraperitoneal insufflation of carbon dioxide (Veress needle).
   1. The aortic bifurcation lies directly beneath the umbilicus, especially if the Trendelenburg position has already been established.
   2. Modern laparoscopic insufflators automatically terminate gas flow when a preset intra-abdominal pressure (IAP) of 10 to 15 mmHg is reached.

B. Patients are usually placed in the Trendelenburg position for laparoscopic gynecologic procedures while laparoscopic cholecystectomy usually involves change to a steep reverse Trendelenburg with left lateral tilt to facilitate retraction of the gallbladder fundus.

III. PHYSIOLOGICAL EFFECTS OF LAPAROSCOPY
(Fig. 38-1)

A. **Cardiovascular Effects**
   1. The principal physiologic responses are an increase in systemic vascular resistance (SVR), mean arterial blood pressure (MAP), and myocardial filling pressures, accompanied by an initial fall in cardiac index (CI), with little change in heart rate.
   2. **Mechanical Effects of Pneumoperitoneum**
      a. Increased IAP associated with pneumoperitoneum may compress venous capacitance vessels causing an initial increase, followed by a sustained decrease in preload.
      b. Compression of the arterial vasculature increases afterload and may result in a marked increase in calculated SVR.
      c. Cardiac index may be significantly reduced and the magnitude of this effect is proportional to the intra-abdominal pressure achieved.
   3. **Neurohumoral Response.** Hypercapnia and pneumoperitoneum are likely to cause stimulation of the sympathetic nervous system and catecholamine release.

B. **CO_2 Absorption**
   1. Significant hypercapnia and acidosis may occur during laparoscopy as a result of CO_2 absorption.
   2. Hypercapnia may cause a decrease in myocardial contractility and lower the cardiac arrhythmia threshold.

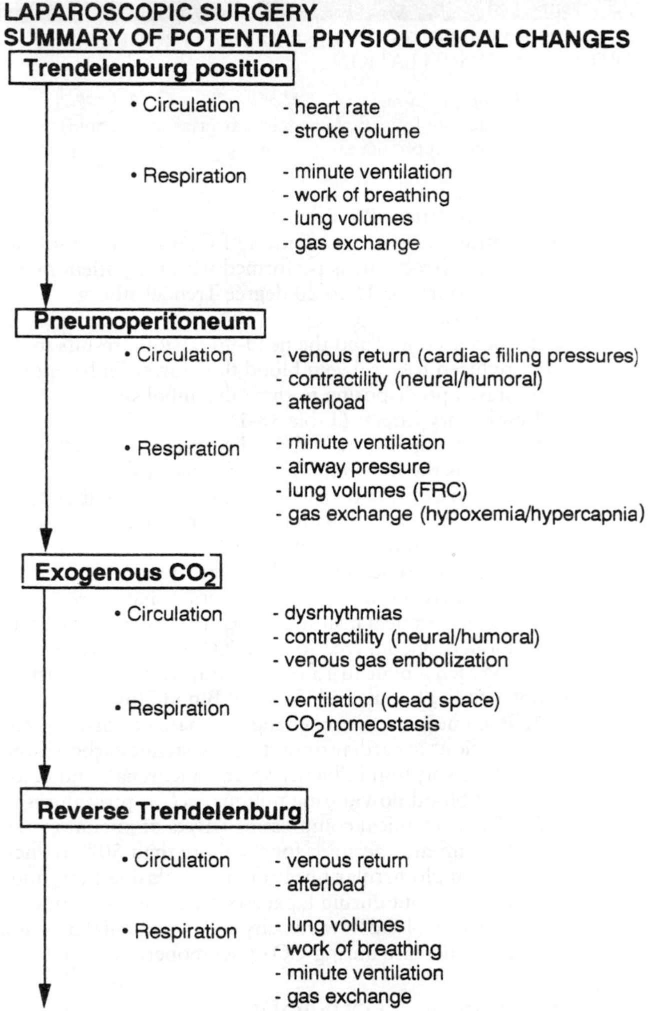

LAPAROSCOPIC SURGERY
SUMMARY OF POTENTIAL PHYSIOLOGICAL CHANGES

| Trendelenburg position |

- Circulation - heart rate
  - stroke volume

- Respiration - minute ventilation
  - work of breathing
  - lung volumes
  - gas exchange

| Pneumoperitoneum |

- Circulation - venous return (cardiac filling pressures)
  - contractility (neural/humoral)
  - afterload

- Respiration - minute ventilation
  - airway pressure
  - lung volumes (FRC)
  - gas exchange (hypoxemia/hypercapnia)

| Exogenous CO_2 |

- Circulation - dysrhythmias
  - contractility (neural/humoral)
  - venous gas embolization

- Respiration - ventilation (dead space)
  - CO_2 homeostasis

| Reverse Trendelenburg |

- Circulation - venous return
  - afterload

- Respiration - lung volumes
  - work of breathing
  - minute ventilation
  - gas exchange

FIGURE 38-1. Physiologic changes that may accompany laparoscopic surgery.

TABLE 38-1

MECHANICAL EFFECTS ON RESPIRATION PRODUCED BY ABDOMINAL INSUFFLATION

Reductions in lung volumes
Decreases in functional residual capacity (arterial hypoxemia)
Decreases in lung compliance

   C. **Effect of Patient Position**
      1. Intraperitoneal insufflation of CO_2 for laparoscopic cholecystectomy is performed with the patient in a horizontal or 15 to 20 degree Trendelenburg position.
      2. Increased IAP and the head-up position results in reduced femoral vein blood flow lower limb venous stasis, predisposing to thromboembolism.
   D. **Respiratory Effects** (Table 38-1)
   E. **Gas Exchange Effects—CO_2 absorption**
      1. CO_2 is the insufflation gas of choice for laparoscopic surgery (unlike nitrous oxide it does not support combustion and therefore can be used safely with diathermy).
      2. Carbon dioxide absorption is greater during extraperitoneal (pelvic) insufflation than during intraperitoneal insufflation. During uneventful pneumoperitoneum creation, $PaCO_2$ progressively rises to reach a plateau 15 to 30 minutes after insufflation.
   F. **Splanchnic, Renal, and Cerebral Blood Flow**
      1. Pneumoperitoneum, changes in patient position, reductions in cardiac output, and systemic carbon dioxide absorption influence splanchnic, renal, and cerebral blood flow during minimal access procedures.
      2. The mechanical compressive effects of pneumoperitoneum may account for the more than 50% reduction in glomerular filtration, renal plasma flow, and urine output during laparoscopic cholecystectomy.
      3. Cerebral blood flow velocity and intracranial pressure both increase during CO_2 pneumoperitoneum.

IV. ANESTHETIC TECHNIQUE

   A. The high level of sympathetic denervation required, the frequent need for change of patient position, and the mandatory pneumoperitoneum may be associated with adverse ventilatory and circulatory responses complicating perioperative management.

B. Airway Management
1. Endotracheal intubation and controlled mechanical ventilation comprise the accepted anesthetic technique to reduce the increase in $PaCO_2$ and avoid ventilatory compromise because of pneumoperitoneum and initial Trendelenburg position.
2. The laryngeal mask airway (LMA) has been used widely during pelvic laparoscopy.
3. Choice of neuromuscular blocking drug depends on anticipated duration of surgery and individual drug side effect profile. Reversal of residual neuromuscular blockade with neostigmine may increase the incidence of postoperative nausea and vomiting.

C. Monitoring
1. $ETCO_2$ is most commonly used as a noninvasive indicator of $PaCO_2$ in assessing the adequacy of ventilation during laparoscopic procedures.
2. Persistent refractory hypercapnia or acidosis may require deflation of the pneumoperitoneum, lowering of the insufflation pressure, or conversion to an open procedure.

D. Nitrous Oxide
1. The use of nitrous oxide (N_2O) during laparoscopic procedures is controversial because of concerns regarding its ability to diffuse into bowel lumen causing distension and to increase postoperative nausea (not a consistent observation).
2. Avoidance of N_2O is balanced against the increased risk of awareness.

E. Analgesia
1. Opioids remain an important component of a balanced general anesthetic technique for minimal access procedures.
   a. Opioid-induced spasm of the sphincter of Oddi may be antagonized by including glucagon and naloxone.
   b. Reduction of opioid dose with multimodal analgesia regimes may reduce the incidence of PONV.

V. SPECIFIC INTRAOPERATIVE COMPLICATIONS
(Table 38-2)

VI. POSTOPERATIVE CONSIDERATIONS

A. Laparoscopic surgery may reduce postoperative pulmonary complications by avoiding the restrictive

TABLE 38-2

INTRAOPERATIVE COMPLICATIONS DURING MINIMAL ACCESS PROCEDURES

Major vascular injuries (unexplained hypotension)
Gastrointestinal tract perforations
Hepatic and splenic tears
Cardiac arrhythmias
Inadvertent extraperitoneal insufflation (extensive
  subcutaneous emphysema; increased CO_2 absorption)
Pneumothorax, Pneumomediastinum and Pneumopericardium
Gas Embolism
  Venous CO_2 embolism is associated with profound
  hypotension, cyanosis, and asystole after creation of the
  pneumoperitoneum.
  Signs and severity of effects of CO_2 embolism may include
  hypotension with cardiovascular collapse, hypoxemia, and
  an associated decrease in $ETCO_2$

TABLE 38-3

VIDEO-ASSISTED THORACIC SURGERY

Lungs
  Pneumonectomy
  Lobectomy
  Wedge, subsegmental, segmental resection
  Resection of pulmonary metastases
  Excision of blebs and bullae
Heart
  Pericardiocentesis
  Pericardiectomy
  Insertion of implantable cardioverter defibrillator
Esophagus
  Esophagectomy
  Repair of esophageal perforation
  Fundoplication
Mediastinum
  Excision of tumors/cysts
Sympathetic nervous system
  Transthoracic endoscopic sympathectomy
Vagus
  Truncal vagotomy
Thoracic spine
  Disc herniation
  Deformity correction
  Abscess drainage

pattern of respiration that usually follows upper abdominal surgery.
B. Increased IAP during pneumoperitoneum may cause venous stasis, which can increase the potential for deep vein thrombosis and pulmonary embolism.

VII. AMBULATORY LAPAROSCOPIC CHOLECYSTECTOMY

A. The minimally invasive nature of laparoscopic surgery facilitating earlier mobilization, and feeding, and reduced hospital stay has extended the range of procedures that can be performed on a day-case basis to include laparoscopic cholecystectomy.
B. Early discharge will lead to occasional delays in diagnosis and management of postoperative complications.

VIII. VIDEO-ASSISTED THORACIC SURGERY (VATS)
(Table 38-3)

A. Most VATS are performed under general anesthesia with one-lung ventilation (OLV) provided through a double-lumen endobronchial tube placed in the left mainstem bronchus and verified bronchoscopically.
B. Continuous pulse oximetry and end-tidal carbon dioxide tension ($PETCO_2$) are measured.

CHAPTER 39 ■ ANESTHESIA AND THE LIVER

The liver occupies the center of a diverse spectrum of vital physiologic functions and plays an essential role in maintaining perioperative homeostasis (Kaufman BS, Roccaforte JD. Anesthesia and the liver. In Barash PG, Cullen BF, Stoelting RK [eds]: *Clinical Anesthesia*, pp 1072–1111. Philadelphia, Lippincott Williams & Wilkins, 2006). The liver is a remarkably resilient organ, with unparalleled regenerative capacity and substantial physiologic reserves (normal function may be present in humans when as much as 80% of the organ has been resected). A careful preoperative history and physical examination will help identify patients in whom laboratory evaluation of liver function is appropriate.

I. **HEPATIC ANATOMY.** The liver is the largest gland in the human body with a median weight of 1.8 kg in men and 1.4 kg in women.

A. **Lobes Versus Segments of the Liver**
   1. The customary division of the liver into the right, left, caudate, and quadrate lobes is derived from the topographic anatomy, with the falciform ligament separating the right and left lobes (Fig. 39-1). This anatomic description does not correspond to the branches of the liver's vascular supply and therefore is of limited clinical and physiologic significance.
   2. The liver can be divided on a different plane into right and left hemi-livers, which have their own blood supplies and duct drainage (this anatomic arrangement facilitates limited segmental resection of the liver with relatively bloodless surgical dissection along the planes between segments and thereby prevents major disruption of hepatobiliary function).

B. **Vascular Supply of the Liver**
   1. The liver receives about 25% of the cardiac output, and therefore has an average blood flow between 100 and 130 mL/min/100 g (sources of blood flow are hepatic artery and portal vein).

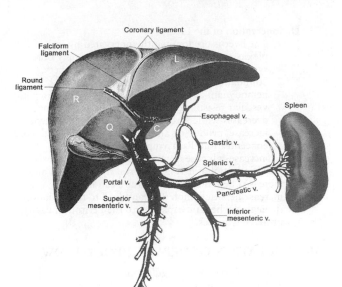

FIGURE 39-1. Schematic representation depicting the lobar classification of the liver and the extrahepatic portal venous circulation.

2. The hepatic artery provides about 25% of total hepatic blood flow but nearly 50% of hepatic oxygen delivery.
3. The portal vein provides the remaining 75% of total hepatic blood flow (partially deoxygenated) and 50% of hepatic oxygen delivery.

C. **Intrahepatic Circulation**
1. The portal vein and hepatic artery enter the liver at the porta hepatis, where the larger bile ducts join and accompany them.
2. Hepatic arterial pressure is similar to aortic pressure while the mean portal vein pressure is approximately 6 to 10 mm Hg.
3. Blood drains from the hepatic sinusoids into the central vein and then flows through sublobular veins that join to form one of the three major hepatic veins (right, middle, and left).

D. Innervation of the Liver
1. The liver is predominantly innervated by two plexuses that enter at the hilum and supply both sympathetic and parasympathetic nerve fibers.
2. Stimulation of the sympathetic fibers alters hemodynamics and metabolism in the liver. Hepatic vascular resistance increases and blood volume decreases while glycogenolysis and gluconeogenesis increase, producing an increase in the blood glucose concentration. Parasympathetic stimulation increases glucose uptake and glycogen synthesis.

E. Hepatic Lymphatic System. Portal hypertension and increased hepatic venous pressure can markedly increase hepatic lymph flow and lead to transudation through the hepatic capsule into the peritoneal cavity, producing ascites.

II. REGULATION OF HEPATIC BLOOD FLOW

A. Intrinsic Circulatory Regulation
1. Hepatic arterial flow varies reciprocally with changes in portal venous flow (response appears to be mediated via adenosine).
2. The hepatic arterial system undergoes flow autoregulation when the liver is very active metabolically (postprandial), but not during the fasted state (thus hepatic flow autoregulation is not likely to be an important mechanism during most anesthetics).

B. Extrinsic Circulatory Regulation
1. Extrinsic factors regulate blood flow through the portal vein indirectly by modulating the tone of arterioles in the preportal splanchnic organs.
2. Stimulation of alpha-1 adrenergic receptors increases vascular tone, leading to constriction and a reduction in both blood flow and blood volume in the sinusoids.
3. Hepatic arteriolar tone is the main determinant of resistance in the hepatic arterial tree.

C. Humoral Regulators
1. During activation of the sympathetic nervous system, the hepatic circulatory effects of epinephrine and norepinephrine exceed those of dopamine, which probably has little if any importance as a physiologic modulator of the hepatic circulation.

2. Glucagon induces a graded, long-lasting dilation of hepatic arterioles; it also antagonizes arterial constrictor responses to a wide range of physiologic stimuli, including stress-induced sympathoadrenal outflow.

3. Angiotensin II markedly constricts both hepatic arterial and portal beds, and significantly reduces mesenteric outflow; the result is a substantial decrease in total hepatic blood flow.
   a. Vasopressin also intensely constricts splanchnic vessels, markedly reducing flow into the portal vein.
   b. This action accounts for the efficacy of high-dose vasopressin (0.2 to 0.4 U/min iv) to alleviate portal hypertension and decrease bleeding from esophageal varices. The splanchnic and hepatic effects of low-dose (0.02 to 0.04 U/min iv) vasopressin for endogenous vasopressin deficiency replacement therapy in sepsis remains controversial.

III. MAJOR PHYSIOLOGIC FUNCTIONS OF THE LIVER (Table 39-1)

IV. ASSESSMENT OF HEPATIC FUNCTION

A. **Laboratory Evaluation of Hepatic Function** (Table 39-2). Liver function tests (LFT) can be classified into several broad categories.
   1. **Indices of Hepatocellular Damage.** Increased serum activities of AST (formerly serum glutamic oxalacetic transaminase, SGOT) and ALT (formerly serum glutamic pyruvic transaminase, SGPT) are detected when there is hepatocellular injury and necrosis.
   2. **Indices of Obstructed Bile Flow**
      a. Alkaline phosphatase (AP) elevations that are disproportionate to changes of AST and ALT occur with intrahepatic or extrahepatic obstruction to bile flow (highly sensitive test for assessing the integrity of the biliary system).
      b. Hyperbilirubinemia is classified as either predominantly unconjugated or predominantly conjugated (Table 39-3).
   3. **Indices of Hepatic Synthetic Function**

TABLE 39-1

MAJOR PHYSIOLOGIC FUNCTIONS OF THE LIVER

Blood reservoir (liver contains nearly 25 to 30 mL of blood per 100 g of tissue)

Regulator of blood coagulation (synthesis of procoagulation factors and anticoagulant factors)

Endocrine organ (synthesizes insulin-like growth factor-1, angiotensinogen, and thrombopoietin; principal site of hormone biotransformation and catabolism)

Erythrocyte breakdown and bilirubin excretion (bilirubin is an end product of heme degradation).

Metabolic functions

  Carbohydrate metabolism (liver can maximally store approximately 75 g of glycogen; in patients with chronic liver disease, hyperglycemia occurs commonly because portosystemic shunting allows direct entry of glucose-rich portal venous blood into the systemic circulation; hypoglycemia is a late manifestation of advanced liver disease)

  Lipid metabolism (fatty acids in the liver are esterified to form triglycerides, cholesterol esters, and phospholipids)

  Amino acid metabolism

Synthesis of important proteins (albumin, coagulation factors and their inhibitors with exception of factor VIII)

Immunologic function (Kupffer cells produce a variety of inflammatory mediators and cytokines)

Pharmacokinetics (by converting lipophilic substances to excretable metabolites, hepatic enzymes detoxify drugs and terminate their pharmacologic activity)

a. Measurement of serum albumin level and assays of coagulation function are the most widely used methods for assessing hepatic synthetic function.

b. Because the half-life in serum is as long as 20 days, the serum albumin level is not a reliable indicator of hepatic protein synthesis in acute liver disease.

c. The prothrombin time (PT) and international normalized ratio (INR) are sensitive indicators of severe hepatic dysfunction whether patients have acute or chronic liver disease because of the short half-life of factor VII. A progressively increasing PT is usually ominous in patients with acute hepatocellular disease, suggesting an increased likelihood of acute hepatic failure.

TABLE 39-2
LABORATORY EVALUATION OF HEPATIC FUNCTION

	Bilirubin overload (hemolysis)	Parenchymal dysfunction	Cholestasis
Aminotransferases	Normal	Increased (may be normal or decreased in advanced stages)	Normal (may be increased in advanced stages)
Alkaline phosphatase	Normal	Normal	Increased
Bilirubin	Unconjugated	Conjugated	Conjugated
Serum proteins	Normal	Decreased	Normal (may be decreased in advanced stages)
Prothrombin time	Normal	Prolonged (may be normal in early stages)	Normal (may be prolonged in advanced stages)
Blood urea nitrogen	Normal	Normal (may be decreased in advanced stages)	Normal
Sulfobromophthalein/indocyanine green	Normal	Retention	Normal or retention

   4. **Indices of Hepatic Blood Flow and Metabolic Capacity**
      a. Elimination of the dye indocyanine green (ICG) from the blood provides an estimate of hepatic perfusion and hepatocellular function because it is highly extracted (70 to 95%) by the liver following an intravenous injection.
      b. Hepatic function can also be assessed with substances that are metabolized selectively by the liver (lidocaine is metabolized by oxidative N-demethylation to monoethylglycinexylidide [MEGX]).

TABLE 39-3

CAUSES OF HYPERBILIRUBINEMIA

Unconjugated (Indirect)
Conjugated (Direct)
  Hepatocellular disease (hepatitis, cirrhosis, drugs)
  Intrahepatic cholestasis (drugs, pregnancy)
  Benign postoperative jaundice, sepsis
  Congenital conjugated hyperbilirubinemia
    Dubin-Johnson syndrome
    Rotor's syndrome
Excessive bilirubin production (hemolysis)
Immaturity of enzyme systems
  Physiologic jaundice of newborn
  Jaundice of prematurity
Inherited defects
  Gilbert's disease
  Crigler-Jajjar syndrome
Obstructive jaundice
  Extrahepatic (calculus, stricute, neoplasm)
  Intrahepatic (selerosing cholangitis, neoplasm, primary
    biliary cirrhosis)

- B. **Hepatobiliary Imaging**
  1. Ultrasonography is the primary screening test for hepatic disease, gallstones, and biliary tract disease.
  2. Computed tomography provides better and more complete anatomic definition than ultrasonography.
  3. Percutaneous transhepatic cholangiography may be used to determine the level and cause of biliary obstruction, confirm the presence of cholestasis without obstruction, and evaluate whether a proximal cholangiocarcinoma is surgically resectable.
  4. Endoscopic retrograde cholangiopancreatography (ERCP) uses endoscopy to visualize the ampulla of Vater and guide insertion of a guidewire and catheter through the ampulla to permit selective injection of contrast material into the pancreatic and common bile ducts, which are then imaged radiographically. ERCP is the imaging technique of choice in patients with choledocholithiasis, as a sphincterotomy and stone extraction can often be performed.
- C. **Liver biopsy** has a central role in the evaluation of patients with suspected liver disease because it provides the only means of determining the precise nature of

hepatic damage (necrosis, inflammation, steatosis, or fibrosis). The presence of coagulopathy (PT that is 3 seconds greater than control, platelet count <60,000 cells/mL) contraindicates percutaneous liver biopsy, although transjugular liver biopsy can be performed safely in these patients.

V. HEPATIC AND HEPATOBILIARY DISEASES. Liver diseases are divided into parenchymal diseases and cholestatic diseases (Table 39-4).

TABLE 39-4

CLASSIFICATION OF LIVER DISEASE

Parenchymal Diseases
Viral Hepatitis
  Hepatitis C (accounts for 40% of chronic liver disease; because of the use of serologic testing in screening donated blood, hepatitis C has almost been eliminated as a cause of posttransfusion hepatitis)
  Cytomegalovirus
  Epstein-Barr
  Herpes simplex
Nonviral Hepatitis
  Toxin and drug-induced hepatitis
    Acetaminophen
    Nonsteroidal anti-inflammatory drugs
    Antibiotics
    Volatile anesthetics (metabolism to trifluoroacyl metabolites may result in cross-sensitivity between fluorinated volatile anesthetics, exception is sevoflurane which is not metabolized to trifluoroacyl metabolites)
    Nonopioid sedative–hypnotic agents (rare)
    Opioids (increase tone of common bile duct and sphincter of Oddi but unlikely to be hepatotoxic)
Inflammation and sepsis
Hypoxia and ischemia
  Severe congestive heart failure
  Surgical stress
Chronic hepatitis
Fatty liver disease
Alcoholic liver disease

Cholestatic diseases
Biliary obstruction

TABLE 39-5
PATHOPHYSIOLOGY OF HEPATIC CIRRHOSIS

Cardiovascular Abnormalities
Hyperdynamic circulation
Hypervolemia
Arteriovenous collateralization
Cardiomyopathy

Hepatic Circulatory Dysfunction
Portal hypertension
Ascites
Variceal hemorrhage
Sepsis and infection

Pulmonary Dysfunction
Arterial hypoxemia (intrapulmonary vascular dilations)
Hydrothorax
Portopulmonary hypertension

Ascites

Renal Dysfunction and the Hepatorenal Syndrome

Spontaneous Bacterial Peritonitis

Hematologic and Coagulation Disorders
Hyperfibrinolysis
PT and INR elevated and serve as prognostic indicators
Thrombocytopenia

Endocrine Disorders
Abnormal glucose utilization (prone to hypoglycemia)
Abnormal metabolism of sex hormones (gonadal dysfunction in
    both men and women)

Hepatic Encephalopathy (treatment is orthotopic liver
    transplantation)

VI. CIRRHOSIS: A PARADIGM FOR END-STAGE PARENCHYMAL LIVER DISEASE (Tables 39-5, 39-6, and 39-7)

VII. UNCOMMON CAUSES OF CIRRHOSIS (Table 39-8)

VIII. HEPATOCELLULAR CARCINOMA

A. Primary hepatocellular carcinoma (HCC) is one of the most common tumors in the world and the third most frequent cause of death from cancer.

TABLE 39-6

DIFFERENTIAL DIAGNOSIS OF ACUTE AZOTEMIA IN PATIENTS WITH LIVER DISEASE

Failure	Prerenal azotemia	Hepatorenal syndrome	Acute renal (acute tubular necrosis)
Urinary sodium concentration	<10 mEq/L	<10 mEq/L	>30 mEq/L
Urine-to-plasma creatinine ratio	>30:1	>30:1	<20:1
Urinary osmolality	Exceeds plasma osmolality by at least 100 mOsm	Exceeds plasma osmolality by at least 100 mOsm	Equal to plasma osmolality
Urinary sediment	Normal	Unremarkable	Casts, cellular debris

B. HCC usually arises in a cirrhotic liver. The most common presenting complaint is abdominal pain, and the most frequent finding on physical examination is an abdominal mass.

IX. PREGNANCY-RELATED DISORDERS

A. Acute fatty liver of pregnancy occurs in the late stages of pregnancy.

TABLE 39-7

MODIFIED CHILD-PUGH SCORE

	Points[a]		
	1	2	3
Albumin (g/dL)	>3.5	2.8–3.5	<2.8
Prothrombin time Seconds prolonged	<4	4–6	>6
International normalized ratio	<1.7	1.7–2.3	>2.3
Bilirubin (mg/dL)	<2	2–3	>3
Ascites	Absent	Slight to moderate	Tense
Encephalopathy	None	Grade I–II	Grade III–IV

[a] Class A, 5–6 points; Class B, 7–9 points; Class C, 10–15 points.

TABLE 39-8
UNCOMMON CAUSES OF CIRRHOSIS
Wilson's disease (characterized by hepatic copper accumulation)
Hemochromatosis (characterized by excessive iron absorption)
Primary biliary cirrhosis (positive antimitochondrial antibody test)
Alpha-1 antitrypsin deficiency
Budd-Chiari syndrome (venous outflow obstruction from the liver)

      1. Affected women usually present in the third trimester with symptoms related to hepatic failure.
      2. When acute fatty liver is diagnosed, delivery of the fetus is expedited (disease usually improves in response to termination of pregnancy).
  B. **Preeclampsia and HELLP Syndrome** (hemolysis, increased liver transaminases, thrombocytopenia, hyperbilirubinemia). Prompt delivery is indicated if the syndrome develops beyond 34 weeks of gestation or earlier if life-threatening morbidity develops in the mother.
  C. **Hepatic Rupture, Hematoma, and Infarct.** These conditions occur in preeclampsia and may be the extreme end of the spectrum of HELLP syndrome.

X. CHOLESTATIC DISEASE

  A. **Cardiovascular Dysfunction.** The presence of bile salts in circulating blood (cholemia) can impair myocardial contractility.
  B. **Coagulation Disorders.** Cholestatic disease predisposes the patient toward development of coagulopathy primarily related to vitamin K deficiency. Usually, the coagulation disorders are moderate, and parenteral vitamin K corrects the problem. Should such patients need urgent surgery, the coagulopathy will require immediate treatment with fresh frozen plasma.

XI. PERIOPERATIVE MANAGEMENT (Table 39-9)
(Figs. 39-2 and 39-3)

TABLE 39-9

PERIOPERATIVE MANAGEMENT OF THE PATIENT WITH LIVER DISEASE

Preoperative

Hepatic evaluation and preparation (prior episodes of jaundice, use of alcohol, current medications, easy bruising, episodes of gastrointestinal bleeding, liver function tests only if suspicion of liver dysfunction based on history and physical examination)

Intraoperative

Monitoring and vascular access (arterial cannula, central venous, assessment of coagulation status)

Selection of anesthetic technique (regional anesthesia for peripheral procedures without coagulation abnormalities)

Induction of general anesthesia (all intravenous induction drugs acceptable, decreased cholinesterase activity due to liver disease rarely a problem)

Maintenance of anesthesia (consider adequacy of blood flow and oxygen supply to the liver, opioids are useful, consider clearance mechanisms of muscle relaxants)

Fluids and blood products

Vasopressors (peripheral vasodilation may be resistant to vasopressors)

Postoperative

Liver dysfunction and management (postoperative dysfunction usually transient, jaundice the earliest sign of significant dysfunction)

Hemolysis and transfusion (resorption of surgical hematomas and transfusions a source of jaundice in absence of hepatocellular dysfunction)

XII. CAUSES OF POSTOPERATIVE LIVER DYSFUNCTION UNRELATED TO PERIOPERATIVE FACTORS

A. **Asymptomatic and Preexisting Hepatic Injury.** Although postoperative liver dysfunction can result from anesthetic or surgical interventions, it is often unrelated to perioperative factors (preexisting liver disease).

B. **Congenital Disorders**

1. Gilbert's syndrome (familial unconjugated hyper-bilirubinemia) is the most common cause of jaundice. It is a benign metabolic disorder characterized

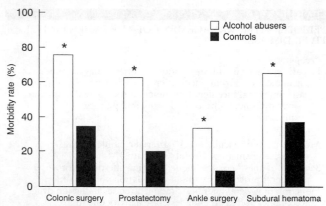

FIGURE 39-2. Postoperative morbidity is increased in patients with a history of alcohol abuse.

by a decrease in the activity of the hepatic enzyme bilirubin glucuronyltransferase, which is required for hepatocyte uptake of unconjugated bilirubin.

2. Crigler-Najjar syndrome (congenital nonhemolytic jaundice) exhibits either an absence (type 1) or marked decrease (type 2) of bilirubin glucuronyltransferase, producing unconjugated hyperbilirubinemia.

3. Surgical and anesthesia-related problems are apparently minimal in patients with either Gilbert's or Crigler-Najjar syndrome.

XIII. CONCLUSION: PREVENTION AND TREATMENT OF POSTOPERATIVE LIVER DYSFUNCTION

A. Identifying patients at high risk for developing liver dysfunction or for having an exacerbation of pre-existing liver disease is of utmost importance for minimizing the morbidity and mortality in such patients (careful preoperative evaluation).

1. When liver abnormalities are recognized preoperatively, it is prudent to defer elective procedures until the course of the disease can be determined.

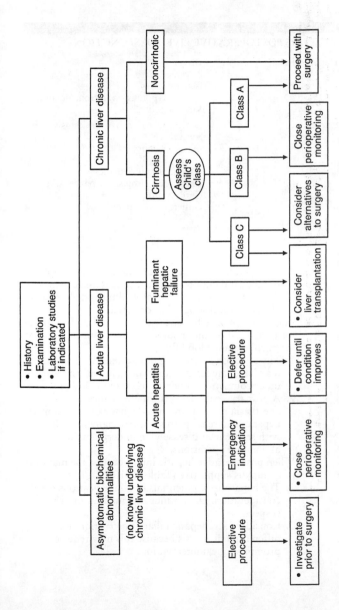

FIGURE 39-3. Preoperative approach to a patient with known or suspected liver disease.

658 Management of Anesthesia

TABLE 39-10
CAUSES OF POSTOPERATIVE LIVER DYSFUNCTION

Hepatocellular	Drugs
	Anesthetics
	Ischemia
	Shock, hypotension, iatrogenic injury
	Viral hepatitis
Cholestasis	Benign postoperative cholestasis
	Sepsis
	Bile duct injury
	Drugs
	Antibiotics, antiemetics
	Choledocholithiasis or pancreatitis
	Cholecystitis
	Gilbert syndrome

    2. For operations that cannot be deferred, clinically significant pathophysiologic changes associated with the liver disease (coagulopathy, fluid and electrolyte abnormalities) should be corrected.

B. The choice of anesthesia is usually an insignificant issue for peripheral or minor surgery (operations that do not affect splanchnic blood flow).

    1. The selection of pharmacologic anesthetic agents may have important implications in patients undergoing major operations (avoid halothane).

    2. A primary goal during the maintenance of anesthesia is to ensure the adequacy of splanchnic, hepatic, and renal perfusion, especially in patients with severe liver disease who undergo major abdominal operations.

C. When postoperative hepatic injury occurs, the mainstay of therapy is supportive (Table 39-10).

    1. The hepatotoxic potentials of all medications merit consideration. Discontinue any medication that is suspect.

    2. Consider extrahepatic biliary obstruction in the differential diagnosis because this may require prompt surgical intervention.

CHAPTER 40 ■ ANESTHESIA FOR ORTHOPAEDIC SURGERY

Anesthesia for orthopedic surgery requires an understanding of special positioning requirements (risk of peripheral nerve injury), appreciation of the possibility of large intraoperative blood loss and techniques to limit the impact of this occurrence, and recognition of the importance of postoperative analgesia and early ambulation (Horlocker TT, Wedel DJ: Anesthesia for orthopaedic surgery. In Barash PG, Cullen BF, Stoelting RD [eds]: *Clinical Anesthesia*, pp 1112–1128. Philadelphia, Lippincott Williams & Wilkins, 2006). Many orthopedic surgical procedures lend themselves to the use of regional anesthesia, which offers both intraoperative surgical anesthesia as well as postoperative pain relief. Patients undergoing orthopedic surgical procedures are at risk for deep venous thrombosis, emphasizing the need for the anesthesiologist to consider the interaction of anticoagulants and antiplatelet drugs with anesthetic drugs or techniques (especially regional anesthesia).

I. **PREOPERATIVE ASSESSMENT** (Table 40-1). The patient is evaluated for preexisting medical problems, previous anesthetic complications, potential airway difficulties, and considerations relating to intraoperative positioning.

II. **CHOICE OF ANESTHETIC TECHNIQUE** (Table 40-2)

III. **SURGERY TO THE SPINE**

A. **Spinal Cord Injuries**
   1. Spinal cord injuries must be considered in any patient who has experienced trauma (cervical spine injuries are associated with head and thoracic injuries, lumbar spine injuries are associated with abdominal injuries and long bone fractures).
   2. **Tracheal Intubation**
      a. Airway management is critical because the most common cause of death with acute cervical spinal cord injury is respiratory failure.

TABLE 40-1

PREOPERATIVE ASSESSMENT OF THE ORTHOPEDIC SURGICAL PATIENT

Coexisting Medical Problems
Coronary artery disease (consider perioperative beta-blockade)
Rheumatoid arthritis (steroid therapy, airway management)

Physical Examination
Mouth opening/neck extension
Evidence of infection and anatomic abnormalities at proposed
    sites for introduction of regional anesthesia
Arthritic changes and limitations to positioning

b. All patients with severe trauma or head injuries
   should be assumed to have an unstable cervical
   fracture until proven otherwise radiographically.
c. Awake fiberoptic-assisted intubation may be
   necessary, with general anesthesia induced only
   after voluntary upper and lower extremity
   movement is confirmed.
d. In a truly emergent situation, oral intubation of
   the trachea with direct laryngoscopy (minimal
   flexion or extension of the neck) is the usual
   approach.
3. **Respiratory considerations** include inability to
   cough and clear secretions, which may result in
   atelectasis and infection.
4. **Cardiovascular considerations** are based on loss of
   sympathetic nervous system innervation ("spinal

TABLE 40-2

ADVANTAGES OF REGIONAL VERSUS GENERAL ANESTHESIA FOR ORTHOPEDIC SURGICAL PROCEDURES

Improved postoperative analgesia
Decreased incidence of nausea and vomiting
Less respiratory and cardiac depression
Improved perfusion because of sympathetic nervous system
    block
Decreased intraoperative blood loss
Decreased blood pressure
Blood flow redistribution to large caliber vessels
Locally decreased venous pressure

shock") below the level of spinal cord transection (cardioaccelerator fiber [T1–4] loss results in bradycardia and possible absence of compensatory tachycardia if blood loss occurs).

5. **Succinylcholine-Induced Hyperkalemia.** It is usually safe to administer succinylcholine within the first 48 hours after spinal cord injury (avoid in all spinal cord injuries after 48 hours).

6. **Temperature Control.** Loss of vasoconstriction below the level of spinal cord transection causes patients to become poikilothermic (maintain body temperature by increasing ambient air temperature, warming intravenous fluids and inhaled gases).

7. **Maintaining Spinal Cord Integrity**
   a. An important component of anesthetic management is preservation of spinal cord blood flow (maintain perfusion pressure and avoid extreme hyperventilation of the lungs).
   b. Neurophysiologic monitoring (somatosensory or motor evoked potentials) and/or a "wake-up test" are used to recognize neurologic ischemia before it becomes irreversible.

8. **Autonomic Hyperreflexia** (Table 40-3)

B. **Scoliosis**
   1. **Pulmonary Considerations.** Postoperative ventilation of the patient's lungs is likely to be necessary if the vital capacity is <40% of the predicted value. Prolonged arterial hypoxemia, hypercapnia, and pulmonary vascular constriction may result in right ventricular hypertrophy and irreversible pulmonary hypertension.

TABLE 40-3

CHARACTERISTICS OF AUTONOMIC HYPERREFLEXIA

Occurs in 85% of patients with spinal cord transection above T5
Paroxysmal hypertension with bradycardia (baroreceptor reflex)
Cardiac dysrhythmias
Cutaneous vasoconstriction below and vasodilation above level of transection
Precipitated by any noxious stimulus (distention of a hollow viscus)
Treatment is removal of stimulus, deepening of anesthesia, administration of vasodilator

2. **Cardiovascular Considerations.** Prolonged alveolar
   hypoxia as a result of hypoventilation and
   ventilation-perfusion mismatch eventually causes
   irreversible vasoconstriction and pulmonary
   hypertension.
3. **Surgical Approach and Positioning**
   a. The prone position is used for the posterior
      approach to the spine (consideration of the
      hazards of the prone position including brachial
      plexus stretch injury [rotate head toward
      abducted arm], tape eyes closed).
   b. The anterior approach is achieved with the
      patient in the lateral position usually with the
      convexity of the curve uppermost (removal of a
      rib may be necessary, double lumen endotracheal
      tube to collapse lung on operative side).
   c. Combined anterior and posterior approach (one
      or two stages, increased morbidity [blood loss,
      nutritional deficits]) yield higher union rates.
4. **Anesthetic Management**
   a. Respiratory reserve is assessed by exercise
      tolerance, vital capacity measurement, and arterial
      blood gas analysis. Autologous blood donation
      is often recommended (usually 4 or more units
      can be collected in the month before surgery).
   b. Anesthetic considerations for surgical correction
      of scoliosis by spinal fusion and instrumentation
      must be considered (Table 40-4).
5. **Monitoring** (Table 40-5)
C. **Degenerative Vertebral Column Disease**
   1. Spinal stenosis, spondylosis, and spondylolisthesis
      are forms of degenerative vertebral column disease

TABLE 40-4

ANESTHETIC CONSIDERATIONS FOR SURGICAL CORRECTION OF SCOLIOSIS

Management of the prone position
Hypothermia (long procedure and extensive exposed area)
Extensive blood and fluid losses
Maintenance of spinal cord integrity
Prevention and treatment of venous air embolism
Reduction of blood loss through hypotensive anesthetic
   techniques

TABLE 40-5

MONITORING OF THE PATIENT UNDERGOING SCOLIOSIS SURGERY

Cannulation of radial artery (direct blood pressure measurement and assessment of blood gases)
Central venous catheter (evaluate blood and fluid management and aspirate air should venous air embolism occur)
Pulmonary artery catheter (pulmonary hypertension)
Neurophysiologic monitoring (prompt diagnosis of neurologic changes and early intervention)
   Somatosensory evoked potentials
   Motor evoked potentials
   Wake-up test

that may lead to neurologic deficit necessitating surgical intervention.

2. **Surgical Approach and Positioning**
   a. Cervical laminectomy is most often performed with patients in the prone position (Fig. 40-1).
   b. Fiberoptic-assisted intubation may be necessary in patients with severely limited cervical movement.
   c. The anterior approach places the surgical incision (anterior border of the sternocleidomastoid muscle) near critical structures (carotid artery, esophagus, trachea [edema, recurrent nerve injury]).
   d. The use of the sitting position for cervical laminectomy allows a more blood-free surgical

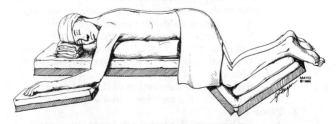

FIGURE 40-1. Prone position with the patient's head turned and the dependent ear and eye protected from pressure. Chest rolls are in place, the arms are extended forward without hyperextension, and the knees are flexed.

field but introduces the risk of venous air
embolism (incidence less than for sitting posterior
fossa craniotomy but still need to monitor with a
precordial Doppler).

3. **Anesthetic Management**
   a. General anesthesia is most often selected for spinal
   surgery (ensures airway access, acceptable for prolonged operations). Patients undergoing cervical
   laminectomy should be assessed preoperatively
   for cervical range of motion and the presence of
   neurologic symptoms during flexion, extension,
   or rotation of the head (awake fiberoptic
   intubation of the trachea may be necessary).
   b. Succinylcholine is avoided if there is evidence of a
   progressive neurologic deficit.

D. **Spinal Cord Monitoring**
   1. Paraplegia is a feared complication of spine surgery.
   The two methods to detect intraoperative
   compromise of spinal cord function are the
   "wake-up test" and neurophysiologic monitoring.
   2. **The wake-up** test consists of intraoperative
   awakening of patients after completion of spinal
   instrumentation. Surgical anesthesia (often includes
   opioids) and neuromuscular blockers are allowed to
   dissipate and the patient is asked to move the hands
   and feet before anesthesia is again reestablished.
   Recall may occur but is rarely viewed as unpleasant
   especially if the patient is fully informed
   preoperatively.
   3. Neurophysiologic monitoring (adjunct or alternative
   to wake-up test) includes somatosensory evoked
   potentials (waveforms may be altered by volatile
   anesthetics, hypotension, hypothermia, hypercarbia),
   motor evoked potentials (neuromuscular blocking
   drugs cannot be used), and electromyography.
   a. Somatosensory evoked potentials reflect the dorsal
   columns of the spinal cord (proprioception and
   vibration) supplied by the posterior spinal artery.
   b. Motor evoked potentials reflect the motor
   pathways and the portion of the spinal cord
   supplied by the anterior spinal artery.

E. **Blood Loss**
   1. A combination of intravenous hypotensive agents
   and volatile anesthetics is frequently used in an
   attempt to decrease blood loss during surgery.

2. Perioperative coagulopathy from dilution of coagulation factors and/or platelets or fibrinolysis may be predicted from measurement of either the prothrombin time or activated partial thromboplastin time.

F. **Visual Loss After Spine Surgery.** Most cases are associated with complex instrumented fusions often associated with prolonged intraoperative hypotension, anemia, large intraoperative blood loss, and prolonged surgery.

G. **Venous Air Embolus**
   1. Venous air embolism can occur in all positions used for laminectomies because the operative site is above the heart level.
   2. Presenting signs are usually unexplained hypotension and an increase in the end-tidal nitrogen concentration.

H. **Postoperative Care**
   1. Most patients' tracheas can be extubated immediately following posterior spinal fusion operations if the procedure was relatively uneventful and preoperative vital capacity values were acceptable. The presence of severe facial edema may prevent prompt tracheal extubation.
   2. Aggressive postoperative pulmonary care, including incentive spirometry, is necessary to avoid atelectasis and pneumonia.
   3. Continued hemorrhage in the postoperative period is a concern.

I. **Epidural and Spinal Anesthesia After Major Spine Surgery**
   1. Postoperative anatomic changes make needle or catheter placement more difficult after major spine surgery (Table 40-6).
   2. Spinal anesthesia may be a more reliable technique than epidural anesthesia if a regional technique is selected.
   3. The presence of postoperative spinal stenosis or other degenerative changes in the spine and/or preexisting neurologic symptoms may preclude the use of regional anesthesia in these patients.

IV. SURGERY TO THE UPPER EXTREMITIES

A. Orthopedic surgical procedures to the upper extremities are well suited to regional anesthetic

TABLE 40-6

CHANGES AFTER MAJOR SPINE SURGERY THAT MAY INFLUENCE ABILITY TO PERFORM EPIDURAL OR SPINAL ANESTHESIA

Degenerative changes (spondylothesis below level of fusion) that increase chance for spinal cord ischemia and neurologic complications with regional anesthesia

Ligamentum flavum injury from prior surgery results in adhesions and possible obliteration of the epidural space or interference with spread of local anesthetic solution ("patchy block")

Increased incidence of accidental dural puncture if epidural space altered by prior surgery (blood patch difficult to perform if needed)

Prior bone grafting or fusion may prevent midline insertion of needle

techniques. Upper extremity peripheral nerve blocks may be used in the treatment and prevention of reflex sympathetic dystrophy. Continuous catheter techniques provide postoperative analgesia and facilitate early limb mobilization.

1. The patient should be examined preoperatively to document any neurologic deficits as orthopedic surgical procedures often involve peripheral nerves with preexisting deficits (ulnar nerve transposition at the elbow, carpal tunnel release of the median nerve at the wrist) or may be adjacent to neural structures (total shoulder arthroplasty or fractures of the proximal humerus). Improper surgical positioning, the use of a tourniquet, and constrictive casts or dressings may also result in perioperative neurologic ischemia.

2. Local anesthetic selection should be based on the duration and degree of sensory and/or motor block required (prolonged anesthesia in the upper extremity in contrast to the lower extremity is not a contraindication to hospital discharge).

B. **Surgery to the Shoulder and Upper Arm**

1. A significant incidence of neurologic deficits in patients undergoing this type of surgery demonstrates the importance of clinical examination before performance of regional anesthetic techniques in these patients.

a. Total shoulder arthroplasty may be associated with a postoperative neurologic deficit (brachial plexus injury) that is at the same level of the nerve trunks at which an interscalene block is performed (impossible to determine a surgical or anesthetic etiology). Most of these injuries represent a neurapraxia and resolve in 3 to 4 months.

b. Radial nerve palsy is associated with humeral shaft fractures and axillary nerve injury is associated with proximal humeral shaft fractures.

2. **Surgical Approach and Positioning**

   a. Typically the patient is flexed at the hips and knees ("beach chair position") and placed near the edge of the operating table to allow unrestricted access by the surgeon to the upper extremity.

   b. The head and neck are maintained in a neutral position because excessive rotation or flexion of the head away from the side of surgery may result in stretch injury to the brachial plexus.

3. **Anesthetic Management**

   a. Surgery to the shoulder and humerus may be performed under regional (interscalene or supraclavicular brachial plexus block) or general anesthesia.

   b. The ipsilateral diaphragmatic paresis and 25% loss of pulmonary function produced by interscalene block contraindicates this block in patients with severe pulmonary disease.

C. **Surgery to the Elbow**

   1. Surgical procedures to the distal humerus, elbow, and forearm are suited to regional anesthetic techniques.

   2. Supraclavicular block of the brachial plexus is more reliable than the axillary approach (may miss the musculocutaneous nerve) but introduces the risk of pneumothorax (typically manifests 6 to 12 hours after hospital discharge such that a postoperative chest x-ray may not be useful).

D. **Surgery of the Wrist and Hand**

   1. Brachial plexus block (axillary approach) is most commonly used for surgical procedures of the forearm, wrist, and hand. The interscalene approach is seldom used for wrist and hand procedures because of possible incomplete block of the ulnar nerve (15 to 30% of patients), whereas the

supraclavicular approach introduces the risk of pneumothorax.

2. Intravenous regional anesthesia ("Bier block") permits the use of a tourniquet but has disadvantages of limited duration (90 to 120 minutes), possible local anesthetic systemic toxicity, and rapid termination of anesthesia (and postoperative analgesia) on tourniquet deflation.

E. **Continuous Brachial Plexus Anesthesia**
   1. Catheters placed in the sheath surrounding the brachial plexus permit continuous infusion of local anesthetic solution (bupivacaine 0.125% prevents vasospasm and improves circulation after limb replantation or vascular repair and higher concentrations permit analgesia and early joint mobilization [painful surgical procedures to elbow]) for prolonged upper extremity anesthesia and postoperative analgesia.
   2. Indwelling catheters may be left in place for 4 to 7 days postoperatively.

V. SURGERY TO THE LOWER EXTREMITIES

A. Orthopedic procedures to the lower extremity may be performed under general or regional anesthesia although regional anesthesia may provide some unique advantages (see Table 40-2).

B. **Surgery to the Hip**
   1. **Surgical Approach and Positioning.** The lateral decubitus position is frequently used to facilitate surgical exposure for total hip arthroplasty, and a fracture table is often used for repair of femur fractures. The patient must be carefully monitored for hemodynamic changes during positioning when under general or regional anesthesia (adequate hydration and gradual movement minimize blood pressure decreases). Care is taken to pad and position the arms and to avoid compression of the brachial plexus ("chest roll" is placed caudad to the axilla to support the upper part of the dependent thorax).
   2. **Anesthetic Technique.** Spinal or epidural anesthesia is well suited to procedures involving the hip. Deliberate hypotension can also be used with general anesthesia as a means of decreasing surgical blood loss.

C. **Total Knee Arthroplasty**
   1. Patients undergoing total knee arthroplasty (TKA) experience significant postoperative pain, which impedes physical therapy and rehabilitation.
   2. Regional anesthetic techniques that can be used for surgical procedures on the knee include epidural, spinal, and peripheral leg blocks. Spinal anesthesia is often selected while an advantage of a continuous epidural is postoperative pain management (aggressive postoperative regional analgesic techniques for 48 to 72 hours shorten the rehabilitation period more than systemic opioids)
   3. The patient undergoing amputation of a lower limb often benefits from the use of regional anesthesia, although adequate sedation is imperative.
D. **Knee Arthroscopy and Anterior Cruciate Ligament (ACL) Repair**
   1. Diagnostic knee arthroscopy may be performed under local anesthesia with sedation (single dose or continuous lower extremity block is not warranted in most patients).
   2. ACL repair requires postoperative analgesia (consider peripheral blocks).
E. **Surgery to the Ankle and Foot** (Table 40-7)
   1. The selection of a regional technique is based on the surgical site, use of a tourniquet (use of a high tourniquet for longer than 15 to 20 minutes necessitates a neuraxial or general anesthetic), and need for postoperative analgesia.
   2. Peripheral nerve blocks (femoral and sciatic nerve) provide acceptable anesthesia for surgery on the foot and ankle.
F. **Postoperative Analgesia**
   1. **Systemic Analgesics.** Delivery of opioids using patient-controlled analgesia is commonly utilized but pain after total joint replacement (especially total knee replacement) is severe and achievement of adequate analgesia is often accompanied by side effects (sedation, nausea, pruritus).
   2. **Neuraxial and Peripheral Blockade.** Epidural analgesia provides better pain relief and faster postoperative rehabilitation than patient-controlled analgesia. Continuous femoral nerve block may be an alternative to epidural analgesia.

TABLE 40-7

ANESTHETIC TECHNIQUES FOR COMMON FOOT AND
ANKLE OPERATIONS

	Surgical procedures	Regional technique	Comments
Forefoot	Hallux valgus	Metatarsal, ankle, popliteal blockade	Sural nerve block necessary for surgery
	Amputations	Ankle, popliteal blockade	Popliteal blockade is the technique of choice in the presence of infection or swelling
Midfoot	Transmetatarsal amputations	Popliteal, ankle blockade	
Hindfoot	Ankle arthroscopy	Spinal, epidural, or general anesthesia	Operation typically requires good muscle relaxation for manipulation; thigh tourniquet
	Achilles tendon repair	Spinal, epidural, or popliteal blockade	Spinal or epidural anesthesia whenever thigh tourniquet is required
	Ankle fractures	Spinal, epidural, or popliteal blockade	Epidural block requires blockade of L5–S1
	Triple arthrodesis	Spinal or epidural	Neuraxial technique preferred for bone graft harvesting; popliteal blockade for postoperative analgesia

3. **Intra-articular injection** of local anesthetics and/or opioids is common after arthroscopic knee surgery.

VI. MICROVASCULAR SURGERY (Table 40-8)

VII. PEDIATRIC ORTHOPEDIC SURGERY

A. Regional anesthetic techniques are adaptable to the pediatric patient especially in those over 7 years of age.

TABLE 40-8

ANESTHETIC CONSIDERATIONS FOR MICROVASCULAR SURGERY FOR LIMB REPLANTATION

Maintenance of blood flow through microvascular anastomoses (critical for graft viability)
  Prevent hypothermia (increase temperature of operating room to 21°C; warm intravenous solutions and inhaled gases)
  Maintain perfusion pressure
  Avoid vasopressors
  Use vasodilators (volatile anesthetics, nitroprusside) and sympathetic nervous system block (regional anesthesia)
  Consider normovolemic hemodilution
  Administer antithrombotics (heparin) and/or fibrinolytics low-molecular weight dextran
Positioning considerations associated with long surgical procedures
Replacement of blood and fluid losses
Choice of anesthesia (often a combination of regional and general anesthesia)
  Regional anesthesia
    Sympathectomy helpful but long duration of surgery may limit use of single-shot techniques (option is a continuous technique)
  General anesthesia
    Ensures airway access and patient immobility

  B. Intravenous regional anesthesia is particularly useful in the pediatric patient for minor procedures such as closed reduction of forearm fractures.
   1. The use of local anesthetic creams minimizes patient discomfort during placement of an intravenous catheter.
   2. The size of the upper arm often precludes the use of a double tourniquet in pediatric patients, thus limiting the duration of the surgical procedure to 45 to 60 minutes (tourniquet pain typically develops by this time).

VIII. OTHER CONSIDERATIONS

  A. Anesthesia for Nonsurgical Orthopedic Procedures.
     Some minor procedures (cast and dressing changes in pediatric patients, pin removal) require only light sedation, whereas procedures involving bone and joint

manipulation (hip and shoulder relocation, closed reduction of fractures) usually require a general or regional anesthetic.

B. **Regional Anesthesia in the Outpatient Setting.** Hospital discharge criteria generally include successful oral intake, ambulation, and voiding by the patient. Thus patients who have undergone a neuraxial technique will not be discharged until complete block resolution (requirement to void is controversial).

C. **Tourniquets**
   1. Opinions differ as to the pressure required in tourniquets to prevent bleeding (usually 100 mm Hg above patient's systolic blood pressure for the leg and 50 mm Hg above systolic blood pressure for the arm). Before the tourniquet is inflated, the limb should be elevated for about 1 minute and tightly wrapped with an elastic bandage distally to proximally. Oozing despite tourniquet inflation is most likely because of intramedullary blood flow in long bones.
   2. The duration of safe tourniquet inflation is unknown (1 to 2 hours is not associated with irreversible changes). Five minutes of intermittent perfusion between 1 and 2 hours may allow more extended use.
   3. Transient systemic metabolic acidosis and increased $PaCO_2$ (1 to 8 mm Hg) may occur after tourniquet deflation.
   4. Tourniquet pain despite adequate operative anesthesia typically appears after about 45 minutes (may reflect more rapid recovery of C fibers as block wanes). During surgery this pain is managed with opioids and hypnotics.

D. **Fat Embolus Syndrome**
   1. Patients at risk include those with multiple traumatic injuries and surgery involving long bone fractures and intramedullary instrumentation and/or cementing, and those undergoing total knee surgery. The incidence of fat embolism syndrome in isolated long bone fractures is 3 to 4% and the mortality rate is 10 to 20%.
   2. Clinical and laboratory signs usually occur 12 to 40 hours after injury and can range from mild dyspnea to coma (Table 40-9).

TABLE 40-9
CRITERIA FOR DIAGNOSIS OF FAT EMBOLISM SYNDROME

Major	Minor
Axillary/subconjunctival petechiae	Tachycardia (>100 beats/min)
Hypoxemia (PaO$_2$ <60 mm Hg)	Hyperthermia
Central nervous system depression (disproportionate to hypoxemia)	Retinal fat emboli
	Urinary fat globules
Pulmonary edema	Decreased platelets
	Increased erythrocyte sedimentation rate
	Disseminated intravascular coagulation

    3. Treatment includes early stabilization of fractures and support of oxygenation. Steroid therapy may be instituted.

E. Methylmethacrylate

    1. Insertion of this cement may be associated with hypotension, which has been attributed to absorption of the volatile monomer of methylmethacrylate and/or embolization of air (discontinue nitrous oxide before cement is placed) and bone marrow during femoral reaming.

    2. Adequate hydration and maximizing oxygenation will minimize the hypotension and arterial hypoxemia that can accompany cementing of the prosthesis.

F. Deep Venous Thrombosis and Pulmonary Embolus

    1. The risk of deep vein thrombosis associated with total hip arthroplasty is 20 to 80% (pulmonary embolism is the major cause of death after this surgery) and 50% with total knee replacement. Prophylactic measures (oral anticoagulants, intravenous dextran, external pneumatic compression devices, adjusted-dose heparin) have decreased but not abolished this life-threatening complication.

2. The incidence of deep vein thrombosis and pulmonary embolism in patients undergoing total hip arthroplasty or total knee replacement is decreased when epidural or spinal anesthesia is used (see Table 40-11). It is not proven that the benefit of regional anesthesia is additive to pharmacologic prophylaxis with anticoagulants.

3. Venous thromboembolism is a major cause of death after surgery or trauma to the lower extremities. Without prophylaxis 40 to 80% of orthopedic patients will develop venous thrombosis (incidence of fatal pulmonary embolism highest in patients who have undergone surgery for hip fracture).

G. **Antithrombotic prophylaxis** is based on identification of risk factors (Table 40-10).

TABLE 40-10

ANTITHROMBOTIC REGIMENS TO PREVENT THROMBOEMBOLISM IN ORTHOPEDIC SURGICAL PATIENTS

Hip and Knee Arthroplasty and Hip Fracture Surgery
Low-molecular weight heparin (LMWH)[a] started 12 hours before surgery or 12 to 24 hours after surgery, or 4 to 6 hours after surgery at half the usual dose and then increasing to the usual high-risk dose the following day
Fondaparinux (2.5 mg started 6 to 8 hours after surgery)
Adjusted-dose warfarin started preoperatively or the evening after surgery (INR target 2.5 and range 2.0 to 3.0)
Intermittent pneumatic compression is an alternative to anticoagulant prophylaxis in patients undergoing total knee (but not hip) replacement

Spinal Cord Injury
LMWH once primary hemostasis is evident
Intermittent pneumatic compression is an alternative when anticoagulation is contraindicated early after surgery
During the rehabilitation phase, conversion to adjusted-dose warfarin (INR target 2.5 with range 2.0 to 3.0).

Elective Spine Surgery
Routine use of thromboprophylaxis, apart from early and persistent mobilization, not recommended

Knee Arthroscopy
Routine use of thromboprophylaxis, apart from early and persistent mobilization, not recommended

[a] Use with caution in patients receiving neuraxial anesthesia/analgesia. INR, international normalized ratio.

TABLE 40-11

POSSIBLE EXPLANATIONS FOR DECREASED INCIDENCE OF DEEP VEIN THROMBOSIS IN PATIENTS RECEIVING REGIONAL ANESTHESIA

Rheologic changes resulting in hyperkinetic lower extremity blood flow and associated decrease in venous stasis and thrombus formation

Beneficial circulatory effects from epinephrine added to local anesthetic solution

Altered coagulation and fibrinolytic responses to surgery under neural blockade resulting in decreased tendency for blood to clot

Absence of positive-pressure ventilation and its effects on circulation

Direct local anesthetic effects (decreased platelet aggregation)

    1. Several studies show a decreased incidence of deep vein thrombosis and pulmonary embolism in patients undergoing hip surgery and knee surgery under epidural and spinal anesthesia (Table 40-11).

  H. **Neuraxial Anesthesia and Analgesia in the Patient Receiving Antithrombotic Therapy**

    1. Despite perceived advantages of neuraxial techniques for hip and knee surgery (decreased incidence of deep vein thrombosis), patients receiving perioperative anticoagulants and antiplatelet medications are often not considered candidates for spinal or epidural anesthesia because of the risk of neurologic deficit from a spinal or epidural hematoma (Table 40-12).

    2. The patient should be closely monitored in the perioperative period for signs of paralysis. If a spinal hematoma is suspected, the treatment is immediate decompressive laminectomy (recovery of neurologic function is unlikely if >10 to 12 hours elapse).

TABLE 40-12

NEURAXIAL ANESTHESIA AND ANALGESIA IN THE ORTHOPEDIC PATIENT RECEIVING ANTITHROMBOTIC THERAPY

Low-Molecular Weight Heparin (LMWH)
Needle placement should occur 10 to 12 hours after a dose
Indwelling neuraxial catheters are acceptable with once (but not twice daily) dosing of LMWH
Optimal to place/remove indwelling catheters in the morning and administer LMWH in the evening to allow normalization of hemostasis to occur prior to catheter manipulation

Warfarin
Adequate levels of all vitamin-K dependent factors should be present during catheter placement and removal
Patients chronically on warfarin should have a normal international normalized ratio (INR) prior to performance of the regional technique
Monitor prothrombin time (PT) and INR daily
Remove catheter when INR <1.5

Fondaparinux
Neuraxial techniques are not advised in patients who are anticipated to receive fondaparinux

Nonsteroidal Anti-Inflammatory Drugs
No significant risk of regional anesthesia–related bleeding is associated with aspirin-type drugs
For patients receiving warfarin or LMWH, the combined anticoagulant and antiplatelet effects may increase the risk of perioperative bleeding
Other medications affecting platelet function (thienophyridine derivatives and glycoprotein IIb/IIIa platelet receptor inhibitors) should be avoided

CHAPTER 41 ■ ANESTHESIA AND THE ENDOCRINE SYSTEM

An understanding of the pathophysiology of endocrine function is important in the management of anesthesia for patients with disorders of hormone-producing glands (Schwartz JJ, Rosenbaum SH: Anesthesia and the endocrine system. In Barash PG, Cullen BF, Stoelting RK [eds]: *Clinical Anesthesia*, pp 1129–1151. Philadelphia, Lippincott Williams & Wilkins, 2006).

I. THYROID GLAND

A. Thyroid Metabolism and Function

1. Thyroxine (T_4) and triiodothyronine (T_3) are the major regulators of cellular metabolic activity. The thyroid gland is solely responsible for the daily secretion of T_4 (80 to 100 μg daily, elimination half-time 6 to 7 days). About 80% of T_3 is produced by extrathyroidal deiodination of T_4 (elimination half-time 24 to 30 hours). Thyroid hormone synthesis occurs in four stages (Fig. 41-1).

2. Most of the excess effects of thyroid hormones (hyperadrenergic state) are mediated by T_3 (Table 41-1).

B. Tests of Thyroid Function (Table 41-2)

C. Hyperthyroidism

1. Treatment and Anesthetic Considerations (Table 41-3)

   a. A combination of propranolol (effective in attenuating the manifestations of excessive sympathetic nervous system activity, as evidenced by a heart rate <90 beats/min) and potassium iodide (inhibits hormone release) is effective in rendering patients "euthyroid" before anesthesia and surgery. Esmolol may be administered as a continuous intravenous infusion to maintain the heart rate <90 beats/min.

   b. The goal of intraoperative management is achievement of a depth of anesthesia (often with isoflurane or desflurane) that prevents an

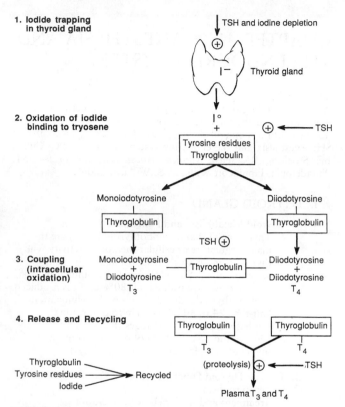

1. Iodide trapping in thyroid gland

TSH and iodine depletion

Thyroid gland

2. Oxidation of iodide binding to tryosene

Tyrosine residues
Thyroglobulin

← TSH

Monoiodotyrosine

Diiodotyrosine

Thyroglobulin

Thyroglobulin

TSH ⊕

3. Coupling (intracellular oxidation)

Monoiodotyrosine
+
Diiodotyrosine
T_3

Thyroglobulin

Diiodotyrosine
+
Diiodotyrosine
T_4

4. Release and Recycling

Thyroglobulin

Thyroglobulin

T_3

T_4

Thyroglobulin
Tyrosine residues → Recycled
Iodide

(proteolysis) ⊕ ← TSH

Plasma T_3 and T_4

FIGURE 41-1. Schematic depiction of the four stages in synthesis and release of thyroid hormone. TSH = thyroid-stimulating hormone.

TABLE 41-1

EFFECTS OF TRIIODOTHYRONINE ON RECEPTOR CONCENTRATIONS

Increased number of beta-receptors
Decreased number of cardiac cholinergic receptors

TABLE 41-2

TESTS OF THYROID FUNCTION

	Serum thyroxine	Serum triiodothyronine	Thyroid hormone binding	Thyroid stimulating hormone rate
Hyperthyroidism	Elevated	Elevated	Elevated	Normal or low
Primary hypothyroidism	Low	Normal to low	Low	Elevated
Secondary hypothyroidism	Low	Low	Low	Low
Sick euthyroidism	Normal	Low	Normal	Normal
Pregnancy	Elevated	Normal	Low	Normal

TABLE 41-3

PREPARATION OF HYPERTHYROID PATIENTS

Propylthiouracil (inhibits synthesis and decreases peripheral
conversion of T_4 to T_3)
Inorganic iodide (inhibits hormone release)
Beta-adrenergic antagonists (propranolol administered over
12–24 hr decreases heart rate to <90 beats/min)
Iopanoic acid (radiographic contrast agent that decreases
peripheral conversion of T_4 to T_3)
Glucocorticoids (decrease hormone release and peripheral
conversion of T_4 to T_3)

exaggerated sympathetic nervous system response
to surgical stimulation. Drugs that activate the
sympathetic nervous system (ketamine) or increase
the heart rate (pancuronium) are not likely to be
recommended.
  c. If a regional anesthetic is selected, epinephrine
  should not be added to the local anesthetic
  solution.
2. **Anesthesia for thyroid surgery** (subtotal
  thyroidectomy) is an alternative to prolonged
  medical therapy. Complications associated with
  surgery occur more frequently when preoperative
  preparation is inadequate (Tables 41-4 and 41-5).
  a. It is useful to evaluate vocal cord function in the
  early postoperative period by asking patients to
  say the letter "e."
  b. Unexpected difficult intubation is increased in the
  presence of goiter (consider inhalation induction

TABLE 41-4

COMPLICATIONS FOLLOWING THYROID SURGERY

Thyroid storm (distinguish from malignant hyperthermia,
pheochromocytoma, inadequate anesthesia; most often develops
in undiagnosed or untreated hyperthyroid patients because of
the stress of surgery)
Airway obstruction (computed tomography of the neck)
Recurrent laryngeal nerve damage (hoarseness if unilateral and
aphonia if bilateral)
Hypoparathyroidism (symptoms of hypocalcemia develop in
24–48 hr and include laryngospasm)

TABLE 41-5
MANAGEMENT OF THYROID STORM

Intravenous fluids
Sodium iodide (250 mg orally or iv every 6 hr)
Propylthiouracil (200–400 mg orally or via a nasogastric tube
every 6 hr)
Hydrocortisone (50–100 mg iv every 6 hr)
Propranolol (10–40 mg orally every 4–6 hr) or esmolol (titrate)
Cooling blankets and acetaminophen (meperidine, 25–50 mg iv
every 4–6 hr may be used to treat or prevent shivering)
Digoxin (congestive heart failure with atrial fibrillation and rapid
ventricular response)

or awake fiberoptic intubation if evidence of
significant airway obstruction or tracheal
deviation or narrowing).
  c. Postoperative airway obstruction caused by
hematoma or tracheomalacia may require urgent
reintubation of the trachea.
  d. Operating on an acutely hyperthyroid patient may
provoke thyroid storm.
D. Hypothyroidism
  1. Hypothyroidism is a relatively common disease (0.5
to 0.8% of the adult population) that results from
inadequate circulating levels of T_4 and/or T_3
(Table 41-6).
  2. Treatment and Anesthetic Considerations
    a. There is no evidence to support postponement of
elective surgery (including coronary artery bypass

TABLE 41-6
MANIFESTATIONS OF HYPOTHYROIDISM

Lethargy
Cold intolerance
Decreased cardiac output and heart rate
Peripheral vasoconstriction
Heart failure (unlikely unless coexisting cardiac disease)
Decreased platelet adhesiveness
Anemia (gastrointestinal bleeding)
Impaired renal concentrating ability
Adrenal cortex suppression
Decreased gastrointestinal motility (may compound effects of
postoperative ileus)

TABLE 41-7
MANAGEMENT OF MYXEDEMA
Tracheal intubation and controlled ventilation of the lungs as needed
Levothyroxine (200–300 mg iv over 5–10 min)
Cortisol (100 mg iv and then 25 mg iv every 6 hr)
Fluid and electrolyte therapy as guided by serum electrolyte measurements
Warm environment to conserve body heat

     graft surgery) in the presence of mild to moderate hypothyroidism.

    b. There is no evidence to support choice of a specific anesthetic technique or selection of drugs with hypothyroid patients, although opioids and volatile anesthetics are often considered to have increased depressant effects in these patients. There appears to be little if any decrease in anesthetic requirements as reflected by the minimum alveolar concentration.

    c. Meticulous attention must be paid to maintaining body temperature.

  3. Myxedema coma is a medical emergency that requires aggressive therapy (Table 41-7).

II. PARATHYROID GLANDS

A. Calcium Physiology. Parathyroid hormone secretion is regulated by the serum ionized calcium concentration (negative feedback mechanism) to maintain calcium levels in a normal range (8.8 to 10.4 mg/dL).

B. Hyperparathyroidism

  1. Hypercalcemia is responsible for a broad spectrum of signs and symptoms (nephrolithiasis, confusion).

  2. Treatment and Anesthetic Considerations. Preoperative intravenous administration of normal saline and furosemide can lower serum calcium concentrations. There is no evidence that a specific anesthetic drug or technique is preferred. A cautious approach to the use of muscle relaxants is suggested by the unpredictable effect of hypercalcemia at the neuromuscular junction. Careful positioning of osteopenic patients during

TABLE 41-8

MANIFESTATIONS OF HYPOCALCEMIA

Neuronal irritability
Skeletal muscle spasms
Congestive heart failure
Prolonged Q-T interval on the electrocardiogram

       surgery is necessary to minimize the likelihood of
       pathologic bone fractures.
  C. Hypoparathyroidism. Clinical features are
     manifestations of hypocalcemia, and treatment is with
     calcium gluconate (10 to 20 mL of 10% solution iv)
     (Table 41-8).

III. ADRENAL CORTEX

  A. Biologic effects of adrenal cortex dysfunction reflect
     cortisol or aldosterone excess or deficiency (Table 41-9).
  B. Glucocorticoid Excess (Cushing's Syndrome) (Table
     41-10)
    1. The diagnosis of hyperadrenocorticism is established
       by failure of the exogenous administration of
       dexamethasone to suppress endogenous cortisol
       secretion.
    2. Anesthetic Management (Table 41-11)
    3. Etomidate has been used for temporizing medical
       treatment of severe Cushing's disease because of its
       inhibition of steroid synthesis.
  C. Mineralocorticoid excess should be considered in
     nonedematous hypertensive patients who have
     persistent hypokalemia and are not receiving
     potassium-wasting diuretics.
  D. Adrenal Insufficiency (Addison's Disease)
    1. Clinically, primary adrenal insufficiency is usually
       not apparent until at least 90% of the adrenal cortex
       has been destroyed.
    2. Clinical presentation almost always includes
       hypotension (maintain a high degree of suspicion for
       patients who demonstrate cardiovascular instability
       without a defined cause).
    3. Treatment and Anesthetic Considerations
     a. Immediate therapy consists of electrolyte
       resuscitation (dextrose in normal saline) and

TABLE 41-9
COMPARATIVE PHARMACOLOGY OF CORTICOSTEROIDS[a]

	Anti-Inflammatory	Mineralocorticoid	Approximate equivalent dose (mg)
Short Acting			
Cortisol (hydrocortisone)	1.0	1.0	20.0
Cortisone	0.8	0.8	25.0
Prednisone	4.0	0.25	5.0
Prednisolone	4.0	+/−	5.0
Methylprednisolone	5.0	+/−	4.0
Intermediate Acting			
Triamcinolone	5.0	+/−	4.0
Long Acting			
Dexamethasone	30	+/−	0.75

[a]The glucocorticoid and mineralocorticoid properties of cortisol are considered to be equivalent to 1.

TABLE 41-10

MANIFESTATIONS OF GLUCOCORTICOID EXCESS

Truncal obesity and thin extremities (reflects redistribution of fat and skeletal muscle wasting)
Osteopenia
Hyperglycemia
Hypertension (fluid retention)
Emotional changes
Susceptibility to infection

steroid replacement (100 mg iv every 6 hours for 24 hours).

  b. Inotropic support is indicated if hemodynamic instability persists despite adequate fluid resuscitation.

E. **Steroid Replacement During the Perioperative Period**

  1. Patients with adrenal insufficiency and those with hypothalamic-pituitary adrenal (HPA) axis suppression from chronic steroid use require additional corticosteroids to mimic the increased output of the normal adrenal gland during stress.

  a. Normal adrenal glands can secrete up to 200 mg of cortisol per day and during stress may secrete between 200 and 500 mg per day.

  b. The HPA axis is considered to be intact if plasma cortisol levels are greater than 22 μg/dL during acute stress.

  c. Regional anesthesia postpones the elevation in plasma cortisol levels evoked by surgery and deep general anesthesia suppresses the elevation of stress hormones.

TABLE 41-11

MANAGEMENT OF PATIENTS UNDERGOING ADRENALECTOMY

Regulate hypertension
Control diabetes
Normalize intravascular fluid volume (diuresis with spironolactone helps mobilize fluid and normalize the potassium concentration)
Replace glucocorticoid (cortisol 100 mg iv every 8 hr)
Position patient carefully on operating table (osteopenic)
Decrease initial dose of muscle relaxant if skeletal muscle weakness is present

TABLE 41-12
SUPPLEMENTAL STEROID COVERAGE REGIMENS
Physiologic (low-dose approach) Cortisol 25 mg iv before induction of anesthesia, followed by a   continuous infusion (100 mg iv over 24 hr)
Supraphysiologic Cortisol 200–300 mg iv in divided doses on day of surgery

      d. Despite symptoms of clinically significant adrenal insufficiency during the perioperative period, these findings have rarely been documented in direct association with glucocorticoid deficiency.

  2. Identifying patients who require steroid supplementation is not practical (provocative testing with ACTH stimulation is too costly compared with the risk of brief steroid supplementation).

      a. HPA axis suppression can occur after five daily doses of prednisone of 20 mg or more. Suppression can also occur with topical, regional, and inhaled steroids (alternate day therapy decreases the risk of suppression).

      b. Recovery of HPA axis function occurs gradually and can take up to 9 to 12 months.

  3. There is no proven optimal regimen for perioperative steroid replacement (low-dose versus high-dose replacement) (Table 41-12). Patients who are using steroids at the time of surgery should receive their usual dose on the morning of surgery and are supplemented at a level that is at least equivalent to the usual daily replacement. Cortisol coverage is rapidly tapered to the patient's normal maintenance dosage during the postoperative period.

  4. Although there is no conclusive evidence supporting an increased incidence of infection or abnormal wound healing when supraphysiologic doses of supplemental steroids are used acutely, the goal of therapy is to use the minimal drug dosage necessary to adequately protect the patient.

 F. **Exogenous Glucocorticoid Therapy** (see Table 41-9)

IV. ADRENAL MEDULLA

  A. The adrenal medulla is analogous to a postganglionic neuron, although the catecholamines it secretes function as hormones, not as neurotransmitters.

TABLE 41-13

MANIFESTATIONS OF PHEOCHROMOCYTOMA

Sustained (occasionally paroxysmal) hypertension (headaches)
Masquerade as malignant hyperthermia
Cardiac dysrhythmias
Orthostatic hypotension (decreased blood volume)
Congestive heart failure
Cardiomyopathy

B. **Pheochromocytoma.** These tumors produce, store, and secrete catecholamines that may result in life-threatening cardiovascular effects (Table 41-13)
   1. **Diagnosis** of pheochromocytoma is based on measurement of catecholamines in the plasma and catecholamine metabolites (vanillylmandelic acid) in the urine.
      a. Excess production of catecholamines is diagnostic for pheochromocytoma.
      b. Computed tomography or magnetic resonance imaging may be used to localize these tumors.
   2. **Anesthetic Considerations**
      a. **Preoperative preparation** consists of a blockade (phentolamine, prazosin) initiated before surgery if possible, restoration of intravascular fluid volume, and institution of beta-blockade. Beta-blockade is indicated only if cardiac dysrhythmias or tachycardia persists after institution of alpha-blockade. The goals of medical therapy are to control heart rate, suppress cardiac dysrhythmias, and prevent paroxysmal increases in blood pressure.
      b. **Perioperative Anesthetic Management** (Table 41-14)
      c. Postoperatively, plasma catecholamine levels return to normal over several days, and about 75% of patients become normotensive within 10 days.

V. DIABETES MELLITUS

A. Diabetes mellitus is the most common endocrine disease present in surgical patients (25 to 50% of diabetics will require surgery). It is a disease with a broad range of severity and its manifestations can be altered (unmasked

TABLE 41-14

ANESTHETIC MANAGEMENT OF PATIENTS WITH PHEOCHROMOCYTOMA

Continue preoperative medical therapy

Invasive monitoring (arterial and pulmonary artery catheters, transesophageal echocardiography)

Adequate depth of anesthesia before initiating direct laryngoscopy for tracheal intubation

Maintenance of anesthesia with opioids and a volatile anesthetic that does not sensitize the heart to catecholamines

Select muscle relaxants with minimal cardiovascular effects

Control systemic blood pressure with nitroprusside or phentolamine (magnesium, nitroglycerin, and calcium channel blockers may be alternative vasodilator drugs)

Control tachydysrhythmias with propranolol, esmolol, or labetalol

Anticipate hypotension with ligation of the tumor's venous blood supply (initially treat with intravenous fluids and vasopressors, [continuous infusion of norepinephrine an option] if necessary)

for the first time) in response to stress as produced by surgery.

B. **Classification** (Table 41-15)
C. **Treatment** (Table 41-16)
D. **Anesthetic Management**
   1. **Preoperative** (Table 41-17). It is axiomatic that the patient should be in the best state of metabolic control that is possible preoperatively.

TABLE 41-15

CLASSIFICATION OF DIABETES MELLITUS

Type I (Insulin Dependent)
Childhood onset
Thin
Prone to ketoacidosis
Always requires exogenous insulin

Type II (Noninsulin Dependent)
Maturity onset
Obese
Not prone to ketoacidosis
May be controlled by diet or oral hypoglycemic drugs

Gestational Diabetes
May presage future type II diabetes mellitus

TABLE 41-16

TREATMENT OF DIABETES MELLITUS

Type I	Insulin
Type II	Diet and exercise
	Sulfonylureas (enhance insulin secretion by beta cells)
	Metformin (enhance sensitivity of hepatic and peripheral tissues to insulin)
	Thiazolidinediones (increases insulin sensitivity)
	alpha-Glucosidase inhibitors (decreases postprandial glucose absorption)

2. **Intraoperative.** The details of the anesthetic plan depend ultimately on the presence of end-organ disease. Invasive monitoring may be indicated for the patient with heart disease. Fluid management and drug selection may be influenced by renal function, and aspiration considerations may be affected by the presence of gastroparesis.
   a. Blood glucose levels should be measured preoperatively and postoperatively. The need for additional measurements is determined by the duration and magnitude of surgery and the stability of the diabetes.
   b. Dehydration may be present on arrival in the operating room based on osmotic diuresis.
   c. It is important to note the amount of glucose administered intravenously to avoid an overdose

TABLE 41-17

PREOPERATIVE EVALUATION OF THE PATIENT WITH DIABETES MELLITUS

History and physical examination (detect symptoms of cerebrovascular disease, coronary artery disease, peripheral neuropathy)

Laboratory tests (electrocardiogram, blood glucose, creatinine, and potassium levels; urinalysis [glucose, ketones, albumin])

Evidence of stiff joint syndrome (difficult to perform laryngoscopy)

Evidence of cardiac autonomic nervous system neuropathy (resting tachycardia, orthostatic hypotension)

Evidence of vagal autonomic nervous system neuropathy (gastroparesis slows emptying of solids [metoclopramide may be useful] but probably not clear fluids)

Autonomic neuropathy predisposes to intraoperative hypothermia

(standard glucose dose for an adult is 5 to 10 g/hr; 100 to 200 mL of 5% glucose/hr).

   d. Another area of patient monitoring that is extremely important in the diabetic patient is positioning on the operating table. The peripheral nerves of diabetics may already be partly ischemic and therefore are uniquely susceptible to pressure or stretch injuries.

3. **Glycemic Goals**
   a. Even mild hyperglycemia is associated with increased perioperative morbidity and tight control to achieve euglycemia can reduce complications (hyperglycemia exacerbates neuronal ischemic damage).
   b. It is reasonable to keep perioperative glucose levels between 110 and 200 mg/dL.

4. **Management Regimens**
   a. There is no consensus about the optimal way to manage perioperative metabolic changes in diabetic patients and many options are available. Several factors will influence the regimen selected (Table 41-18).
   b. The goal of any regimen is to minimize metabolic derangements and avoid hypoglycemia (Table 41-19).

E. **Emergencies**
   1. **Hyperosmolar Nonketotic Coma** (Table 41-20)
   2. **Diabetic Ketoacidosis**
      a. Manifestations of diabetic ketoacidosis reflect insufficient insulin to block the metabolism of fatty acids, resulting in the accumulation of acetoacetate and beta-hydroxybutyrate (Table 41-21). Because leukocytosis, abdominal

---

TABLE 41-18

FACTORS THAT INFLUENCE SELECTION OF DIABETIC MANAGEMENT REGIMEN

Type of diabetes mellitus
How aggressively euglycemia will be sought
Whether patient takes insulin
Whether surgery is minor and in an ambulatory unit
Whether surgery is elective or emergency
Ability of hospital resources to administer a complex regimen plan

TABLE 41-19

INTRAOPERATIVE MANAGEMENT REGIMENS FOR PATIENTS WITH DIABETES MELLITUS

Type I Diabetes Mellitus
Administer two-thirds of patient's usual intermediate-acting insulin subcutaneously on the morning of surgery
Titrate regular insulin (sliding scale) based on blood glucose measurement or infuse insulin (0.5–2.0 units/hr, 100 units of regular insulin in 1,000 mL of normal saline at 5–20 mL/hr) adjusted to maintain blood glucose at desired level
Glucose infusion (5% at 75–125 mL/hr) to prevent hypoglycemia while fasting

Type II Diabetes Mellitus
Hold sulfonylureas while patient is NPO (decreases risk of hypoglycemia and these drugs interfere with cardioprotective effect of ischemic preconditioning)
Hold metformin (especially if risk of decreased renal function perioperatively and associated risk of lactic acidosis)
Continue thiazolidinediones (do not predispose to hypoglycemia)
Hold alpha-glucosidase inhibitors (only work with meals)
Patients receiving insulin are treated as type I

Postoperative
Transition to chronic regimen as resume oral intake
Type II diabetics who undergo gastric bypass surgery may have rapid resolution of glucose intolerance (need for oral agents or insulin reduced)

TABLE 41-20

MANIFESTATIONS OF HYPEROSMOLAR NONKETOTIC COMA

Elderly patients with impaired thirst mechanism
Minimal or mild diabetes
Profound hyperglycemia (>600 mg/dL)
Absence of ketoacidosis
Hyperosmolarity (seizures, coma, venous thrombosis)

TABLE 41-21

MANIFESTATIONS OF DIABETIC KETOACIDOSIS

Metabolic acidosis
Hyperglycemia (300–500 mg/dL)
Dehydration (osmotic diuresis and vomiting)
Hypokalemia (manifests when acidosis is corrected)
Skeletal muscle weakness (hypophosphatemia with correction of acidosis)

TABLE 41-22
MANAGEMENT OF DIABETIC KETOACIDOSIS

Regular insulin 10 U iv followed by a continuous intravenous
  infusion (insulin in U/hr = blood glucose/150)
Intravenous fluids (isotonic) as guided by vital signs and urine
  output (anticipate a 4- to 10-liter deficit)
Potassium chloride 10–40 mEq/hr iv when urine output exceeds
  0.5 mL/kg/hr
Glucose 5% 100 mL/hr when serum glucose concentration drops
  below 250 mg/dL
Consider intravenous sodium bicarbonate to correct pH <6.9

pain, ileus, and mildly elevated amylase levels are
common in the presence of diabetic ketoacidosis,
an occasional patient is misdiagnosed as having an
intra-abdominal surgical problem.
  b. **Treatment** (Table 41-22)
3. **Hypoglycemia** produces signs of sympathetic nervous
  systemic stimulation (tachycardia, hypertension,
  diaphoresis), which in the anesthetized patient may
  be masked or misdiagnosed as an inadequate level of
  anesthesia relative to the surgical stimulation.
  a. Diabetic surgical patients are more likely to
    develop hypoglycemia if insulin or sulfonylureas
    are given without supplemental glucose.
  b. Renal insufficiency prolongs the action of insulin
    and oral hypoglycemic drugs.

VI. PITUITARY GLAND

  A. The pituitary gland is divided into the anterior pituitary
    (thyroid-stimulating hormone, adrenocorticotrophic
    hormone, gonadotropins, growth hormone) and
    posterior pituitary (vasopressin, oxytocin). Both are
    under the control of the hypothalamus.
  B. Acromegaly poses several problems for the
    anesthesiologist (Table 42-23).
  C. **Diabetes insipidus** reflects a relative or absolute
    deficiency of antidiuretic hormone (ADH), resulting in
    hypovolemia (inability to concentrate urine) and
    hypernatremia. ADH is also used in vasodilatory shock
    as an adjuvant to other pressors.
  D. **Inappropriate secretion of antidiuretic hormone**
    manifests as dilutional hyponatremia and decreased

TABLE 41-23
ANESTHETIC PROBLEMS ASSOCIATED WITH ACROMEGALY

Hypertrophy of skeletal, connective, and soft tissues
    Enlarged tongue and epiglottis (upper airway obstruction)
    Increased incidence of difficult intubation
    Thickening of vocal cords (hoarseness, consider awake tracheal
       intubation)
    Paralysis of recurrent laryngeal nerve (stretching)
    Dyspnea or stridor (subglottic narrowing)
    Peripheral nerve or artery entrapment
Hypertension
Diabetes mellitus

serum osmolarity. These changes typically occur in the presence of head injury or an intracranial tumor. Initial treatment is restriction of daily fluid intake to 800 mL.

VII. ENDOCRINE RESPONSES TO SURGICAL STRESS

A. Anesthesia, surgery, and trauma elicit a generalized endocrine metabolic response (increased plasma levels of cortisol, ADH, renin, catecholamines, endorphins) and metabolic changes (hyperglycemia, negative nitrogen balance).

B. Regional anesthesia may block part of the metabolic stress response during surgery (blockade of neural communications from the surgical area).

CHAPTER 42 ■ OBSTETRIC ANESTHESIA

During pregnancy, alterations occur in nearly every maternal organ system, with associated implications for the anesthesiologist (Table 42-1) (Santos AC, Braveman FR, Finster M: Obstetric anesthesia. In Barash PG, Cullen BF, Stoelting RK [eds]: *Clinical Anesthesia*, pp 1152–1180. Philadelphia: Lippincott Williams & Wilkins, 2006).

I. PHYSIOLOGIC CHANGES OF PREGNANCY

A. Increased alveolar ventilation along with decreased functional residual capacity enhances maternal uptake and elimination of inhaled anesthetics.

B. Decreased functional residual capacity and increased basal metabolic rate may predispose the parturient to arterial hypoxemia during periods of apnea, as associated with endotracheal intubation.

C. Vascular engorgement of the airway may predispose the patient to bleeding on insertion of nasopharyngeal airways, nasogastric tubes, or endotracheal tubes.

D. Controversy exists as to when a pregnant woman becomes at risk for aspiration. Earlier studies showing delayed emptying in the first trimester may have been a result of subjects' pain, anxiety or opioid administration.

II. PLACENTAL TRANSFER AND FETAL EXPOSURE TO ANESTHETIC DRUGS

A. Most drugs (opioids, local anesthetics, inhaled anesthetics) readily cross the placenta.

1. Placental transfer depends on several factors (Table 42-2).

2. Rapid transfer of inhalational agents result in detectable arterial and venous concentrations after 1 minute.

B. **Fetus and Newborn.** Several characteristics of the fetal circulation delay equilibration between fetal arterial and venous blood and thus delay the onset and/or

TABLE 42-1
PHYSIOLOGIC CHANGES OF PREGNANCY

Hematologic Alterations
Increased plasma volume (40–50%)
Increased total blood volume (25–40%)
Dilutional anemia (hematocrit 35%)

Cardiovascular Changes
Increased cardiac output (30–50%)
Aortocaval compression (supine hypotensive syndrome occurs in about 50% of parturients)

Ventilatory Changes
Increased alveolar ventilation (70%)
Decreased functional residual capacity (20%)
Airway edema

Gastrointestinal Changes
Delayed gastric emptying
Decreased lower esophageal sphincter tone (heartburn)

Altered Drug Responses
Decreased requirements for inhaled anesthetics (minimum alveolar concentration [MAC]) by 8–12 weeks (parallels increased progesterone levels)
Decreased local anesthetic requirements (engorgement of veins resulting in decreased volume of the epidural and subarachnoid space versus progesterone-induced increased sensitivity of nerves to local anesthetics)

TABLE 42-2
DETERMINANTS OF DRUG PASSAGE ACROSS THE PLACENTA

Physical and Chemical Characteristics of the Drug
Molecular weight (<500)
Lipid solubility
Nonionized versus ionized

Concentration Gradient
Dose administered
Timing of intravenous administration relative to uterine contraction
Use of vasoconstrictors

Hemodynamic Factors
Aortocaval compression
Hypotension from regional blockade

TABLE 42-3

CHARACTERISTICS OF FETAL CIRCULATION THAT DELAY
DRUG EQUILIBRATION

Fetal liver is the first organ perfused by the umbilical vein
Dilution of umbilical vein blood by fetal venous blood from the
gastrointestinal tract, head, and extremities (explains why
thiopental, 4 mg/kg iv, administered to the mother does not
produce significant depressant effects in the fetus)

magnitude of depressant effects of anesthetic drugs
(Table 42-3).

C. Neurobehavioral studies in neonates born in the
presence of epidural anesthesia may reveal subtle
changes in newborn neurologic and adaptive function
(changes are minor and transient, lasting only 24 to 48
hours).

III. ANESTHESIA FOR LABOR AND VAGINAL DELIVERY

A. Analgesia for the first stage of labor (pain caused by
uterine contractions) is provided by block of T10–L1,
whereas analgesia for the second stage of labor (pain
caused by distention of the perineum) is provided by
block of S2–4.

B. **Psychoprophylaxis.** Parturients who are educated in the
physiology of childbirth often require (request) less
systemic medication.

C. **Systemic Medication.** Time and method of
administration must be chosen carefully to avoid
maternal and neonatal depression.

  1. Opioids

    a. **Meperidine** appears to produce less neonatal
ventilatory depression than does morphine.
Meperidine administered intravenously
(analgesia in 5 to 10 minutes) or intramuscularly
(peak effect in 40 to 50 min) rapidly crosses the
placenta.

    b. **Fentanyl,** 1 μg/kg iv, provides prompt pain relief
(forceps application) without severe neonatal
depression. For more analgesia, fentanyl or
remifentanil can be administered with
patient-controlled delivery devices.

    c. **Naloxone,** 10 μg/kg iv, may be administered
       directly to newborns to reverse excessive opioid
       depression.
  2. **Ketamine** provides adequate analgesia (0.2 to 0.4
     mg/kg iv) without producing neonatal depression.
D. **Regional Anesthesia**
  1. Regional techniques (central neuraxial blockade
     [spinal, epidural, combined spinal-epidural])
     provide excellent analgesia with minimal depressant
     effects in mother and fetus.
  2. **Hypotension** resulting from sympathectomy is the
     most frequent complication that occurs with central
     neuraxial blockade (maternal systemic blood
     pressure is typically monitored every 2 to 5 minutes
     for about 15 to 20 minutes after the initiation of the
     block and at regular intervals thereafter).
  3. Regional analgesia may be contraindicated in the
     presence of a coagulopathy, acute hypovolemia, or
     infection at the needle insertion site
     (chorioamnionitis without frank sepsis is not a
     contraindication).
E. **Epidural analgesia** may be used for pain relief during
   labor and vaginal delivery and converted to anesthesia
   for cesarean delivery if required.
  1. Effective analgesia during the first stage of labor
     may be achieved by blocking the T10–L1
     dermatomes with dilute concentrations of local
     anesthetic and/or use of opioids, which have their
     effect at the opioid receptors in the dorsal horn of
     the spinal cord (Table 42-4). For the second stage of
     labor and delivery, because of pain as a result of
     vaginal distention and perineal pressure, the block
     should be extended to include the S2–4 segments.
  2. The first stage of labor may be slightly prolonged by
     epidural analgesia but this is not clinically significant

TABLE 42-4

**TESTS TO RULE OUT INTRATHECAL OR INTRAVASCULAR
PLACEMENT OF THE LUMBAR EPIDURAL CATHETER**

Aspiration (may not be diagnostic)
Local anesthetic (bupivacaine 7.5 mg or lidocaine 45 mg)
Epinephrine 15 μg (false-positive reaction with uterine
  contractions; may decrease uteroplacental perfusion)

provided aortocaval compression is avoided. Epidural analgesia initiated during the latent phase of labor (2 to 4 cm cervical dilation) does not result in a higher incidence of dystocia or cesarean section.

3. Prolongation of the second stage of labor by epidural analgesia (presumably related to loss of the maternal urge to push) may be minimized by the use of an ultradilute concentration of local anesthetic in combination with an opioid.

4. Analgesia for the first stage of labor may be achieved with 5 to 10 mL of bupivacaine, ropivacaine, or levobupivacaine (0.125 to 0.25%) followed by continuous infusion (8 to 12 mL/hr) of 0.0625% bupivacaine or levobupivacaine, or 0.1% ropivacaine. Addition of 1 to 2 μg/mL of fentanyl (or sufentanil 0.3 to 0.5 μg/L mL) permits a more dilute local anesthetic solution to be administered. During delivery the sacral dermatomes may be blocked with 10 mL of 0.5% bupivacaine, 1% lidocaine, or if a rapid effect is needed, 2% chloroprocaine, administered in the semirecumbent position.

5. Patient-controlled epidural analgesia is an alternative to bolus or infusion techniques.

F. **Spinal Analgesia**
   1. A single subarachnoid injection for labor analgesia has the advantages of a reliable and rapid onset of neuraxial blockade.
   2. Spinal analgesia with fentanyl 10 μg or sufentanil 2 to 5 μg alone or in combination with 1 mL of isobaric bupivacaine, 0.25%, may be appropriate in the multiparous patients whose anticipated course of labor does not warrant a catheter technique.
   3. Spinal anesthesia ("saddle block") is a safe and effective alternative to general anesthesia for instrument delivery.
   4. There is a risk of postdural puncture headache and the motor block may be undesirable.

G. **Combined Spinal-Epidural Analgesia**
   1. Combined spinal-epidural analgesia is an ideal analgesic technique for use during labor because it combines the rapid onset of profound analgesia (spinal injection) with the flexibility and longer duration of epidural techniques.

2. After identification of the epidural space a long pencil-point spinal needle is advanced into the subarachnoid space through the epidural needle. Following intrathecal injection (fentanyl 10 to 20 μg or sufentanil 2.5 to 5 μg alone or in combination with 1 mL of bupivacaine 0.25% produces profound analgesia lasting 90 to 120 minutes with minimal motor block), an epidural infusion of bupivacaine 0.03 to 0.625% with added opioid is started.
   a. Women with hemodynamic stability and preserved motor function, who do not require continuous fetal monitoring, may ambulate with assistance (walking has little effect on the course of labor).
   b. The most common side effects of intrathecal opioids are pruritus, nausea, vomiting, and urinary retention. The risk of postdural puncture headache does not seem to be increased. Fetal bradycardia may occur.
   c. The potential exists for epidurally administered drug to leak into the subarachnoid space following dural puncture, particularly if large volumes of drug are rapidly injected.
   d. This technique should be used with caution in those women who may require an urgent cesarean section and are at increased risk (morbidly obese, difficult airway) for difficult anesthetic management.
H. **Inhalation analgesia** makes the pain of uterine contractions more tolerable and is useful for delivery in combination with a pudendal block (S2–4).

IV. ANESTHESIA FOR CESAREAN SECTION

A. The choice of anesthesia often is influenced by the urgency of the operative procedure and condition of the fetus.
B. **Regional anesthesia** offers the advantages of decreased risk of pulmonary aspiration of gastric contents, avoidance of depressant drugs, and fulfillment of the mother's wishes to remain awake.
   1. The risk of hypotension is greater than during vaginal delivery because the block must extend to at least the T4 dermatome.
   2. Proper positioning and prehydration with up to 20 mL/kg of crystalloid solution is recommended. If

hypotension occurs despite these measures, left uterine displacement is increased, the rate of infusion is augmented, and ephedrine 10 to 15 mg iv or phenylephrine, 20 to 50 μg, iv is injected.

C. **Spinal anesthesia** is provided most often with hyperbaric, 0.75%, bupivacaine, 1.6 to 1.8 mL lasting approximately 120 to 180 minutes. Improved perioperative analgesia can be provided by addition of fentanyl (6.25 μg) or preservative-free morphine (100 μg) to the local anesthetic solution. It is probably not necessary to adjust the dose of local anesthetic based on the parturient's height.
   1. Despite a block extending to T4, parturients often experience visceral discomfort, particularly with exteriorization of the uterus and traction on abdominal viscera (fentanyl, 25 μg iv, may be useful).
   2. Oxygen should be routinely administered by face mask to optimize maternal and fetal oxygenation.

D. **Lumbar Epidural Anesthesia.** Compared with spinal anesthesia, lumbar epidural anesthesia requires more time and drug to establish an adequate sensory level, but there is a lower risk of postdural puncture headache, and the level of anesthesia can be adjusted by titration of local anesthetic solution injected through the indwelling catheter.
   1. Adequate anesthesia is usually achieved with injection through the lumbar epidural catheter of 15 to 25 mL of local anesthetic solution (Table 42-5).
   2. Addition of morphine (0.3 to 0.5 mg) to the local anesthetic solution provides postoperative analgesia.

E. **General anesthesia** may be necessary when contraindications exist to regional anesthesia or when time precludes central neuraxial blockade. Situations in which uterine relaxation facilitates delivery (multiple

---

TABLE 42-5

EPIDURAL ANESTHESIA FOR CESAREAN SECTION

2-Chloroprocaine 3%
Lidocaine 2% with epinephrine 1:200,000
0.5% bupivacaine, ropivacaine, or levobupivacaine

TABLE 42-6
GENERAL ANESTHESIA FOR CESAREAN SECTION

Preoperative evaluation of airway (inability to intubate is the leading cause of maternal death related to anesthesia)

Premedication with a nonparticulate antacid, 15–30 mL within 30 minutes of induction and an H2 receptor antagonist iv

Maintain parturient in left uterine displacement position while on operating table

Preoxygenation

Defasciculating dose of nondepolarizing muscle relaxant is not necessary

Thiopental, 4 mg/kg iv (propofol 2 mg/kg or ketamine 0.5 mg/kg iv), plus succinylcholine, 1–1.5 mg/kg iv, during cricoid pressure (inject at the onset of contraction if patient is in labor)

Skin incision after confirmation of tracheal tube placement

Rocuronium, 0.6 mg/kg iv, is an acceptable alternative when succinylcholine is contraindicated

Consider use of a laryngeal mask airway if tracheal intubation cannot be accomplished

Maintenance in the predelivery interval with 50% nitrous oxide and 0.5 MAC of a volatile anesthetic (temporarily increased to 2 MAC a few minutes before delivery if uterine relaxation is needed to facilitate delivery, alternatively nitroglycerin will relax the uterus)

Avoid extreme hyperventilation of the lungs (may reduce uterine blood flow)

Add oxytocin to the infusion after delivery and deepen anesthesia (opioids?)

Extubate the trachea when patient awakens

gestations, breech) are most often managed with general anesthesia (Table 42-6).

1. A newborn's condition after cesarean section with general anesthesia is comparable to that when regional techniques are used. The uterine incision to delivery time (<180 seconds) is more important to fetal outcome than is the anesthetic technique.

2. The usual amount of blood loss during cesarean section is 750 to 1,000 mL, and transfusion is rarely necessary.

3. When tracheal intubation is unexpectedly difficult, it may be prudent to permit the parturient to awaken and then to pursue alternative approaches (awake fiberoptic tracheal intubation, regional anesthesia) rather than to persist with repeated unsuccessful and traumatic attempts at tracheal intubation.

TABLE 42-7

ANESTHETIC COMPLICATIONS

Maternal Mortality
Most often related to arterial hypoxemia during airway management difficulties
Pregnancy-induced anatomic changes (decreased functional residual capacity, increased oxygen consumption, oropharyngeal edema may expose the parturient to increased risk of arterial oxygen desaturation during periods of apnea and hypoventilation)

Pulmonary Aspiration

Hypotension
Regional anesthesia (related to degree and rapidity of local anesthetic–induced sympatholysis)
Prehydration (up to 20 mL/kg of lactated Ringers solution) prior to initiation of regional anesthesia and avoidance of aortocaval compression may decrease the incidence of hypotension
Treatment is increased displacement of the uterus, rapid intravenous fluid infusion, titration of ephedrine (5–10 mg) or phenylephrine (20–50 μg), oxygen administration, and placement in the Trendelenburg position

Total Spinal Anesthesia

Local Anesthetic–Induced Seizures
Treatment is with intravenous administration of thiopental (50–100 mg) or diazepam (5–10 mg)

Postdural Puncture Headache
Incidence is less with pencil-point needles (Whitacre or Sprotte) compared with diamond-shaped (Quincke) cutting needles
Treatment of a severe headache is with a blood patch (10–15 mL of the patient's blood is injected into the epidural space close to the site of dural puncture)

Nerve Injury
Consider possible role of compression of maternal lumbosacral trunk by the fetus

V. ANESTHETIC COMPLICATIONS (Table 42-7)

VI. MANAGEMENT OF HIGH-RISK PARTURIENTS

A. **Preeclampsia** (pregnancy-induced hypertension) or **eclampsia** (seizures) is characterized by hypertension, proteinuria, and edema that may progress to oliguria, congestive heart failure, and seizures (eclampsia) (Table 42-8).

TABLE 42-8
SYMPTOMS OF SEVERE PREECLAMPSIA

Systolic blood pressure >160 mmHg
Diastolic blood pressure >110 mmHg
Proteinuria >5 g/24 hours
Evidence of end organ damage
    Oliguria (<400 mL/24 hours)
    Cerebral or visual disturbances
    Pulmonary edema
    Epigastric pain
    Intrauterine growth retardation
Thrombocytopenia (steroids may prevent)

1. Many of the symptoms associated with preeclampsia may result from an imbalance between the placental production of prostacyclin and thromboxane.
2. The HEELP syndrome is a form of severe preeclampsia characterized by hemolysis, elevated liver enzymes, and low platelet count. In contrast to preeclampsia, elevations in blood pressure and proteinuria may be mild.
3. **General Management** (Table 42-9)
4. **Anesthetic Management**
    a. Epidural anesthesia or combination spinal-epidural analgesia for labor and delivery should not be considered contraindicated, provided there is no clotting abnormality or plasma volume deficit. In volume-repleted parturients positioned with left uterine displacement, the institution of epidural anesthesia does not typically cause an

TABLE 42-9
CONSIDERATIONS IN THE MANAGEMENT OF PARTURIENTS WITH PREECLAMPSIA OR ECLAMPSIA

Prevent or control seizures (magnesium sulfate potentiates muscle relaxants and may increase the severity of hypotension under regional anesthesia)
Restore intravascular fluid volume (central venous or pulmonary capillary wedge pressure 5–10 mmHg; urine output 0.5–1 mL/kg/hr)
Normalize blood pressure (hydralazine, nitroprusside)
Correct coagulation abnormalities

unacceptable decrease in blood pressure and may result in significant improvements in placental blood flow.

  b. Spinal anesthesia may produce severe alterations in cardiovascular dynamics, resulting from sudden sympathetic nervous system blockade. The incidence of hypotension, perioperative fluid administration, and neonatal conditions are similar in preeclamptic parturients who receive either spinal or epidural anesthesia.

  c. General anesthesia is often chosen for acute emergencies, remembering the probable exaggerated blood pressure responses to induction of anesthesia and intubation of the trachea and possible interactions of muscle relaxants with magnesium sulfate therapy.

  d. Decreased doses of ephedrine are recommended to treat hypotension, as parturients with preeclampsia or eclampsia may exhibit increased sensitivity to vasopressors.

B. **Antepartum Hemorrhage**
  1. Placenta previa (painless bright red bleeding after the seventh month of pregnancy) is the most common cause of postpartum hemorrhage.
  2. Abruptio placentae typically manifests as uterine hypertonia and tenderness with dark red vaginal bleeding. Maternal and fetal mortality rates are increased.
  3. General anesthesia (often with ketamine induction of anesthesia, 0.75 mg/kg iv) is used in view of the increased risk of hemorrhage and clotting disorders.

C. **Heart Disease.** Cardiac decompensation and death occur most commonly at the time of maximum hemodynamic stress. For example, cardiac output increases during labor, with the greatest increase immediately after delivery of the placenta. These changes in cardiac output are blunted by regional anesthesia.

D. **Preterm delivery** is defined as birth before the thirty-seventh week or term weight of the infant as more than two standard deviations below the mean (small for gestational age). Such infants account for 8 to 10% of all births and nearly 80% of early neonatal deaths.

TABLE 42-10
PROBLEMS ASSOCIATED WITH PREMATURITY

Respiratory distress syndrome (glucocorticoids administered to the mother for 24–48 hours may enhance fetal lung maturity)
Intracranial hemorrhage
Hypoglycemia
Hypocalcemia
Hyperbilirubinemia

1. Several problems are likely to develop in preterm infants (Table 42-10).
2. Beta-2 agonists (ritodrine, terbutaline) used to inhibit labor may interact with anesthetic drugs or produce undesirable changes before induction of anesthesia (Table 42-11).
   a. Delay of anesthesia for at least 3 hours after the cessation of tocolysis allows beta-mimetic effects of beta-2 agonists to dissipate, and potassium supplementation is not necessary.
   b. Preterm infants are more sensitive to the depressant effects of anesthetic drugs. Regardless of the technique or drugs selected, the most important goal is prevention of asphyxia of the fetus.

VII. HUMAN IMMUNODEFICIENCY VIRUS INFECTION (HIV) AND ACQUIRED IMMUNODEFICIENCY SYNDROME (AIDS)

A. Prevention of vertical transmission to the fetus is based on antiretroviral therapy to decrease maternal viral load and elective cesarean delivery prior to rupture of membranes/labor.

TABLE 42-11
SIDE EFFECTS OF BETA-2 AGONISTS ADMINISTERED TO STOP PREMATURE LABOR

Hypokalemia (cardiac dysrhythmias)
Hypotension (accentuated by regional anesthesia)
Tachycardia (avoid atropine, pancuronium)
Pulmonary edema (cautious prehydration)

TABLE 42-12
COCAINE ABUSE AND MANAGEMENT OF ANESTHESIA

Tachycardia (avoid beta-blockers as leaves alpha effects
  unopposed)
Hypertension
Cardiac dysrhythmias (sudden death)
Seizures
Myocardial infarction
Pulmonary edema
Subarachnoid hemorrhage
Congenital anomalies
Premature labor
Intrauterine growth retardation
Enhanced local anesthetic toxicity (additive effects with local
  anesthetic effects of cocaine)
Thrombocytopenia (chronic abuse)

    B. Spread of HIV to the central nervous system occurs
rapidly after initial infection and there is no evidence
linking the use of regional anesthesia to progression of
the disease.

    C. Blood patch to treat postdural puncture headache does
not seem to accelerate HIV symptoms.

VIII. SUBSTANCE ABUSE of amphetamines, ectasy, opioid,
marijuana, or cocaine is not uncommon among women of
reproductive age. Cocaine abuse has the greatest
implications for anesthetic management (Table 42-12).

IX. FETAL AND MATERNAL MONITORING

    A. Biophysical Monitoring. Ultrasonographic
cardiography and measurement of uterine activity with
a tocodynamometer provide noninvasive monitoring of
fetal well-being (Table 42-13 and Fig. 42-1). Prolonged

TABLE 42-13
BIOPHYSICAL MONITORING OF THE FETUS

Baseline heart rate (normal 120–160 beats/min)
Beat-to-beat variability (reflects variations in autonomic nervous
  system tone; disappears with fetal distress, opioids, local
  anesthetics)
Fetal heart rate deceleration

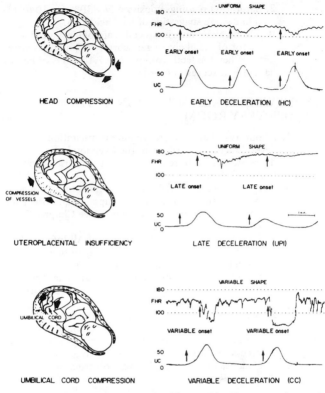

FIGURE 42-1. Relationship and significance of fetal heart rate changes in association with uterine contractions. FHR = fetal heart rate; UC = uterine contraction.

deceleration is present when fetal heart rate decreases below baseline for >2 but <10 minutes. All decelerations should be quantified based on deviation from baseline and duration.

B. **Fetal pulse oximetry** is an adjunct to fetal heart rate monitoring as a reflection of intrapartum fetal oxygenation.
   1. Fetal oxygen saturation between 30 and 70% is considered normal.

2. Saturation readings consistently <30% for 10 to 15 minutes are suggestive of fetal acidemia.

C. **Biochemical Monitoring.** Fetal scalp pH is a good predictor of the likely Apgar score 1 to 2 minutes after birth. When the fetal scalp pH is <7.16, 80% of babies have Apgar scores of 6 or less.

X. NEWBORN RESUSCITATION IN THE DELIVERY ROOM

A. About 6% of all neonates require resuscitation. Several factors contribute to the likelihood of depression at birth, requiring neonatal resuscitation (Table 42-14).

B. **Resuscitation.** Every delivery room must be equipped with appropriate resuscitation equipment and drugs for newborn and maternal resuscitation (see Chapter 58 and Appendix C).

1. **Initial Treatment and Evaluation of All Infants.** The pharynx is suctioned, heart rate is quantified, and ventilation is assessed. The scoring system introduced by anesthesiologist Dr. Virginia Apgar is a useful method of clinically evaluating newborns (Table 42-15).

2. Meconium staining is treated by oropharyngeal suctioning at the time of delivery; tracheal intubation and airway suctioning are probably only necessary in the presence of a low Apgar score and evidence of mechanical airway obstruction.

TABLE 42-14

EVENTS ASSOCIATED WITH NEONATAL DEPRESSION AT BIRTH

Prematurity (80% <1,500 g need resuscitation)
Drugs used during labor or delivery
Trauma or precipitated labor
Birth asphyxia (reflects interference with placental perfusion)
Tight umbilical cord
Prolapsed cord
Premature separation of placenta
Uterine hyperactivity
Maternal hypotension

TABLE 42-15
CALCULATION OF APGAR SCORE

	0	1	2
Heart rate	Absent	<100 beats/min	>100 beats/min
Respiratory effort	Absent	Slow and irregular	Crying
Muscle tone	Limp	Some flexion of extremities	Moving
Reflex irritability	No response	Grimace	Crying, cough
Color	Pale, blue	Body pink, extremities blue	Pink

3. **Use of cardiac massage** (chest compressions of the middle third of the sternum) should be provided if heart rate is <60 beats/min despite adequate ventilation for 30 seconds. The ratio of chest compression to ventilation should be approximately 3:1 or 100 compressions to 30 breaths/min.
4. **Rapid Correction of Acidosis**
   a. Sodium bicarbonate is not recommended during brief cardiopulmonary resuscitation as hyperosmolarity and carbon dioxide generation may be detrimental to cardiac and cerebral function.
   b. After ensuring adequate ventilation and perfusion, severe acidosis (pH <7.0) may need to be corrected promptly by infusion of sodium bicarbonate into the umbilical vein.
5. **Other Drugs and Fluids** (Table 42-16)

TABLE 42-16
OTHER DRUGS AND FLUIDS USED IN NEONATAL RESUSCITATION

Naloxone (avoid in infants born to opioid-addicted mothers)
Epinephrine (to treat asystole or persistent bradycardia; administer intravenously or by tracheal tube)
Lactated Ringers solution (10 mL/kg iv)
Type O-negative blood (10 mL/kg iv)

TABLE 42-17

CONSIDERATIONS IN THE MANAGEMENT OF ANESTHESIA FOR NONOBSTETRIC SURGERY IN THE PREGNANT WOMAN

Physiologic changes of pregnancy
  Decreased requirements for local and inhaled anesthetics
  Low functional residual capacity
  High basal metabolic rate
  Slowed gastric emptying
  Aortocaval compression
Teratogenicity of anesthetic drugs (period of organogenesis is
  15–56 days; single exposure seems unlikely to cause
  abnormalities)
Adequacy of uteroplacental circulation
Initiation of premature labor

XI. ANESTHESIA FOR NONOBSTETRIC SURGERY IN THE PREGNANT WOMAN

A. When the necessity for surgery in the pregnant patient arises, anesthetic considerations are related to multiple factors (Table 42-17).

B. Perform only emergency surgery during pregnancy, especially in the first trimester. It is logical to select drugs with a long history of safety (opioids, muscle relaxants, thiopental, nitrous oxide). The fetal heart rate should be monitored after the 16th week.

CHAPTER 43 ■ NEONATAL ANESTHESIA

The neonatal period is defined as the first 30 days of extrauterine life (Berry FA, Castro BA: Neonatal anesthesia. In Barash PG, Cullen BF, Stoelting RK [eds]: *Clinical Anesthesia*, pp 1181–1204. Philadelphia, Lippincott Williams & Wilkins, 2006). The most significant part of the change from fetal to extrauterine life (period of transition or adaptation) occurs during the first 24 to 72 hours. All systems of the body change during transition, but the most important to the anesthesiologist are the circulatory, pulmonary, hepatic, and renal systems.

I. TRANSITION OF THE CARDIOPULMONARY SYSTEM

A. **Fetal circulation** is characterized by three shunts (placenta, foramen ovale, ductus arteriosus), with oxygenated blood leaving the placenta through the umbilical vein. After the lungs expand and the umbilical cord is clamped, dramatic circulatory changes follow, including decreases in pulmonary vascular resistance (Table 43-1).
   1. Pulmonary vascular resistance declines in 3 to 4 days to the eventual level that it will achieve during the neonatal period. Nitric oxide (endothelial-derived relaxing factor) is an integral part of the decrease in pulmonary vascular resistance.
   2. The foramen ovale usually closes permanently over the first several months of life. Nevertheless, about 30% of individuals <30 years of age and 20% of those >30 years of age have a foramen ovale that may become patent if the right atrial pressure exceeds the left atrial pressure.
B. **Transition of the Pulmonary System**
   1. The primary initial event in the transition of the pulmonary system is initiation of ventilation, which changes the alveoli from a fluid-filled to an air-filled state. The initial negative intrathoracic pressures may be 40 to 60 mm H_2O.

TABLE 43-1

CIRCULATORY CHANGES ASSOCIATED WITH INITIAL EXPANSION OF THE NEONATE'S LUNGS

Pulmonary blood flow increases
Foramen ovale closes (left atrial pressure > right atrial pressure)
Patient ductus arteriosus closes

2. By 10 to 20 minutes, a newborn has achieved its almost normal functional residual capacity and arterial blood gas concentrations are stabilized (Table 43-2).

C. **Patent Ductus Arteriosus**
   1. Patency of the ductus arteriosus beyond day 4 of life is abnormal regardless of gestational age.
   2. The incidence of patent ductus arteriosus in premature infants with a history of respiratory distress syndrome is increased.

D. **Persistent Pulmonary Hypertension**
   1. Hypoxemia and acidosis may cause pulmonary hypertension to persist or recur (Table 43-3).
   2. Treatment is characterized as noninterventionist or interventionist (Table 43-4). In both situations, if it is evident that treatment is not effective, a rescue treatment of ventilation with high frequency oscillation, extracorporeal membrane oxygenation (ECMO), or nitric oxide is used. Successful treatment with nitric oxide may allow ECMO to be avoided.
   3. Designation of persistent pulmonary hypertension as persistent fetal circulation is a misnomer because fetal circulation is characterized by a placental shunt that is no longer present.

TABLE 43-2

ARTERIAL BLOOD GAS VALUES FOR NEONATES

Age	PaO_2 (mm Hg)	$PaCO_2$ (mm Hg)	pH
10 min	50	48	7.20
1 hr	70	35	7.35
1 week	75	35	7.40

TABLE 43-3
EVENTS ASSOCIATED WITH PERSISTENT PULMONARY HYPERTENSION

Meconium aspiration (hypoxia during delivery)
Respiratory failure
Congenital diaphragmatic hernia

   E. Meconium Aspiration
      1. Chronic fetal hypoxia leads to the passage of meconium in utero, which enters the pulmonary system when the fetus breathes (serves as a marker of fetal hypoxia in the third trimester).
      2. Meconium aspiration at delivery is different from meconium aspiration in utero. Meconium at birth is often thick and tenacious and mechanically obstructs the tracheobronchial system (may result in fatal asphyxia).
        a. Treatment of meconium aspiration at birth is no longer routine tracheal intubation and suctioning.
        b. The recommended treatment of meconium aspiration or staining (found in approximately 10% of newborns) is routine oropharyngeal suctioning at the time of delivery, with tracheal intubation and suctioning performed selectively based on the condition of the infant.

TABLE 43-4
TREATMENT OF PERSISTENT PULMONARY HYPERTENSION

Noninterventionist
Accept modest hypercapnia ($PaCO_2$ 40–60 mm Hg) and ventilatory settings that maintain $PaCO_2$ 50–70 mm Hg and pH >7.25
Vasodilator therapy if failure to respond to conventional ventilator therapy
Avoid sedatives and muscle relaxants

Interventionist
Aggressive ventilator management (inflation pressures up to 50 cm H_2O and breathing rates 100–150/min) in an attempt to maintain pH >7.5 with $PaCO_2$ 20–30 mm Hg
Risk of volutrauma and increased incidence of residual lung disease

II. TRANSITION AND MATURATION OF THE RENAL SYSTEM

A. The limited ability of the neonate's kidneys to concentrate or dilute urine results from the low glomerular filtration rate at birth. By 3 to 4 days, this limited ability is largely overcome.

   1. The kidneys are approximately 70% mature by 1 month, and renal function is sufficient to handle almost any contingency.
   2. Immature renal tubular cells do not respond optimally to aldosterone (neonates cannot conserve sodium even with severe sodium deficits [obligate sodium losers]).

B. **Fluid and Electrolyte Therapy in Neonates**

   1. Fluids must contain sodium, as in Lactated Ringers solution.
   2. Infants of diabetic mothers and those small for gestational age are at risk for development of hypoglycemia.

III. ANATOMIC AND MATURATIONAL FACTORS OF NEONATES AND THEIR CLINICAL SIGNIFICANCE (Fig. 43-1)

A. **The Pulmonary System** (Table 43-5)

   1. Airway obstruction, breath holding, coughing, or apnea (as during laryngoscopy) leads to rapid desaturation because of high oxygen consumption.
   2. A rapid breathing rate (necessary because of high oxygen consumption) results in increased alveolar ventilation with associated rapid induction of and recovery from anesthesia.

B. **The Cardiovascular System**

   1. **Heart and Sympathetic Nervous System.** The ability of the neonate's immature cardiovascular system to respond to stress is limited by the relatively low contractile mass per gram of cardiac tissue, which results in a limited ability to increase myocardial contractility and a decrease in compliance of the ventricle.

      a. As a result, the neonate's ability to increase stroke volume is limited, and any increase in cardiac output must be accomplished by an increase in heart rate (rate-dependent cardiac output).

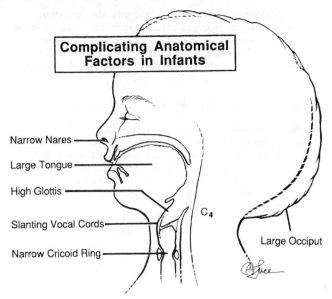

FIGURE 43-1. Complicating anatomic factors in infants.

      b. Bradycardia (hypoxia is a prominent cause) has serious consequences (decreased cardiac output) in the neonate.

      c. The sympathetic nervous system is immature, and the cardiac output can increase only by 30 to 40% (300% in the adult).

TABLE 43-5

COMPARISON OF VENTILATION IN NEONATES AND ADULTS

	Neonate	Adult
Oxygen consumption (mL/kg/min)	7–9	3
Tidal volume (mL/kg)	7	7
Breathing rate (times/min)	30–50	12–16
Functional residual capacity (mL/kg)	27–30	30
Alveolar ventilation (mL/kg/min)	100–150	60

2. **Baroresponse** (reflex tachycardia that occurs in response to hypotension) is immature in the neonate, resulting in a limited ability to compensate for hypotension. In addition, the baroresponse of the neonate is more depressed than that of the adult at the same level of anesthesia.

IV. ANESTHETIC DRUGS FOR THE NEONATE

A. **Anticholinergic Drugs.** An anticholinergic drug (atropine, 0.02 mg/kg im) may be recommended to decrease secretions. It is also common to administer atropine intravenously just prior to the injection of succinylcholine. There is little need to administer sedatives or opioids to neonates.

B. **Inhalational Agents**
   1. Nitrous oxide has mild depressant effects on systemic hemodynamics in sedated infants similar to those reported in adults but does not increase pulmonary artery pressure and pulmonary vascular resistance.
   2. Isoflurane, desflurane, and sevoflurane decrease systemic vascular resistance so that the major effect is a decrease in peripheral vascular resistance.

C. **Neuromuscular Blocking Drugs (NMBDs)**
   1. **Succinylcholine.** The neonate and infant have a larger extracellular fluid volume, leading to a larger volume of distribution and an increased dose requirement (3 mg/kg) compared to children (2 mg/kg) and adults.
      a. Hyperkalemia and cardiac arrest following administration of succinylcholine is very rare and succinylcholine is still recommended for rapid sequence induction and airway emergencies.
      b. When it is evident that a neonate's airway is obstructed by either laryngospasm or any other reason and no progress is made in ventilation, then either intramuscular or intravenous succinylcholine should be administered.
   2. **Nondepolarizing Agents**
      a. The neonate's neuromuscular junction is more sensitive to nondepolarizing relaxants but the larger extracellular fluid volume tends to balance this effect so the dose requirements are similar in neonates and children.
      b. Rocuronium (0.6 mg/kg iv) is intermediate acting but if a larger dose (1.0 to 1.2 mg/kg iv) is

administered to avoid succinylcholine during a rapid sequence induction, then rocuronium will be a relatively long-acting relaxant.

3. **Reversal Agents.** It is a common practice to reverse all nondepolarizing NMBDs in neonates utilizing edrophonium (1 mg/kg iv achieves 90% reversal in 2 minutes) or neostigmine (0.07 mg/kg iv achieves 90% reversal in 10 minutes). The onset of edrophonium is so rapid that atropine (0.01 to 0.02 mg/kg iv) should be administered before the edrophonium.

D. **Opioids** are mild vasodilators but if the infant is adequately volume resuscitated, the administration of opioids should have little effect on the blood pressure.

1. Metabolism of fentanyl may be prolonged particularly in those with increased intra-abdominal pressure.

2. Morphine has a longer half-life and decreased plasma clearance in neonates compared to children and adults. Failure to detect morphine-6-glucuronide, a metabolite of morphine with analgesic properties, may reflect immaturity of the neonate's liver.

E. **Intravenous Agents.** Ketamine (1 to 2 mg/kg iv followed by 0.5 to 1 mg/kg every 15 to 30 minutes) is useful in infants with an unstable cardiovascular system or in whom there is a question about volume repletion.

V. ANESTHETIC MANAGEMENT OF THE NEONATE

A. Factors to consider in selecting an anesthetic technique are (1) whether it is anticipated that the neonate will be extubated at the end of surgery, (2) the need to control blood pressure, and (3) the need for postoperative pain relief.

1. These goals may be achieved with inhalational anesthetics, regional techniques, muscle relaxants, opioids, and ketamine.

2. Caudal anesthesia reduces the need for inhalational agents, opioids, and muscle relaxants

B. **Tracheal intubation** is not mandatory for brief, noninvasive operations. Decisions to intubate the trachea while the neonate is awake must be tempered by the possibility that associated hypertension could place excessive stress on fragile cerebral blood vessels. The neonate's trachea is typically extubated only after signs of awakening and reacting to the tracheal tube are present.

C. **Impact of Surgical Requirements on Anesthetic Technique**
    1. Blood replacement is indicated if the neonate has demonstrated circulatory instability and considerable blood loss is anticipated.
    2. If the neonate is healthy and the anticipated blood loss is 25 to 30% of the blood volume and final hemoglobin is in the range of 8 to 9 g/dL, then blood transfusion probably can be avoided.

D. **Uptake and Distribution of Anesthetics in Neonates**
    1. The faster uptake of anesthetics in infants may reflect the ratio of alveolar ventilation to FRC (5:1 in the infant and 1.5:1 in the adult) and the greater distribution of the cardiac output to vessel-rich group of organs.
    2. It is possible that nonrebreathing systems deliver higher inhaled concentrations of volatile anesthetics.

E. **Anesthetic Dose Requirements of Neonates**
    1. Neonates and premature infants have lower anesthetic requirements than older infants and children (Table 43-6).
    2. Possible explanations for lower minimum alveolar concentration (MAC) (Table 43-7).

F. **Regional Anesthesia** (Table 43-8)
    1. Caudal epidural block is frequently used in combination with general anesthesia, especially for abdominal and thoracic surgery.
        a. Caudal anesthesia decreases the requirements for injected or inhaled anesthetic drugs and muscle relaxants and provides postoperative analgesia, which permits early tracheal extubation.

TABLE 43-6
ANESTHETIC REQUIREMENTS (MAC) IN INFANTS

	Halothane MAC[a]
Premature infant	0.6%
Full-term neonate	0.89%
Neonate 2–4 mo	1.12%

[a]Similar directional changes for isoflurane MAC.

TABLE 43-7

EXPLANATIONS FOR DECREASED ANESTHETIC REQUIREMENTS (MAC) IN NEONATES

Immature central nervous system
Progesterone
Increased endorphins (which enter central nervous system across an immature blood-brain barrier)

---

   b. A single-shot epidural (1 to 1.25 mL/kg of 0.25% bupivacaine or 0.2% ropivacaine with 1:200,000 epinephrine) can provide postoperative analgesia for 6 to 8 hours. The risk of cardiac and central nervous system toxicity may be less with ropivacaine than bupivacaine.
  2. Accidental total spinal anesthesia is manifested as a decreasing arterial oxygen saturation rather than hypotension and tachycardia (reflects an immature sympathetic nervous system).
  3. Ring block of the penis (0.25 to 0.5% bupivacaine subcutaneously at the base of the penis) provides anesthesia for circumcision.

VI. SPECIAL CONSIDERATIONS

  A. **Maternal Drug Use During Pregnancy**
    1. Maternal cocaine and marijuana use during pregnancy result in a reduced catecholamine uptake and accumulation of catecholamines.
    2. Problems affecting the infant are premature birth, intrauterine growth retardation, and cardiovascular abnormalities including low cardiac output.
  B. **Respiratory distress syndrome** reflects a deficiency of surfactant.

TABLE 43-8

REASONS FOR MORE RAPID INDUCTION OF ANESTHESIA IN NEONATES

Greater alveolar ventilation relative to the functional residual capacity
Greater proportion of the cardiac output goes to vessel-rich group tissues (brain, heart)
Lower blood/gas solubility
Lower MAC requirement

C. **Postoperative Apnea.** Infants at highest risk are those born prematurely, those with multiple congenital anomalies, those with a history of apnea and bradycardia, and those with chronic lung disease.
   1. Hypothermia and anemia may contribute to the development of postoperative apnea.
   2. Infants with life-threatening apnea and bradycardia before surgery may be on central nervous system stimulants (caffeine and theophylline).
   3. Infants at high risk for development of postoperative apnea may benefit from the use of a regional anesthetic as opposed to general anesthesia.
   4. The most widely accepted guideline is to monitor all infants younger than 50 weeks postconceptual age for at least 12 hours after surgery.

D. **Retinopathy of Prematurity**
   1. Neonates weighing <1,000 g are at the greatest risk, whereas the likelihood of developing this entity is low in neonates weighing >1,500 g and without other complicating medical conditions.
   2. An arbitrary recommendation is to maintain the arterial oxygen saturation near 95% in infants <40 weeks postconceptual age.

E. **Sudden infant death syndrome** is the most frequent cause of death in infants 1 to 12 months of age. The causes are unknown, but premature infants may be at increased risk. There is no evidence that general anesthesia triggers this syndrome. The American Academy of Pediatrics recommends that prone positioning of infants during sleep be avoided.

F. **Neurodevelopment effects of anesthetic agents** on the developing brain are inconclusive.

VII. SURGICAL PROCEDURES IN NEONATES

A. Except for gastroschisis, which should be repaired within 12 to 24 hours, there are no acute emergency operations in the neonate. This means that a period of 2 to 3 days can be allowed for stabilization and/or transport to an appropriate pediatric center for treatment.

B. **Surgical Procedures in the First Week of Life**
   1. **Congenital diaphragmatic hernia** is present in about 1 in every 4,000 live births, and mortality (despite surgery) remains near 50%, principally because of

TABLE 43-9

MANIFESTATIONS OF CONGENITAL DIAPHRAGMATIC HERNIA

Scaphoid abdomen
Decreased to absent breath sounds on side of hernia
Arterial hypoxemia
Radiographic confirmation

severe underdevelopment of the neonatal lungs. Abdominal contents compress the developing lung buds and often result in hypoplastic lungs.

a. **Clinical presentation** depends on the degree of the hernia and its interference with breathing (Table 43-9). Immediate supportive care is **tracheal intubation** and **decompression of the stomach.** Delivery of excessive airway pressure may result in a **pneumothorax.** Associated congenital anomalies (often cardiac) should be sought.

b. **Antenatal diagnosis.** Polyhydramnios is present in 30%, and ultrasonography can be used to make the diagnosis in utero.

c. **Preoperative care.** Surgery is delayed to allow stabilization of the infant. Conventional ventilation with permissive hypercapnia avoids the risk of iatrogenic lung injury.

d. **Perioperative care.** Despite a period of preoperative stabilization, some infants will still have a component of reactive pulmonary hypertension. Any sudden deterioration of arterial oxygenation should arouse suspicion of a pneumothorax. Maintenance of intravascular fluid volume is essential to avoid the development of acidosis, which could precipitate pulmonary hypertension. Nitrous oxide is avoided.

e. **Postoperative care.** The majority of infants will require some form of ventilatory support in the postoperative period (occasionally nitric oxide, ECMO). Cardiac development may be impaired in these infants.

2. **Omphalocele-Gastroschisis**

a. An **omphalocele** is covered with a membrane (amnion), which protects against infection and loss of extracellular fluid. Affected neonates have

TABLE 43-10

PERIOPERATIVE CARE ASSOCIATED WITH OMPHALOCELE-GASTROSCHISIS

Fluid loss (requires balanced salt solutions; monitor central venous pressure and urine output)

Control infection

Avoid nitrous oxide

Skeletal muscle relaxation (primary closure and ventilation; Dacron silo a consideration if intragastric pressure >20 mm Hg)

Hypertension (renin release in response to mechanical decrease in renal blood flow)

Leg edema

Anticipate the need for postoperative ventilation of the lungs

a high incidence (about 20%) of other congenital anomalies, especially cardiac defects.

b. **Gastroschisis** is not covered with a membrane (infection, hypothermia, and fluid loss are likely), but associated congenital anomalies are less likely.

c. **Antenatal diagnosis.** High levels of α-fetoprotein in the maternal serum (closure of the abdominal wall and neural tube decreases release into the amniotic fluid) suggest the diagnosis, which may be confirmed by ultrasonography. Cesarean section may be considered when the diagnosis is known.

d. **Perioperative care** (Table 43-10)

3. **Tracheoesophageal fistula** occurs in about 1 in every 3,000 live births, and 87% have a fistula from the distal trachea to the esophagus and a blind proximal esophageal pouch. About 50% have associated congenital anomalies (especially cardiac), and prematurity may be associated with respiratory distress syndrome.

a. **Clinical presentation** (Table 43-11)

TABLE 43-11

MANIFESTATIONS OF TRACHEOESOPHAGEAL FISTULA

Polyhydramnios

Inability to pass a nasogastric tube into the stomach

Cyanosis and choking with oral fluids

Aspiration pneumonitis

TABLE 43-12

ANESTHETIC CONSIDERATIONS IN THE PRESENCE OF A TRACHEOESOPHAGEAL FISTULA

Leave the gastrostomy tube open to the atmosphere
Awake versus anesthetized tracheal intubation
Position the tracheal tube distal to the fistula (breath sounds; gas bubbles out of gastrostomy tube cease)
Consider migration of the tracheal tube into the fistula with sudden changes in compliance of the lungs or oxygen saturation
Anticipate the needs for postoperative ventilation of the lungs

>   **b. Anesthetic considerations.** A gastrostomy may be performed initially to protect the lungs from aspiration and to allow the infant's general condition to improve before surgery (Table 43-12).
>   **4. Intestinal Obstruction**
>   **a. Upper gastrointestinal tract obstruction** usually manifests in the first 24 hours of life (Table 43-13).
>   **b. Lower gastrointestinal tract obstruction** usually manifests 2 to 7 days after birth (Table 43-14).
>   **5. Meningomyelocele** introduces unique management problems (Table 43-15).
> **C. Surgical Procedures in the First Month of Life**
>   **1. Necrotizing enterocolitis** in premature infants introduces numerous considerations for anesthetic management if surgery is needed to resect gangrenous bowel (Table 43-16).
>   **2. Inguinal hernia repair** is indicated to prevent incarceration or intestinal obstruction.

TABLE 43-13

PERIOPERATIVE CONCERNS ASSOCIATED WITH UPPER GASTROINTESTINAL OBSTRUCTION

Vomiting and electrolyte losses (sodium)
Awake tracheal intubation (consider topical anesthesia if a concern is that associated hypertension could cause intracranial hemorrhage in a premature infant)
Adequate skeletal muscle relaxation
Nitrous oxide is acceptable if minimal preexisting intestinal gas is present
Anticipate the need for postoperative ventilation of the lungs

TABLE 43-14

PERIOPERATIVE CONCERNS ASSOCIATED WITH LOWER GASTROINTESTINAL OBSTRUCTION

Fluid loss into the gastrointestinal tract (delay anesthesia and surgery until plasma sodium concentration >130 mEq/L and urine output is adequate)
Consider awake tracheal intubation if patient is vomiting
Avoid nitrous oxide
Provide adequate skeletal muscle relaxation
Anticipate the need for postoperative ventilation of the lungs

TABLE 43-15

MANAGEMENT PROBLEMS ASSOCIATED WITH MENINGOMYELOCELE

Infection
Fluid and electrolyte losses
Positioning for tracheal intubation
Hydrocephalus

TABLE 43-16

ANESTHETIC CONSIDERATIONS IN THE PRESENCE OF NECROTIZING ENTEROCOLITIS

Peritonitis
Sepsis
Acidosis
Hypovolemia (replace with balanced salt solution; whole blood)
Tolerate minimal anesthesia (ketamine 0.5–1 mg/kg iv; avoid nitrous oxide)
Invasive monitoring (blood pressure, central venous pressure, arterial blood gases)
Anticipate the need for postoperative ventilation of the lungs

TABLE 43-17

INDICATIONS THAT PATIENTS WITH PYLORIC STENOSIS ARE ADEQUATELY PREPARED FOR SURGERY

Normal skin turgor
Plasma sodium >130 mEq/L
Plasma potassium >3 mEq/L
Plasma chloride >85 mEq/L
Urine output 1–2 mL/kg/hr

3. **Pyloric stenosis** is a medical emergency, and surgical correction is considered only after correction of fluid and electrolyte deficits (Table 43-17). **Anesthetic management** must consider the risk of aspiration (Table 43-18).
4. **Ligation of a patent ductus arteriosus** may be necessary in a small premature infant with congestive heart failure and respiratory distress syndrome.
   a. Administration of fentanyl (20 to 25 μg/kg iv) and pancuronium provides adequate analgesia and surgical working conditions.
   b. In low-birth-weight infants, video-assisted ligation of the patent ductus is accomplished without spreading the ribs or cutting muscles.
5. **Placement of a central venous catheter** requires tracheal intubation, a motionless patient, and a high index of suspicion for bleeding and pneumothorax.

TABLE 43-18

PERIOPERATIVE CONCERNS ASSOCIATED WITH PYLORIC STENOSIS

Orogastric tube (empty the stomach and instill 5–7 mL sodium bicarbonate)
Awake versus anesthetized (inhalation or intravenous) intubation of the trachea
Skeletal muscle relaxation (anesthesia or short-acting muscle relaxant)
Extubate the trachea when the neonate is awake and responding to the tracheal tube
Consider caudal epidural (1.25 mL/kg of 0.25% bupivacaine) after the induction of general anesthesia

CHAPTER 44 ■ PEDIATRIC ANESTHESIA

I. INTRODUCTION

A. The provision of safe anesthesia for the pediatric patient requires a clear understanding of the psychological, physiologic, and pharmacologic differences between patients in different age epochs from newborn to adolescent (Cravero JP, Kain ZN: Pediatric anesthesia. In Barash PG, Cullen BF, Stoelting RK [eds]: *Clinical Anesthesia*, pp 1205–1218. Philadelphia, Lippincott Williams & Wilkins, 2006).

B. There are numerous specific anatomic, physiologic, and psychological issues that should be understood prior to anesthetizing pediatric patients (Table 44-1).

II. THE PREOPERATIVE EVALUATION (Table 44-2)

A. **Coexisting Health Conditions**
   1. **Upper Respiratory Infection (URI)**
      a. A child with a URI or who is recovering from a URI is at increased risk to develop laryngospasm, bronchospasm, oxygen desaturation, and postoperative atelectasis and croup.
      b. It is unclear how long surgery should be delayed following a URI (bronchial hyperreactivity may exist for up to 7 weeks after a URI).
      c. The final decision should take into account the risk-to-benefit ratio of the surgical procedure.
      d. Mask anesthesia, but not laryngeal mask airway, was clearly shown to be associated with a significantly lower rate of perioperative complications as compared to endotracheal tube anesthesia and thus should be used whenever possible with these children.
   2. **Obstructive Sleep Apnea (OSA)**
      a. Severe adenotonsillar hypertrophy with OSA is a frequent indication for children to undergo tonsillectomy and adenoidectomy.

TABLE 44-1

ANATOMICAL AND PHYSIOLOGICAL DISTINCTIONS BETWEEN ADULTS AND PEDIATRIC PATIENTS

Physical/physiologic variable	Contrast between child and adult	Anesthetic implications
Head size	Much larger head size relative to body	Consider roll under shoulders or neck for optimal intubation positioning
Tongue size	Larger size relative to mouth	Makes airway appear slightly anterior. Oral airways particularly helpful during mask ventilation
Airway shape	Narrowest diameter is below the glottis in children under 8 years old	Uncuffed tubes can make a seal when appropriately sized
Respiratory physiology	Oxygen consumption is 2–3 times greater in infants than adults	Oxygen desaturation is extremely rapid following apnea
Cardiac physiology	Relatively fixed stroke volume in neonates and infants	Bradycardia must be treated aggressively in young age groups. Consider atropine prior to airway management. Heart rates under 60 require circulatory support
Renal function	Limited GFR at birth—does not reach adult levels until late infancy. Total body water and percentage extracellular fluid are increased in infants	Prolonged duration of action for hydrophilic drugs—particularly those that are renally excreted

(continued)

TABLE 44-1

CONTINUED

Physical/physiologic variable	Contrast between child and adult	Anesthetic implications
Hepatic function	P-450 system not fully developed in neonates and infants. Liver blood flow is decreased in newborns.	Prolonged excretion of drugs depending on hepatic metabolism
Body surface area	Larger surface to body ratio in newborns/infants/toddlers	Heat loss more prominent problem for these age groups
Psychological development	0–6 months—stress on family 8 months–4 years—separation anxiety 4–6 years—misconceptions of surgical mutilation 6–13 years—fear of not waking up 13 years and older—fear of loss of control, body image issues	Changes the manner in which each patient and family should be approached. Must address issues with personal and systemic strategies.

TABLE 44-2

PREOPERATIVE EVALUATION AND PREPARATION OF CHILD FOR SURGERY

Pertinent maternal history, birth and neonatal history
Review of systems
Physical examination (height, weight, vital signs)
Drugs (bronchodilators, steroids, chemotherapeutic drugs, herbal medicines)
Congenital malformations
Discussion of anesthetic risks, anesthetic plans, postoperative analgesia
Address preoperative anxiety (child and parents)

    b. Children with OSA may experience upper airway obstruct during the induction process and thus muscle relaxants should be used carefully.

    c. Postoperatively, patients with severe OSA may exhibit worsening of their obstructive symptoms secondary to tissue edema, altered response to carbon dioxide, and residual anesthetic and analgesic agents.

    d. Children with severe OSA may require postoperative observation in the hospital.

3. Asthma

    a. Children with asthma should be under optimal medical care prior to undergoing general anesthesia and surgery.

    b. All oral and inhaled medications, such as corticosteroids and beta agonists, should be continued up to and including the day of surgery.

4. The Former Preterm Infant

    a. Three frequent problems are the impact bronchopulmonary dysplasia might have on the patient's perioperative course, the presence of anemia, and the possibility of postoperative apnea.

    b. Risk of postoperative apnea is inversely related to postconceptual age, and infants with a history of apnea and bradycardia, respiratory distress, and mechanical ventilation may be at increased risk.

    c. Overnight hospital monitoring should be planned for any child considered to be at significant risk for postoperative apnea.

B. Laboratory Evaluation

1. Healthy children undergoing elective minor surgery require no laboratory evaluation and thus can be spared the anxiety and pain of blood drawing. Routine chest X rays and urinary analysis is also unnecessary.

2. Coagulation testing should only be considered in children in whom either the history or medical condition suggests a possible hemostatic defect, in patients undergoing surgical procedures that might induce hemostatic disturbances (cardiopulmonary bypass), when the coagulation system is particularly needed for adequate hemostasis, and in patients for whom even minimal postoperative bleeding could be critical.

3. Pregnancy screening (anesthetics may be teratogenic) of female patients of childbearing age before the administration of anesthesia is a matter of policy at individual facilities.

C. Preoperative Fasting Period

1. Solids are prohibited within 6 to 8 hours of surgery (generally after midnight), formula within 6 hours of surgery, breast milk within 4 hours of surgery, and clear liquids within 2 hours of surgery.

2. Liquids such as apple or grape juice, flat cola, and sugar water may be encouraged up to 2 hours prior to the induction of anesthesia.

3. Fasting time is of importance as the younger the child, the smaller are the glycogen stores and the more likely is the occurrence of hypoglycemia with prolonged intervals of fasting.

D. Preoperative Sedatives (Table 44-3). The primary goals of premedication in children are to facilitate a smooth and anxiety-free separation from the parents and induction of anesthesia.

III. ANESTHETIC AGENTS

A. Potent Inhalation Agents

1. **Mask Induction Pharmacology.** The incidence of bradycardia, hypotension, and cardiac arrest during inhalation induction is higher in infants younger than 1 year of age (reflects rapid uptake of inhalation agents and high inspired concentrations used early in induction).

TABLE 44-3
PREOPERATIVE SEDATIVES IN CHILDREN

Oral
Midazolam (0.5–0.75 mg/kg, onset in 30 minutes and lasts approximately 30 minutes)
Ketamine (5–6 mg/kg)
Transmucosal fentanyl (facial pruritus, nausea and vomiting, oxygen desaturation)
Clonidine (4 μg/kg)

Nasal
Midazolam (0.2 mg/kg, rapid absorption as avoids first pass metabolism, disadvantage is transient nasal irritation)

Rectal
Midazolam (0.5–1.0 mg/kg)

Intramuscular
Midazolam (0.3 mg/kg, anxiolysis in 5–10 minutes)
Ketamine (3–4 mg/kg)

2. **Minimal Alveolar Concentration (MAC)** of anesthetic required in pediatric patients differs with age (small increase in MAC between birth and 2 to 3 months and after that time, MAC slowly decreases with age).
3. **Intracardiac Shunts.** Although intracardiac shunts can, in theory, alter the uptake of anesthetic agents and affect the speed of induction, this is rarely clinically evident.
4. **Inhaled Agents for Induction of Anesthesia** Sevoflurane produces a rapid onset and relatively less frequent junctional bradycardia than halothane.

B. **Inhaled Agents—General Points on Maintenance and Recovery in Pediatric Patients**
1. The safety and efficacy of sevoflurane for maintenance of anesthesia in children has been established in hundreds of studies.
2. While emergence from anesthesia is more rapid with sevoflurane than with more soluble agents such as halothane or isoflurane, there is a growing literature supporting the fact that agitation behaviors in children on emergence are more common with this agent.

IV. INTRAVENOUS AGENTS

A. **Sedative-hypnotics** may be employed after inhaled induction of anesthesia or they may be used as primary induction and maintenance agents in children who have an iv in place.
1. Doses of intravenous agents used in infants and toddlers will often need to be increased by 25 to 40% in order to obtain the same level of sedation/anesthesia in children as compared to adults.
2. Propofol induction doses range from 3 to 4 mg/kg iv for children younger than 2 years to approximately 2.5 to 3 mg/kg iv for older children while maintenance of anesthesia requires 200 to 300 μg/kg/min.
   a. Emergence from deep propofol sedation/anesthesia is faster than that from most other sedative agents and most inhaled agents, especially after prolonged administration.
   b. Emergence from propofol is associated with less nausea and vomiting and it is accompanied by less emergence agitation, so readiness for discharge is rapid.
3. Ketamine offers both hypnosis and analgesia, preserves airway reflexes, maintains respiratory drive, increases endogenous catecholamine release, and results in bronchodilation as well as pulmonary vasodilation.
   a. Induction doses of 1 mg/kg iv yield effective analgesia and sedation with rapid onset.
   b. Intramuscular (IM) doses of 3 to 4 mg/kg results in a similar state with significant analgesia—appropriate for minor procedures such as iv catheterplacement or fracture manipulation.
   c. Simultaneous administration of an anticholinergic will minimize oral secretions.
   d. Emergence can be marked by diplopia, occasional disturbing dreams, and nausea/vomiting, although these are less common in children than adults.
B. **Opioids** are important elements of balanced anesthesia and sedation in children.
1. Use of opioids for surgical anesthesia will decrease MAC of inhaled agents, smooth hemodynamics

during airway management or stimulating procedures, and provide postoperative analgesia.

2. Opioids depress central respiratory effort, and newborns and infants younger than 6 months are particularly susceptible to this effect because of the immature blood brain barrier and increased levels of free drug.

C. **Muscle Relaxants**

1. Succinylcholine (1.5 to 2.0 mg/kg iv) produces excellent intubating conditions in 60 seconds with recovery in 6 to 7 minutes.

   a. Succinylcholine can also be given im (4 mg/kg) in emergencies when iv access is not available.

   b. Succinylcholine is contraindicated in a variety of patients (Table 44-4).

   c. Succinylcholine can only be recommended in situations where ultrarapid onset and short duration of action is of paramount importance (laryngospasm) or when relaxation is required or when iv access is not available and im administration is required.

2. All nondepolarizing muscle relaxants used in adults are effective for pediatric patients (Table 44-5).

   a. Neonates and infants have a larger percentage of total body water and larger extracellular fluid volume and thus a larger volume of distribution for these hydrophilic drugs than older children and adults. On the other hand, these patients are slightly more sensitive to these drugs.

   b. The result is a pharmacokinetic and pharmacodynamic profile where the recommended doses of these agents are identical for children and adults but the duration of action tends to be slightly longer.

TABLE 44-4

CONTRAINDICATIONS TO ADMINISTRATION OF SUCCINYLCHOLINE TO CHILDREN

Muscular dystrophy
Recent burn injury
Spinal cord transection and/or immobilization
Family history of malignant hyperthermia
Relative contraindication based on FDA warning

TABLE 44-5

COMPARATIVE PHARMACOLOGY OF NONDEPOLARIZING NEUROMUSCULAR BLOCKING AGENTS IN CHILDREN

	Dose (μg/kg)[a]	Onset	Duration	Cardiovascular effects	Cost
Atracurium	500	Intermediate	Intermediate	Rare hypotension	Intermediate
Cisatracurium	80–120	Slow to intermediate	Intermediate to long	Absent	Inexpensive to intermediate
Mivacurium	250–400	Intermediate	Short	Rare hypotension	Intermediate
Pancuronium	100	Intermediate	Intermediate to long	Tachycardia, occasional hypertension	Inexpensive
Rocuronium	500–1200	Rapid	Intermediate	Slight increase in heart rate	Intermediate
Vecuronium	100–400	Intermediate (rapid with large doses)	Intermediate (long with doses >150 μg/kg)	Absent	Intermediate

[a]Personal recommendations of author.

  c. Rocuronium has the fastest onset of action in this class (60 to 90 seconds for a 1 mg/kg iv dose) and is generally the choice for rapid sequence intubation.

 3. Muscle twitch should be monitored and reversal agents (neostigmine 0.05 mg/kg with 0.015 mg/kg of atropine or 0.01 mg/kg glycopyrrolate) administered iv if residual weakness is detected.

V. ANTIEMETICS

 A. Postoperative nausea and vomiting (PONV) are among the most common causes of prolonged recovery stays and unanticipated hospitalization in children.

  1. Ondansetron (0.05 to 0.15 mg/kg) orally is effective in tonsillectomy and strabismus models but its effectiveness as a "rescue" medication is not proven.

  2. Dexamethasone (0.15 to 1.0 mg/kg iv) appears to be effective in limiting PONV after oral pharyngeal surgery (tonsillectomy).

  3. Droperidol is effective in children as an antiemetic but concern regarding prolonged QT syndrome and possible torsades de pointes with its use has impacted the frequency of administration of this drug.

 B. A practice of requiring patients to eat and/or drink prior to discharge will only increase PONV.

 C. The use of pain control modalities in lieu of opioids (acetaminophen or nonsteroidal anti-inflammatory drugs [NSAIDs] and regional anesthesia) will likely decrease the overall risk of PONV.

VI. FLUID AND BLOOD PRODUCT MANAGEMENT

 A. Perioperative fluid and blood product management for pediatric patients must take into account fluid deficits (calculated maintenance requirement times number of hours NPO), translocation of fluids and blood loss during surgery, and maintenance fluid requirements (Table 44-6).

 B. Immediate intravascular volume expansion may be accomplished with a 10 mL/kg iv bolus of isotonic fluid. The balance of the calculated fluid deficit can be

TABLE 44-6

MAINTENANCE FLUID REQUIREMENTS FOR PEDIATRIC PATIENTS

Weight (kg)	Hourly fluids (mL)	24-Hour fluids (mL)
<10	4 mL/kg	100 mL/kg
11–20	40 mL + 2 mL/kg >10 kg	1000 mL + 50 mL/kg >10 kg
>20	60 mL + 1 mL/kg >20 kg	1500 mL + 20 mL/kg >20 kg

provided over 1 or 2 hours and is often provided in the form of an isotonic fluid or a 5% dextrose solution in 0.9% normal saline.

1. Liberalized recommendations for intake of clear fluids (generally up to 2 hours prior to surgery) means hypoglycemia is unlikely in children as a result of fasting prior to surgery.
2. Administration of 5% dextrose solutions to replace deficits or fluid losses intraoperatively may result in hyperglycemia (problematic for patients with intracranial injury).
3. Intraoperative monitoring of blood glucose is appropriate for newborns, former premature infants, and any high-risk pediatric patients.

C. Surgical manipulation is associated with the isotonic transfer of fluids from the extracellular fluid compartment to the nonfunctional interstitial compartment (third-space loss).

1. Estimated third-space loss during intra-abdominal surgery varies from 6 to 15 mL/kg/hour, whereas in intrathoracic surgery it is less (4 to 7 mL/kg/hour) and during intracranial or cutaneous surgery it is negligible (1 to 2 mL/kg/hr).
2. These third-space losses should be estimated and replaced on an hourly basis.
   a. These losses are derived from extracellular fluid, therefore, it is important to replace with a balance/salt solution to avoid hyponatremia that would result from using hypotonic replacement.
   b. Lactated Ringers solution is frequently used, as normal saline contains an excessive chloride and acid load for infants.

D. Indications for blood or blood component therapy in pediatric patients are based on considerations of the patient's blood volume, preoperative hematocrit, general medical condition, ability to provide oxygen to tissues, the nature of the surgical procedure, and the risks versus benefits of transfusion.

1. All blood loss should be measured as accurately as possible and accounted for with some form of volume replacement in order to maintain intravascular volume and perfusion.

2. If an isotonic solution is chosen to replace some element of blood loss it should be given in a ratio of 3:1 (crystalloid:blood lost).

E. The concept of the maximum allowable blood loss (MABL) takes into account the patient's total blood volume, starting hematocrit, and estimated "target" hematocrit—that which represents the lowest acceptable hematocrit for this patient considering age and comorbid conditions.

1. In general, blood volume is estimated at 100 mL/kg for the preterm infant, 90 mL/kg for the term infant, 80 mg/kg for the child 3 to 12 months of age, and 70 mg/kg for the patient older than 1 year.

2. These estimates of blood volume can be used in calculating the individual patient's blood volume by multiplying the child's weight by the estimated blood volume (EBV) per kilogram.

F. The end point of fluid and blood therapy is adequate blood pressure, tissue perfusion, and urine volume (0.5 to 1.0 mL/kg/hour).

VII. AIRWAY MANAGEMENT

A. The choice of airway will depend on the age of the child, the time since last oral intake, coexisting illness, and the procedure to be performed.

1. Endotracheal tubes are preferred for premature infants and most neonates because of the slightly greater difficulty of providing effective face mask ventilation under appropriate levels of anesthesia and the risk of filling the stomach with air while providing mask ventilation.

2. Laryngeal mask airways (LMAs) come in a range of sizes and half sizes and can be employed in infants, toddlers, and older children for almost any

procedure that does not involve opening the abdomen or thoracic cavity.

3. Because the narrowest portion of the pediatric airway is at the level of the cricoid cartilage, uncuffed tubes can be used and will create a functional seal when appropriately sized. Air should leak out at no higher than 20 to 25 cm H_2O to minimize risk of postextubation croup.

4. Intubation in children can be safely accomplished after inhaled induction with or without the use of muscle relaxant.

VIII. PEDIATRIC BREATHING CIRCUITS

A. Nonrebreathing circuits minimize the work of breathing because they have no valves to be opened by the patient's respiratory effort. A number of combinations of the simple T-piece tubing, reservoir bag, and sites of fresh gas entry and overflow are possible.

B. Circle breathing systems can also be used very effectively in infants and children.

IX. MONITORING

A. The pediatric patient should be monitored continuously with precordial or esophageal stethoscope.

B. Pulse oximetry, capnography, blood pressure (measured with appropriately sized cuffs), temperature, and electrocardiogram should also be monitored routinely in children as in adults.

C. Low tidal volumes, rapid respiratory rates, and changing intrapulmonary shunts make $ETCO_2$ measurements inaccurate for infants and premature neonates with respiratory distress syndrome.

X. PAIN MANAGEMENT AND REGIONAL ANESTHESIA

A. Children experience pain, just like adults, regardless of their age.

B. The most common oral analgesic used in children is acetaminophen (10 to 15 mg /kg orally every 4 hours). The rectal route of administration can be particularly effective for children with no intravenous access.

  1. Ketorolac (0.75 mg/kg im) is effective but has the disadvantage of prolonging bleeding time because of its effect on platelet aggregation.

  2. Ibuprofen (10 mg/kg orally) is the most popular NSAID given to children.

C. Regional Anesthesia

  1. Ilioinguinal-iliohypogastric nerve block, ring block of the penis, or caudal block can be very useful for common pediatric surgical procedures.

  2. Strict attention must be paid to the dose of local anesthetic, dose of epinephrine, and technique of administration.

  3. Caudal block is the most commonly used form of regional anesthesia in children.

  a. This technique can provide postoperative analgesia following a wide variety of lower abdominal and genitourinary surgical procedures.

  b. Bupivacaine 0.175% solution in a dose of 1 mg/kg is used and if larger volumes are needed, the use of 0.125% is recommended. Postoperative analgesia typically lasts 4 to 6 hours and is not associated with a motor paralysis.

  4. Spinal anesthesia may be used for procedures involving surgical dermatomes below T6.

  a. It is important to note that the dural sac migrates cephalad during the first year of life and in a neonate it is at S3 while over the age of 1 year it is at the S1 level.

  b. Spinal anesthesia is an option for premature infants who undergo surgery as the incidence of postoperative apnea is reduced in these infants with the use of this technique.

  5. Epidural anesthesia can be used in order to provide postoperative analgesia for thoracic, lumbar, and sacral dermatomes. In young children, the epidural space can be reached easily by the caudal approach with less risk of dural puncture than with thoracic or lumbar approaches.

XI. POSTANESTHESIA CARE (Table 44-7)

TABLE 44-7

CHALLENGES DURING RECOVERY OF THE YOUNG CHILD IN THE POSTANESTHESIA CARE UNIT

Hypothermia

Nausea and vomiting (prophylactic ondansetron)

Postoperative pain (self reported or physiologic signs including hypertension, tachycardia, agitation, nausea and vomiting; treat severe pain with fentanyl or morphine iv)

Fear associated with awakening in a strange environment (permit parents to be present)

CHAPTER 45 ■ ANESTHESIA FOR THE GERIATRIC PATIENT

Advances in nutrition, public health, education, and social services have produced major changes in longevity (almost one-third of all surgical patients are 65 years of age or older and elderly patients account for more than one-half of all hospital care days) in industrialized societies (Muravchick S: Anesthesia for the geriatric patient. In Barash PG, Cullen BF, Stoelting RK [eds]: *Clinical Anesthesia*, pp 1219–1228. Philadelphia, Lippincott Williams & Wilkins, 2006).

I. CONCEPTS OF AGING AND GERIATRICS

A. There is no consensus as to when the geriatric (elderly) years begin (establishing a rigid chronologic definition has little value other than for administrative purposes). Nevertheless, elderly is accepted as 65 years of age or older and "aged" as older than 80 years.

B. Many changes because of age-related disease have been erroneously attributed to aging.

C. Mechanisms that control aging remain unknown.
   1. Age-related declines in organ function may be the inevitable accumulation of nonspecific, degenerative phenomena (declining mitochondrial bioenergetics).
   2. Throughout adulthood, increasing levels of oxygen-derived free radicals within the mitochondria appear to disrupt the structural and enzymatic machinery of oxidative phosphorylation. As the ability to scavenge these byproducts of aerobic metabolism declines, it creates a "vicious cycle of aging" within the mitochondria (Fig. 45-1).

II. AGING AND ORGAN FUNCTION

A. Organs and tissues undergo a complex and nonlinear change in function (previously depicted as a linear process) that first becomes apparent following the years that represent the peak of somatic maturation (about the fourth decade of life, which is somewhat later than once thought) (Fig. 45-2). Age-related loss of tissue elasticity is ubiquitous.

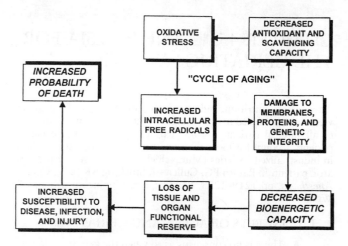

FIGURE 45-1. At a cellular level, there may be a self-sustaining "cycle of aging" within mitochondria in which oxidative stress damages the metabolic machinery needed to provide adequate bioenergetic capacity for full organ system functional reverse.

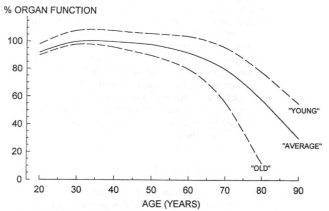

FIGURE 45-2. Interindividual variability in the rate at which the function of organ systems change with increasing age, and, to a lesser extent, initial functional levels explain the presentation of geriatric patients as physiologically "younger" or "older" than "average."

1. Elderly patients who maintain greater than average functional capacities (maximum organ system function that is greater than basal demands) can be considered "physiologically young."
2. When organ function declines at an earlier age than usual or at a more rapid rate, elderly patients appear to be "physiologically old."
3. Changes in organ function with aging are highly variable among individuals even in the absence of disease. This change is significantly altered by activity level, social habits, diet, and genetic background.

B. Organ system functional reserve reflects a "safety margin" of organ capacity available to meet additional demands (increased cardiac output, carbon dioxide excretion, protein synthesis) that may be imposed by trauma, disease, or surgery and convalescence (Fig. 45-3).
   1. It is reasonable to assume that the functional reserve of all organ systems is progressively and significantly decreased in elderly patients.

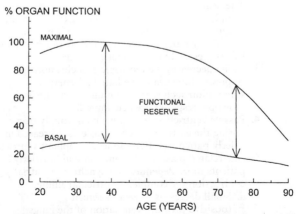

FIGURE 45-3. For any organ system, "functional reserve" represents the difference between basal (minimal) and maximal organ system function. The age-related decrease in functional reserve may not be apparent until demands made on the organ system are increased by stress, disease, polypharmacy, or surgical intervention.

2. Increased susceptibility of elderly patients to stress- and disease-induced organ system decompensation is a defining characteristic of physiologic aging. Therefore, preoperative testing in the elderly patient is most effective when it provides the anesthesiologist with a quantifiable assessment of organ system reserve and is clinically directed according to symptoms and complaints referable to age-related disease and the deterioration of physiologic homeostasis.

III. CARDIOPULMONARY FUNCTION

A. Modest decrease in resting cardiac index observed in most elderly patients is not evidence of degenerative cardiovascular change but rather represents an appropriate integrated response to the decreased needs for perfusion and metabolism that occur with age-related atrophy of skeletal muscle and loss of tissue mass.

1. Under conditions of submaximal demand, myocardial contractility appears to remain uncompromised by increasing age until at least the eighth decade.

2. The heart, unlike other major organs, does not atrophy with age. Short-term increases in cardiac output are accomplished in the elderly patient initially by modest increases in heart rate and then by progressively larger stroke volumes.

3. Aging decreases the inotropic and chronotropic responses to neurally mediated adrenergic stimulation such that maximum heart rate and inotropic response are age limited.

4. Passive ventricular filling, which normally occurs during the early phase of diastole, is decreased in elderly patients (stiffer and less compliant ventricle).

5. Age-related diastolic dysfunction makes elderly patients more dependent on synchronous atrial contraction for complete ventricular filling.

    a. Small decreases in venous return (positive-pressure ventilation of the lungs, hemorrhage, vasodilator drugs) may significantly compromise stroke volume, especially when cardiac dysrhythmias are present.

b. For these reasons, perioperative arterial hypotension is predictably more common in elderly than in young patients.

6. Systolic arterial hypertension reflects fibrotic replacement of elastic tissues within the cardiovascular system (produces the "overshoot" characteristics of radial artery waveform tracings in elderly patients as well as the discrepancies between blood pressure measured invasively versus by cuff).

7. Even sedentary geriatric subjects benefit dramatically from programmed increases in aerobic activity.

B. Loss of lung elastic recoil because of an increase in fibrous connective tissue in the lung parenchyma (inevitable emphysema-like changes) is a primary anatomic mechanism by which aging exerts deleterious effects on pulmonary gas exchange.

1. Vital capacity is progressively compromised as residual volume increases at the expense of inspiratory and expiratory reserve volumes.

2. Costochondral calcification makes the thorax more rigid, which increases the work of breathing and predisposes elderly patients to postoperative ventilatory failure.

3. Overall, pulmonary function in older adults during general anesthesia is best described as progressive ventilation-to-perfusion mismatching as a result of deterioration of alveolar architecture and anesthetic-induced depression of active hypoxic pulmonary vasoconstriction.

4. The threshold stimulus needed for vocal cord closure is increased in the elderly, thus increasing the risk of aspiration of gastric contents.

IV. HEPATORENAL AND IMMUNE FUNCTION

A. Hepatic enzyme activities are comparable to those of young adults but liver tissue mass declines about 40% by the age of 80 years and hepatic blood flow is proportionally reduced.

1. Loss of perfused hepatic tissue mass largely explains the reduced rates of plasma clearance and prolonged clinical effects of many drugs.

2. Nevertheless, hepatic metabolism and drug biotransformation are unpredictable because of

sustained exposure to the intense polypharmacy of age-related chronic diseases.

B. Renal tissue mass (including glomeruli and nephrons) decreases by about 30% by the eighth decade of life (atrophy is especially marked in the renal cortex).

1. Serum creatinine concentration usually remains within the normal range in elderly patients because their declining skeletal muscle mass generates a progressively smaller creatinine load.

2. Geriatric surgical patients do not appear to require a unique fluid replacement protocol but their renal functional reserve is rarely adequate to withstand gross disruptions of water and electrolyte balance.

3. Diminished thirst, poor diet, and the use of diuretics to decrease age-related hypertension predispose elderly patients to intravascular and intracellular dehydration (meticulous monitoring and management of fluid and electrolyte balance is needed in the perioperative period).

C. Elderly patients exhibit decreased immune responsiveness. Older adults are particularly predisposed to streptococcal pneumonia, meningitis, and septicemia (sepsis is second only to respiratory failure as a cause of morbidity and mortality in elderly trauma patients).

V. METABOLISM, BODY COMPOSITION, AND PHARMACOKINETICS

A. Aging in men results in a progressive and generalized loss of skeletal muscle mass and reciprocal increases in the lipid fraction (Fig. 45-4).

1. These changes in body composition decrease the basal metabolic requirements, and the corresponding decrease in heat production puts elderly surgical patients at special risk for intraoperative hypothermia.

a. In the geriatric patient, intraoperative decreases in core body temperature average almost 1°C per hour (about twice that observed in young adults).

b. The time needed for postoperative spontaneous rewarming may be prolonged in elderly patients.

2. Because skeletal muscles and the liver normally provide storage for carbohydrates, aging is

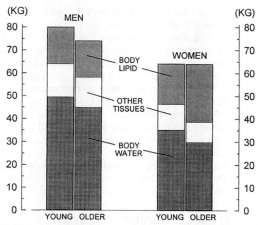

FIGURE 45-4. Age-related changes in body composition are gender specific. Increases in body fat offset bone loss and intracellular dehydration in women, whereas in men accelerated loss of skeletal muscle mass and other components of lean tissue mass produces contraction of intracellular water and a decrease in total body weight.

associated with progressive impairment of the ability to handle an intravenous glucose challenge.

B. After the young adult years, men gain adipose tissue and lose skeletal muscle mass, which ultimately may result in a decline in body weight. In women, muscle and bone loss (osteoporosis) are largely offset by increasing body fat and total body weight is less impacted.

C. Plasma volume, red cell mass, and extracellular fluid volumes are well maintained in nonhypertensive elderly individuals who maintain daily physical activity. Decreases in circulating blood volume typically occur only in bed-ridden and deconditioned elderly or in those with essential hypertension.

VI. CENTRAL NERVOUS SYSTEM

A. Aging decreases brain size, with most of the loss reflecting attrition of neurons, particularly in the gray matter. Neurons that synthesize neurotransmitters seem to be most affected.

B. Cerebral blood flow decreases in proportion to decreased brain tissue mass.
  1. Mechanisms that couple regional cortical and subcortical perfusion to local variation in metabolic demands are maintained and the blood-brain barrier is intact. Aging does not change autoregulation or cerebrovascular resistance to alterations in arterial blood pressure.
  2. Most neurodegenerative disorders and normal aging neurons share declining mitochondrial bioenergetics and rising levels of oxidative stress as common characteristics.
  3. Language skills, personality, general knowledge, and long-term memory are well maintained in aged individuals if they remain physically fit.

VII. PERIPHERAL NERVOUS SYSTEM

A. The threshold intensities of stimuli needed to initiate all forms of perception are increased in elderly individuals. There is an almost exponential decline in the density of pain-sensing Meissner's corpuscles in the skin of elderly individuals.
B. Aging is associated with a gradual but significant deterioration of electrical conduction along efferent motor pathways.
C. An increase in the total number of cholinoceptors at the skeletal muscle membrane offsets the age-related decrease in the density of motor neuron endplates (dose requirements for neuromuscular blocking drugs are not decreased despite loss of skeletal muscle mass).

VIII. AUTONOMIC NERVOUS SYSTEM

A. Neurons in the sympathoadrenal pathways undergo significant cellular attrition, and adrenal tissue and cortisol secretion decline by at least 15% by 80 years of age. Nevertheless, plasma concentrations of norepinephrine are significantly increased in elderly compared with young adults.
  1. Effects of increased plasma concentrations of catecholamines are not apparent clinically because aging markedly and progressively depresses beta-adrenergic end-organ responsiveness (response

to isoproterenol is markedly reduced). Aging produces endogenous beta-blockade.

2. Aging appears to produce little change in alpha-adrenergic or muscarinic cholinoceptor activity.

B. Autonomic reflex responses (baroreceptors) that maintain cardiovascular homeostasis are progressively impaired in elderly patients. This may explain an increased incidence of hypotension in elderly patients following induction of anesthesia.

C. The autonomic nervous system in elderly patients is "underdamped," permitting wider variation from homeostasis set points and delayed restabilization during hemodynamic stress.

IX. ANALGESIC AND ANESTHETIC REQUIREMENTS

A. The net effect of age-related structural and functional changes within the nervous system on pain-related neurological function is controversial.

1. Perceived intensity of pain perioperatively is unpredictable and appears to be more dependent on anxiety, personality, and the prospect of long-term debility than age itself.

2. Nevertheless, parenteral morphine requirements are inversely related to patient age and essentially independent of body weight. Similarly, slightly higher levels of sensory blockade occur in elderly patients undergoing spinal anesthesia.

B. Anesthetic requirements for inhaled anesthetics (minimum alveolar concentration [MAC]) decrease predictably as much as 30% with increasing age (Fig. 45-5). The consistency of this decrease for anesthetic agents with markedly different chemical characteristics suggests that it reflects a fundamental neurophysiological process (declining neuronal bioenergetics because of mitochondrial genetic mutation or oxidative stress).

C. Data on the effect of aging on the pharmacodynamics of opioids (systemic morphine requirements are inversely related to patient age), barbiturates, and benzodiazepines are less consistent than those for inhaled anesthetics.

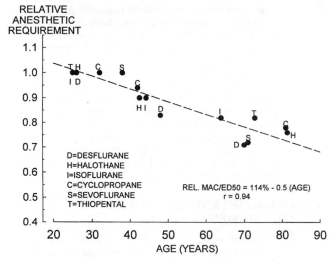

FIGURE 45-5. The linear age-related decrease in relative anesthetic requirements (MAC) for a variety of inhaled and injected anesthetics suggests a pharmacodynamic mechanism rather than a pharmacokinetic explanation.

1. Poor drug mixing as a result of delayed intercompartmental transfer of drugs and not a decreased initial volume of distribution may explain "decreased" drug requirements in elderly patients (a pharmacokinetic explanation rather than a pharmacodynamic mechanism).
2. Analysis of electroencephalographic recordings confirms that aging increases brain sensitivity to injected drugs (opioids, barbiturates), but the median effective plasma concentration is not altered (dose required to produce the same plasma concentration in elderly patients is less than the dose required in young patients).

D. Despite the loss of skeletal muscle mass, doses of muscle relaxants and steady-state plasma concentrations required to produce a given degree of neuromuscular blockade are not changed by aging. In fact, neurogenic atrophy at the neuromuscular junction allows proliferation of extrajunctional cholinoceptors and may increase doses of neuromuscular blocking drugs needed to produce competitive blockade.

1. The clinical duration of action is prolonged if the elimination of the muscle relaxant is dependent on hepatic or renal clearance mechanisms.
2. The intensity of neuromuscular blockade at the time of pharmacologic antagonism plus the anticholinesterase drug selected, and not patient age, ultimately determine the speed and completeness of return of neuromuscular transmission.

X. PERIOPERATIVE MANAGEMENT AND OUTCOME

A. Age-related disease and not aging is primarily responsible for the progressive increase in morbidity and mortality of elderly surgical patients (Table 45-1). The greater need for invasive surgical procedures and high prevalence of polypharmacy associated with chronic disease and its treatment also produces an age-related increase in adverse drug reactions (Table 45-2).

1. The probability of a serious pulmonary or hemodynamic complication after surgery in the elderly, as in the young adult, is largely determined by the site of operation and by the patient's physical status.
2. In the absence of severe ventricular dysfunction or incapacitating lung disease, an elderly patient can be an excellent candidate for any kind of surgery. For the elderly surgical patient at high cardiac risk,

TABLE 45-1
AGE-RELATED DISEASES
Hypertension
Ischemic heart disease
Congestive heart failure
Peripheral vascular disease
Obstructive pulmonary disease
Renal disease
Diabetes mellitus
Arthritis
Dementia

TABLE 45-2
DRUGS LIKELY TO BE TAKEN BY ELDERLY PATIENTS

Antihypertensives
Antidepressants
Anticoagulants
Oral hypoglycemics
Corticosteroids
Beta-blockers
Nighttime sedatives
Alcohol

coronary angiography prior to elective surgery may be indicated.

B. Adverse surgical outcomes in elderly patients show a predominance of dysfunction of cardiac (dysrhythmias, myocardial ischemia), pulmonary (infection), and renal mechanisms, emphasizing the importance of preoperative evaluation and preparation as it relates to these organ systems.

C. The choice of anesthetic drug or technique does not seem to influence the overall outcome in elderly patients. Neither regional anesthesia nor general anesthesia has clearly demonstrable superiority of outcome in elderly patients.

1. There may be value in careful titration of the depth of surgical anesthesia in selected elderly patients to the minimum value needed to prevent awareness.

2. Prompt and complete postoperative recovery of mental function is particularly important in elderly patients (Table 45-3). The use of newer intravenous agents such as remifentanil and cisatracurium minimize dependence on organ function for elimination. Sevoflurane and desflurane provide rapid recovery of consciousness.

   a. Elderly patients are less likely to experience nausea and vomiting but more likely to experience mental confusion following outpatient surgery compared with younger adults.

   b. Full recovery of psychomotor function is somewhat delayed in older patients even after typically brief outpatient anesthesia.

   c. Nerve palsies as a result of regional anesthesia seem to occur more often in elderly patients compared with younger adults.

TABLE 45-3

ADJUSTMENTS OF ANESTHETIC AND ADJUVANT DRUGS IN ELDERLY PATIENTS

Drug group	Adjustment needed
Volatile anesthetics	Decrease inspired concentration
Barbiturates, etomidate, propofol	Small to moderate decrease in initial dose; lower maintenance infusion rate
Opioids	Marked decrease in initial dose; anticipate increased duration of systemic and epidural effects; greater incidence of skeletal muscle rigidity; greater incidence of respiratory depression (?)
Local anesthetics (spinal or epidural anesthesia)	Small to moderate decrease in segmental dose requirement; anticipate prolonged effects
Benzodiazepines	Modest decrease in initial dose; anticipate marked increase in duration of action (except midazolam)
Succinylcholine	Slightly decreased dose in elderly men
Nondepolarizing muscle relaxant	Same or slight increase in initial dose; anticipate increased duration of action (except atracurium or mivacurium)
Neostigmine, edrophonium	No change in dose or efficacy; slightly prolonged duration of action
Atropine	Increased dose for equal heart rate response; anticipate central anticholinergic syndrome
Isoproterenol (and other beta agonists)	Increased doses required for equal cardiovascular responses

D. **Postoperative Cognitive Dysfunction.** Even when anesthetic management of the elderly patient is appropriate and surgical convalescence uncomplicated, after a prolonged general anesthetic full return of cognitive function to preoperative levels may require up to 2 weeks.

  1. Perioperative environmental factors such as chronic medication and drug interactions, disorientation because of sensory deprivation, or the disruption of normal routine needed to maintain implicit memory may predispose elderly patients to delirium.

2. Overall, the neurophysiological or pharmacological explanation for persistent disruption of nervous system function remains unknown.

3. Postoperative cognitive dysfunction can be demonstrated 3 months after apparently uncomplicated surgery in 10 to 15% of patients 60 years of age or older who have had major procedures or a hospital stay of 4 or more days. This suggests that, in adults with reduced central nervous system functional reserve, either the process of general anesthesia or drugs used to produce it may produce residual neurological dysfunction.

E. Physical management of elderly patients in the operating room and postoperatively requires special precautions.

1. Aged skin and bones are fragile and joints are stiff, and their range of motion may be limited by arthritic changes (gentle and careful positioning is required).

2. Active heating devices in contact with poorly perfused skin, connective tissue, or pressure points can quickly produce ischemic lesions.

F. Postoperative bleeding and bacterial infection are more likely to occur in elderly patients compared with younger adults.

G. Because of diastolic dysfunction and increased ventricular stiffness, rates of intravenous fluid administration that would be modest for young adults may precipitate pulmonary edema in elderly patients.

H. Untreated pain and related emotional stress may significantly impair immune responsiveness in elderly patients and increase the risk of postoperative infection. An anesthetic plan that includes postoperative sympathectomy and analgesia may be of special value in elderly patients.

CHAPTER 46 ■ ANESTHESIA FOR AMBULATORY SURGERY

In March 30, 1842, the first ether anesthetic was administered for ambulatory surgery, and today the majority of patients return home within 24 hours of an operative procedure (Lichtor JL: Anesthesia for ambulatory surgery. In Barash PG, Cullen FB, Stoelting RK [eds]: *Clinical Anesthesia*, pp 1229–1245. Philadelphia, Lippincott Williams & Wilkins, 2006). Patient selection today is based on the desire to decrease costs while maintaining quality of care, so that morbidity from the procedure or preexisting disease is no greater than if the patient had been hospitalized. Unanticipated hospital admission rates after ambulatory surgery are usually lower than 3%.

I. PLACE, PROCEDURES, AND PATIENT SELECTION

A. Ambulatory surgery occurs in a variety of settings (hospital, satellite facility, doctor's office). By 2005, it is estimated that 20% of all surgical procedures will be performed in doctors' offices.

B. Appropriate procedures for ambulatory surgery are those associated with postoperative care that is easily managed at home and with low rates of postoperative complications (lists of acceptable procedures and/or patients on whom to perform ambulatory surgery quickly become outdated) (Table 46-1).

   1. Length of surgery is not a criterion for ambulatory procedures because there is little relationship between length of anesthesia and recovery time (Fig. 46-1).

      a. Long operations should be scheduled early in the day.

      b. A variable often correlated with unanticipated hospital admission is completion of surgery late in the day.

   2. The need for transfusion is not a contraindication for ambulatory surgery.

TABLE 46-1

UNLIKELY CANDIDATES FOR AMBULATORY SURGERY

Infants at risk
    Premature birth and <50 weeks postconceptual age
    Apneic episodes
    Failure to thrive
    Respiratory distress syndrome at birth requiring ventilatory
      support
    Bronchopulmonary dysplasia
    Family history of sudden infant death syndrome and <12
      months of age
Susceptibility to malignant hyperthermia
Uncontrolled seizure activity
Medically unstable
Morbidly obese and other systemic diseases
Acute substance abuse
Presence of infection
Uncooperative and/or unreliable patient
No responsible adult at home

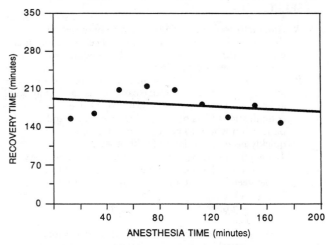

Slope = -0.1092; **intercept** = 190.5; *r* = 0.2360.

FIGURE 46-1. Effect of anesthesia time on recovery time.

3. **Preterm infants** (gestational age <37 weeks) who are younger than 50 weeks postconceptual age should not leave an ambulatory surgery center for at least 23 hours after a surgical procedure because they are at risk for developing apnea even in the absence of a past history of this disorder.
   a. **Anemia** (hematocrit <30 mL/dL) is also associated with an increased incidence of apnea in preterm infants <60 conceptual weeks.
   b. **Caffeine,** 10 mg/kg, administered immediately after induction of general anesthesia and unsupplemented spinal anesthesia has not been associated with postoperative apnea in preterm infants <44 conceptual weeks.
4. Advanced age is not a reason to disallow surgery (such as transurethral resection of the prostate) on an ambulatory basis, recognizing the increased likelihood of preexisting medical diseases (evaluate with preoperative history and physical examination) and altered drug pharmacokinetics (decreased clearance of drugs such as midazolam and propofol).
5. Patients who are classified as ASA physical status III or IV are appropriate candidates for ambulatory surgery, provided that their systemic diseases are medically stable.

C. Patients undergoing ambulatory surgery should be accompanied by a responsible adult to take them home and to stay with them to provide any necessary care.

II. PREOPERATIVE EVALUATION AND REDUCTION OF PATIENT ANXIETY

A. Reducing Patient Anxiety

1. Each outpatient facility should develop its own method of preoperative screening to be conducted before the day of surgery (telephone interview, automated history taking, pre-anesthesia clinic) (Table 46-2).
   a. The process also provides the staff with the opportunity to remind patients of arrival time, suitable attire, and dietary restrictions.
   b. Screening may uncover additional problems such as the need for transportation to the facility or the need for child care.

TABLE 46-2

QUESTIONNAIRE BEFORE OUTPATIENT ANESTHESIA

Do you feel sick?
Do you have any serious illnesses (hypertension, diabetes)?
Do you become short of breath from climbing one flight of stairs?
Do you cough?
Do you wheeze?
Do you experience chest pain from climbing stairs or with other
  forms of exertion?
Do you have ankle swelling?
Have you taken medications in the past 3 months?
Do you have any allergies?
Have you or any of your relatives experienced difficulties with
  anesthesia?
Could you be pregnant?

---

   2. An important reason for preoperative screening is to
      help alleviate the patient's anxiety. For children,
      information-modeling and coping-based programs
      decrease anxiety and enhance coping during the
      preoperative period.
B. Upper Respiratory Tract Infection (URI)
   1. Children with active or recent URIs have more
      episodes of breath holding, incidences of desaturation
      to <90%, and more respiratory events compared to
      children without symptoms (Table 46-3).
   2. It is probably acceptable to proceed with the planned
      surgical procedure if the patient with a URI has a
      normal appetite, is afebrile, has a normal breathing
      rate, and does not appear toxic.

TABLE 46-3

INDEPENDENT RISK FACTORS FOR ADVERSE RESPIRATORY
EVENTS IN CHILDREN WITH UPPER RESPIRATORY TRACT
INFECTIONS

Tracheal intubation versus laryngeal mask airway or face mask
History of prematurity
History of reactive airway disease
History of paternal smoking
Surgery involving the airway
Presence of copious secretions
Nasal congestion

C. **Restriction of Food and Liquids Before Ambulatory Surgery**
   1. To decrease the risk of pneumonitis and airway obstruction should aspiration of gastric contents occur, patients are routinely asked not to eat solid food for at least 6 to 8 hours before surgery. Prolonged fasting may be detrimental.
   2. Practice guidelines published by the American Society of Anesthesiologists allow a light meal up to 6 hours before an elective procedure. The guidelines support a fasting period for clear fluids of 2 hours.
      a. Coffee is not transparent but is free of particulate matter and is accepted as a clear fluid (ingestion before surgery may prevent caffeine withdrawal headache).
      b. Patients may take their chronic medications with water up to 2 hours before surgery.

III. MANAGING THE ANESTHETIC: PREMEDICATION

A. The outpatient is not that different from the inpatient undergoing surgery, so that premedication is useful to control anxiety, postoperative pain, nausea, and vomiting and to decrease the risk of pneumonitis if aspiration of gastric contents occurs during surgery. Most premedications do not prolong recovery when given in appropriate doses (fentanyl, 1 μg/kg iv; midazolam, 0.04 mg/kg iv).

B. **Controlling Anxiety** (Table 46-4)

TABLE 46-4

PROVISION OF PREOPERATIVE SEDATION FOR AMBULATORY SURGERY

Recognize that not every patient requires pharmacologic premedication

Pharmacologic premedication (adult patient):
  Diazepam 2–5 mg orally night before and 6:00 AM on day of surgery
    or
  Midazolam, 2 mg iv or propofol, 5 mg iv

Pharmacologic premedication (children):
  Midazolam, 0.5 mg/kg orally
    or
  Transmucosal fentanyl

1. If in doubt about patient anxiety, ask the patient; predictive accuracy in determining whether patients are anxious increases when they are asked.
2. Children are more likely to demonstrate problematic behavior around the time of separation from parents, especially if they have not received information about what is going to happen preoperatively.
3. **Benzodiazepines** are the drugs used most often to decrease anxiety and induce sedation prior to ambulatory surgery (oral transmucosal fentanyl may be useful for decreasing anxiety in children).
   a. Oral midazolam (0.5 mg/kg) is a useful premedication for children, usually allowing separation from parents within 10 minutes of its administration. When short-acting inhaled anesthetics (sevoflurane, desflurane) are administered to patients premedicated with oral midazolam, the initial recovery time may be prolonged but the time to discharge is not affected.
   b. Routine administration of supplemental oxygen with or without continuous monitoring or arterial oxygen saturation is recommended whenever benzodiazepines are given intravenously.
   c. The potential for amnesia after premedication with a benzodiazepine is a concern, especially for patients undergoing ambulatory surgery (no study has documented that retrograde amnesia occurs).
4. **Opioids and Nonsteroidal Analgesics**
   a. Opioids may be useful preoperatively to sedate patients, and they are also useful to control hypertension during tracheal intubation and to decrease pain following surgery (nonsteroidal analgesics such as ketorolac are also useful and meperidine may decrease postoperative shivering).
   b. The effectiveness of opioids in relieving anxiety is controversial.
   c. Preoperative administration of opioids or nonsteroidal anti-inflammatory drugs is useful in controlling postoperative pain.
   d. Preoperative sedation is not needed for every patient. For patients seen at least 24 hours before the scheduled procedure and expressing a desire for medication to relieve anxiety, oral diazepam the night before and at 6:00 AM on the morning of surgery is useful. For patients seen for the first time

TABLE 46-5

PHARMACOLOGIC PROPHYLAXIS AGAINST ASPIRATION PNEUMONITIS

H_2-receptor antagonists	Cimetidine, ranitidine, famotidine, nizatidine
Substituted benzimidazole	Omeprazole
Nonparticulate antacid	Sodium citrate
Gastrokinetic drug	Metoclopramide

in the preoperative holding area who seem to need medication, midazolam 0.1 mg/kg iv is helpful or the patient is brought to the operating room and propofol 0.7 mg/kg iv is administered. For children, when necessary, oral midazolam, 0.5 mg/kg, is administered in the preoperative holding area.

C. Controlling the Risk of Aspiration

1. Patients who undergo ambulatory surgery may be at some small risk for aspiration of gastric contents, although this risk is no greater than for inpatients. Preoperative anxiety probably has no effect on gastric acidity for individuals without a history of duodenal ulcer.

2. Pharmacologic prophylaxis may be considered for selected patients (those with hiatal hernia, those who are obese, or parturients) (Table 46-5).

IV. INTRAOPERATIVE MANAGEMENT: CHOICE OF ANESTHETIC METHOD

A. Many considerations are involved in the selection of the anesthetic technique (general anesthesia, regional anesthesia, block with sedation) (Table 46-6).

TABLE 46-6

CONSIDERATIONS INFLUENCING CHOICE OF TECHNIQUES AND DRUGS FOR MANAGEMENT OF ANESTHESIA

Cost
Time to recovery (pharmacokinetics)
Incidence of postoperative nausea and vomiting
Cardiopulmonary effects
Time in operating room necessary to induce/institute anesthesia (success rate)
Likelihood of myalgia, backache, headache, sore throat

TABLE 46-7

REGIONAL TECHNIQUES FOR AMBULATORY ANESTHESIA

Spinal anesthesia (lidocaine and mepivacaine are ideal for
  ambulatory surgery because of their short duration of action;
  lidocaine may be associated with postoperative backache
  [transient neurologic symptoms])
Epidural anesthesia
Caudal anesthesia
Peripheral nerve block anesthesia (axillary nerve block for hand
  surgery, interscalene nerve block for shoulder surgery,
  ilio-inguinal-hypogastric nerve block to decrease pain after
  inguinal hernia repair)

---

    1. No study has shown that regional anesthesia or
       conscious sedation is "safer" than general anesthesia.
    2. Outcome studies are needed to show the value of new
       drugs (propofol, desflurane, sevoflurane, intermediate-
       and short-acting nondepolarizing muscle relaxants)
       and techniques (spinal anesthesia with Sprotte
       needles).

  B. **Regional Techniques** (Table 46-7). Patients usually
    experience less postoperative pain when local or regional
    anesthesia has been used. Patients may have a numb
    extremity (after brachial plexus block) but otherwise
    meet all criteria for discharge (protect the extremity with
    a sling).

    1. **Spinal anesthesia** is useful for ambulatory procedures
       in children born prematurely.
      a. The use of spinal needles with pencil-point,
         noncutting tips has prompted a resurgence of
         spinal anesthesia for ambulatory surgery in adults.
         Nausea is less after epidural or spinal anesthesia
         than after general anesthesia.
      b. Use of smaller-gauge needles results in a lower
         incidence of headache (must follow up with
         telephone calls to ensure that no disabling
         symptoms of headache have developed).
      c. Spinal anesthesia need not be avoided in
         ambulatory patients (bed rest does not decrease the
         incidence of headache and early ambulation may
         decrease the incidence).

    2. **Epidural and Caudal Anesthesia.** An advantage of
       epidural block is that it can be performed outside the

operating room and the problem of postdural puncture headache is obviated.

3. **Nerve Blocks.** Placement of a catheter (paravertebral somatic nerve block after breast surgery, perineural catheters through the popliteal fossa, interscalene perineural catheters) is useful for controlling postoperative pain.

C. **Sedation and Analgesia.** Many patients who undergo surgery with local or regional anesthesia prefer to be sedated and to have no recollection of the procedure. Levels of sedation vary from light, during which a patient's consciousness is minimally depressed, to very deep, in which protective reflexes are partially blocked and the response to physical stimulation or verbal command may not be appropriate.

D. **General Anesthesia**

1. **Induction** of anesthesia is most often accomplished with propofol based on its short duration of effect and antiemetic qualities (pain on injection may be lessened by using a large vein or preceding the injection with lidocaine).

   a. Inhalation induction of anesthesia with sevoflurane is an alternative to propofol especially when intravenous catheter placement is deferred until after the start of anesthesia (children may prefer this approach).

   b. Parental presence is becoming more accepted during induction of anesthesia in children although documentation of its advantages (separation anxiety, behavioral changes after surgery) is not conclusive.

   c. Tracheal intubation may be facilitated by succinylcholine (may be associated with hyperkalemia and malignant hyperthermia in male children with unrecognized muscular dystrophy) or a nondepolarizing drug such as mivacurium or rocuronium

2. **Maintenance** of anesthesia is influenced by selection of drugs (desflurane, sevoflurane, propofol) that are perceived to permit the most rapid and complete awakening (time to discharge has not been consistently shown to be sooner compared with patients receiving inhaled anesthetics of intermediate blood solubility).

**...S OF THE LARYNGEAL MASK AIRWAY FOR
...ATORY ANESTHESIA**

Coughing is less than with tracheal intubation
Muscle relaxants not needed for tracheal intubation
Anesthetic requirements decreased
Hoarseness and sore throat less

a. Postoperative nausea and vomiting are usually less in patients who have received propofol as the maintenance drug or as a supplement to the inhaled drug (propofol is more expensive than other injected and some inhaled anesthetics but the cost may be offset by fewer patient side effects).

b. Desflurane is not recommended for induction of anesthesia in children because it causes a high incidence of coughing and laryngospasm (sevoflurane is not as irritating to the airways).

c. The use of nitrous oxide for ambulatory anesthesia is controversial based on the perception of some (but not a consistent observation) that the incidence of nausea and vomiting is increased.

d. Opioids (most often fentanyl) are useful to supplement analgesia intraoperatively (postoperative nausea and vomiting are concerns).

e. Reversal of nondepolarizing muscle relaxants must be performed if there is any question about lingering neuromuscular blockade at the conclusion of surgery (nausea and vomiting may be less if reversal drugs are not required; this has led some to favor selection of mivacurium, especially for surgeries lasting <30 minutes).

f. Bispectral index monitoring may permit a decrease in anesthetic dose requirements necessary for sedation and amnesia yet use of muscle relaxants may be increased to prevent patient movement.

g. Laryngeal mask airway is an alternative to tracheal intubation (Table 46-8).

V. MANAGEMENT OF POSTANESTHESIA CARE

A. **Reversal of drug effects** (muscle relaxants, opioids, benzodiazepines) may be necessary in selected patients.

TABLE 46-9

DRUGS USED IN THE PHARMACOLOGIC PROPHYLAXIS AGAINST POSTOPERATIVE NAUSEA AND VOMITING

Droperidol	Large doses (>1.25 mg iv) may produce restlessness and/or delayed recovery
Propofol	Include as part of anesthetic induction and/or maintenance
Promethazine	
Ondansetron	Doses of 4–8 mg iv (100 g/kg iv in children) as administered at the conclusion of surgery are superior to metoclopramide and droperidol
Accupressure	Preoperative placement of a band 5 cm proximal to the distal wrist crease may reduce postoperative nausea and vomiting

Flumazenil should not be used routinely (only when sedation seems excessive).
B. **Nausea and Vomiting**
   1. This complication is the most common morbidity in the postanesthesia care unit (PACU) and the most common reason for unscheduled admission to the hospital after planned ambulatory surgery.
   2. Much research has been undertaken to study prophylactic treatment of this problem; treatment after the problem has developed has received less attention (Table 46-9).
      a. Drugs that may be effective after the onset of nausea and vomiting include droperidol, ondansetron, metoclopramide, and propofol.
      b. Anxiety and pain may be the explanations for nausea and vomiting.
C. **Pain**
   1. It is important to distinguish postsurgical pain from hypoxemia, hypercapnia, or a distended bladder.
   2. Medication for pain includes opioids given in small intravenous doses (adults receive morphine, 1 to 3 mg, or fentanyl, 10 to 25 mcg, every 5 minutes until pain is controlled) or nonsteroidal anti-inflammatory drugs (ketorolac, 30–60 mg iv or im).
D. **Preparation for Discharging the Patient**
   1. Scoring systems have been developed to guide transfer from the PACU to phase II recovery to home (Table 46-10). The need for ingestion of fluids or to void

TABLE 46-10

POSTANESTHETIC DISCHARGE SCORING SYSTEM[a]

Vital Signs
2 = within 20% of preoperative value
1 = 20–40% of preoperative value
0 = 40% of preoperative value

Ambulation and Mental Status
2 = oriented times 3 and gait is steady
1 = oriented times 3 or gait is steady
0 = neither

Pain or Nausea and Vomiting
2 = minimal
1 = moderate
0 = severe

Surgical Bleeding
2 = minimal
1 = moderate
0 = severe

Intake and Output
2 = oral fluids and has voided
1 = oral fluids or has voided
0 = neither

[a] Score equal to 9 or higher indicates readiness for discharge.

(especially following epidural or spinal anesthesia) before discharge is unproved and with respect to fluids may actually increase the incidence of nausea.

2. Patients should be advised against driving, operating power tools, making important decisions, and ingesting alcohol for at least 24 hours after the procedure.

3. Patients should be advised that they may experience pain, headache, nausea, vomiting, dizziness, and skeletal muscle aches and pains that cannot be attributed to the surgical incision.

4. It must be confirmed that a responsible adult will accompany (drive) the patient home and if appropriate remain with the patient for some period of time.

5. At some facilities, staff members telephone the patient the next day to determine the progress of recovery.

CHAPTER 47 ■ MONITORED ANESTHESIA CARE

Anesthesiologists typically provide monitored anesthesia care (MAC) to patients undergoing therapeutic or diagnostic procedures that would otherwise be uncomfortable or unsafe (Hillier SC, Mazurek MS: Monitored anesthesia care. In Barash PG, Cullen BF, Stoelting RK [eds]: *Clinical Anesthesia*, pp 1246–1261. Philadelphia, Lippincott Williams & Wilkins, 2006). MAC usually involves intravenous administration of drugs with anxiolytic, hypnotic, analgesic, and amnestic properties either alone or as a supplement to a local or regional anesthetic.

I. TERMINOLOGY

A. It is important to distinguish between the terms MAC and sedation/analgesia.

B. MAC implies the potential for a deeper level of sedation than that provided by sedation/analgesia and is always administered by an anesthesia professional.

C. Conceptually, MAC is attractive because it should invoke less physiologic disturbance and allow a more rapid recovery than general anesthesia.

   1. MAC often includes the administration of medications for which the loss of protective reflexes or consciousness is likely.

   2. Because MAC is a physician service provided to an individual patient and is based on medical necessity, it should be subject to the same level of reimbursement as general or regional anesthesia.

   3. MAC always includes a preoperative assessment and evaluation and intraoperative monitoring. The facilities and expertise to secure the patient's airway and provide general anesthesia should be immediately available.

II. PREOPERATIVE ASSESSMENT

A. The preoperative assessment for a patient scheduled for surgery under MAC should be as comprehensive as that performed prior to a general anesthetic.

B. Additional considerations in the preoperative assessment of the patient scheduled to undergo MAC include evaluation of the patient's ability to remain immobile and cooperative.

1. Verbal communication between the anesthesiologist and patient is important so as to evaluate the level of sedation, to reassure the patient, and to provide a mechanism when the patient is required to cooperate.

2. The presence of a persistent cough may make it difficult for the patient to remain immobile (attempts to attenuate the cough with sedation are not likely to be successful).

3. Orthopnea may make it impossible for the patient to lie flat.

III. TECHNIQUES OF MONITORED ANESTHESIA CARE

A. The appropriate regimen frequently involves the administration of either individual drugs or combinations of analgesic, amnestic, and hypnotic drugs.

B. The drug(s) selected should allow rapid and complete recovery with a minimal incidence of nausea and vomiting or residual cardiorespiratory depression.

1. MAC may or may not involve the provision of sedation ranging from a minimally depressed level of consciousness (patient retains the ability to independently and continuously maintain an upper airway and respond appropriately to physical stimulation and verbal commands) to deep sedation (verbal communication is lost and risks of the technique may be likened to those of general anesthesia with an unprotected and uncontrolled airway).

2. Increased patient agitation may be a result of pain or anxiety (Table 47-1).

   a. Pain may be treated with systemic analgesics, regional techniques, or removal of the painful stimulus.

   b. Anxiety may be treated with reassurance and/or a benzodiazepine.

TABLE 47-1

CAUSES OF PATIENT AGITATION DURING MONITORED ANESTHESIA CARE

Pain or anxiety
Life-threatening factors
  Hypoxemia
  Hypoventilation
  Impending local anesthetic toxicity
  Cerebral hypoperfusion
Less ominous but often overlooked factors
  Distended bladder
  Hypothermia or hyperthermia
  Pruritus
  Nausea
  Positional discomfort
  Uncomfortable oxygen masks or nasal cannulas
  Intravenous cannulation site infiltration
  Member of surgical team leaning on patient
  Prolonged pneumatic tourniquet inflation

IV. PHARMACOLOGIC BASIS OF MONITORED ANESTHESIA CARE TECHNIQUES—OPTIMIZING DRUG ADMINISTRATION

A. The ability to predict the effects of drugs requires an understanding of their pharmacokinetic and pharmacodynamic properties (context-sensitive half-time, effect-site equilibration time, drug interactions).

B. To avoid excessive levels of sedation, drugs should be titrated in increments rather than administered in larger doses according to predetermined notions of efficacy.

C. Continuous infusions (propofol) are superior to intermittent bolus dosing because they produce less fluctuation in drug concentration, thus reducing the number of episodes of inadequate or excessive sedation and contributing to a more prompt recovery (Fig. 47-1).

V. DISTRIBUTION, ELIMINATION, ACCUMULATION, AND DURATION OF ACTION. Following the administration of intravenous drugs, the immediate distribution phase causes a rapid

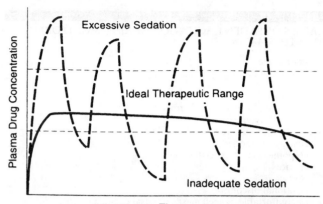

FIGURE 47-1. Schematic depiction of the changes in drug concentration during continuous infusion of the drug (heavy line indicates maintenance of a therapeutic concentration) or intermittent bolus injection of the drug (lighter line indicates that the drug concentration is often above or below the desired therapeutic concentration).

decrease in plasma levels as the drug is quickly transported to the vessel-rich group of rapidly equilibrating tissues. Accumulation of drug in poorly perfused tissues during prolonged intravenous infusion may contribute to delayed recovery when the drug is released back into the central compartment after drug administration is discontinued.

A. **Elimination half-life** is often cited as a determinant of a drug's duration of action, when, in fact, it is often difficult to predict the clinical duration of action from this value.
   1. The elimination half-life represents a single-compartment model in which elimination is the only process that can alter drug concentration.
   2. Nevertheless, most drugs used by anesthesiologists for MAC are lipophilic and much more suited to multicompartmental modeling than single-compartment modeling.
   3. In multicompartmental models, the metabolism and excretion of some intravenous drugs may make only a minor contribution to changes in plasma concentration when compared with the effects of intercompartmental distribution.

B. **Context-sensitive half-time** describes the time required for the plasma drug concentration to decline by 50% after terminating an intravenous infusion of a particular duration. It is calculated by computer simulation of multicompartmental pharmacokinetic models of drug disposition.

 1. The context-sensitive half-time increases as the duration of the infusion increases (particularly for fentanyl and thiopental).

    a. This confirms that thiopental is not an ideal drug for continuous infusion during ambulatory procedures.

    b. The context-sensitive half-time of propofol is prolonged to a minimal extent as the infusion duration increases (after the infusion ends, the drug that returns to the plasma from the peripheral compartments is rapidly cleared by metabolic processes and is therefore not available to retard the decay in plasma levels).

 2. The context-sensitive half-times of drugs bear no constant relationship to their elimination half-times.

 3. **How Does the Context-Sensitive Half-Time Relate to the Time to Recovery?**

    a. Context-sensitive half-time does not directly describe how long it will take for the patient to recover from sedation/analgesia but rather how long it takes for the plasma concentration or drug to decrease by 50%.

    b. The time to recovery depends on how far the plasma concentration must decrease to reach levels compatible with awakening (Fig. 47-2).

 4. **Effect-site equilibration** describes the time from rapid intravenous administration of a drug until its clinical effect is manifest (delay occurs because the blood is not usually the site of action but is merely the route by which the drug reaches its effect site. The half-time of equilibration between drug concentration in the blood and the drug effect (brain) is designated as t1/2keo.

    a. Thiopental, propofol, and alfentanil have a short t1/2keo compared with midazolam, sufentanil, and fentanyl. (This is an important consideration when determining bolus spacing of doses.)

    b. A distinct time lag between the peak serum fentanyl concentration (important consideration

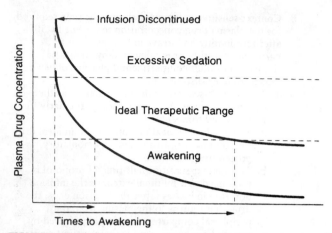

FIGURE 47-2. The time to awakening is determined by the duration of infusion (context-sensitive half-time), the difference in the plasma concentration at the end of the procedure, and the plasma concentration below which awakening will occur.

when determining bolus spacing of doses) and the peak electroencephalographic slowing can be seen, whereas following administration of alfentanil, the electroencephalographic spectral edge changes closely parallel serum concentrations. (If an opioid is required to blunt the response to a single brief stimulus, alfentanil might represent a more logical choice than fentanyl.)

VI. DRUG INTERACTIONS IN MONITORED ANESTHESIA CARE

A. No one inhaled iv drug can provide all the components of MAC. Patient comfort is usually maintained by a combination of drugs that act synergistically to enable reductions in the dose requirements of individual drugs.

B. It is likely that a rapid recovery in the ambulatory setting can be achieved by using an opioid in combination with other drugs (especially a benzodiazepine) rather than by using an opioid as the sole anesthetic.

1. Opioid and benzodiazepine combinations are frequently used to achieve the components of hypnosis, amnesia, and analgesia.
2. The opioid-benzodiazepine combination displays marked synergism in producing hypnosis.
3. This synergism also extends to unwanted effects of these drugs (midazolam alone produces no significant effects on ventilation, whereas the combination with fentanyl produces apnea in many patients).
4. The advantage of synergy between opioids and benzodiazepines should be carefully weighed against the disadvantages of the potential adverse effect of this drug combination on the cardiovascular system and breathing.

VII. SPECIFIC DRUGS USED FOR MONITORED ANESTHESIA CARE

A. **Propofol** has many of the ideal properties of a sedative-hypnotic for use in sedation/analgesia.
   1. The context-sensitive half-time of propofol remains short even after prolonged intravenous infusions (in contrast to midazolam), and the short effect-site equilibration time makes propofol an easily titratable drug that has an excellent recovery profile.
   2. The prompt recovery combined with a low incidence of nausea and vomiting make propofol well suited to ambulatory sedation/analgesia procedures.
   3. Propofol in typical sedation/analgesia doses (25 to 75 μg/kg/min iv) has minimal analgesic properties and does not reliably produce amnesia.
B. **Benzodiazepines** are commonly used during sedation/analgesia for their anxiolytic, amnestic, and hypnotic properties.
   1. **Midazolam** has many advantages over diazepam and is the most commonly used benzodiazepine for sedation/analgesia.
      a. Despite a short elimination half-time, there is often prolonged psychomotor impairment following sedation/analgesia techniques using midazolam as the main component.
      b. Midazolam may be better used in a modified role by administering lower doses prior to the start of

RECOMMENDED REGIMEN FOR USE OF FLUMAZENIL

Initial recommended dose is 0.2 mg iv
If desired level of consciousness is not achieved in 45 seconds, repeat 0.2 mg dose iv
If necessary, repeat 0.2 mg iv every 60 seconds to a maximum of 1.0 mg
Recognize the potential for resedation

a propofol infusion to provide the specific amnestic and anxiolytic component of a balanced sedation technique.
  c. The analgesic component of a balanced sedation technique could be provided by regional/local techniques or opioids (risk of significant respiratory depression when a benzodiazepine is combined with an opioid).
  d. The dose of benzodiazepine required to reach a desired clinical end point is decreased in the elderly compared to younger patients (reflects pharmacodynamic factors) (Fig. 47-3).

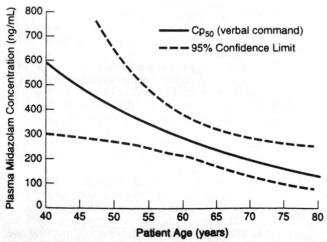

FIGURE 47-3. The plasma concentration of midazolam at which 50% of subjects will fail to respond to verbal command (Cp50) is a function of age.

TABLE 47-3

INDICATIONS FOR ADMINISTRATION OF AN OPIOID DURING MONITORED ANESTHESIA CARE

Initial injection of a local anesthetic
   Retrobulbar block
Patient discomfort unrelated to procedure
   Uncomfortable position
   Propofol injection
   Pneumatic tourniquet pain

    2. Flumazenil antagonism of benzodiazepines (see Table 47-2). Routine use of flumazenil-antagonized benzodiazepine sedation is not cost-effective.
  C. Opioids
    1. The analgesic component of "balanced sedation/analgesia" is provided by an opioid, whereas sedation is provided by drugs (propofol, midazolam) with specific and potent hypnotic and amnestic properties (Tables 47-3 and 47-4).

TABLE 47-4

DOSE RANGES FOR DRUGS USED TO PRODUCE SEDATION/ANALGESIA

Drug	Typical adult intravenous dose (titrated to effect in increments)
Benzodiazepines	
Midazolam	1–2 mg prior to propofol or remifentanil infusion
Diazepam	1.5–10 mg
Opioids	
Alfentanil	5–20 μg/kg bolus 2 minutes prior to stimulus
Fentanyl	0.5–2.0 μg/kg bolus 2–4 minutes prior to stimulus
Remifentanil	0.5 μg/kg/min infusion 5 minutes prior to stimulus and then wean to 0.5 μg/kg/min as tolerated (adjust up or down in increments of 0.025 μg/kg/min; decrease dose accordingly when coadministered with midazolam or propofol)
Propofol	250–500 μg/kg boluses 25–75 μg/kg/min infusion
Ketamine	4–6 mg/kg orally, 2–4 mg/kg im, 0.25–1.0 mg/kg iv
Dexmedetomidine	0.5–1.0 μg/kg iv over 10–20 minutes followed by 0.2–0.7 μg/kg/hr iv

2. **Remifentanil** is a μ-opioid agonist with a rapid onset (brain-equilibration time 1.0 to 1.5 minutes) and offset (ester hydrolysis) that facilitate titration to effect during MAC.

   a. The likelihood of depression of ventilation and/or chest wall rigidity is decreased by administering remifentanil over 30 to 90 seconds or using a continuous intravenous infusion technique.

   b. A bolus dose (1 μg/kg iv) administered over 30 seconds, administered 90 seconds before placement of a retrobulbar block, is effective in preventing pain during subsequent placement of the block.

   c. Administration of midazolam (2 mg iv) in combination with remifentanil results in decreased dose requirements for the opioid and relieves patient anxiety.

   d. Because most painful stimuli are of unpredictable duration and because the risk of depression of ventilation is increased following bolus administration, the most logical method for administration of remifentanil during monitored anesthetic care is by adjustable intravenous infusion (see Table 47-4).

   e. Discontinuation or accidental interruption of the remifentanil infusion will result in abrupt offset of effect, which may result in patient discomfort, hemodynamic instability, and patient movement.

D. **Ketamine** is an intense analgesic and is frequently used as a component of pediatric sedation techniques (0.25 to 1.0 mg/kg iv produces minimal respiratory and cardiovascular depression) (see Table 47-4).

   1. Increased oral secretions make laryngospasm more likely (administer an antisialagogue).

   2. Ketamine is frequently combined with a benzodiazepine to reduce the incidence of hallucinations.

   3. Patient movement may make ketamine less than ideal for procedures requiring a motionless patient.

E. **Dexmedetomidine** stimulates alpha-2 receptors to produce sedation, analgesia, decreases in sympathetic outflow, and an increase in cardiac vagal activity (bradycardia and hypotension) (see Table 47-4).

1. Respiratory function is not depressed to the same extent as with other sedatives and patients sedated with dexmedetomidine are more easily aroused from a given level of sedation

VIII. PATIENT-CONTROLLED SEDATION AND ANALGESIA

A. Techniques that allow the patient some direct control on the level of sedation increases patient satisfaction and eliminates the unpredictable variability in dose requirements between patients.

B. A conventional patient-controlled analgesia delivery system, set to deliver 0.5 mg midazolam and 25 μg fentanyl with a 5-minute lockout interval, is useful. Alfentanil as a 5-μg/kg iv bolus with a 3-minute lockout period results in patient acceptability and an outcome comparable to physician-controlled analgesia.

IX. RESPIRATORY FUNCTION AND SEDATIVE-HYPNOTICS

A. During MAC, there is a risk of depression of ventilation as a result of drug-induced effects (opioids, hypotension resulting in brainstem hypoperfusion). During sedation, it is likely that protective upper airway reflexes will be attenuated.

B. Sedation and the Upper Airway

1. The coordinated activation of the diaphragm and upper airway muscles (important for maintaining airway patency) is extremely sensitive to sedative–hypnotic drug administration.

2. Elderly patients and those with preexisting chronic obstructive pulmonary disease often have limited respiratory reserve and are unable to increase their respiratory muscle activity in response to the increased work of breathing induced by sedation; they may become hypercarbia, acidotic, and hypoxemic.

C. Sedation and Protective Airway Reflexes

1. Protective laryngeal and pharyngeal (swallowing) reflexes are depressed by drugs that produce sedation.

      a. Aspiration of gastric contents may occur either in the operating room or during recovery, particularly if oral intake is allowed before the return of adequate upper airway protective reflexes.

      b. Advanced age and debilitation may compromise protective upper airway reflexes, placing these patients at increased risk for aspiration during sedation.

    2. Ideally, patients should be awake enough to recognize the regurgitation of gastric contents and be able to protect their own airways.

D. Sedation and Respiratory Control

    1. It is likely that during regional anesthesia there is a degree of deafferentation that will potentiate the respiratory depressant effects of sedative–hypnotic drugs, especially opioids.

    2. When used in combination, opioids and benzodiazepines appear to have the potential to produce marked depressant effects on respiratory responsiveness.

E. Supplemental Oxygen Administration

    1. Arterial hypoxemia as a result of alveolar hypoventilation is a risk following the administration of sedatives, hypnotics, or analgesics.

    2. In the absence of significant lung disease, the administration of only modest concentrations of supplemental oxygen is usually effective in restoring oxygenation to an acceptable level.

      a. A patient who is receiving minimal supplemental oxygen may have acceptable oxygenation despite significant alveolar hypoventilation.

      b. Before making the decision to discharge a patient to a less well-monitored environment without supplemental oxygen, it is useful to measure oxygen saturation with a pulse oximeter while the patient is breathing room air.

X. MONITORING DURING MONITORED ANESTHESIA CARE

A. ASA Standards for **Basic Anesthetic Monitoring** are applicable to all levels of anesthesia care, including MAC (see Appendix D).

TABLE 47-5

MONITORING TECHNIQUES AND DEVICES DURING MONITORED ANESTHESIA CARE

Visual, Tactile, and Auditory Assessment
Rate, depth, and pattern of breathing
Palpation of the arterial pulse
Peripheral perfusion based on temperature of extremities and
 capillary refill
Diaphoresis
Pallor
Shivering
Cyanosis
Acute changes in neurologic status

Auscultation
Heart and breath sounds (precordial stethoscope)

Pulse Oximetry (an ASA Standard)

Capnography (most effective in intubated patients but can be
 adapted [side-stream] to MAC)

Electrocardiogram

Temperature (forced-air heating an effective means of
 maintaining normothermia)

Bispectral Index (value <80 minimizes the possibility of recall
 during sedation)

   B. Communication and Observation
      1. The presence of a vigilant anesthesiologist is the
         single most important monitor in the operating
         room.
      2. The effectiveness of this vigilance is enhanced by
         monitoring techniques and devices (Table 47-5).
      3. It is important that the anesthesiologist continually
         evaluate the patient's **response to verbal stimulation**
         to titrate the level of sedation and to allow the early
         detection of neurologic or cardiopulmonary
         dysfunction.
   C. Preparedness to Recognize and Treat Local Anesthetic
      Toxicity
      1. Because MAC is often provided in the context of
         regional or local anesthetic techniques, it is
         important that the anesthesiologist maintain a high
         index of suspicion for the risk of local anesthetic
         toxicity, especially in elderly and debilitated patients.

2. Even if the anesthesiologist does not perform the block, he or she is in a unique position to advise the surgeon about the most appropriate volume, concentration, and type of local anesthetic drug or technique to be used.

3. The clinically recognizable toxic effects of local anesthetics on the central nervous system and the cardiovascular system are concentration dependent. Cardiovascular toxicity usually occurs at a higher plasma concentration than neurotoxicity, but when it does occur it is usually more difficult to manage than neurotoxicity (see Chapter 17).

   a. At low plasma concentrations, sedation and numbness of the tongue and circumoral tissues and a metallic taste are prominent features of local anesthetic toxicity.

   b. As plasma concentrations increase, restlessness, vertigo, tinnitus, and difficulty in focusing may occur.

   c. Higher plasma concentrations result in slurred speech and skeletal muscle twitching, which often herald the onset of tonic-clonic seizures.

   d. Cardiotoxicity may manifest before neurotoxicity when **bupivacaine** local anesthetic toxicity occurs.

4. The conduct of MAC may modify the individual's response to the potentially toxic effects of local anesthetic administration and adversely affect the margin of safety of a regional or local anesthetic technique.

   a. Any decrease in cardiac output and hepatic blood flow during sedation may decrease the clearance of local anesthetics that are dependent on metabolism in the liver.

   b. Drug-induced depression of ventilation during sedation leads to **acidosis,** which increases delivery of local anesthetic to the brain *via* increases in cerebral blood flow, increases intracellular concentrations of the active nonionized form of the local anesthetic, and potentiates the cardiovascular toxicity of local anesthetics.

   c. Administration of sedative–hypnotic drugs may interfere with the patient's ability to communicate the symptoms of impending local anesthetic toxicity.

d. The anticonvulsant properties of benzodiazepines and barbiturates may attenuate the seizures associated with local anesthetic toxicity.

XI. SEDATION AND ANALGESIA BY NONANESTHESIOLOGISTS

A. The ASA has developed practice guidelines to guide the level of sedation that should be provided by nonanesthesiologist providers.
   1. Four levels of sedation are defined in the ASA practice guidelines (minimal sedation, moderate sedation, deep sedation, general anesthesia).
   2. These practice guidelines emphasize that sedation and analgesia represent a continuum of sedation where patients can easily pass into a level of sedation deeper than intended.
B. A patient whose only response is reflex withdrawal is sedated to a greater degree than defined by the term "sedation and analgesia" and may be at risk for cardiopulmonary compromise.
C. The routine administration of supplemental oxygen is recommended.
D. The responsible individual should be able to recognize airway obstruction, establish an airway, and maintain oxygenation and ventilation.

CHAPTER 48 ▪ TRAUMA AND BURNS

Injuries are the most common cause of death in Americans under the age of 45 years, and more than 50% of all deaths in people between the ages of 5 and 34 years result from trauma (Capan LM, Miller SM: Trauma and burns. In Barash PG, Cullen BF, Stoelting RK [eds]: *Clinical Anesthesia*, pp 1262–1294. Philadelphia, Lippincott Williams & Wilkins, 2006). Approximately 75% of the hospital mortality from trauma occurs within 48 hours of admission, most commonly from thoracic, abdominal, retroperitoneal, vascular, or central nervous system injuries.

I. INITIAL EVALUATION AND RESUSCITATION

A. The general approach to evaluation of the acute trauma victim includes three sequential components: rapid overview, primary survey, and secondary survey (Fig. 48-1).
   1. During this period, the anesthesiologist identifies injuries, preexisting conditions, and the resulting functional abnormalities that require either immediate treatment or provision for resuscitative and anesthetic management.
   2. Universal infection control precautions are the standard, because many trauma victims are carriers of hepatitis B, hepatitis C, or human immunodeficiency virus.
B. **Airway Evaluation and Intervention**
   1. If the patient can speak, serious airway obstruction is unlikely.
      a. Signs of upper and lower airway obstruction include dyspnea, hoarseness, stridor, dysphoria, subcutaneous emphysema, and hemoptysis.
      b. Cervical deformity, edema, crepitation, tracheal deviation, or jugular venous distention may be present before appearance of symptoms.
   2. The initial steps in airway management are chin lift, jaw thrust, clearing of the oropharyngeal cavity, and placement of an oral or nasopharyngeal airway

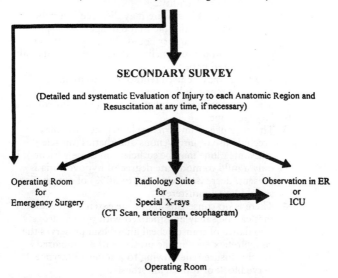

RAPID OVERVIEW

(Differentiation between stable, unstable, and dead or dying patient)

PRIMARY SURVEY

(Evaluation and Concurrent Resuscitation)

1) Airway
2) Breathing
3) Circulation
4) Neurologic function
5) Examination of undressed patient

(Essential Laboratory and Radiologic Examination)

SECONDARY SURVEY

(Detailed and systematic Evaluation of Injury to each Anatomic Region and Resuscitation at any time, if necessary)

Operating Room
for
Emergency Surgery

Radiology Suite
for
Special X-rays
(CT Scan, arteriogram, esophagram)

Observation in ER
or
ICU

Operating Room

FIGURE 48-1. The general approach to evaluation of the acute trauma victim includes the sequential steps of rapid overview, primary survey, and secondary survey.

following immobilization of the cervical spine and administration of oxygen by face mask.

    a. Ventilation is supported in inadequately breathing patients by a self-inflating bag.

    b. If these measures do not provide adequate ventilation, the trachea must be intubated using either direct laryngoscopy or cricothyroidotomy.

    c. Proper placement of devices such as a laryngeal mask airway (LMA), esophageal-tracheal combitube, or endotracheal tube by paramedics should be confirmed by capnometry as soon as possible after the patient enters the hospital.

C. **Full stomach** is a background condition in acute trauma and the urgency of securing the airway often does not permit time for pharmacologic measures to decrease gastric volume and acidity.

    1. Excessive cricoid pressure may displace a vertebral bone fragment with potential damage to the spinal cord. Spinal cord injury could also accompany cricoid pressure and manual incline stabilization to cervical spine injured patients.

    2. The LMA may be used temporarily to maintain airway patency (full stomach precludes its sustained use) or to facilitate intubation aided by a fiberoptic laryngoscope.

    3. The presence of uncorrectable hypotension may preclude use of intravenous anesthetics (muscle relaxants alone may be sufficient in these patients). If only a mild to moderate degree of hypovolemia is present, decreased doses (30 to 50%) of anesthetics should be administered.

    4. There is no consensus about the extent of the airway that can be safely anesthetized with topical drugs. Avoidance of transtracheal anesthesia preserves the cough reflex even in the presence of an impaired glottic closure reflex owing to a superior laryngeal nerve block or topical anesthesia.

    5. Agitated and uncooperative patients (topical anesthesia is not possible) may require a rapid sequence induction of anesthesia followed by direct laryngoscopy to secure the airway.

D. **Head, Open Eye, and Contained Major Vessel Injuries**

    1. These conditions require deep anesthesia (opioids and intravenous anesthetics) and profound skeletal muscle

relaxation before airway manipulation (this assumes a difficult tracheal intubation is not anticipated and the patient is not hypotensive).
2. Hypertension, coughing, and reacting to the tracheal tube may adversely increase systemic blood pressure, intracranial pressure, and intraocular pressure.
3. Hypotension dictates either reduced or no intravenous anesthetic administration.
E. Cervical Spine Injury
1. Immobilization of the neck in a neutral position is indicated in all unconscious patients, in conscious patients with cervical pain and/or tenderness, and whenever the pain of other injuries is likely to mask neck pain.
2. Orotracheal intubation with direct laryngoscopy is more desirable than nasotracheal intubation, although stabilization of the neck may make glottic visualization difficult (flexible fiberoptic laryngoscopy is an alternative but difficult to perform in uncooperative patients).
F. Direct Airway Injuries (Table 48-1)
G. Management of Breathing Abnormalities
1. Of the several causes that may alter breathing after trauma, tension pneumothorax, flail chest, and open pneumothorax are immediate threats to life and therefore require rapid diagnosis and treatment.

TABLE 48-1

MECHANISMS OF DIRECT AIRWAY INJURY

Maxillofacial Injuries
Soft tissue edema of the pharynx (hematoma or edema may expand during the 6–12 hours after injury, liberal fluid administration may contribute to edema)
Blood and debris in the oropharyngeal cavity
Mandibular condylar fractures (if bilateral, prevents opening of the mouth)

Cervical Airway Injuries
Blunt or penetrating trauma (hoarseness, dysphagia, flattening of the thyroid cartilage protuberance)

Thoracic Airway Injuries
Blunt injury usually involves the posterior membranous portion of the trachea and the mainstem bronchi (suspect when a seal around the tracheal tube cuff cannot be obtained)

2. A flail chest results from comminuted fractures of at least three adjacent ribs or rib fractures with associated costochondral separation or sternal fracture.

   a. An underlying pulmonary contusion with increased elastic recoil of the lung and work of breathing is the main cause of respiratory insufficiency or failure and resulting hypoxemia.

   b. Respiratory failure often develops over a 3- to 6-hour period, causing gradual deterioration of the chest radiography and arterial blood gases.

3. Tracheal intubation is often necessary in patients with pulmonary contusion, respiratory insufficiency, or failure despite adequate analgesia.

   a. Positive end-expiratory pressure is used if ventilation is controlled.

   b. In intubated spontaneously breathing patients, airway pressure release ventilation provides improved arterial oxygenation and maintenance of blood pressure, lower sedation requirements, and shorter periods of intubation.

   c. In bilateral severe contusions with life-threatening hypoxemia, high-frequency jet ventilation may enhance oxygenation as well as cardiac function, which may be compromised by concomitant myocardial contusion.

4. The definitive diagnosis of tension pneumothorax is with a chest roentgenogram. When there is no time for radiologic confirmation, a 14-gauge angiocath can be placed through the fourth intercostal space in the midaxillary line.

5. In the absence of significant gas exchange abnormalities, chest wall instability alone is not an indication for tracheal intubation and mechanical ventilation (Table 48-2). Effective pain relief (continuous epidural analgesia) by itself can improve respiratory function and often prevent the need for mechanical ventilation.

6. Hypoxia and hypercarbia result from an open pneumothorax (occlusive dressing is the initial treatment).

H. **Management of Shock**

   1. In the initial phase of trauma, hypotension has many causes, but hemorrhage is the most common etiology (Table 48-3).

TABLE 48-2

INDICATIONS FOR MECHANICAL VENTILATION IN PATIENTS WITH FLAIL CHEST

Clinical evidence of respiratory failure
  Progressive fatigue or deterioration
  Respiratory rate >35 breaths/min
  PaO_2 <60 mm Hg breathing at least 50% oxygen
  $PaCO_2$ >55 mm Hg
  Vital capacity <15 mL/kg
Clinical evidence of shock
Associated severe head injury with need to hyperventilate the
  patient's lungs
Severe associated injury requiring surgery
Airway obstruction
Significant preexisting chronic pulmonary disease

TABLE 48-3

CAUSES OF HYPOTENSION IN THE INITIAL PHASE OF TRAUMA

Hemorrhage or Extensive Tissue Injury
Tachycardia, narrow pulse pressure, peripheral vasoconstriction
Crystalloid solution initially and transfuse if 2000 mL in
  15 minutes does not improve blood pressure

Cardiac Tamponade
Tachycardia, dilated neck veins, muffled heart sounds
Pericardiocentesis

Myocardial Contusion
Tachycardia, cardiac dysrhythmias
Crystalloids, vasodilators, inotropes

Pneumothorax or Hemothorax
Tachycardia, dilated neck veins, absent breath sounds, dyspnea,
  subcutaneous emphysema
Chest tube

Spinal Cord Injury
Hypotension without tachycardia, narrow pulse pressure or
  vasoconstriction
Crystalloids, vasopressor, inotropes

Sepsis
Develops typically a few hours after colon injury (in normovolemic
  patients manifests as modest tachycardia, wide pulse pressure,
  fever)
Antibiotics, crystalloids, inotropes

2. Evaluation of the severity of hemorrhagic shock in the initial phase is based on a few relatively insensitive and nonspecific clinical signs (Table 48-4).

   a. Although tachycardia is one of the earliest signs of hemorrhagic shock, the heart rate does not necessarily correlate with the blood loss. Tachycardia may be absent in up to 30% of hypotensive trauma patients because of increased vagal tone or chronic cocaine use.

   b. Equating a normal systemic blood pressure with normovolemia during initial resuscitation may lead to loss of valuable time for treating underlying hypovolemia.

3. The response of the heart rate and blood pressure to initial fluid therapy also aids in assessment of the degree of hypovolemia (Table 48-5).

4. Markers of organ perfusion to guide resuscitation include base deficit, blood lactate level, and sublingual capnometry (gut perfusion).

5. During the initial phase of treatment, serial measurements of the hematocrit (helpful if the first sample is obtained before administration of large volumes of fluid) help to determine the need for transfusion.

   a. A low hemoglobin determination (<8 g/dL) immediately after injury is a strong indicator of ongoing blood loss and poor prognosis.

   b. During fluid infusion, a reasonable transfusion threshold is a hematocrit <25 mL/dL for young, healthy patients and <30 mL/dL for older patients or those with coronary or cerebrovascular disease.

   c. The control of active bleeding has a higher priority than restoration of blood volume or placement of invasive monitors in the initial resuscitation.

6. Rapid establishment of venous access with large-bore cannulas placed in peripheral veins that drain both above and below the diaphragm is essential for adequate fluid resuscitation in the severely injured patient.

II. EARLY MANAGEMENT OF SPECIFIC INJURIES

A. Head Injury

1. Approximately 40% of deaths from trauma are caused by head injury.

TABLE 48-4

ADVANCED TRAUMA LIFE SUPPORT CLASSIFICATION OF HEMORRHAGIC SHOCK

	Class I	Class II	Class III	Class IV
Blood loss (mL)	Up to 750	750–1,500	1,500–2,000	>2,000
Blood loss (% of blood volume)	Up to 15%	15–30%	20–40%	>40%
Heart rate (beats/min)	<100	>100	>120	>140
Systemic blood pressure	Normal	Normal	Decreased	Decreased
Pulse pressure	Normal or increased	Decreased	Decreased	Decreased
Capillary refill test	Normal	Positive	Positive	Positive
Respiratory rate (breaths/min)	14–20	20–30	30–40	<35
Urine output (mL/hr)	>30	20–30	5–15	Negligible
Mental status	Slightly anxious	Mildly anxious	Anxious and confused	Confused and lethargic
Fluid replacement (3:1 rule)	Crystalloid	Crystalloid	Crystalloid and blood	Crystalloid and blood

TABLE 48-5

ASSESSMENT OF THE DEGREE OF HYPOVOLEMIA IN HYPOTENSIVE AND TACHYCARDIC PATIENTS

Decrease in Circulating Blood Volume Equivalent to 10–20%
Administration of lactated Ringers solution (2,000 mL over 15 minutes in adults or 20 mL/kg in children) should normalize blood pressure

Decrease in Circulating Blood Volume Equivalent to 20–40%
Administration of lactated Ringers solution produces a transient increase in blood pressure
More crystalloids and/or blood transfusions are needed

Decrease in Circulating Blood Volume Exceeds 40%
Administration of lactated Ringers solution does not improve blood pressure
Rapid infusion of crystalloids, colloids, and blood is needed
Blood typing and cross-matching requires 45 minutes versus type specific, which can be available in about 15 minutes, versus immediate transfusion with type O blood (Rh-negative preferred for women of child-bearing age)

2. Prevention of progression of brain injury beyond the initial area is the primary objective of early management of brain trauma. Of all the possible insults to the injured brain, hypotension has the greatest detrimental impact, followed by hypoxia.
3. A baseline neurologic examination should be performed before any sedative or muscle relaxant drugs are administered or the trachea is intubated. The examination should be repeated at frequent intervals because the patient's condition may change rapidly (Table 48-6).
   a. If consciousness remains depressed despite treatment of shock and hypoxia, it is assumed that a head injury is present.
   b. Dilatation and sluggish response of the pupil is a sign of compression of the oculomotor nerve by the medial portion of the temporal lobe (uncus). A maximally dilated and unresponsive ("blown") pupil suggests uncal herniation.
4. **Computed tomographic** scanning is used for the diagnosis (midline shift, distortion of the ventricles, presence of a hematoma, depressed skull fractures) of most head injuries (magnetic resonance imaging has advantage of being able to demonstrate ischemia but

TABLE 48-6

BASELINE NEUROLOGIC EXAMINATION OF TRAUMA PATIENT

Level 1—AVPU System	
A	Alert
V	Responds to verbal stimuli
P	Responds to painful stimuli (motor activity of extremities)
U	Unresponsive
Level 2—Glasgow Coma Scale	
Score 8	Deep coma, severe head injury, poor outcome
Score 9–12	Conscious patient with moderate injury
Score 13–15	Mild injury

is rarely used because of its cost and impracticality in injured patients). Patients in coma (Glasgow coma score <8) have a 40% likelihood of having an intracranial hematoma.

5. **Management** includes therapeutic maneuvers intended to maintain cerebral perfusion pressure and oxygen delivery (Table 48-7).

   a. Whether active normalization of hyperglycemia (common in head-injured patients) has any salutary effect is not known.

   b. Measurement of jugular bulb oxygen saturation (<50% is considered critical desaturation) is a useful guide for treatment of head-injured patients (reflects demand of the brain for oxygen and its

TABLE 48-7

UNIVERSALLY ACCEPTED ASPECTS OF TREATMENT FOR HEAD-INJURED PATIENTS

Normalization of systemic blood pressure (mean cerebral perfusion pressure >60 mm Hg)

Normalization of arterial oxygenation (SaO_2 >95%)

Sedation and skeletal muscle paralysis as necessary

Mannitol and possibly a loop diuretic to shrink the brain and decrease intracranial pressure

Drainage of cerebrospinal fluid

Mechanical hyperventilation of the lungs if intracranial pressure remains increased (otherwise maintain normal ventilation)

High-dose barbiturates used only for refractory intracranial hypertension

Immediate surgical decompression if indicated (epidural hematoma)

supply; AvDO2 >6 is a sign of insufficient blood flow).

c. Hyperventilation could enhance increased cerebral vascular resistance that is responsible for the initial cerebral hypoperfusion likely to occur during the first 6 hours following head trauma. Use of hyperventilation is ideally guided by monitoring intracranial pressure and AvDO2.

d. Mannitol (0.25 to 0.5 g/kg iv) produces an osmotic diuretic effect to decrease intracranial pressure and may improve cerebral blood flow by decreasing blood viscosity. There is a risk of hypovolemia and hypotension when therapeutic doses of mannitol are used. Hyponatremia reflects intravascular volume expansion.

e. Because of a synergistic action between mannitol and loop diuretics, addition of furosemide may be preferred to increasing doses of mannitol when intracranial hypertension persists.

f. Steroids are no longer viewed as a necessary part of treatment of severe head injury.

g. Maintenance of normovolemia rather than fluid restriction is desirable.

6. **Anesthetic considerations** include the likely occurrence of hypotension and the risk of administering succinylcholine to patients with spine injury.

B. **Spine and Spinal Cord Injury**

1. **Initial Evaluation.** The objective of the evaluation is to diagnose instability of the spine and extent of neurologic injury. Often the urgency of the associated injuries precludes a definitive assessment, necessitating spine protection until a satisfactory diagnosis is established.

a. In a comatose patient, flaccid areflexia, loss of rectal sphincter tone, diaphragmatic breathing, and bradycardia suggest the diagnosis of spinal cord injury.

b. In cervical spine trauma, an ability to flex but not to extend the elbow and response to painful stimuli above but not below the clavicle suggest neurologic injury.

c. Neurogenic shock describes the hypotension and bradycardia caused by the loss of vasomotor tone and sympathetic innervation of the heart as a result of functional depression of the descending sympathetic pathways of the spinal cord (usually present after high thoracic and cervical spine injuries and improves within 3 to 5 days).

2. **Radiologic Evaluation**
    a. For radiologic diagnosis of the cervical spine the recommendation is a standard three-view (anteroposterior, lateral, and open mouth) series of radiographs and examination of suspect areas with CT scans.
    b. The cross-table lateral view is capable of detecting <70% of fracture dislocations.
    c. The computed tomographic scan is the most reliable diagnostic technique (sensitivity nearly 100%). CT scans are more effective at diagnosing ligamentous injuries than at detecting fractures.

3. **Immobilization and Intubation.** If a cervical spine fracture is suspected, immobilization or manual in-line stabilization of the neck is of paramount importance.

4. **Steroids.** Treatment with methylprednisolone for 24 to 48 hours is an option.

5. **Respiratory complications** are common in all phases of the care of spinal cord–injured patients (accessory respiratory muscle paresis may cause a significant loss of expiratory reserve; pulmonary edema may follow catecholamine surge associated with spinal cord injury, aspiration).
    a. Paradoxical respiration in the quadriplegic patient is aggravated when the patient is placed in the upright position.
    b. Unopposed vagal activity during tracheal intubation may result in severe bradycardia and cardiac dysrhythmias (precede instrumentation with oxygen and atropine, 0.4 to 0.6 mg iv).
    c. **Hemodynamic management** may include assessment with a pulmonary artery catheter. Left ventricular dysfunction may contribute to hypotension in quadriplegic patients.

C. **Neck Injury.** Penetrating and blunt trauma may injure major structures in the neck (vessels, respiratory, digestive, nervous system).

D. **Chest Injury**
    1. **Chest wall injury** (ribs, sternum, and scapula) to a certain extent can predict the likelihood and severity of internal injuries. For example, patients with three

or more fractured ribs have a greater likelihood of hepatic and splenic injury.

2. **Pleural injury** manifesting as a closed pneumothorax most commonly develops as a result of lung puncture by a displaced rib fracture. (Diagnosis is made by upright or supine chest film [this position may be contraindicated in hypovolemic patients or those with suspected spine or head injury] that is obtained routinely in evaluation of all trauma victims). CT is more reliable for detecting a small pneumothorax and should be performed in patients who require general anesthesia or mechanical ventilation of the lungs after thoracoabdominal trauma.
   a. Subcutaneous emphysema is suggestive of a coexisting pneumothorax.
   b. Once diagnosed, a traumatic pneumothorax, no matter how small, should be treated with thoracostomy drainage.
   c. Bleeding intercostal vessels are responsible for most hemothoraces. Initial drainage of more than 1,000 mL of blood or collection of more than 200 mL/hr is an indication for thoracotomy.

3. **Penetrating cardiac injury** may result in **pericardial tamponade** (diagnose with transesophageal echocardiography).

4. **Blunt Cardiac Injury.** Diagnosis of myocardial contusion is based on clinical history (blunt chest trauma, angina, cardiac dysrhythmias) and results of transesophageal echocardiography (segmental wall motion abnormalities), CPK-MB isoenzymes, and the electrocardiogram.

5. **Thoracic aortic injury** is suspected in patients with a history of high-impact trauma with deceleration, especially to the chest (widened mediastinum should prompt search for this injury). Transesophageal echocardiography, contrast-enhanced CT, and ultrasound techniques are important tools for evaluating aortic trauma.

6. **Diaphragmatic injury** is suggested on the chest radiograph when the nasogastric tube is above the diaphragm.

E. **Abdominal and Pelvic Injuries**
   1. Liver and spleen lacerations are the most common abdominal injuries following both blunt and

penetrating abdominal trauma, presenting most often with signs of hemorrhage.
- **a.** Because of the unpredictable course of bullets in the body, exploratory laparotomy or laparoscopy (selected cases) is required after any gunshot wound to the abdomen.
- **b.** Abdominal ultrasonography and CT are useful for the evaluation of abdominal and pelvic injuries.
2. **Fractures of the pelvis** may result in major hemorrhage, especially if there is disruption of the pubic symphysis.

F. **Extremity Injuries**
1. Surgical repair of extremity fractures (open or closed) should be performed as soon as possible to decrease the risk of deep vein thrombosis, fat embolism syndrome, pulmonary complications, and sepsis (likely when repair is delayed longer than 6 hours).
2. **Compartment syndrome** is suggested by severe pain in the affected extremity, swelling, and tenseness. Profound analgesia in the presence of an extremity fracture may delay the diagnosis of this syndrome.

III. BURNS

A. Determination of the size of the burned area (rule of nines) and depth of burn (a partial-thickness burn is red, blanches to the touch, and is painful, whereas a full-thickness burn does not blanche and is insensate) set the guidelines for resuscitation as well as the timing of surgical intervention.
B. Information about the mechanism of the injury (closed space is associated with airway damage; electrocution shows little external injury despite internal injury) facilitates the diagnosis of associated clinical abnormalities.
C. **Airway Complications**
1. Singed eyebrows and/or eyelashes and black soot in and around the nose or mouth should increase the suspicion of airway injury.
2. The initial chest radiograph, arterial blood gases, and pulmonary function tests are usually normal in the immediate post-burn period, followed by the appearance of clinical symptoms reflecting pulmonary edema.

TABLE 48-8	
SYMPTOMS OF CARBON MONOXIDE TOXICITY	
Blood carboxyhemoglobin level (%)	**Symptoms**
<15–20%	Headache
	Dizziness
	Occasional confusion
20–40%	Disorientation
	Visual impairment
40–60%	Agitation
	Combativeness
	Hallucinations
	Coma and shock
60%	Death

      3. Fiberoptic bronchoscopy is the best way to evaluate large airways.

  D. Ventilation and Intensive Care. Hypoxemia may persist despite tracheal intubation and ventilation, in the first 36 hours reflects pulmonary edema while after 2 to 5 days reflects atelectasis and bronchial pneumonia.

  E. Carbon Monoxide Toxicity

      1. An increased inhaled oxygen concentration promotes elimination of carbon monoxide (100% oxygen decreases the blood half-time of carboxyhemoglobin from 4 hours to <1 hour) (Table 48-8).

      2. A normal oxygen saturation from a pulse oximeter does not exclude the possibility of carbon monoxide toxicity.

      3. Increased carboxyhemoglobin levels do not cause tachypnea because the carotid bodies are sensitive to arterial PaO_2 and not arterial oxygen content.

  F. Cyanide toxicity (manifests as metabolic acidosis) is a possibility when cyanide or hydrocyanic acid is produced by incomplete combustion of synthetic materials. Pulse oximetry readings will be accurate in the absence of carbon monoxide toxicity and nitrate therapy–induced methemoglobinemia.

  G. Fluid Replacement

      1. Fluid resuscitation is essential in the early care of burn patients, although overaggressive resuscitation may be deleterious (causing airway edema, pulmonary edema, or abdominal edema).

2. If fluid resuscitation is successful, edema formation stops within 18 to 24 hours.
3. Administration of fluids during the initial phase should be titrated to specific goals such as urine output of about 0.5 mL/kg/hr, a heart rate of 110 to 120 beats/min, a normal blood lactate level, and a mixed venous oxygen partial pressure of >35 mm Hg. An increase in the hematocrit during the first day of burn suggests inadequate fluid resuscitation.

IV. OPERATIVE MANAGEMENT (Tables 48-9 and 48-10)

A. Monitoring (Table 48-11)

1. **Hemodynamic Monitoring**
   a. There is no effective substitute for direct intra-arterial monitoring, which permits beat-to-beat assessment of blood pressure (a hemodynamically stable patient may suddenly become hypotensive when the chest or abdomen is opened) and facilitates sampling for measurement of blood gases. During mechanical ventilation of the patient's lungs, the extent of systolic blood pressure variation can provide reliable information about the status of the intravascular fluid volume (Fig. 48-2).
   b. Placement of a central venous pressure or pulmonary artery catheter is not necessary in young patients in the absence of heart disease (a reasonable assessment of the patient's blood volume can be made by repeated observation of systemic blood pressure, hematocrit, arterial blood gases, and urine output).
   c. **Transesophageal echocardiography** provides valuable diagnostic information in myocardial contusion, cardiac valvular dysfunction, pericardial fluid accumulation, intravascular fluid volume, cardiac output, myocardial contractility, and large vessel injury (do not place probe if there is a possibility of esophageal injury).

2. **Urine Output**
   a. As a rough guideline, urine output should be maintained at >0.5 mL/kg/hr (after prolonged shock renal failure may already be present on arrival in the operating room).

TABLE 48-9

IMPLICATIONS OF PREEXISTING DISEASES FOR INTRAOPERATIVE MANAGEMENT OF THE TRAUMA PATIENT

Substance Abuse
Alcohol
  Delayed gastric emptying
  Vasodilation and myocardial depression
  Potentiation of trauma-induced hypothermia
  Hemostatic defect
  Postoperative alcohol withdrawal
Cocaine
  Unpredictable hemodynamic response to hemorrhage
  Cardiac dysrhythmias
Opioids
  Delayed gastric emptying
  Vasodilation
  Postoperative opioid withdrawal

Hypertension
Decreased tolerance to hypovolemia
Exaggerated hypertensive response to pain
Increased likelihood of myocardial ischemia and cardiac
  dysrhythmias

Ischemic Heart Disease
Increased likelihood of myocardial ischemia because of
  trauma-induced changes

Anemia

Sickle Cell Disease

Coagulation Disorders

Diabetes Mellitus
Delayed gastric emptying
Decreased response to resuscitative measures in patients with
  autonomic neuropathy
Increased likelihood of ischemic heart disease
Electrolyte abnormalities

Asthma

    b. Osmotic diuresis produced by preoperative radiopaque dye or mannitol decreases the value of urine output as a monitor of organ perfusion.
    c. Cola-colored urine suggests hemoglobinuria from incompatible blood transfusion (associated with pink-stained plasma) or myoglobinuria caused by

TABLE 48-10

SPECIALIZED EQUIPMENT, SUPPLIES, AND DRUGS THAT MAY BE NEEDED FOR MANAGEMENT OF THE TRAUMA PATIENT

Equipment
Fiberoptic bronchoscope with a light source
Mechanical ventilator that is effective in patients with decreased pulmonary compliance (lung contusion, aspiration)
Jet ventilator system
Positive end-expiratory pressure valves
Blood and fluid bag pressurizing systems
Fluid warming system
Rapid infusion system
Forced air warming device and heated humidifier for inspired gases
Calibrated infusion pumps
Transesophageal echocardiography
Pneumatic tourniquet
Cardiopulmonary bypass

Supplies
Material for special airway management
Material for arterial and pulmonary artery catheter placement

Drugs
Vasopressors
Inotropes
Calcium chloride
THAM intravenous infusion
Sodium bicarbonate
Topical anesthetics

skeletal muscle destruction, as after blunt or electrical trauma. Both of these conditions may result in acute renal failure (prevent with mannitol diuresis). Red-colored urine usually indicates urinary tract injury in the trauma patient.

3. **Organ Perfusion and Oxygen Utilization**
    a. Occult hypoperfusion may not be detected by traditional hemodynamic monitoring such as systemic blood pressure, heart rate, and urine output.
    b. Intestinal mucosa is particularly vulnerable to occult hypoperfusion (passage of luminal microorganisms into the circulation and release of inflammatory mediators causing sepsis and multiorgan failure).

TABLE 48-11
MONITORING OF THE TRAUMA PATIENT

Physiologic parameter	Degree of importance	Monitoring equipment	Specific intraoperative uses
Cardiac rate, rhythm, and ischemia	Essential	Electrocardiogram	Routine
Arterial blood pressure	Essential	Indirect (cuff, Doppler, oscillometric system)	Routine
		Direct (intra-arterial catheter)	
Central venous pressure	Useful		Hypovolemia
			Pericardial tamponade
			Myocardial contusion
			Air embolism
Pulmonary artery and capillary wedge pressures	Selected patients	Pulmonary artery catheter	Blunt chest injury
			Acute respiratory distress syndrome
			Blunt cardiac injury (contusion)
			Pulmonary edema
Cardiac output	Useful	Computer	Same as pulmonary artery catheter

Parameter	Importance	Device/Test	Indication
Cardiac wall motion abnormalities, myocardial ischemia	Useful	Transesophageal echocardiograph	Blunt cardiac injury (contusion) Major vessel injuries
Ventilation	Essential	End-tidal carbon dioxide monitor	Routine Head injury Air embolism
Arterial oxygenation	Essential	Pulse oximeter Arterial blood gases	Routine
Tissue oxygenation	Useful	Oximeter pulmonary artery catheter	Low perfusion states
Renal function	Essential	Foley catheter and graduated container	All major trauma patients
Temperature	Essential	Esophageal or rectal probe	Routine
Neuromuscular function	Essential	Peripheral nerve stimulator	Routine
Neurologic function	Useful	Bolt, catheter, or fiberoptic sensor	Head injury
Coagulation	Useful	Prothrombin time/partial thromboplastin time/ platelets/fibrinogen Tube test Thromboelastograph	Shock Massive transfusions

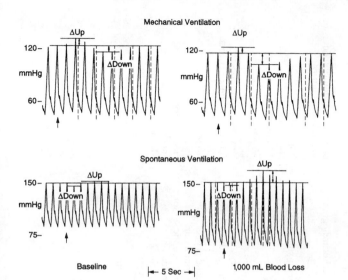

FIGURE 48-2. The magnitude of systolic blood pressure variation can provide valuable information about the status of the intravascular fluid volume.

    c. Markers of organ perfusion and oxygen utilization include oxygen transport variables (oxygen delivery, oxygen consumption, oxygen extraction ratio), base deficit, and blood lactate.

   4. **Coagulation**

    a. Conventional blood coagulation monitoring involves determination of prothrombin time, activated plasma thromboplastin time, platelet count, blood fibrinogen level, and fibrin degradation products.

    b. The "tube test," which involves obtaining a plain tube of blood with no anticoagulant, is a practical intraoperative method of coagulation monitoring (Table 48-12).

    c. Thromboelastography provides quantitation of coagulation data that is reflected by the tube test (Fig. 48-3).

    d. The results of coagulation tests have little primary impact on treatment (platelet and factor replacement are likely to be necessary when more than one blood volume is replaced).

TABLE 48-12

INFORMATION OBTAINED FROM "TUBE TEST"

Coagulation
Clotting factor deficiency is likely if clot does not form or does so
only after 10–20 minutes

Clot Retraction
Platelet depletion or dysfunction is likely if clot fails to contract
within 1 hour

Clot Lysis
Fibrinolysis is likely if clot lysis occurs earlier than 6 hours

    B. **Anesthetic and Adjunct Drugs.** From the standpoint of
       anesthetic management, injuries may be placed in one of
       five categories.
       1. **Airway Compromise.** The primary issue is whether to
          manage the airway with or without the use of
          anesthetic drugs and muscle relaxants. As a general
          precaution, these drugs may be avoided if there is
          significant airway obstruction or if there is doubt as to
          whether the patient's trachea can be intubated because
          of anatomic limitations.
       2. **Hypovolemia.** Inhaled and intravenous anesthetics
          will predictably further decrease blood pressure in the

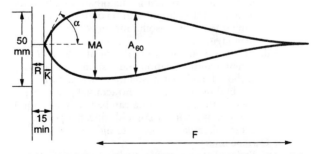

FIGURE 48-3. Thromboelastogram. R = time interval from blood deposition in the cuvette to an amplitude of 1 mm on the thromboelastogram;
K = time interval between the end of R and a point with an amplitude of
20 mm on the thromboelastogram; MA = maximum amplitude of thromboelastogram; α angle = slope of the external divergence of the tracing from
the R value point; A_{60} = amplitude of thromboelastogram 60 minutes after
maximum amplitude; F = time from MA to return to 0 amplitude (normal
>300 minutes).

presence of hypovolemia. Two important principles in the use of anesthetic drugs are accurate estimation of the extent of hypovolemia and decrease of the dose accordingly. Intraoperative use of the bispectral index (BIS) monitor and, whenever possible, titrating anesthetics to levels <60 may prevent recall in trauma patients.

3. **Head and Open Eye Injuries**
   a. Deep anesthesia and adequate skeletal muscle relaxation for tracheal intubation are important principles.
   b. Drugs selected for management of patients with head injury should produce the least increase in intracranial pressure, the least decrease in mean arterial pressure, and the greatest decrease in cerebral metabolic requirements for oxygen. With the exception of ketamine, all intravenous drugs produce similar degrees of cerebral vasoconstriction and suppression of cerebral metabolism. The disadvantage of these drugs is depression of cerebral perfusion pressure.
   c. All inhaled anesthetics have the potential to increase cerebral blood flow, cerebral blood volume, and intracranial pressure while decreasing cerebral metabolic requirements for oxygen (the uncoupling between blood flow and metabolism is greatest for halothane and least for isoflurane). Desflurane and sevoflurane have effects similar to those of isoflurane on cerebral hemodynamics.
   d. In severe head injury with associated loss of cerebral autoregulation and responsiveness to carbon dioxide, even isoflurane may increase cerebral blood flow and intracranial pressure. In these patients, anesthesia can be maintained until the skull is open with opioids plus thiopental, propofol, midazolam, or etomidate.

4. **Cardiac Injury**
   a. **Pericardial tamponade.** Preload, myocardial contractility, and heart rate should be maintained. If possible, the evacuation of the pericardial blood should be accomplished under local anesthesia (all anesthetics decrease myocardial contractility and may cause peripheral vasodilation). Ketamine is

often recommended if anesthesia must be induced before evacuation of the tamponade.

   b. Blunt myocardial injury may put the patient at risk for drug-induced decreases in myocardial contractility (inotropes may be necessary).

5. Burns

   a. Extensive escharotomies may necessitate massive transfusions, temperature control, and management of fluid, electrolyte, and coagulation abnormalities.

   b. A hypermetabolic state necessitates increased oxygen, ventilation, and nutrition.

   c. Hypothermia is a risk in the operating room (maintain room temperature at 28°C to 32°C, use fluid and blood-warming devices, humidify inspired gases).

   d. After the first 24 hours, succinylcholine must be avoided for as long as 1 year, because hyperkalemia may follow administration of this drug (large increases in serum potassium levels occur when the burn size exceeds 10% of the body surface area).

   e. Resistance to nondepolarizing muscle relaxants develops in patients with >30% burns starting about 1 week after the burn injury and peaking in 5 to 6 weeks.

   f. For serial wound debridement, ketamine in intermittent doses, neuraxial or peripheral nerve blocks via an indwelling catheter, or sedation with opioids and intravenous agents may be employed.

C. Management of Intraoperative Complications

   1. Persistent hypotension is suggestive of bleeding, tension pneumothorax, neurogenic shock, or cardiac injury.

   2. Hypothermia that accompanies trauma is associated with increased mortality.

      a. Convective warming forced dry air (Bair Hugger) can prevent a temperature drop in most trauma patients but cannot effectively treat severe hypothermia.

      b. Administration of warm intravenous fluids is the most effective way to prevent and treat hypothermia in the trauma patient.

   3. Coagulation abnormalities may reflect dilutional effects from transfusions, tissue thromboplastin release, and hypothermia-induced platelet dysfunction. Hypothermia may also enhance fibrinolytic activity.

  a. Prompt platelet administration should be considered when abnormal clinical bleeding is noted (assuming surgical bleeding is controlled).
  b. Once the replacement with coagulation-deficient fluids exceeds 1 blood volume, clinical coagulopathy is likely even in the absence of shock, hypothermia, or other aggravating factors.

4. **Electrolyte and Acid-Base Disturbances**
  a. Hyperkalemia may develop as a result of shock-induced alteration in permeability of cell membranes, release from ischemic tissues, or rapid transfusion of blood (faster than 1 unit every 4 minutes).
  b. Metabolic acidosis is caused by shock in the majority of patients after trauma. Treatment of metabolic acidosis includes correction of the underlying cause (hypoxemia, hypovolemia, decreased cardiac output). Symptomatic treatment with sodium bicarbonate has several disadvantages (leftward shift of the oxyhemoglobin dissociation curve, hyperosmolar state, alkalosis).
  c. Base deficit parallels the degree of hypovolemia.

5. **Intraoperative death** is more likely during emergency trauma surgery than it is in any other operative procedure.

TABLE 48-13

NEEDS AND CONCERNS IN THE EARLY POSTOPERATIVE PERIOD IN THE TRAUMA PATIENT

Sedation and analgesia (improves pulmonary function)
Propofol (1.5–6 mg/kg/h) and/or midazolam (0.1–0.2 mg/kg/h)
Morphine (0.02–0.04 mg/kg/h) or fentanyl (1–3 μg/kg/h)
Acute renal failure (decreased urine output is not a good indicator and blood urea nitrogen does not increase until at least 24 hours postoperatively)
Abdominal compartment syndrome (intra-abdominal hypertension from edema of abdominal organs produced by inflammatory mediators, fluid resuscitation, surgical manipulation; suspect if tense abdomen; suggests need to measure intravesical pressure)
Thromboembolism

VI. EARLY POSTOPERATIVE CONSIDERATIONS

(Table 48-13). Reevaluation and optimization of the circulation, oxygenation, temperature, central nervous system function, coagulation, electrolyte and acid-base status, and renal function are the hallmarks of postoperative management.

CHAPTER 49 ■ THE ALLERGIC RESPONSE

Allergic reactions during anesthesia represent an important cause of perioperative complications (Levy JH: The allergic response. In Barash PG, Cullen BF, Stoelting RK [eds]: *Clinical Anesthesia*, pp 1298–1312. Philadelphia, Lippincott Williams & Wilkins, 2006). Anesthesiologists routinely manage patients during their perioperative medical care during which time exposure to foreign substances (drugs including injected anesthetics, antibiotics, neuromuscular blocking drugs, protamine, blood products) and environmental antigens (latex) occurs.

I. BASIC IMMUNOLOGIC PRINCIPLES

A. Host defense systems can be divided into cellular (T-cell lymphocytes) and humoral (antibodies, complement, cytokines) elements.

B. **Antigens** are molecules capable of stimulating an immune response (antibody production or lymphocyte stimulation) (Table 49-1).

C. **Thymus-Derived Lymphocytes (T-Cell Lymphocytes) and Bursa-Derived Lymphocytes (B-Cell Lymphocytes)**

1. **Thymus-derived lymphocytes** contain receptors that are activated by binding with antigens and subsequently secrete mediators that regulate the immune response. Acquired immunodeficiency syndrome is a result of infection of helper T lymphocytes with a retrovirus known as the immunodeficiency virus.

2. **Bursa-derived lymphocytes** differentiate into plasma cells that synthesize antibodies.

   a. **Antibodies** are specific proteins (immunoglobulins) that can recognize and bind to a specific antigen (see Table 49-1).

   b. Antibodies function as specific receptor molecules for immune cells and proteins.

   c. **Opsonization** is the deposition of antibody or complement fragments on the surface of foreign cells, leading to the destruction of those cells.

TABLE 49-1
BIOLOGIC CHARACTERISTICS OF IMMUNOGLOBULINS

	IgG	IgM	IgA	IgE	IgD
Molecular weight	160,000	900,000	170,000	188,000	184,000
Serum concentration (mg/dL)	6–14	0.5–1.5	1–3	$<0.5 \times 10^3$	<0.1
Complement activation	All but IgG4	+	–	–	–
Placental transfer	+	–	–	–	–
Serum half-time (days)	23	5	6	1–5	2–8
Cell binding	Mast cells, neutrophils, lymphocytes, mono-nuclear cells, platelets	Lymphocytes	Mast cells, basophils, lymphocytes	Neutrophils, lymphocytes	–

TABLE 49-2
CELLS THAT PARTICIPATE IN THE IMMUNE RESPONSE

Macrophages (ingest antigens)
Polymorphonuclear leukocytes (neutrophils) are the first cells to
appear in an acute inflammatory reaction
Eosinophils (function unknown)
Basophils (granulocytes in blood; cell surfaces contain IgE
receptors)
Mast cells (located in perivascular spaces of skin, lungs, and
intestine; cell surfaces contain IgE receptors)

II. EFFECTOR CELLS AND PROTEINS OF THE IMMUNE RESPONSE CELLS (Table 49-2)

A. Monocytes, neutrophils (polymorphonuclear leukocytes), and eosinophils are effector cells that migrate into areas of inflammation in response to chemotactic factors.
B. **Opsonization** is deposition of antibody or complement fragments on surfaces of foreign cells with subsequent facilitation of the process that allows the effector cells to destroy the foreign cell.

III. CYTOKINES/INTERLEUKINS

A. Cytokines (**interleukin-1, tumor necrosis factor**) are inflammatory cell activators that are synthesized by macrophages to act as secondary messengers that activate endothelial cells and white blood cells (produce an inflammatory response) (Table 49-3).
B. T-cell lymphocytes produce interleukins.

IV. COMPLEMENT

A. The primary humoral response to antigen and antibody binding is activation of the complement system (about

TABLE 49-3
SYMPTOMS PRODUCED BY RELEASE OF CYTOKINES

Fever
Hypotension
Myocardial depression
Catabolism

20 different proteins that are activated by antigen–antibody interactions, plasmin, and endotoxins).
B. A series of inhibitors regulate the complement system (angioneurotic edema [may be activated by surgery manifesting as laryngeal obstruction] is because of a deficiency of an inhibitor of the C1 complement system).
C. **Effects of Anesthesia on Immune Function**
  1. Anesthesia and surgery depress both T-cell and B-cell responsiveness as well as nonspecific host resistance mechanisms, including phagocytosis.
  2. The significance, if any, of these responses is not known (probably of minor importance compared with the hormonal aspects of the stress response).

V. HYPERSENSITIVITY RESPONSES (ALLERGY)
(Table 49-4 and Fig. 49-1)

VI. INTRAOPERATIVE ALLERGIC REACTIONS

A. More than 90% of the allergic reactions evoked by drugs administered intravenously occur within 3 minutes of administration. It is estimated that allergic reactions occur once in every 5,000–25,000 anesthetics administered.

TABLE 49-4
CLASSIFICATION OF HYPERSENSITIVITY

Type I Reaction
Immediate type hypersensitivity reaction (anaphylaxis) with release of chemical mediators (Table 49–6) from mast cells and basophils in response to binding of IgE antibodies to the surfaces of these cells

Type II Reaction
Mediated by IgG or IgM antibodies directed against antigens on surfaces of foreign cells (ABO incompatibility reactions)

Type III Reaction
Antigen–antibody complexes that form insoluble complexes that deposit in the microvasculature (poststreptococcal infections)

Type IV Reaction
Delayed hypersensitivity reaction of cell-mediated immunity (tissue rejection, tuberculin immunity)

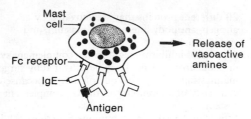

FIGURE 49-1. Type I immediate hypersensitivity reactions (anaphylaxis) involve IgE antibodies binding to mast cells or basophils at the Fc receptors. On encountering immunospecific antigens, the IgE becomes cross-linked, inducing degranulation, intracellular activation, and release of chemical mediators.

TABLE 49-5

RECOGNITION OF ANAPHYLAXIS DURING REGIONAL AND GENERAL ANESTHESIA

Systems	Symptoms	Signs
Respiratory	Dyspnea	Coughing
		Wheezing
		Sneezing
		Laryngeal edema
		Decreased pulmonary compliance
		Fulminant pulmonary edema
		Acute respiratory failure
Cardiovascular	Dizziness	Disorientation
	Malaise	Diaphoresis
	Retrosternal discomfort	Hypotension
		Tachycardia
		Cardiac dysrhythmias
		Decreased systemic vascular resistance
		Pulmonary hypertension
		Cardiac arrest
Cutaneous	Itching	Urticaria
	Burning	Flushing
	Tingling	Periorbital edema
		Perioral edema

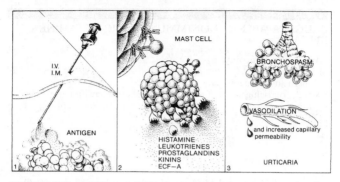

FIGURE 49-2. During a type I allergic reaction, antigen enters a patient during anesthesia via a parenteral route (intravenous or intramuscular) (*Panel 1*). The antigen bridges two IgE antibodies on the surface of mast cells or basophils, causing degranulation (*Panel 2*). The released chemical mediators produce the characteristic clinical symptoms of an allergic reaction (*Panel 3*).

   B. The only manifestation of an intraoperative allergic reaction may be **refractory hypotension** (Table 49-5 and Fig. 49-2).
   C. Anaphylactic Reactions: IgE-Mediated Pathophysiology
     1. Antigen binding to IgE antibodies (reflects prior exposure to the antigen) initiates anaphylaxis.
     2. The antigen binds by bridging two immunospecific antibodies located on the surfaces of mast cells and basophils, resulting in the release of **histamine** and other chemicals.

TABLE 49-6

CHEMICAL MEDIATORS OF ANAPHYLAXIS

Histamine
Peptide mediators
Eosinophilic chemotactic factor
Neurotrophilic chemotactic factor
Arachidonic acid metabolites (leukotrienes and prostaglandins are synthesized following mast cell activation from arachidonic acid metabolism of phospholipid cell membranes)
Kinins
Platelet-activating factor
Tryptase

TABLE 49-7

DRUGS CAPABLE OF NONIMMUNOLOGIC HISTAMINE
RELEASE

Antibiotics (vancomycin)
Basic compounds (protamine)
Hyperosmotic agents
Nondepolarizing skeletal muscle relaxants (atracurium and
  mivacurium > pancuronium, vecuronium and rocuronium)
Opioids (morphine)
Thiobarbiturates (?)

   3. **Chemical Mediators of Anaphylaxis** (Table 49-6)
   4. **Recognition of Anaphylaxis** (see Table 49-5)
      a. Individuals vary greatly in their manifestations
         and course of anaphylaxis (spectrum ranges from
         minor clinical significance to death).
      b. The enigma of anaphylaxis lies in the
         unpredictability of its occurrence, the severity of
         the attack, and the lack of a prior patient allergic
         history.
   D. **Nonimmunologic Release of Histamine**
      1. Many diverse molecules administered during the
         perioperative period release histamine in a
         dose-dependent, nonimmunologic fashion (Table
         49-7).
      2. Nonimmunologic histamine release differs from
         antigen-mediated histamine release in that histamine
         appears to be the only mediator released.
      3. Aminosteroid muscle relaxants (rocuronium) when
         administered at clinically recommended doses have
         minimal effects on histamine release.
      4. **Antihistamine pretreatment** does not inhibit
         histamine release but instead competes with
         histamine at the receptor and attenuates the
         resulting physiologic effects.
   E. **Treatment Plan** (Table 49-8)
      1. All patients who have experienced life-threatening
         allergic reactions should be admitted to the hospital
         for 24 hours of monitoring, because manifestations
         may recur following successful treatment.
      2. **Epinephrine** is the drug of choice for resuscitation of
         patients experiencing an allergic reaction
         (alpha-adrenergic effects reverse hypotension, and
         beta-adrenergic stimulation produces

TABLE 49-8

MANAGEMENT OF ANAPHYLAXIS DURING GENERAL ANESTHESIA

Initial Treatment
Stop administration of antigen
Maintain upper airway and administer 100% oxygen
Discontinue all anesthetic drugs
Initiate intravascular volume expansion (2–4 liters of crystalloid or colloid solution in presence of hypotension)
Administer epinephrine (5–10 μg iv with hypotension and titrate as needed; 0.1–1.0 mg iv with cardiovascular collapse)

Secondary Treatment
Antihistamines (0.5–1 mg/kg diphenhydramine iv)
Catecholamine infusions (starting doses: epinephrine, 4–8 μg/min; norepinephrine, 4–8 μg/min; isoproterenol, 0.5–1 μg/min, as continuous infusion and titrated to effect)
Albuterol (4–8 puffs by metered-dose inhaler)
Corticosteroids (cortisol, 250–1000 mg; methylprednisolone, 1–2 g, especially if suspect complement activation)
Airway evaluation prior to extubation

bronchodilation and inhibits continued release of chemical mediators).
3. Arterial blood gases should be monitored during resuscitation.
4. Up to 40% of intravascular fluid volume may be translocated into the interstitial space during an allergic reaction.
5. The beta agonists (metered-dose inhaler) have replaced aminophylline as the recommended treatment of bronchospasm.
6. If there is any evidence of upper airway edema (facial edema, absence of air leak when tracheal tube cuff is deflated), direct laryngoscopic examination should be performed before the trachea is extubated.
7. **Refractory hypotension** may be treated with arginine vasopressin and use echocardiography to evaluate cardiac function and hypovolemia.

VII. PERIOPERATIVE MANAGEMENT OF THE PATIENT WITH ALLERGIES

A. **Allergic drug reactions** account for 6 to 10% of all adverse drug reactions. It is estimated that 5% of adults in the United States are allergic to one or more drugs.

B. **Immunologic Mechanisms of Drug Allergy**

1. Most drugs administered to patients by anesthesiologists have been reported to produce allergic reactions (Table 49-9).

2. Muscle relaxants are the most common drugs responsible for evoking intraoperative allergic reactions (cross-sensitivity is present between succinylcholine and nondepolarizing muscle relaxants).

3. Unexplained intraoperative cardiovascular collapse has been attributed to anaphylaxis triggered by latex (natural rubber).

   a. Patients with **spina bifida** have an increased incidence of allergy to latex.

   b. Symptoms as a result of latex allergy may not occur until several minutes after exposure and thus may be erroneously attributed to other causes.

4. Life-threatening allergic reactions are more likely to occur in patients with a history of allergy, atopy, or asthma. Because the incidence of allergic reactions is so rare, even this history does not mandate further evaluation or pharmacologic pretreatment.

TABLE 49-9

DRUGS IMPLICATED IN ALLERGIC REACTIONS DURING ANESTHESIA

Anesthetic Drugs
Muscle relaxants (cross-sensitivity among all drugs is possible)
Induction drugs (barbiturates, propofol)
Local anesthetics (para-aminobenzoic acid ester drugs)
Opioids

Other Drugs
Antibiotics (cephalosporins, penicillin, vancomycin)
Blood products (whole blood, packed cells, platelets, fresh frozen plasma, fibrinogen, gamma globulin)
Aprotinin
Methylmethacrylate
Protamine
Radiocontrast dye
Latex (natural rubber)
Drug preservatives/additives
Colloid volume expanders
Vascular graft material

VIII. EVALUATION OF PATIENTS WITH ALLERGIC REACTIONS

A. Identifying the drug responsible for a suspected allergic reaction still depends on circumstantial evidence indicating the temporal sequence of drug administration.

1. Direct challenge of a patient with a test dose of the suspected offending drug is potentially hazardous and not recommended.

2. A small test dose of drug given during anesthesia more accurately reflects a **pharmacologic test dose** and has nothing to do with immunologic dosages.

3. The demonstration of drug-specific antibodies is generally accepted as evidence that the patient may be at risk for anaphylaxis if the drug is administered.

B. Testing for Allergy

1. Following an allergic reaction, it is important to identify the offending allergen so as to prevent readministration (often patients have simultaneously received multiple different drugs with or without preservatives).

2. In vitro tests are available for anesthetic drugs (Table 49-10).

IX. AGENTS IMPLICATED IN ALLERGIC REACTIONS

A. Any agent a patient received as either an injection, infusion, or environmental antigen has the potential to produce an allergic reaction.

TABLE 49-10

TESTS FOR DRUG ALLERGY

Leukocyte histamine release (incubate patient's leukocytes with the drug in question and measure histamine release as a marker for basophil activation)

Radioallergosorbent test (RAST) (commercially available antigens [few anesthetic drugs are available] are incubated with the patient's plasma for detection of specific IgE antibodies)

Enzyme-linked immunosorbent assay (ELISA) (measures antigen-specific antibodies; similar to the RAST test)

Intradermal testing (histamine release from mast cells causes vasodilation [flare] and localized edema)

B. **Latex Allergy.** Health care workers and children with spina bifida and urogenital abnormalities are at increased risk. Patients allergic to bananas, avocados, and kiwis may cross-react with latex. It is a complex task to create a latex-free environment for care of sensitized patients (should be identified by a Medic Alert Bracelet).

C. **Muscle Relaxants** possess molecular features that make them potential allergens.

1. Prick tests are often used for authenticating neuromuscular blocking drugs as causes of allergic reactions. There is the potential for cross-sensitivity between muscle relaxants because of similarity of the active site (quaternary ammonium molecule).

2. An alternative muscle relaxant cannot be chosen without some degree of immunologic testing.

CHAPTER 50 ■ DRUG INTERACTIONS

Modern drug regimens often involve use of multiple drugs in combination, which introduces the risk of drug interactions (Rosow CE, Levine WC: Drug interactions. In Barash PG, Cullen BF, Stoelting RK [eds]: *Clinical Anesthesia*, pp 1313–1330. Philadelphia, Lippincott Williams & Wilkins, 2006).

I. PROBLEMS CREATED BY DRUG-DRUG INTERACTION

A. The probability of a drug-drug interaction increases with the number of drugs administered.

B. Drug interactions are uncommon despite the fact many patients are taking multiple drugs preoperatively (antihypertensives, antidepressants, gastrointestinal drugs) and then receive 5 to 10 drugs during anesthesia (many reactions are not significant, drugs have a large safety margin, many interactions are not recognized).

C. **Why Combine Drugs?** The goal of combining drugs is to decrease toxicity while maintaining efficacy (hypertension, chemotherapy, prophylaxis against grand mal seizures).

II. PHARMACEUTICAL INTERACTIONS

A. A chemical or physical interaction may occur between drugs before they are administered to form a precipitate (thiopental or ketamine injected with succinylcholine, epinephrine injected with sodium bicarbonate as during cardiopulmonary resuscitation).

B. A chemical or physical interaction may occur between drugs before they are administered to form a toxic compound (desflurane or isoflurane in contact with dry soda lime to form carbon monoxide, nitric oxide in contact with oxygen forms nitrogen dioxide).

III. PHARMACOKINETIC INTERACTIONS

A. A pharmacokinetic interaction occurs when one drug alters the absorption, metabolism, or elimination of another drug.

B. **Absorption** may be altered because of direct chemical or physical interaction between drugs in the body (orally administered tetracycline is inactivated by chelation with antacids, opioids slow gastric emptying) or changes in regional blood flow (local administration of epinephrine retards absorption of local anesthetics; congestive heart failure or shock may alter the onset and intensity of drug effect by decreasing tissue perfusion).

C. **Distribution**-related drug interactions occur when distribution of a second drug is altered by hemodynamics (drug-induced changes in cardiac output), drug ionization ("ion trapping"), or binding to plasma and tissue proteins (alpha-1 acid glycoprotein concentrations increase postoperatively and following myocardial infarction or trauma, albumin concentrations may be decreased by hepatic cirrhosis).

   1. A drug that is highly bound to plasma protein effectively exists in a depot (similar to a drug given by intramuscular administration).
   2. Altered protein binding or displacement from protein-binding sites has been dogma for many years but the true clinical relevance of this type of interaction is not clear.

D. **Metabolism**
   1. Drugs administered to inhibit acetylcholinesterase (as for reversal on nondepolarizing neuromuscular blocking drugs) will also inhibit pseudocholinesterase and prolong the duration of action of succinylcholine.

E. **Monoamine Oxidase (MAO) Interactions**
   1. Inhibition of MAO, which is present in tissues throughout the body, by MAO inhibitors may produce interactions with drugs that affect sympathetic neurotransmission (ephedrine produces an exaggerated response as more presynaptic transmitters are available for release, "wine and cheese" interaction because of tyramine content of foods) or interactions that involve central nervous system depressants (hyperpyrexia and hypertension that may progress to seizures and coma in patients receiving meperidine).

2. Current clinical opinion favors continuing MAO inhibitor therapy up to the time of surgery.
3. Patients taking MAO inhibitors have the potential for perioperative hemodynamic instability, yet beta-blockers, direct vasodilators, and direct-acting vasopressors appear to be safe and effective treatments in most circumstances.

F. **Hepatic Biotransformation**
1. Many anesthetic drugs undergo oxidative metabolism by one of the isoforms of cytochrome P-450 found in liver microsomes.
   a. P-450 isoforms have low substrate specificity such that drugs of diverse structures (general anesthetics, opioids, barbiturates, benzodiazepines) can be biotransformed by a single group of enzymes.
   b. Inhibitors or inducers of these enzymes can also affect the clearance of broad groups of drugs (Table 50-1).

TABLE 50-1

CLASSIFICATION OF PHARMACODYNAMIC DRUG INTERACTIONS

Additive Interactions (most likely to occur when drugs with identical mechanisms of action are combined)
Administration of two aminosteroid nondepolarizing muscle relaxants
Administration of nitrous oxide with a volatile anesthetic

Antagonistic Drug Interactions
Deliberate
  Administration of neostigmine, naloxone, flumazenil
Unintended
  Succinylcholine and a nondepolarizing muscle relaxant
  Epidural opioid administered after establishing a block with chloroprocaine

Synergistic Drug Interactions (most likely to occur when drugs of different classes or mechanisms are administered to produce the same effect)
Potentiation of opioids by nonsteroidal anti-inflammatory drugs
Potentiation of nondepolarizing muscle relaxants by volatile anesthetics
Potentiation between hypnotics that have related mechanisms of action (act on gamma-aminobutryic acid-A chloride ionophore)

2. Removal of a drug from the blood by hepatic biotransformation (hepatic clearance) is dependent on hepatic blood flow and intrinsic clearance (maximal ability of the liver to metabolize that drug or extraction ratio).

   a. For drugs with a high extraction ratio (lidocaine, morphine, propranolol), hepatic blood flow is the rate-limiting factor in overall hepatic clearance. Decreases in hepatic blood flow (anesthesia, congestive heart failure) result in increased plasma concentrations.

   b. For drugs with a low extraction ratio (diazepam, alfentanil), hepatic enzyme activity is the rate-limiting factor.

3. The most common reason for increased intrinsic clearance is enzyme induction of cytochrome P-450 enzymes (microsomal or CYP enzymes). The most important subfamily appears to be CYP3A, which is found in greatest abundance in the human liver and is responsible for the metabolism of a large number of drugs.

4. Drugs may also inhibit the hepatic biotransformation of other drugs by competing for the same P-450 enzymes (protease inhibitors can inhibit the metabolism of midazolam and fentanyl by inhibiting CYP3A4.

G. **Drug elimination** may result in pharmacokinetic drug interactions via alterations in renal or pulmonary clearance.

IV. PHARMACODYNAMIC INTERACTIONS

A. A pharmacodynamic interaction occurs when one drug

TABLE 50-2

DRUGS THAT INDUCE OR INHIBIT HEPATIC DRUG METABOLISM

Inhibitors	Inducers
Phenobarbital	Cimetidine
Phenytoin	Ketoconazole
Rifampicin	Erythromycin
Carbamazepine	Disulfiram
Ethanol	Ritonavir

alters the sensitivity of a target receptor or tissue to the effects of a second drug (pharmacokinetic interaction is a change in the amount of active drug reaching receptor sites).

B. The dose-response curve or concentration-response curve for one drug is shifted by another drug (Table 50-2).

V. PHARMACODYNAMIC INTERACTIONS AFFECTING HEMODYNAMICS

A. Prior recommendations that cardiovascular stimulant or depressant drugs should be discontinued preoperatively because they interfered with protective responses to the trauma of anesthesia and surgery are no longer advocated.
   1. Hypertensive patients who remain well controlled are less likely to have wide swings in systemic blood pressure during surgery.
   2. Abrupt discontinuation of vasoactive medications can actually increase cardiovascular instability (rebound hypertension, cardiac dysrhythmias).

B. The majority of cardiovascular drug interactions are extensions of the known pharmacology of the drugs (Table 50-3).
   1. There is currently no consensus on the preoperative management of patients taking angiotensin-converting enzyme inhibitors.
      a. Continuation through the perioperative period may be associated with an increased incidence of hypotension during induction of general anesthesia.
      b. Withholding these drugs for 24 hours may decrease intraoperative hypotension but also make blood pressure extremely labile during surgery.
      c. Chronic blockade of the angiotensin system reduces the vasoconstrictor response to norepinephrine (may explain why drug-induced hypotension is resistant to sympathetic drugs).

C. **Acute cocaine intoxication** may present as hypertension, tachycardia, and myocardial ischemia (resembles pheochromocytoma). Administration of a beta-blocker alone may allow unopposed alpha-adrenergic stimulation and large increases in systemic vascular resistance.

TABLE 50-3
EFFECTS OF ANTIHYPERTENSIVE DRUGS DURING ANESTHESIA

Class	Drugs	Effects
alpha-blockers	Phenoxybenzamine	Hypotension/vasodilation
	Phentolamine	Reflex tachycardia
	Prazosin	
beta-blockers	Propranolol	Hypotension
	Metoprolol	Decreased myocardial contractility
	Atenolol	Bradycardia
		Heart block
Mixed alpha/beta-blocker	Labetalol	Hypotension/vasodilation
		Bradycardia
		Heart block
Calcium channel blockers	Verapamil	Hypotension/vasodilation
	Diltiazem	Decreased myocardial contractility
	Nifedipine	
	Nicardipine	Heart block
Direct vasodilators	Nitroglycerin	Hypotension/vasodilation
	Isosorbide	Reflex tachycardia
	Hydralazine	
Angiotensin-converting enzyme inhibitors	Captopril	Hypotension/vasodilation
	Enalapril	Hyperkalemia
	Lisinopril	
Angiotensin II blocker	Losartan	Hypotension/vasodilation
	Valsartan	Hyperkalemia
Diuretics	Thiazides	Hypovolemia
	Furosemide	Hypokalemia
	Bumetanide	Vasodilation (?)

VI. PHARMACODYNAMIC INTERACTIONS AFFECTING ANALGESIA OR HYPNOSIS
(Table 50-4)

VII. HERBAL PREPARATIONS AND DRUG INTERACTIONS (Table 50-5)

TABLE 50-4

DRUG INTERACTIONS BETWEEN COMBINATIONS OF CENTRAL NERVOUS SYSTEM DEPRESSANTS

Opioid—Hypnotic
Fentanyl decreases dose requirements for thiopental (more rapid awakening after short surgical procedures)
Opioids potentiate propofol
Infusions of remifentanil or alfentanil decrease the needed infusion rate of propofol

Opioid—Benzodiazepine
Alfentanil (weak hypnotic but highly selective depressant of central nervous system [sedation]) decreases the hypnotic (sleep) dose of midazolam

Benzodiazepine—Hypnotic
Midazolam potentates the hypnotic effects of propofol

Volatile Anesthetic—Opioid
Opioids produce dose-dependent decreases in minimum alveolar concentration

α2-Agonist Interactions
Clonidine and dexmedetomidine potentiate opioid analgesia and decrease minimum alveolar concentration (may reflect depression of the locus ceruleus, which is the main adrenergic nucleus in the brain as well as being important for sleep, memory, and analgesia)

TABLE 50-5

EVIDENCE FOR HERBAL TOXICITY

Herb	Common use	Claimed toxicity	Evidence supporting
Ephedra adverse	Weight loss Antitussive Bacteriostatic	Cardiac dysrhythmias Enhanced sympathomimetic effects Stroke Hypertension	Oral ephedra known to cause CNS and cardiac events
Echinacea	Common cold prevention Urinary tract infections Bronchitis	Hepatotoxicity Decrease corticosteroid effect	No evidence Lab evidence of macrophage activation
Garlic	Lipid lowering Hypertension Antiplatelet Antioxidant	Potentiates warfarin	No evidence of interaction with warfarin Decreased platelet aggregation in vitro
Ginger	Nausea Antispasmodic	Inhibits thromboxane synthetase	In vitro evidence of thromboxane synthetase inhibition Inhibits platelet function when dose exceeds 5 g
Ginkgo	Circulatory stimulant	Inhibits platelet-activating factor	Reports of increased bleeding

(continued)

CONTINUED

Herb	Common use	Claimed toxicity	Evidence supporting
Goldenseal	Diuretic Anti-inflammatory Laxative Hemostatic	Oxytocic Paralysis in overdose Edema Hypertension	No evidence
Kava	Anxiolytic	Hepatotoxicity Potentiates barbiturates and benzodiazepines	Reports of hepatotoxicity Clinical studies demonstrating sedation and anxiolysis
Licorice	Gastric/duodenal ulcer Gastritis Bronchitis	Hypokalemia Hypertension Edema	Hypokalemia with abuse
St John's Wort	Depression	Decreased digoxin level Enzyme induction Prolonged anesthesia	Supportive clinical data Supportive clinical data Reports of prolonged emergence
Valerian	Sedative Anxiolytic	Potentiates barbiturates	Small clinical trial shows decreased sleep latency
Vitamin E	Anti-aging Prevent stroke Prevent pulmonary vitro emboli Prevent atherosclerosis Promote wound healing	Hypertension Bleeding	No evidence Decreased platelet aggregation

CHAPTER 51 ■ ANESTHESIA PROVIDED AT ALTERNATIVE SITES

I. **INTRODUCTION.** Alternate sites may be defined as locations that are remote from the main operating room complex (radiology department or endoscopy) (Souter KJ: Anesthesia provided at alternative sites. In Barash PG, Cullen BF, Stoelting RK [eds]: *Clinical Anesthesia*, pp 1331–1344. Philadelphia, Lippincott Williams and Wilkins, 2006).

II. **GENERAL PRINCIPLES.** Standards introduced by The Joint Commission on Accreditation of Healthcare Organizations (JCAHO) require that the anesthesia service of a hospital participate with nonanesthesiology departments in setting up a uniform quality of care for patients undergoing sedation in all parts of the hospital. Anesthesiologists undertake most of their training in the operating room, surrounded by familiar equipment and staff experienced in the care of the anesthetized patient. Away from the operating room these facilities may not be taken for granted and a simple three-step paradigm can be used to approach an anesthetic assignment in an alternate site (Table 51-1).

A. **The Environment.** The American Society of Anesthesiologists (ASA) has developed guidelines to apply to anesthesia in remote locations (Table 51-2).
   1. **Anesthesia Equipment and Monitors.** Anesthesia machines and monitors that remain in an outside location need to be routinely serviced along with anesthesia equipment used in the main operating rooms. This equipment is not often used on a daily basis (attention should be paid to the freshness of the soda lime).
   2. **Technical Equipment.** The complex technical equipment used in alternate sites, particularly in the radiology suites is often bulky and fixed to the floor. Magnetic resonance imaging creates its own environmental concerns related to magnetic fields.

TABLE 51-1

A THREE-STEP APPROACH TO ANESTHESIA AT ALTERNATE SITES

1. **Environment**
   Anesthetic equipment
   Anesthesia monitors
   Suction
   Resuscitation equipment
   Personnel
   Technical equipment
   Radiation hazard
   Magnetic fields
   Ambient temperature
2. **Procedure**
   Diagnostic or therapeutic
   Duration
   Level of discomfort/pain
   Position of patient
   Special requirements (functional monitoring)
   Potential complications
   Surgical support
3. **Patient**
   Ability to tolerate sedation versus general anesthesia
   ASA grade and co-morbidity
   Airway assessment
   Allergies—iv contrast
   Monitoring requirements—simple versus advanced
   Warming blankets

   B. **Procedures** (Table 51-3). It is vital that the anesthesiologist understands the nature of the procedure, the position the patient will be in, how painful it is, and how long it will last (allows the development of an anesthesia plan to provide safe patient care and facilitate the procedure).
   C. **Patients** (Table 51-4). Children represent a special group of patients who are more likely to require sedation or anesthesia for various diagnostic and therapeutic procedures.

III. **ANESTHESIA CARE.** JCAHO defined anesthesia care as the administration of intravenous (iv), intramuscular (im), or inhalational agents that may result in the loss of the patient's protective reflexes. Patients who receive anesthesia or sedation at alternate sites should expect the

TABLE 51-2

ASA GUIDELINES FOR NONOPERATING ROOM ANESTHETIZING LOCATIONS

1. **Oxygen**
   Reliable source
   Backup E cylinder—full
2. **Suction**
   Adequate and reliable
3. **Scavenging system if inhalational agents are administered**
4. **Anesthetic equipment**
   Back up self-inflating bag to deliver positive-pressure ventilation
   Adequate anesthetic drugs and supplies
   Anesthesia machine with equivalent function to those in the operating rooms and maintained to the same standards
   Adequate monitoring equipment to allow adherence to the ASA Standards for Basic Monitoring
5. **Electrical outlets**
   Sufficient for anesthesia machine and monitors
   Isolated electrical power or ground fault circuit interrupters if "wet location"
6. **Adequate illumination**
   Battery-operated backups
7. **Sufficient space for**
   Personnel and equipment
   Easy and expeditious access to patient, anesthesia machine, and monitoring
8. **Resuscitation equipment immediately available**
   Defibrillator
   Emergency drugs
   Cardiopulmonary resuscitation equipment
9. **Adequate trained staff to support anesthesia team**
10. **All building and safety codes and facility standards should be observed**
11. **Postanesthesia care facilities**
    Adequately trained staff to provide postanesthesia care
    Appropriate equipment to allow safe transport to main PACU

same standard of care as they would receive in the operating room. The ASA has published guidelines and standards and definitions of general anesthesia and levels of sedation (Table 51-5). At the conclusion of the procedure patients should recover from anesthesia or sedation in a postanesthesia care unit (PACU) or similar setting supervised by personnel who are trained to take care of

TABLE 51-3

COMMON PROCEDURES REQUIRING ANESTHESIA AT ALTERNATE SITES RADIOLOGY

Computed tomography (CT)
Magnetic resonance imaging (MRI)
Interventional radiology (vascular and nonvascular)
Interventional neuroradiology (INR)
Functional brain imaging

Radiotherapy
Radiation therapy
Intraoperative radiotherapy
Radiosurgery

Gastroenterology
Upper GI endoscopy
Endoscopic retrograde cholangiopancreatography (ERCP)
Colonoscopy
Liver biopsy
Transjugular intraheptaic portosystemic shunt (TIPS)

Cardiology
Cardiac catheterization
Radiofrequency ablation
Cardioversion

Psychiatry
Electroconvulsive therapy (ECT)

TABLE 51-4

PATIENT FACTORS REQUIRING SEDATION OR GENERAL ANESTHESIA AT ALTERNATE SITES

Anxiety and panic disorders
Claustrophobia
Developmental delay and learning difficulties
Cerebral palsy
Seizure disorders
Movement disorders
Severe pain
Acute trauma with unstable cardiovascular, respiratory, or
    neurological function
Significant co-morbidity
Children

TABLE 51-5
DEFINITION OF GENERAL ANESTHESIA AND LEVELS OF SEDATION/ANALGESIA

	Minimal sedation "anxiolysis"	Moderate sedation/analgesia "conscious sedation"	Deep sedation/analgesia	General anesthesia
Responsiveness	Normal response to verbal stimulation	Purposeful response to verbal or tactile stimulation	Purposeful response following repeated or painful stimulation	Unarousable even with painful stimulus
Airway	Unaffected	No interventions required	Interventions may be required	Intervention often required
Spontaneous ventilation	Unaffected	Adequate	May be inadequate	Frequently inadequate
Cardiovascular function	Unaffected	Usually maintained	Usually maintained	May be impaired

unconscious patients and with appropriate monitoring and resuscitation equipment immediately to hand.

IV. RADIOLOGY AND RADIATION THERAPY.

Interventional radiologists now perform an increasing number of procedures that were once in the domain of surgeons. Two important aspects of the radiological environment are the side effects of contrast media, which are commonly used to enhance radiological images and the hazards of ionizing radiation.

A. **Intravenous contrast agents** are iodinated compounds that are eliminated via the kidneys, and contrast-induced nephropathy is a concern (accounts for 10% of hospital-acquired renal failure and is more likely to occur in patients with preexisting renal insufficiency, diabetes, and those taking nonsteroidal anti-inflammatory drugs). Adequate hydration, careful monitoring of urine output, and the use of low osmolarity contrast media helps to reduce the risk of contrast-induced nephropathy. Sodium bicarbonate is effective in preventing contrast-induced nephropathy when given by iv infusion 1 hour before contrast administration.

B. **Protection from Ionizing Radiation.** Patients, physicians, and other health care workers are frequently exposed to ionizing radiation, usually in the form of X-rays. With the routine use of a lead apron, protective goggles, and thyroid shield, exposure to radiation can be kept to a low level.

C. **Specific Radiological Procedures.** Cerebral and spinal angiography cause minimal discomfort and may be performed under local anesthesia with or without light sedation administered by nonanesthesiologists. Patients are required to remain completely motionless during these procedures.

D. **Interventional Neuroradiology.** Endovascular treatment of intracranial aneurysms with detachable platinum coils has become an acceptable alternative to surgery for reducing the risk of spontaneous recurrent hemorrhage following subarachnoid hemorrhage. Endovascular treatment avoids the need for craniotomy and reduces cognitive impairment and frontotemporal brain damage associated with craniotomy.

TABLE 51-6

COMPLICATIONS OF INTERVENTIONAL
NEURORADIOLOGICAL PROCEDURES

Air embolism via femoral artery sheath
Hematoma or hemorrhage from femoral artery puncture
Pulmonary embolism
Bradycardia during carotid artery stent placement
Intracranial hemorrhage
Thromboemboic stroke

    Arteriovenous malformations (AVMs) are increasingly
being treated endovascularly.

E. **Anticoagulation** is required during and up to 24 hours
after interventional radiological procedures to prevent
thromboemboli.

F. **Complications** (Table 51-6)

G. **Anesthetic Technique.** General anesthesia is usually
conducted with endotracheal intubation and
intermittent positive-pressure ventilation although the
laryngeal mask airway is a suitable alternative to an
endotracheal tube. Propofol and thiopental are the
most commonly used induction agents. Invasive
monitoring is used less often in patients undergoing
interventional neuroradiology compared to those
having neurosurgical procedures. Controlled
hypotension is often requested to facilitate
embolization of AVMs. Certain procedures require
patients to be awake at least for part of the procedure.
A sleep-awake-sleep anesthetic technique using a
propofol infusion allows the patient to be rapidly
awakened for appropriate neurological testing and once
this is complete the patient is resedated or anesthetized
while the definitive procedure is carried out.

H. **Computed Tomography (CT) and Magnetic Resonance
Imaging (MRI)** are used for a wide array of diagnostic
imaging and an increasingly large number of
therapeutic procedures such as aspiration of masses and
needle placement for nerve blockade. The procedures
are similar in that they are relatively painless and most
adults can tolerate them without the need for sedation
or anesthesia. There is, however, an absolute
requirement for the patient to remain motionless.

Children and adults with a variety of psychological or neurological disorders may require sedation or anesthesia to allow them to tolerate the procedures (see Table 51-4). Patients with acute thoracic, abdominal, and head trauma often require urgent imaging to facilitate diagnosis. It is not unknown for these patients to develop hemorrhagic shock, raised ICP, depression of conscious level and cardiac arrest in the CT scanner. Patients must be adequately resuscitated and stabilized before transportation to the radiology department.

1. **Computerized Tomography.** Modern CT scanners obtain a cross-sectional image in just a few seconds, and spiral scanners can image a slice of the body in less than 1 second, minimizing the problems with motion artifacts.

2. **Magnetic Resonance Imaging.** Deaths and adverse outcomes in MRI scanners are entirely because of the presence of ferrometallic foreign bodies such as cerebral aneurysm clips or implanted devices such as pacemakers. Before entering the vicinity of the magnet, patients and staff need to complete a rigorous checklist to make sure they have no ferrometallic objects in their bodies. Ferromagnetic anesthetic gas cylinders, if brought within the 50 Gauss line, become potentially lethal projectiles. Standard pulse oximeters will work in the MRI scanner but have been reported to produce burns and nonferrous or fiberoptically cabled pulse oximeters should be used. The EKG is sensitive to the changing magnetic signals and it is nearly impossible to eliminate all artifacts. Noninvasive blood pressure monitors and transducers for invasive pressure monitoring are available. In the absence of MRI compatible monitors, long sampling tubes can be connected to standard capnographs and anesthetic agent monitors. Resuscitation attempts should take place outside the scanner since laryngoscopes, oxygen cylinders, and cardiac defibrillators cannot be taken close to the magnet.

3. **Anesthetic Techniques.** Fourteen percent of adult patients require some form of sedation in order to tolerate MRI scanning. In most cases this may be provided as either oral sedation with benzodiazepines or intravenous sedation administered under the supervision of the

TABLE 51-7
GOALS OF ANESTHETIC MANAGEMENT OF PEDIATRIC PATIENTS UNDERGOING RADIATION THERAPY

Rapid onset
Brief duration of action
Not painful to administer
Prompt recovery
Minimal interference with eating or drinking and playing
Avoidance of tolerance to the anesthetic agents
Maintenance of a patent airway in a variety of body positions

radiologist. Anesthesiologists are usually only involved in more complex patients; such as those with obesity, obstructive sleep apnea, raised intracranial pressure, movement disorders, developmental delay and the potential for a difficult airway. Most children under the age of 5 and many up to the age of 11 require sedation or general anesthesia to tolerate MRI and CT scanning.

I. **Radiation Therapy.** Two different types of radiation therapy commonly require anesthesia care—external beam radiation treatments, usually for children with malignancies, and intraoperative radiation to tumor masses that cannot be completely resected (Table 51-7). Patients with central nervous system (CNS) tumors should be assessed for signs of raised intracranial pressure. Many children receive cytotoxic or immunosuppressive chemotherapy as well as radiotherapy. This may result in increased risk of sepsis, thrombocytopenia, and anemia. General anesthesia or deep sedation techniques with propofol are preferable to prevent patient movement (see Table 51-7). Portable monitors and methods for delivery of oxygen and agents to maintain general anesthesia during transport are all required. After treatment, patients must be transported back to the operating room for surgical closure.

V. CARDIAC CATHETERIZATION is performed in
children with congenital heart disease (CHD) for both hemodynamic assessment and interventional procedures. Patients often present with cyanosis, dyspnoea, congestive

heart failure, and intracardiac shunts. Hypoxia, hypercarbia, and sympathetic stimulation as a result of anxiety may all exacerbate cardiopulmonary abnormalities. In patients with a patent ductus arteriosus high oxygen tension can lead to premature closure and should be avoided. Prostaglandin infusions are often used to maintain duct patency. Meticulous attention must be paid to preventing air bubbles entering intravenous lines since they may cross to the arterial circulation via a right to left shunt. General anesthesia is necessary when children cannot tolerate sedation techniques; when the child has significant cardiac or other morbidity and when the procedure involves severe hemodynamic disturbances such as ventricular septal defect occlusion. Ketamine is useful in children with myocardial depression and can be used as an infusion together with propofol.

A. **Electrophysiological Procedures.** Electrophysiological (EP) studies and ablation of abnormal conduction pathways are performed increasingly for treatment of arrhythmias caused by aberrant conduction pathways. The volatile anesthetic agents and propofol have been shown not to interfere with cardiac conduction during these procedures. EP studies are lengthy and can be painful; children usually require general anesthesia.

B. **Automatic implantable cardiac defibrillators (AICDs)** are usually implanted in the EP lab rather than in the operating room, under general anesthesia or sedation.

VI. **CARDIOVERSION.** Transthoracic cardioversion is an accepted, often used treatment for atrial fibrillation and atrial flutter. Two strategies are employed to prevent thromboembolism following cardioversion in patients who have been in atrial fibrillation (AF) for longer than 48 hours. The conventional approach is to initiate anticoagulation 3 weeks before cardioversion, usually with coumadin, and to continue for 4 weeks after cardioversion. Transesophageal echocardiography (TEE) has been recommended to determine whether patients are at low or high risk of thromboembolism, and in low-risk patients the dose of anticoagulants can be reduced.

A. **Anesthetic Technique.** Cardioversion is a brief but distressing procedure and should be carried out using sedation. The usual anesthetic technique for cardioversion is a small bolus of intravenous induction agent (propofol, etomidate, midazolam). In general patients do not require intubation for cardioversion unless there is a risk of regurgitation. During TEE, a bite block is inserted to prevent the patient from biting down on the probe, which might damage both the patient's teeth and the probe. The anesthesia team can often assist the cardiologists by deepening the level of sedation in the initial stages to allow the TEE probe to be inserted more easily.

VII. **GASTROENTEROLOGY.** In the majority of cases, gastroenterologists provide their own sedation for GI endoscopy (Table 51-8). Propofol has been used by gastroenterologists and found to provide excellent conditions for GI endoscopy and endoscopic retrograde cholangiopancreatography (ERCP).

A. **Upper GI endoscopy** is tolerated without sedation in the majority of patients and in the rest conscious sedation is usually sufficient.

B. **Endoscopic Retrograde Cholangiopancreatography** is important in the diagnosis and treatment of both biliary and pancreatic disease. Patients usually experience discomfort during ERCP, particularly with instrumentation and stenting of the biliary and pancreatic ducts. Conscious or deep sedation techniques are recommended. If sphincter opening pressure is being measured opioids, glycopyrrolate, atropine, and glucagon should be avoided because they

TABLE 51-8

COMMON GASTROENTEROLOGICAL PROCEDURES

Upper endoscopy
Sigmoidoscopy
Colonoscopy
Endoscopic retrograde cholangiopancreatography (ERCP)
Esophageal dilatation
Esophageal stenting
Percutaneous endoscopic gastrostomy (PEG) tube placement
Transjugular intrahepatic portosystemic shunt (TIPS)

TABLE 51-9

PREOPERATIVE CONSIDERATIONS IN PATIENTS
PRESENTING FOR THE TRANSJUGULAR INTRAHEPATIC
PORTOSYSTEMIC SHUNT PROCEDURE

Airway (risk of aspiration)	Recent GI bleeding
	Raised intragastric pressure
	Decreased level of consciousness because of hepatic encephalopathy
Respiratory system	Decreased functional residual capacity because of ascites
	Pleural effusion
	Intrapulmonary shunts
	Pneumonia
Cardiovascular system	Associated alcoholic cardiomyopathy
	Altered volume status
	Acute hemorrhage from esophageal varices
	Intraperitoneal hemorrhage
Hematological system	Coagulopathy
	Thrombocytopenia
Neurological system	Hepatic encephalopathy

affect sphincter pressure. Patients presenting for
emergency ERCP may have significant co-morbidity
including acute cholangitis with septicemia, jaundice
with liver dysfunction and coagulaopathy, and bleeding
from esophageal varices, resulting in hypovolemia or
biliary stricture following major hepatobiliary surgery
including liver transplantation.

C. **Transjugular intrahepatic portosystemic shunt** (TIPS)
connects the right or left portal vein through the liver
parenchyma to one of the three hepatic veins (purpose
is to decompress the portal circulation in patients with
portal hypertension). The TIPS procedure causes
minimal stimulation, lasts between 2 to 3 hours, and
may be performed under sedation or general
anesthesia. Patients presenting for a TIPS procedure,
in general, have significant hepatic dysfunction and
require careful preoperative assessment (Table 51-9).

VIII. **ELECTROCONVULSIVE THERAPY** (ECT) is used
to treat depression, mania, and affective disorders in
schizophrenic patients as well as a number of other

TABLE 51-10

PHYSIOLOGICAL RESPONSES TO ELECTROCONVULSIVE
THERAPY

Grand mal seizure (10- to 15-second tonic phase followed by a
   clonic phase lasting 30 to 60 seconds)
Cardiovascular responses
Increased cerebral blood flow
Increased intracranial pressure
Initial bradycardia
Hypertension and tachycardia
Cardiac dysrhythmias
Myocardial ischemia
Short-term memory loss
Muscular aches
Fracture dislocations
Emergence agitation
Status epilepticus
Sudden death

psychiatric disorders. Typically ECT is performed
3 times a week for 6 to 12 treatments followed by
weekly or monthly maintenance therapy to prevent
relapses.

A. **The Physiological Response to ECT** (Table 51-10)
B. **Anesthetic Considerations.** Patients with depression
   presenting for ECT are often elderly with a number of
   coexisting conditions and a thorough preoperative
   assessment and work-up should be performed before
   the patient begins treatment. Patients may be taking a
   variety of drugs, which can have important interactions
   with an anesthetic agent. The anesthetic requirements
   for ECT include amnesia, airway management,
   prevention of bodily injury from the seizure, control of
   hemodynamic changes, and a smooth, rapid emergence.
   Propofol is more effective at attenuating the acute
   hemodynamic responses to ECT and recovery is rapid.
   Propofol has anticonvulsant effects, although with a
   small dose (0.75 mg/kg iv), seizure duration is usually
   acceptable. The short-acting opioids alfentanil and
   remifentanil can be used to decrease the dose of
   induction agent and prolong seizure duration without

reducing the depth of anesthesia. Muscle relaxants are used to prevent musculoskeletal complications such as fractures or dislocations during the seizure. Succinylcholine 0.75 to 1.5 mg/kg iv is the most commonly used agent and is preferable to the longer acting nondepolarizing agents. Before inducing the seizure a bite guard is placed to protect the teeth. In younger patients 15 to 30 mg of intravenous ketorolac helps to reduce ECT-induced myalgia. The parasympathetic effects of ECT (salivation, transient bradycardia, and asystole) can be prevented by premedication with glycopyrrolate or atropine. Labetalol (0.3 mg/kg iv) and esmolol (1 mg/kg iv) both ameliorated the hemodynamic responses, although esmolol has a lesser effect on seizure duration than labetalol, controlling blood pressure without affecting seizure duration.

IX. **DENTAL SURGERY.** General anesthesia may be required during more complicated or prolonged cases and when patients are uncooperative, phobic, or mentally challenged. Down's syndrome is commonly encountered and the anesthesia team should be aware of cardiac abnormalities including conduction abnormalities and structural defects; the risk of atlantooccipital dislocation and a variety of potential airway problems including macroglossia, hypoplastic maxilla, palatal abnormalities, or mandibular protrusion. If the patient is head-up in the dental chair, vasodilation and myocardial depressant effects of anesthetics can be pronounced, especially in patients with cardiovascular diseases.

A. **Anesthetic Management.** Ketamine is a useful induction agent. Orally (1 to 2 mg/kg iv, 5 to 10 mg/kg iv, 2 to 4 mg/kg im with an onset time of 5 to 10 minutes). Oral midazolam is popular. EMLA cream facilitates the placement of intravenous lines. Tracheal intubation, often via the nasal route, is required to protect the airway, although recently the laryngeal mask airway has been used successfully. The immediate postoperative complications include bleeding, airway obstruction, and laryngeal spasm.

X. TRANSPORT OF PATIENTS. Patients who receive anesthesia or sedation at alternate sites need to be transported to the PACU at the end of the procedure; this may be some distance away. During transport patients should be accompanied by a member of the anesthesia team who should continue to evaluate, monitor, and support the patient's medical condition.

CHAPTER 52 ■ OFFICE-BASED ANESTHESIA

Office-based anesthesia (OBA) describes anesthesia that is performed in a location, usually an office or procedure room, that is not accredited by a state agency as an ambulatory surgery center (ASC) and may, in some states, have no accreditation at all (Hausman LM, Rosenblatt MA: Office-based anesthesia. In Barash PG, Cullen BF, Stoelting RK [eds]: *Clinical Anesthesia*, pp 1345–1357. Philadelphia, Lippincott Williams & Wilkins, 2006). It is estimated that by 2005 approximately 82% of all procedures will be outpatient and of these, 24% will be office-based.

I. **ADVANTAGES/DISADVANTAGES** (Table 52-1)

II. **OFFICE SAFETY.** Injuries and deaths occurring in offices are often multifactorial in their causation (they include overdosages of local anesthetics, prolonged surgery with occult blood loss, accumulation of multiple anesthetics, hypovolemia, hypoxemia, and the use of reversal drugs with short half-lives). Both the Anesthesia Patient Safety Foundation (APSF) and the American Society of Anesthesiologists (ASA) have emerged as leaders in the field of OBA safety and have advocated that the quality of care in an office-based practice be no less than that of a hospital or ASC. Reports of morbidity and mortality within office-based practices vary dramatically. The challenge of acquiring accurate morbidity and mortality data for OBA is complicated by the fact that many offices are not required to report adverse events. There are reported cases of injuries to patients in offices resulting from obsolete and malfunctioning anesthesia machines, as well as resulting from alarms that have not been serviced and/or are not functioning properly. The ASA has created guidelines for defining obsolete anesthesia machines (Table 52-2).

III. **PATIENT SELECTION.** Prior to presenting for an office-based procedure, the patient must be medically optimized. The patient should have a preoperative history

844 Management of Anesthesia

TABLE 52-1

ADVANTAGES AND DISADVANTAGES OF OFFICE-BASED ANESTHESIA

Advantages
Cost containment (facility fee)
Ease of scheduling
Patient and surgeon convenience
Decreased patient exposure to nosocomial infections
Improved patient privacy
Continuity of care

Disadvantages
Issues of patient safety and peer review
 May be absence of regulations regarding certification of surgeon
 or anesthesiologist
 May be absence of documentation, policies, and procedures and
 reporting of adverse outcomes

and physical examination recorded within 30 days, all pertinent laboratory tests obtained, and any medically indicated specialist consultation(s) completed. The ideal patient for an office-based procedure has an ASA physical status of 1 or 2. The ASA also has developed recommendations regarding patient selection. When determining whether a patient is suitable for OBA it is important to realize that the location is often times remote, and the anesthesiologist may be unable to get assistance should it be required. Anticipated anesthetic problems must be avoided (Table 52-3).

A. Obesity and Obstructive Sleep Apnea. It is estimated that 60 to 90% of all obstructive sleep apnea (OSA) patients are obese. The majority of the patients with

TABLE 52-2

CAUSES OF INJURY IN THE OFFICE

Inadequate resuscitation equipment
Inadequate monitoring (most commonly no pulse oximetry)
Inadequate preoperative or postoperative evaluation
Human error
 Slow recognition of an event
 Slow response to an event
 Lack of experience
 Drug overdosage

TABLE 52-3

CHARACTERISTICS OF PATIENTS WHO MAY NOT BE GOOD CANDIDATES FOR AN OFFICE-BASED PROCEDURE

Poorly controlled diabetes mellitus
Expected significant blood loss or postoperative pain
History of substance abuse
Seizure disorder
Malignant hyperthermia susceptibility
Potential difficult airway
  Morbid obesity
  Obstructive sleep apnea syndrome
NPO less than 8 hours
No escort
Previous adverse outcome from anesthesia
Significant drug allergies
Pulmonary aspiration risk

OSA have not been formally diagnosed. There may be failure to intubate the trachea, or to ventilate the lungs; they may have respiratory distress soon after tracheal extubation or suffer from respiratory arrest with preoperative sedation or postoperative analgesia. These patients tend to be exquisitely sensitive to the respiratory depressant effects of even small dosages of sedation or analgesics.

IV. **SURGEON SELECTION.** The relationship between the surgeon and anesthesiologist must be one of mutual trust and understanding. There have been cases reported of surgeons performing procedures for which they have little or no training. There should be a system in place for monitoring continuing medical education as well as peer review and performance improvement, for both the surgeon and anesthesiologist (Table 52-4).

V. **OFFICE SELECTION.** The office needs to be appropriately equipped and stocked to perform a general anesthetic (Table 52-5). All equipment described in the ASA algorithm for management of the difficult airway should be present. Perioperative monitoring must adhere to the ASA Standards for Basic Anesthetic Monitoring. The office-based anesthesiologist should be prepared to begin

TABLE 52-4

SENTINEL EVENTS THAT SHOULD TRIGGER A CHART REVIEW AND BE PRESENTED AT A PERFORMANCE IMPROVEMENT QUALITY ASSURANCE MEETING

Dental injury
Corneal abrasion
Perioperative myocardial infarction or stroke
Pulmonary aspiration
Reintubation of the trachea
Return to the operating room
Peripheral nerve injury
Adverse drug reaction
Uncontrolled pain or nausea/vomiting
Unexpected hospital admission
Cardiac arrest
Death
Incomplete charts
Controlled substance discrepancy
Patient complaints

TABLE 52-5

EQUIPMENT NEEDED FOR SAFE DELIVERY OF OFFICE-BASED ANESTHESIA

Monitors
    Noninvasive blood pressure with an assortment of cuff sizes
    Heart Rate/ECG
    Pulse oximeter
    Temperature
Airway Supplies
    Nasal cannulas
    Oral airways
    Face masks
    Self-inflating bag-mask ventilation device
    Laryngoscopes multiple sizes and styles
    Various sizes of tracheal tubes
    Intubating stylettes
    Emergency Airway Equipment (laryngeal mask airways [LMAs], cricothyroidotomy kit, means for transtracheal jet ventilation)
    Suction catheters and suction equipment
Cardiac defibrillator
Emergency drugs
    ACLS drugs
    Dantrolene and malignant hyperthermia supplies
Anesthetic drugs
Vascular cannulation equipment

TABLE 52-6

EMERGENCIES THAT MAY OCCUR WITHIN AN OFFICE WHICH REQUIRE CONTINGENCY PLANS

Fire
Bomb/bomb threat
Power loss
Equipment malfunction
Loss of oxygen supply pressure
Cardiac or respiratory arrest in the waiting room or operating room
Earthquake
Hurricane
External disturbance such as a riot
Malignant hyperthermia
Massive blood loss
Emergency transfer of patient to a hospital

the initial treatment of malignant hyperthermia, which requires having at least 12 bottles of dantrolene. Drug accounting must be performed in accordance with state and federal regulations. A medical director, responsible for overall operations, should be identified for every office.

A. **Emergencies** can occur in an office-based setting (Table 52-6). Destinations for a patient in need of hospital admission must be identified with a formal written arrangement with a nearby hospital. There must be contingency plans in the event of a power supply interruption or electrical failure.

B. **Accreditation** (Tables 52-7 and 52-8). The actual improvement in safety conferred by performing surgery in an accredited office has yet to be determined and as long as there is no mandatory reporting system in place, it will be impossible to determine true morbidity rates associated with an office-based practice.

VI. **PROCEDURE SELECTION.** Suitable office-based procedures range from incision and drainage of abscesses to microlaparoscopies. There are very few data regarding procedure length and suitability for an office; however, it has been recommended that procedures not exceed 6 hours in duration and be completed by 3 PM to allow for recovery time. In addition, when determining the

TABLE 52-7

ASA CLASSIFICATION OF SURGICAL OFFICES ACCORDING TO THE ANESTHESIA AND SURGICAL PROCEDURES PERFORMED

Class A
   Minor surgical procedures
   Local, topical infiltration of local anesthetic
   No sedation preoperatively or intraoperatively
Class B
   Minor or major surgical procedures
   Sedation via oral, rectal, or intravenous sedation
   Analgesic or dissociative drugs
Class C
   Minor or major surgical procedures
   General anesthesia
   Major conduction block anesthesia

TABLE 52-8

FACTORS CONSIDERED BY ACCREDITING AGENCIES

Physical layout of the office
Environmental safety/infection control
Patient and personnel records
Surgeon qualification
   Training
   Local hospital privileges (surgical and admission)
Office administration
Anesthesiologist requirements
Staffing intraoperatively and postoperatively
Monitoring capabilities both intraoperatively and postoperatively
Ancillary care
Equipment
Drugs (emergency, controlled substances, routine medications)
BLS, ACLS/PALS certification
Temperature
Neuromuscular functioning
Patient positioning
Pre- and postanesthesia care/documentation
Quality assurance/Peer review
Liability insurance
Discharge evaluation
Emergency procedure (fire/admission/transfer)

suitability of a procedure one must consider the possibility of hypothermia, blood loss, or significant fluid shifts.

A. **Specific Procedures**
   1. **Liposuction** is the most commonly performed plastic surgery procedure and is accomplished by placing hollow rods into small incisions in the skin and suctioning subcutaneous fat into an aspiration canister. Superwet and tumescent techniques utilize large volumes (1 to 4 L) of infiltrate solution that consists of 0.9% saline or lactated Ringers with epinephrine 1:1,000,000 and lidocaine 0.025 to 0.1%. Blood loss is generally 1% of the aspirate with these techniques. The peak serum levels of lidocaine occur 12 to 14 hours after injection. Liposuction is not a benign procedure, with morbidity and mortality as a result of pulmonary embolism, anesthesia, myocardial infarction, infection, and hemorrhage. Risk factors include the use of multiliter wetting solution infiltration, large volume aspiration causing massive third spacing, multiple concurrent procedures, anesthetic sedative effects resulting in hypoventilation, and permissive discharge policies.
   2. **Aesthetics.** Many facial aesthetic procedures such as blepharoplasty, rhinoplasty, and meloplasty are routinely performed in the office, usually under varying depths of sedation (MAC), but occasionally under general anesthesia. Facial plastic procedures that require use of a laser pose a problem for the use of supplemental nasal oxygen to maintain adequate SpO_2 (any supplemental oxygen must be turned off during periods of laser or electrocautery use about the face)
   3. **Breast.** Procedures such as breast biopsy or augmentation, implant exchanges and completion of transverse rectus abdominal muscle (TRAM) flaps are performed in office settings. It is likely that patients undergoing breast surgery will require antiemetic medication and postoperative analgesics.
   4. **GI Endoscopy** includes esophageal, gastric, and duodenal endoscopies (EGD) and colonoscopies. This patient population tends to be older, with significant co-morbid conditions. Insertion of the

endoscope can usually be accomplished with sedation using midazolam and small doses of propofol. Colonoscopy is painful secondary to the insertion and manipulation of the endoscope and may be associated with cardiovascular effects, including dysrhythmias, bradycardia, hypotension, hypertension, myocardial infarction, and death.

5. **Dentistry/Oral and Maxillofacial Surgery.** Nitrous oxide has been used for most of the world's office-based dental anesthetics since 1884, when Horace Wells, himself a dentist, had nitrous oxide administered for a wisdom tooth extraction by a colleague. A high level of safety is attributed to the use of pulse oximetry, blood pressure, and ventilation monitoring, as well as administration of supplemental oxygen.

6. **Orthopedics/Podiatry.** The orthopedic office provides an excellent location for the anesthesiologist who practices regional anesthesia (intra-articular local anesthesia and MAC, three-in-one block of the lumbar plexus, brachial plexus block, ankle block). Spinal anesthetics in the office-based setting must be of short duration. Lidocaine, which provides reliable short-acting analgesia, may be associated with an increased risk of transient neurologic symptoms in the ambulatory patient population.

7. **Gynecology/Genitourinary.** Many procedures, such as dilation and curettage, vasectomy, and cystoscopy have been performed in offices for many years and recently there has been an increase in more invasive procedures such as minilaparoscopies, ovum retrieval, prostate biopsies, and lithotripsy, necessitating an anesthesiologist's expertise.

8. **Ophthalmology/Otolaryngology.** Topical anesthesia or periorbital and retrobulbar blocks are frequently used to provide analgesia. Supplemental sedation may be required.

9. **Pediatrics.** Although no minimum age requirement for a child to undergo OBA has been established, patients greater than 6 months of age and ASA physical status 1 or 2 may be reasonable candidates (dental surgery, lacrimal duct probing, myringotomy) (Table 52-9).

TABLE 52-9

GUIDELINES FOR THE PEDIATRIC PERIOPERATIVE ANESTHESIA ENVIRONMENT

Patient Care Facility and Medical Staff Policies
  Designation of operative procedures
  Categorization of pediatric patients undergoing anesthesia
  Annual minimal case volume to maintain clinical competence
Clinical Privileges of Anesthesiologists
  Regular privileges
  Special clinical privileges
  Pain management
Patient Care Units
  Preoperative evaluation and preparation units
  Operating room
  Anesthesiologists
  Other health care providers involved in perioperative care
  Clinical laboratory and radiologic services availability and capabilities
  Pediatric anesthesia equipment and drugs including resuscitation cart
  $PaCO_2$
  Nursing staff
  Anesthesiologist/physician staff
  Pediatric anesthesia equipment and drugs
Postoperative Intensive Care

VII. ANESTHETIC TECHNIQUES. The ASA recommends that anesthetics be provided or supervised by an anesthesiologist. The ASA has developed definitions regarding depths of anesthesia (Table 52-10). When formulating an anesthetic plan, one must consider that all agents and techniques used should be short-acting, and the patient should be ready for discharge home soon after the completion of the procedure.

  A. Anesthetic Agents. Intravenous sedation (propofol, barbiturates, midazolam, fentanyl, meperidine) is the most often used anesthetic technique in the OBA setting. Drugs should have a short half-life, be inexpensive, and not be associated with undesirable side effects such as nausea and vomiting.

    1. **Remifentanil,** an ultrashort-acting opioid, is an ideal drug for use during many office-based procedures such as facial cosmetic procedures. Remifentanil may cause nausea and vomiting.

TABLE 52-10

DEFINITIONS OF LEVELS OF SEDATION/ANALGESIA BY THE ASA (OCTOBER 13, 1999, BY HOUSE OF DELEGATES)

Minimal Sedation (Anxiolysis)
Drug-induced sedation
Patient responds normally to verbal commands
Cognitive and motor function may be impaired
Ventilatory and cardiovascular function maintained normally

Moderate Sedation/Analgesia (Conscious Sedation)
Drug-induced sedation
Patient responds purposefully to verbal commands either alone or with light tactile stimulation
Patient maintains a patent airway and spontaneous ventilation
Cardiovascular function maintained

Deep Sedation/Analgesia
Drug-induced sedation
Patient cannot be easily aroused but can respond purposefully to repeated or painful stimulation
Ventilatory function may be impaired, requiring assistance in maintaining a patent airway, and spontaneous ventilation may be inadequate
Cardiovascular function is usually maintained

General Anesthesia
Drug-induced loss of consciousness
Patients are not arousable by painful stimulation
Ventilatory function is often impaired; patient may require assistance in maintaining a patent airway
Spontaneous ventilation may be impaired as well as neuromuscular functioning
Positive-pressure ventilation is often required
Cardiovascular function may be impaired

2. **Ketamine** functions as both an anesthetic and an analgesic. It is particularly useful in that it does not depress respirations and is not associated with nausea and vomiting. Ketamine can cause an increase in secretions as well as cause hallucinations. Another advantage of ketamine is that it is relatively inexpensive.
3. **Clonidine** facilitates blood pressure control throughout the perioperative period and it may decrease the total propofol usage.
B. **General anesthesia** can be administered in an office setting safely. The pharmacokinetics and

pharmacodynamics of desflurane and sevoflurane render them good potent inhaled agents for an office-based procedure. Depth of anesthesia monitoring via a processed electroencephalogram has been shown to decrease the time to tracheal extubation and discharge readiness.

VIII. PACU (postanesthesia care unit). Following an office-based procedure, it is expected that the patient will be able to sit in a chair, or ambulate to an examination room to dress, almost immediately. A formal PACU may not be present, and the patient may recover in the surgical suite. Regardless of where the patient recovers, it is important to adhere to all the ASA standards for monitoring and documentation throughout the postoperative period. Problems of postoperative nausea and vomiting (PONV) and pain may become particularly troublesome. It is imperative that every anesthetic administered be designed to maximize patient alertness and mobility and minimize the risks of the need for a prolonged PACU stay.

A. Pain Management. Local anesthesia, conscious sedation supplemented by wound infiltration with local anesthetics, or nerve blocks, often form the basis for a multimodal strategy for postoperative pain management. Opioid analgesics are commonly associated with nausea, vomiting, sedation, dysphoria, pruritus, constipation, urinary retention, and respiratory depression. Nonopioid analgesics (acetaminophen) and nonsteroidal anti-inflammatory drugs (ketorolac) are routinely used. In an effort to minimize the potential for postoperative bleeding and risk of gastrointestinal complications, more specific COX-2 inhibitors are being increasingly used as nonopioid adjuvants for minimizing postoperative pain.

B. Postoperative Nausea and Vomiting. An optimal antiemetic regimen for OBA has yet to be established, but since the causes of PONV are multifactorial, combination therapies may be more beneficial in high-risk patients. Many of the traditional first-line therapies are associated with sedation. Serotonin receptor antagonists and dexamethasone may be valuable.

IX. REGULATIONS. Governmental oversight of office-based surgery varies among states; currently regulations exist in many states, and others are following.

X. BUSINESS AND LEGAL ASPECTS. It is in the anesthesia provider's best interest to seek legal counsel before embarking on a career in OBA. Billing strategies must be legal. In this complex environment of third-party payers it is quite easy to make errors.

CHAPTER 53 ■ ANESTHESIA FOR ORGAN TRANSPLANTATION

Living related organ donation is increasingly common, and 2001 was the first year in which the number of living related kidney donors exceeded the number of cadaveric donors in the United States (Csete M, Glas K: Anesthesia for organ transplantation. In Barash PG, Cullen BF, Stoelting RK [eds]: *Clinical Anesthesia*, pp 1358–1376. Philadelphia, Lippincott Williams & Wilkins, 2006). The use of organs once considered marginal is on the rise, increasing the difficulty of anesthetic management of organ recipients. The United Network of Organ Sharing (www.unos.org) is an important source of information related to organ transplantation for patients and physicians. The United States is divided into 11 regions for purposes of organ distribution, each with its own regional review board. Some 259 transplant centers in the United States perform about 13,000 transplants a year.

Anesthesiologists are involved in the care of organ donors and perioperative management of transplant recipients, and in major transplant centers anesthesiologists with special expertise actively participate in the preoperative assessment and optimization of patients for major organ transplant procedures.

I. ANESTHETIC MANAGEMENT OF ORGAN DONORS

A. **Brain-Dead Donors.** Brain death is declared when the clinical picture is consistent with irreversible cessation of all brain function.
   1. Physicians involved in the transplant recipient process should not be involved in declaration of brain death of the donor (Table 53-1).
   2. Brain death is associated with hemodynamic instability (vasodilation), hormonal chaos (adrenergic surges can cause ischemia, diabetes insipidus), diffuse inflammatory changes, and loss of temperature control.
   3. **Anesthetic management** during organ harvest is guided by the needs of the teams harvesting organs and personnel from organ procurement networks,

TABLE 53-1

DETERMINATION OF BRAIN DEATH

Eliminate potentially reversible causes of coma or
  unresponsiveness (hypothermia, hypotension, drugs, toxins)
Transcranial Doppler confirming no cerebral blood flow
Flat electroencephalogram
Brainstem reflexes absent (absent ventilatory drive with apnea
  testing)

who may come from several centers, and have
discrepant requests depending on the organs
procured.

4. Donated organs are protected by hormone therapy
   (triiodothyronine, methylprednisolone, DDAVP,
   insulin).

5. The mainstay of donor management is maintenance
   of euvolemia. Packed cells are used to maintain
   hematocrit of 30%, fresh frozen plasma to maintain
   the International Normalized Ratio (INR) <1.5.

   a. Arterial catheters and central venous catheters
      are used to guide fluid and vasopressor therapies.

   b. CVP is maintained 6 to 12 mm Hg, and when
      pulmonary artery catheters are used to assess
      cardiac function, PCWP is maintained at
      <12 mm Hg.

6. Transport of ventilated patients often requires PEEP
   valves attached to the Ambu bag to maintain
   oxygenation of the donor. Peak airway pressures
   should be kept below 30 mm Hg.

7. Donor lungs are more susceptible to injury in
   brain-dead patients before procurement than are
   other organs, likely from contusion, aspiration, or
   edema with fluid resuscitation (Table 53-2).

B. Nonheart-Beating Donors

1. These donors usually have severe brain damage but
   are not brain dead, and death is defined by cessation
   of cardiac and respiratory function. Life-support
   measures are used to control the timing of death and
   organ procurement.

2. The donor may be declared dead just outside the
   operating room (OR) then quickly taken into the
   OR for organ procurement without an
   anesthesiologist in attendance. Other hospitals have

TABLE 53-2
IDEAL CADAVERIC LUNG DONOR

Age <55 years
ABO compatibility
Clear chest radiograph
PaO_2 >300 mm Hg on $FIO_2 = 1.0$, PEEP 5 cm H_2O
Tobacco history <20 pack years
Absence of chest trauma
No evidence of aspiration/sepsis
Negative sputum gram stain
Absence of purulent secretions at bronchoscopy

developed protocols that involve preparation of the patient in the OR with an anesthesiologist present, and the anesthesiologist may be responsible for removing the patient from ventilatory support and for declaration of death.

C. **Living Kidney Donors**
   1. Living donors are, by definition, quite healthy and these volunteers deserve exquisite attention to safety and pain management.
   2. General anesthesia is used in many centers, but epidural and combined epidural-spinal techniques (supplemented with intravenous propofol) have also been used successfully.
   3. Laparoscopic (versus open) donor nephrectomy is increasingly the norm and is generally better tolerated by donors in terms of comfort and shorter hospital stay.
      a. Anesthetics and insufflation of the peritoneum with CO_2 decrease renal blood flow, so that fluid repletion is important for maintaining renal perfusion.
      b. Administer crystalloid at 10 mL/kg/hr above calculated losses and to maintain urine output at about 100 mL/hr versus guide fluid replacement with central venous pressure monitoring.
   4. Complications after living donor nephrectomy include atelectasis of the lungs, pneumothorax, cardiac arrhythmias, wound pain or infection, urinary tract infection, and mental status changes.
D. **Living Liver Donors.** Left lobe liver donation is usually done in the context of parent to child donation. Right

lobectomy is a larger procedure and carries a significant mortality risk.

1. Large liver resections may require virtually complete hepatic venous exclusion (cross-clamping of the inferior vena cava above and below the liver and cross-clamping of the hepatic pedicle).

2. Venous return falls by about 50% and without the collaterals developed by patients with liver disease, normal donors may experience significant hypotension when the cava is cross-clamped.

3. Hypothermia is a common reason for not extubating in the OR.

4. Epidural catheters, providing excellent analgesia but with right liver resection, INR rises significantly after surgery, peaking a few days after surgery along with a fall in platelet counts, just when the catheter is usually removed.

E. **Living Lung Donors.** Living donor lobar lung transplantation (LDLLT) procedures are typically reserved for critically ill recipients unlikely to survive until a cadaveric donor becomes available.

II. IMMUNOSUPPRESSIVE DRUGS

A. Suppression of immune responses is used to blunt the reaction to allografts, and drugs powerful enough to suppress the immune system are associated with significant side effects (infections, increased risk of tumors, progressive vascular disease).

1. It is important to review drug regimens with transplant coordinators when post-transplant patients are scheduled for surgery.

2. Immune-suppressed patients coming to the OR deserve special attention to sterile technique, and maintenance of antibiotic/antifungal/antiviral regimens during the perioperative period (Table 53-3).

B. **Calcineurin Inhibitors.** The modern transplant era began with the introduction of cyclosporine, a calcineurin inhibitor. *Tacrolimus* has been particularly important for kidney transplant recipients because of its potency in preventing acute rejection (within 6 months of transplantation), long-term graft survival, and relative lack of side effects compared to historical regimens.

TABLE 53-3

MULTISYSTEM COMPLICATIONS OF CHRONIC IMMUNE SUPPRESSION

System	Complication
Central nervous system	Lowered seizure threshold
Cardiovascular	Diabetes
	Hypertension
	Hyperlipidemia
Renal/electrolyte	Decreased GFR
	Hyperkalemia
	Hypomagnesemia
Hematologic/immune	Increased risk of infections
	Increased risk of tumors
	Pancytopenia
Endocrine/other	Osteoporosis
	Poor wound healing

       1. Calcineurin is associated with significant side effects (hypertension, ischemic cardiac disease, neurologic side effects).

  C. Corticosteroids are used both for maintenance immunosuppression and in pulse dosing for acute rejection.

  D. Antiproliferative drugs rely on the fact that immune activation implies explosive proliferation of lymphocytes.

       1. Azathioprine's major side effect is repression of bone marrow cell cycling, which can cause pancytopenia.

       2. Cardiac arrest and severe upper airway edema are rare complications.

  E. Monoclonal and Polyclonal Antibodies. *OKT3* antibody is directed against a component of the T cell receptor complex, and effects immunosuppression by blocking T cell function. Hypotension, bronchospasm, and pulmonary edema may occur.

III. RENAL TRANSPLANTATION

  A. Preoperative Considerations. Many of the underlying diagnoses treated with renal transplants are also risk factors for coronary artery disease. Dialysis-dependent patients should be dialyzed before surgery (minimizes likelihood of hyperkalemia during surgery). Cadaveric

grafts can be safely transplanted after 24 hours of cold ischemia time.
   B. **Intraoperative Protocols.** Renal transplantation is generally done under general anesthesia and rapid sequence induction of anesthesia is indicated in diabetic patients with gastroparesis.
      1. A central venous catheter (usually triple lumen) is placed for CVP monitoring and drug administration, and a bladder catheter is placed.
      2. Incision is usually in the lower right abdomen to facilitate placement of the graft in the iliac fossa. The recipient iliac artery and vein are used for graft vascularization, followed by connection of the ureter to the recipient bladder.
      3. The major anesthetic consideration is maintenance of renal blood flow. Hemodynamic goals during transplant are systolic pressure >90 mm Hg, mean systemic pressure >60 mm Hg, and CVP >10 mm Hg. These goals are usually achieved without use of vasopressors, using isotonic fluids and adjustment of anesthetic doses. Neuromuscular blockade is usually accomplished with cisatracurium.
      4. Once the first anastomosis is started, a diuresis is initiated (mannitol and furosemide are often both given). For patients with diabetes, intraoperative administration of insulin to normalize blood glucose is utilized to maintain glucose between 80 to 110 mg/dL.
      5. Patient-controlled analgesia is a good choice for postoperative pain management. Nonsteroidal anti-inflammatory agents are contraindicated.
   C. **Pediatric Renal Transplantation.** Adult donors to small children require the graft placement in the retroperitoneum. Although chronic peritoneal dialysis may help expand the abdominal volume, attention to peak inspiratory pressures at closure is important and increased pressures should be reported to the surgical team.

IV. LIVER TRANSPLANTATION

   A. **Preoperative Considerations.** Patients with end-stage liver disease (ESLD) have multisystem dysfunction (Table 53-4). Poor renal function is a major risk factor for poor liver transplant outcome.

TABLE 53-4

MULTISYSTEM COMPLICATIONS OF END-STAGE LIVER DISEASE

System	Complication
Central nervous system	Fatigue
	Encephalopathy (confusion to coma)
	Blood brain barrier disruption and intracranial hypertension (acute liver failure)
Pulmonary	Hypoxemia/hepatopulmonary syndrome
	Respiratory alkalosis
	Pulmonary hypertension
Cardiovascular	Reduced systemic vascular resistance
	Hyperdynamic circulation
	Diastolic dysfunction
	Prolonged QT interval
	Blunted responses to inotropes
	Blunted responses to vasopressors
Gastrointestinal	GI bleeding from varices
	Ascites
	Delayed gastric emptying
	Hematologic
	Hypersplenism (pancytopenia)
	Decreased synthesis of clotting factors
	Impaired fibrinolytic mechanisms
Renal	Hepatorenal syndrome
	Hyponatremia
Endocrine	Glucose intolerance
	Osteoporosis
	Nutritional/metabolic
	Muscle wasting and weakness
	Poor skin integrity
	Increased volume of distribution for drugs
	Decreased citrate metabolism

B. **Intraoperative Procedures.** Intensive preparation for surgery is important since it is difficult to predict which patients are at risk for massive blood loss (place invasive lines and monitors after induction of general anesthesia).
   1. Rapid sequence induction of general anesthesia is indicated since patients with ESLD often have gastroparesis in addition to increased intra-abdominal pressure from ascites.

a. A left radial catheter serves as a monitor of disruption of arterial flow if the axillary vein is used for bypass, and the right femoral arterial line leaves the left groin free for surgical bypass access.

b. Pulmonary artery catheters or continuous echocardiography are used for monitoring volume status, and at least two large-bore catheters are placed for rapid intravenous infusions.

c. A rapid infusion system with the ability to deliver at least 500 mL/min warmed blood is primed and in the OR.

d. Normothermia, essential for optimal hemostasis, is maintained with convective warming blankets.

2. **Coagulation Management.** Fresh frozen plasma (FFP) is used to maintain INR ≤ 1.5 in any patient with anticipated or ongoing bleeding. Platelet transfusion is used to maintain platelet count above 50,000/mm^3. Normal or hypernormal whole blood clotting in the presence of high INR and low platelets should be taken as a caution that the patient may have a clinically significant hypercoagulable state.

3. Perioperative renal dysfunction is a major problem in liver transplantation (hepatorenal syndrome).

4. **Anhepatic phase** begins when the liver is functionally excluded (clamped) from the circulation (vena cava is clamped above and below the liver and the portal vein and hepatic artery are clamped).

a. With complete cava cross clamp, venous return falls by 50 to 60%, often resulting in hypotension.

b. Veno-venous bypass may be used to increase venous return, improve systemic hemodynamics, increase renal perfusion pressure, and to decompress portal pressures for a better surgical field. Most patients can be managed without veno-venous bypass using some volume loading.

5. **Reperfusion** of the graft is associated with hypotension (further drop of already low SVR and increase in CO), which may or may not require treatment. Portal vein reperfusion (despite flushing of the graft) can often result in hemodynamic instability. Hepatic artery unclamping is usually not hemodynamically significant.

6. **Neohepatic Period.** Usually within 30 minutes, the base deficit improves with graft metabolism of citrate. Within the first hour, the CO decreases and SVR increases as the graft metabolizes vasoactive substances.

C. **Pediatric Liver Transplantation.** Indications for pediatric liver transplantation differ considerably from adults, with inherited disorders dominating the pre-op diagnoses. In small children, a radial artery catheter and at least one large (18 g) peripheral intravenous line are placed after induction of anesthesia.

D. **Acute Liver Failure.** Anesthetic considerations for both adults and children with acute liver failure are focused on protection of the brain (intracranial pressure monitoring in presence of vasodilating volatile anesthetics).

V. PANCREAS AND ISLET TRANSPLANTATION

A. The preoperative assessment of pancreas transplant recipients focuses on the end-organ complications of diabetes. Generally patients do not require PA catheters.

1. The major difference between pancreas transplantation and other procedures is that strict attention to control blood glucose is indicated, in order to protect newly transplanted beta-cells from hyperglycemic damage.

B. Islet transplants are generally infused into the portal circulation. Acute portal hypertension is a feared complication.

VI. SMALL BOWEL AND MULTIVISCERAL TRANSPLANTATION

A. Patients who develop liver failure from total parenteral nutrition (TPN) for intestinal failure are candidates for combined liver-intestine transplantation. In general intestinal transplantation should only be considered in patients with life-threatening complications of their intestinal failure.

1. For anesthesiologists, a major hurdle for these transplants is line placement adequate for transfusion of blood products and fluids, which may be substantial during these long cases.

2. Common complications of intestinal failure include dehydration and electrolyte abnormalities, gastric acid hypersecretion, pancreatic insufficiency, bone disease, and TPN-induced liver failure.
3. Intestinal reperfusion is associated with an acute release of acid and potassium from the graft (anticipatory bicarbonate and $CaCl_2$ administration is used to counteract the effects of acid and potassium on the heart).

VII. LUNG TRANSPLANTATION is accepted therapy for end-stage lung and pulmonary vascular disease.

A. **Surgical options** for lung transplantation are single-lung transplant, en-bloc double and sequential double transplants, and heart-lung transplantation.
   1. Single and sequential double lung transplants can be performed without cardiopulmonary bypass (CPB), although CPB is often used, especially for recipients with pulmonary hypertension.
   2. Bilateral lung transplantation is most commonly used in patients with associated pulmonary vascular disease and cystic fibrosis-related bronchiectasis.
B. **Recipient Selection.** Patients are considered for lung transplantation if they exhibit decline in pulmonary function despite maximal medical therapy, and expected lifespan is only 2 to 3 years. Absolute contraindications are significant dysfunction of other organs, particularly kidney and heart, HIV or chronic hepatitis B or C, and malignancy (other than basal cell or squamous cell skin carcinoma).
C. **Pre-anesthetic Considerations**
   1. It is critical to confirm ABO compatibility of donor and recipient prior to surgery.
   2. Medications should be continued in the perioperative period. After determining oxygen saturation, slow, incremental dosing of a short-acting benzodiazepine (0.25 to 1.0 mg midazolam) is used for anxiolysis.
   3. Placement of a PA catheter with continuous cardiac output (CCO) and mixed venous oxygenation monitoring provides both rapid assessment of cardiopulmonary status changes, and minimizes the fluid administration necessary for frequent cardiac output determinations.

D. **Intraoperative Management: Single-Lung Transplantation.**
1. Lung transplant recipients tend to be chronically intravascularly volume depleted, and anesthetic induction can be associated with hypotension.
2. These patients remain intubated for hours to days postoperatively.
3. Nitrous oxide is rarely an anesthetic option, because of bullous emphysematous disease, pulmonary hypertension, or intraoperative hypoxemia.
4. Lung isolation, preferably with a double-lumen endotracheal tube, is necessary for single and bilateral sequential lung transplantation.
   a. During one-lung ventilation, hypoxemia is common.
   b. Lung recipients are susceptible to development of pulmonary hypertension and right ventricular (RV) dysfunction or failure during one-lung ventilation.
5. Cardiopulmonary bypass is indicated during lung transplantation if adequate oxygenation cannot be maintained despite ventilatory and pharmacologic maneuvers and pulmonary artery clamping by the surgeons. Inability to ventilate or development of right ventricular dysfunction are also indications for CPB.
6. Circulation is restored to the donor lung, suture lines are checked for hemostasis, and then ventilation is begun. Systemic hypotension can occur during reperfusion, but it is not as significant as that seen with liver graft reperfusion. Hyperkalemia is also not a common reperfusion event.
   a. Bronchoscopy to suction secretions and blood is recommended to improve ventilation and oxygenation, and to examine bronchial suture lines.
   b. Intraoperative TEE has become a valuable tool in the assessment of lung transplant patients.
7. At the completion of the procedure, the patient should be evaluated for exchange of the double-lumen endotracheal tube to a large (8 mm ID or larger) single-lumen endotracheal tube.

E. **Double-Lung Transplantation.**
1. En-bloc double-lung transplant requires CPB, and a single-lumen endotracheal tube is sufficient.
2. Bilateral sequential transplantation requires lung isolation, preferably via a double-lumen endotracheal

tube. Bilateral sequential transplant is now the preferred procedure, because a tracheal anastomosis is unnecessary, and surgical bleeding is less.

   F. **Pediatric Lung Transplantation.** The most common diagnoses in adolescents are cystic fibrosis, congenital heart disease, and primary pulmonary hypertension. Most pediatric patients receive double lung transplantation with CPB.

   G. **Heart–lung transplant** is the least common intrathoracic transplant procedure. Primary pulmonary hypertension (PPH) and pulmonary hypertension–associated Eisenmenger syndrome are the most common indications for heart-lung transplant. Since a tracheal anastomosis is performed, a single-lumen endotracheal tube is adequate.

VIII. **HEART TRANSPLANTATION.** The most common diagnoses leading to transplantation are ischemic- and idiopathic-dilated cardiomyopathies.

   A. **Recipient Selection.** Patients referred for transplant evaluation should have New York Heart Association (NYHA) Class III or IV heart failure despite optimal medical therapy. Surgical correction of coronary artery disease or valvular heart disease should be undertaken prior to listing. Severe, irreversible pulmonary hypertension is a contraindication to transplant.

   B. **Pre-anesthetic Considerations.** Donor heart function worsens with ischemic times above 6 hours (transplantation must occur when the donor surgery can be done).

   1. Cardiovascular support (inotropic infusions, chronic medications for heart failure, presence of a left ventricular assist device) and presence of hemodynamic monitoring lines or antiarrhythmic devices, such as pacemaker or defibrillator, need to be evaluated.

   2. Patients are frequently taking ACE inhibitors that could increase the risk of intraoperative hypotension (vasopressin infusions may be useful), or coumadin that can increase risk of bleeding.

   3. Differences from nontransplant patients undergoing open heart surgery include the need for strict attention to sterility, presence of immunosuppression, poorer hemodynamic status of transplant

candidates, and issues related to early donor heart function and denervation.

C. **Intraoperative Management**

1. Anesthetic induction in patients with poor ventricular function can be complicated by hemodynamic instability (high-dose opioids often selected with neuromuscular blockade).

2. TEE should be performed intraoperatively and the recipient heart can be monitored prior to CPB for changes in ventricular function or increase in valvular regurgitation. Prior to weaning from CPB, the heart is reevaluated with TEE, looking at ventricular and valvular function.

3. Since the donor heart is denervated, normal physiologic feedback loops controlling inotropy and chronotropy are lost. Isoproterenol is used frequently for its direct effects on cardiac beta receptors, to increase graft heart rate. Use of temporary epicardial pacing is sometimes needed until isoproterenol has had adequate time to reach maximal effect.

4. Residual atrial tissue may continue to have electrical activity, seen clinically as two P waves on ECG. The native P wave has no physiologic activity on the donor heart.

5. The donor right heart is not accustomed to high pulmonary resistance, and may fail acutely (inhaled nitric oxide or prostacyclin).

D. **Pediatric Heart Transplantation**

1. ECMO is used as a bridge to transplant at some centers, although it is acknowledged to be only a short-term option.

2. Although ABO incompatible transplantation is contraindicated in the adult population, it is more successful in infant recipients (hyperacute rejection does not occur as a result of the immaturity of the immune system and absence of antibodies to various antigens).

IX. ANESTHETIC MANAGEMENT OF THE TRANSPLANT PATIENT FOR NONTRANSPLANT SURGERY.

For solid organ recipients, evaluation of patients is centered on function of the grafted organ.

A. **Renal Transplant Patients**
  1. The level of renal dysfunction will determine choice of drugs, particularly neuromuscular blockers, and dose modification of drugs dependent on renal excretion such as antibiotics.
  2. A major consideration for renal transplant recipients is maintenance of renal perfusion with adequate volume replacement.
  3. CVP or TEE is useful to guide fluid replacement, especially in cases where large fluid shifts are anticipated.
  4. For all transplant recipients, antibiotic, antiviral, antifungal, and immune suppression regimens should be disrupted as little as possible in the perioperative period.
  5. Regional and general anesthetic techniques have been used successfully in posttransplant patients.
  6. Invasive monitoring is not indicated solely on the basis of prior transplantation. Nasal intubation should be avoided, because of the potential risk for infection presented by nasal flora.

B. **Lung Transplant Recipients**
  1. If the patient had a lung transplant that included a tracheal anastomosis, denervation has occurred below the level of the suture line, and the cough reflex is diminished or absent. These patients are at increased risk of retained secretions and pneumonia, and have increased airway hyperreactivity and risk of bronchospasm.
  2. Advantages of regional anesthetic techniques in lung transplant patients include minimization of airway manipulation and decreased infectious risk.
  3. ABG in the presence of rejection will show an increased A-a gradient.

C. **Heart Transplant Recipients**
  1. The transplanted heart is denervated and cannot respond to indirect acting agents, such as ephedrine and even dopamine, or to peripheral attempts to induce hemodynamic changes, such as carotid massage, Valsalva maneuver, or laryngoscopy.
     a. Beta effects of epinephrine and norepinephrine are exaggerated in heart transplant recipients.
     b. Isoproterenol is the mainstay of chronotropic therapy in these patients.

    c. ECG analysis may show two P waves, one from the native atrium (does not conduct and should not be confused with complete heart block) and one from the implanted atrium.

    d. Because the denervated heart does not reflexly compensate for hemodynamic changes induced by regional anesthetics, general anesthesia is usually preferred.

2. Preoperative evaluation should focus on cardiac functional status (ECG and TTE).

    a. Significant rejection will present with symptoms of heart failure.

    b. Invasive monitors should be placed only when warranted by the clinical status and surgical procedure. Use of either TEE or CVP monitoring can be helpful in managing fluid resuscitation and inotropic support.

CHAPTER 54 ■ POSTOPERATIVE RECOVERY

An individualized, problem-oriented approach to the assessment of surgical patients is essential to optimize outcome and to minimize risk and expense during postoperative recovery (Mecca RS: Postoperative recovery. In Barash PG, Cullen BF, Stoelting RK [eds]: *Clinical Anesthesia*, pp 1379–1404. Philadelphia, Lippincott Williams & Wilkins, 2006).

I. ASSESSING THE VALUE OF POSTANESTHESIA CARE

A. Indicators of quality in postanesthesia care include not only clinical results and patient satisfaction but also the "value" of the care (improvement in postoperative outcome per dollar spent) per postanesthesia care unit (PACU) admission.

B. As emphasis on cost containment grows, the value of PACU might be defined as the improvement in clinical outcome per dollar spent on a PACU admission (Table 54-1).

C. Selecting the Appropriate Level of Postoperative Care
1. An increasing number of patients exhibit minimal depression on admission to the PACU because of less invasive surgical techniques and improved anesthetic techniques using short-acting drugs with fewer side effects.
2. Providing varying levels of care (separating low-intensity patients from high-intensity patients) could help minimize unnecessary expenditures.

II. ADMISSION TO THE PACU

A. Anesthesiologists should provide an admission report to the PACU nurse and supervise care of patients until vital signs are obtained (Table 54-2).

B. A minimal level of monitoring must be provided in the PACU (Table 54-3).

C. The need for routine supplemental oxygen may be individualized based on pulse oximetry monitoring.

TABLE 54-1

FACTORS THAT DETERMINE COST OF CARE IN THE POSTANESTHESIA CARE UNIT

Admission and discharge policies (regulatory requirements)
Level of routine monitoring required
Nursing staff (number of patients per caregiver)
Physician coverage (dedicated versus on-demand)
Patient mix (monitors, ventilators, infusion pumps)
Standard therapy (oxygen, antiemetics, respiratory therapy)

    D. Postoperative pain management is initiated in the PACU (neuraxial opioids versus intravenous opioids and initiation of patient-controlled analgesia). It is important to distinguish between requirements for analgesia (opioids) and sedation (benzodiazepines).

III. DISCHARGE CRITERIA (Table 54-4). There is no demonstrable benefit from a mandatory minimum

---

TABLE 54-2

ADMISSION REPORT TO POSTANESTHESIA CARE UNIT NURSES

Preoperative History
Chronic medications
Preexisting diseases
Drug allergies
Premedication

Intraoperative Factors
Surgical procedure
Type of anesthetic and drug doses
Muscle relaxant and reversal status
Intravenous fluids
Estimated blood loss
Urine output
Unexpected surgical or anesthetic events
Intraoperative vital signs and laboratory findings
Nonanesthetic drugs (antibiotics, diuretics, vasopressors)

Postoperative Instructions
Pain management
Acceptable vital sign ranges, blood loss, and urine output
Anticipated cardiopulmonary problems
Diagnostic tests (arterial blood gases, hematocrit, electrolytes)
Location of responsible physician

TABLE 54-3

MONITORING IN A POSTANESTHESIA CARE UNIT

Pulse oximetry
Vital signs at least every 15 min
  Blood pressure
  Heart rate
  Breathing rate and airway patency
  Level of consciousness
Electrocardiogram
Body temperature

TABLE 54-4

ASSESSMENT BEFORE DISCHARGE FROM A POSTANESTHESIA CARE UNIT

General Condition
Oriented and follows simple instructions
Adequate skeletal muscle strength
Absence of acute anesthesia/surgical complications (airway edema,
  neurologic compromise, bleeding, nausea, and vomiting)

Cardiovascular System
Blood pressure, heart rate, and cardiac rhythm similar to the
  preoperative value and stable for at least 30 min
Acceptable intravascular fluid volume status

Ventilation and Oxygenation
Acceptable oxygen saturation
Breathing 10–30 times/min
Able to cough and clear secretions

Airway Maintenance
Intact protective reflexes (swallow, gag)
No evidence of airway obstruction (stridor, retraction)
No need for artificial airway support

Control of Pain

Renal Function (urine output >30 mL/hr)

Metabolic and Laboratory
Acceptable hematocrit, electrolytes, glucose, and arterial blood
  gases
Evaluation of electrocardiogram and radiographs

Ambulatory Patients
Ambulate without dizziness or hypotension
Control of nausea and vomiting
Control of pain

duration of PACU care (observe until meet discharge criterion and are no longer at increased risk for cardiorespiratory depression).

IV. CARDIOVASCULAR COMPLICATIONS

A. Postoperative Hypotension
  1. A 20 to 30% decrease in blood pressure from baseline preoperative levels that results in symptoms of organ hypoperfusion (acidosis, myocardial ischemia, oliguria, sympathetic nervous system activation, central nervous system disturbances) requires prompt differential diagnosis and treatment (Table 54-5).
  2. **Treatment** is determined by the mechanism responsible for hypotension.
     a. After confirming the adequacy of oxygenation, it is often most appropriate to administer crystalloid solutions (300 to 500 mL iv over 15 minutes). A transient improvement in blood pressure with this therapy may indicate continued surgical bleeding, whereas the absence of any improvement may reflect cardiac dysfunction.
     b. Vasopressors are a temporizing measure to restore perfusion pressure while the underlying cause for hypotension is corrected.
B. Postoperative Hypertension
  1. A 20 to 30% increase in blood pressure from baseline preoperative levels that produces

TABLE 54-5

DIFFERENTIAL DIAGNOSIS OF HYPOTENSION IN THE POSTANESTHESIA CARE UNIT

Arterial hypoxemia
Hypovolemia (most common cause)
Spurious (cuff too wide, transducer not calibrated)
Pulmonary edema (excess fluids)
Myocardial ischemia
Cardiac dysrhythmias
Decreased systemic vascular resistance (regional blocks, drugs)
Pneumothorax
Cardiac tamponade

874   *Postanesthesia and Consultant Practice*

TABLE 54-6

DIFFERENTIAL DIAGNOSIS OF HYPERTENSION IN PATIENTS IN A POSTANESTHESIA CARE UNIT

Arterial hypoxemia
Spurious (cuff too narrow, transducer not calibrated, transducer overshoot)
Preexisting essential hypertension
Enhanced sympathetic nervous system activity (pain, carinal stimulation, bladder distention, preeclampsia)
Excess fluid administration
Hypothermia

---

symptoms (myocardial ischemia, bleeding, headache) or unusual risk of morbidity (increased intracranial pressure, valvular heart disease) requires prompt differential diagnosis (Table 54-6).

2. **Treatment** is determined by the mechanism responsible for hypertension.

   a. After confirming the adequacy of oxygenation, it is often most appropriate to direct therapy toward correction of events leading to increased sympathetic nervous system activity.

   b. If hypertension persists despite correction of factors promoting sympathetic nervous system activity, it may be necessary to administer antihypertensive medications (hydralazine, labetalol, nitroprusside).

C. **Cardiac Dysrhythmias in the Postoperative Period**

1. Prompt differential diagnosis of cardiac dysrhythmias requires monitoring of the electrocardiogram (Table 54-7).

TABLE 54-7

DIFFERENTIAL DIAGNOSIS OF CARDIAC DYSRHYTHMIAS IN PATIENTS IN A POSTANESTHESIA CARE UNIT

Asymptomatic electrocardiogram abnormalities (nodal rhythms usually resolve spontaneously in 3–6 hr)
Bradycardia (increased parasympathetic nervous system activity reflecting opioids or anticholinesterases; heart block)
Tachycardia (increased sympathetic nervous system activity, paroxysmal atrial tachycardia)
Premature contractions (atrial usually benign; ventricular may be life-threatening)

TABLE 54-8

TREATMENT OF CARDIAC DYSRHYTHMIAS IN PATIENTS IN A POSTANESTHESIA CARE UNIT

Eliminate excessive parasympathetic nervous system activity (atropine, ephedrine)

Eliminate excessive sympathetic nervous system activity (analgesics, beta antagonists)

Decreased ventricular irritability (lidocaine)

Artificial pacemaker insertion versus administration of isoproterenol

2. **Treatment** is determined by the hemodynamic significance of the cardiac dysrhythmias (Table 54-8).

V. POSTOPERATIVE PULMONARY DYSFUNCTION

A. **Inadequate Postoperative Ventilation** (Table 54-9)

B. **Inadequate Postoperative Oxygenation** (Table 54-10)

1. An acceptable PaO_2 must be defined for each individual patient. A common recommendation is to maintain PaO_2 between 70 and 100 mm Hg by adjusting the inspired oxygen concentration (ideally <60%) with or without positive end-expiratory pressure or continuous positive airway pressure (5 to 10 cm H_2O) by face mask.

TABLE 54-9

DIFFERENTIAL DIAGNOSIS OF HYPOVENTILATION IN PATIENTS IN A POSTANESTHESIA CARE UNIT

Inadequate ventilatory drive (residual effects of anesthetics; lack of sensory stimulation)

Ventilatory mechanics

    Increased airway resistance (smokers and patients with bronchospastic disease are at highest risk for bronchospasm after surgery)

    Decreased compliance (obesity, fluid overload)

    Residual neuromuscular blockade

Increased dead space (pulmonary embolus)

Increased carbon dioxide production (hyperthermia, hyperalimentation)

TABLE 54-10

DIFFERENTIAL DIAGNOSIS OF ARTERIAL HYPOXEMIA IN PATIENTS IN A POSTANESTHESIA CARE UNIT

Distribution of ventilation (mismatch of ventilation to perfusion because of loss of functional residual capacity is most likely cause of postoperative hypoxemia)

Distribution of perfusion (mismatch of perfusion to ventilation as a result of impaired hypoxic pulmonary vasoconstriction or altered pulmonary artery pressure)

Inadequate alveolar oxygen partial pressure

Decreased mixed venous oxygen partial pressure (decreased cardiac output; increased tissue oxygen extraction owing to shivering or sepsis)

2. Splinting because of postoperative pain contributes to detrimental loss of lung volume (especially functional residual capacity), reemphasizing the importance of adequate postoperative pain relief.

3. Exposing an intubated trachea to ambient pressures eliminates a patient's ability to create expiratory resistance (physiologic positive end-expiratory pressure), leading to possible loss of functional residual capacity and decreased PaO_2.

4. Patients with abnormal CO_2/pH responses from morbid obesity, chronic airway obstruction, or sleep apnea are more sensitive to respiratory depressants.

C. **Carbon Monoxide Poisoning**

1. During general anesthesia, patients can be exposed to carbon monoxide by a reaction between certain inhaled anesthetics (desflurane, isoflurane) and dry carbon dioxide absorbent.

2. Carbon monoxide poisoning is difficult to recognize in the PACU because a pulse oximeter interprets carboxyhemoglobin as oxyhemoglobin (erroneous false high reading).

D. **Supplemental Oxygen**

1. Clinical observation and assessment of cognitive function do not accurately screen for arterial hypoxemia so monitoring with pulse oximetry is important throughout the PACU stay.

2. If a patient requires PACU admission, it is likely that supplemental oxygen will be administered during the initial recovery from anesthesia.

VI. PERIOPERATIVE ASPIRATION

A. Inhalation of acidic fluid (pH <2.5) in the perioperative period may manifest as varying degrees of arterial hypoxemia and "fluffy" infiltrates (immediately or within 24 hours) on a chest radiograph. Airway obstruction may accompany aspiration of solid food particles.

  1. Suspicion that aspiration has occurred mandates 24 to 48 hours of monitoring for development of aspiration pneumonitis.
  2. If the likelihood of aspiration is small in an ambulatory patient, outpatient follow-up can be done, assuming hypoxemia, cough, wheezing, or radiographic abnormalities do not appear within 4 to 6 hours.

B. Treatment of aspiration is correction of arterial hypoxemia with supplemental oxygen. Tracheal intubation and positive end-expiratory pressure may be required if hypoxemia persists despite supplemental oxygen.

  1. **Pulmonary edema** is usually secondary to pulmonary capillary damage, which may create hypovolemia and necessitate intravascular fluid replacement.
  2. **Antibiotics** are prescribed only if bacterial infection develops.
  3. There is no evidence that corticosteroids improve long-term outcome.
  4. **Bronchoscopy** may be necessary to relieve airway obstruction caused by inhaled food particles.

VII. POSTOPERATIVE RENAL COMPLICATIONS

A. Ability to Void

  1. It is acceptable to discharge adult inpatients to a surgical floor and selected adult ambulatory surgical patients from the facility before they void.
  2. Ambulatory adult patients who are discharged without voiding should be given a specific time interval in which to void (10 to 12 hours).

B. Oliguria (urine output <0.5 mL/kg/hr) despite adequate perfusion pressure, hydration (crystalloid solution 300 to 500 mL iv), and a low-dose furosemide challenge (5 mg iv offsets fluid retention caused by

TABLE 54-11

**CLASSIFICATION AND LIKELY EXPLANATION OF
METABOLIC DERANGEMENTS IN PATIENTS IN A
POSTANESTHESIA CARE UNIT**

Respiratory acidosis (alveolar hypoventilation)
Metabolic acidosis (hypovolemia, tissue hypoxia, hypothermia,
  renal failure, ketoacidosis, sepsis)
Respiratory alkalosis (hyperventilation)
Metabolic alkalosis (prolonged gastric suctioning, potassium
  wasting diuretics)

> antidiuretic hormone) increase the possibility of acute
> tubular necrosis.
>
> C. **Polyuria** is usually self-limited and most often is
>   because of generous intraoperative fluid administration
>   or hyperglycemia (osmotic diuresis). Sustained
>   polyuria (urine output >4 to 5 mL/kg/hr) may result in
>   hypovolemia and electrolyte disturbances.

VIII. METABOLIC COMPLICATIONS (Table 54-11)

IX. GLUCOSE AND ELECTROLYTE DISORDERS
(Table 54-12)

X. MISCELLANEOUS COMPLICATIONS (Table
54-13)

  A. **Nausea and Vomiting**
    1. Nausea and vomiting are common problems in the
       PACU (incidence varies with the surgical procedure,
       anesthetic technique [opioids, neostigmine]), and
       may delay discharge or necessitate overnight
       admission of ambulatory patients.

TABLE 54-12

**GLUCOSE AND ELECTROLYTE CHANGES IN PATIENTS IN A
POSTANESTHESIA CARE UNIT**

Hyperglycemia (<300 mg/dL and usually resolves spontaneously)
Hypoglycemia (masked by residual effects of anesthetics)
Hypokalemia (cardiac dysrhythmias)
Hyperkalemia (hemolyzed sample, renal failure)
Hyponatremia (following transurethral resection of the prostate)

TABLE 54-13

MISCELLANEOUS COMPLICATIONS THAT MAY MANIFEST IN PATIENTS IN A POSTANESTHESIA CARE UNIT

Nausea and vomiting
Incidental trauma
Dental damage
Corneal abrasion
Hearing impairment
Oral soft tissue trauma
Hoarseness/pharyngitis (occurs in 20–50% and is usually benign)
Peripheral nerve compression
Electrical or chemical burns
Extravasation of intravenous fluids
Skeletal muscle pain (usually manifests the day after surgery)
Hypothermia and shivering (usually benign)
Persistent sedation (persistent effects of anesthetic drugs versus residual effects of muscle relaxants)
Altered mental status (emergence reactions more common in children and young adults, whereas elderly may be slower to recover cognitive function; surgical pain must be eliminated as a cause for agitation)
Emergence reactions
Delirium and cognitive decline (elderly patients)

   2. Avoiding gastric distention and providing adequate postoperative analgesia are important, as is limiting postoperative vestibular stimulation by minimizing brisk head motion.
   3. Prior to instituting treatment of postoperative nausea, it is important to consider more serious causes such as hypotension, arterial hypoxemia, increased intracranial pressure, hypoglycemia, or gastric bleeding.
   4. Dexamethasone is a potent antiemetic for postoperative nausea and vomiting prophylaxis (4 to 8 mg iv in adults given before induction of anesthesia).
B. **Temperature** <35°C is an indication for assisted rewarming (radiant lighting, heating blankets, warmed intravenous fluids). As body temperature increases, there may be a need to increase the rate of intravenous fluid administration to offset increased venous capacitance. Resolution of metabolic acidosis often corresponds to rewarming. Supplemental oxygen is administered to offset the increase in oxygen consumption accompanying shivering.

TABLE 54-14
DIFFERENTIAL DIAGNOSIS OF COMA IN PATIENTS IN A
POSTANESTHESIA CARE UNIT

Hypothermia (<33°C)
Hypoglycemia
Electrolyte imbalance (hyponatremia, hypomagnesemia,
　hypocalcemia, hypoosmolarity)
Central nervous system damage (hypoxia, increased intracranial
　pressure, cerebral vascular accident, air embolus)
Drug overdose (treat with naloxone, flumazenil, physostigmine)

    C. **Persistent sedation** is most likely caused by residual
       effects of anesthetics.
       1. Profound skeletal muscle paralysis mimics
          unconsciousness, whereas residual paralysis is ruled
          out by spontaneous ventilation and purposeful
          movement.
       2. Persistence of sedative effects (anesthetic effects
          usually wane in 60 to 90 minutes) requires a
          differential diagnosis of coma (Table 54-14).

CHAPTER 55 ■ MANAGEMENT OF ACUTE POSTOPERATIVE PAIN

Acute postoperative pain is a complex physiologic reaction to tissue injury, viscera distension, or disease (Lubenow TR, Ivankovich AD, Barkin RL: Management of acute postoperative pain. In Barash PG, Cullen BF, Stoelting RK [eds]: *Clinical Anesthesia*, pp 1405–1440. Philadelphia, Lippincott Williams & Wilkins, 2006). Historically, the treatment of postoperative pain has been given a low priority by surgeons and anesthesiologists. As a result, patients previously accepted pain as an unavoidable part of the postoperative experience. With the development of an expanding awareness of the epidemiology and pathophysiology of pain, more attention is being focused on the management of pain in an effort to improve quality of care and decrease postoperative morbidity and mortality.

I. FUNDAMENTAL CONCEPTS

A. **Nociception** refers to the detection, transduction, and transmission of noxious stimuli.
   1. Stimuli generated from thermal, mechanical, or chemical tissue damage may activate nociceptors, which are free nerve endings.
   2. Although nociceptors are free nerve terminals, they are adjacent to small blood vessels and mast cells with which they operate as a functional unit.
   3. As a result of chronic inflammation or repeated tissue injury, nociceptors may be sensitized and thereby become responsive to innocuous stimuli.
B. **Peripheral nerve afferent fibers** are categorized into three groups (A, B, and C), depending on diameter, degree of myelination, rapidity of conduction, and distribution of fibers.
   1. **A delta fibers** are large myelinated fibers that mediate pain sensation.
   2. **B fibers** are medium-size myelinated fibers. Postganglionic, sympathetic, and visceral afferents belong to this group.
   3. **C fibers** are slowly conducting unmyelinated fibers that modulate nociceptive stimuli.

C. **Spinal Cord and Brain Pathways**
1. The peripheral afferent neuron (first-order neuron) sends axonal projections into the dorsal horn and other areas of the spinal cord (relay centers for nociceptive activity), where a synapse occurs with a second-order afferent neuron.
2. Projections from the second-order afferent neuron cross to the contralateral hemisphere of the spinal cord and ascend from that level in the lateral spinothalamic tract to synapse in the thalamus.

D. **Modulation of nociception** can occur in the periphery or at any point where synaptic transmission occurs.
1. **Peripheral modulation** occurs by the liberation of substances (potassium, lactic acid, bradykinin, serotonin, histamine, and prostaglandins) that sensitize and excite nociceptors.
   a. Peripheral terminals of nociceptive sensory neurons contain an excitatory calcium ion channel and are sensitive to the compound capsaicin.
   b. Tetrodotoxin-insensitive sodium channels in pain-sensing neurons modulate increased pain hyperexcitability following inflammation.
2. **Spinal modulation** results from the action of excitatory neurotransmitter substances (glutamate, aspartate) that modulate transmission of nociceptive afferent signals.
   a. Substance P is an important neuromodulator that can enhance or aggravate pain.
   b. Inhibitory neurotransmitter substances involved in the regulation of afferent impulses in the dorsal horns include enkephalins, beta endorphins, norepinephrine, dopamine, adenosine, and perhaps somatostatin.
3. **Neuroplasticity: The Dynamic Modulation of Neural Impulses**
   a. Neural activity–dependent plasticity reflects the dynamic nature of the nociceptive response to injury.
   b. As peripheral nociceptors are sensitized by local tissue mediators of injury, the excitability and frequency of neural discharge increase. This primary hyperalgesia permits previously subnoxious stimuli to generate action potentials that are transmitted to the spinal cord.

   c. The central sensitization to afferent impulses is a result of a functional change in spinal cord processing termed plasticity or neuroplasticity.
4. **Supraspinal modulation** occurs via descending inhibitory tracts (opioid pathways and alpha-adrenergic pathways) that originate at the brainstem level (cell bodies located in the periaqueductal gray matter and reticular formation) and descend and synapse in the dorsal horn where they release inhibitory neurotransmitters (endorphins, norepinephrine).
   a. These inhibitory neurotransmitters regulate synaptic transmission between primary and secondary afferent neurons.
   b. **Cognitive** modulation of pain (pain experienced in a pleasant environment elicits less discomfort) and attention (biofeedback based on premise that only a fixed number of afferent stimuli can reach cortical centers) influence the perception of pain.

II. PATHOPHYSIOLOGY OF PAIN

A. **Components of Surgical Stress.** There is increasing understanding of the deleterious effects of postoperative pain on specific organ systems (Table 55-1).

TABLE 55-1
ADVERSE PHYSIOLOGIC SEQUELAE OF PAIN

Organ system	Clinical effect
Pulmonary	Arterial hypoxemia
	Hypoventilation
	Atelectasis
	Pneumonia
Endocrine	Protein catabolism
	Hyperglycemia
	Sodium and water retention
Cardiovascular	Dysrhythmias
	Myocardial ischemia/infarction
	Congestive heart failure
Immunologic	Decreased immune function
Coagulation effects	Hypercoagulability (thromboembolic phenomena)
Gastrointestinal	Ileus
Genitourinary	Urinary retention

B. **Influence of Anesthesia on the Surgical Stress Response**
   1. **General anesthesia** does not reliably attenuate the neuroendocrine stress response (exception may be high doses of opioids or >1.5 minimum alveolar concentration [MAC] of volatile anesthetics).
   2. **Regional anesthesia and analgesia** may block the cortisol response to stress if the site of surgery is well below the level of sensory block. Improved outcome associated with regional anesthesia is dependent on continuation of intraoperative central neuraxial blockade into the postoperative period.

III. PHARMACOLOGY OF POSTOPERATIVE PAIN MANAGEMENT

A. **Nonopioid analgesics** are represented by aspirin, acetaminophen, and the nonsteroidal anti-inflammatory drugs (NSAIDs), COX-1, COX-2 inhibitors, and acetaminophen, which are most effective for treatment of minor to moderate postoperative pain (Table 55-2).
   1. Although these drugs represent diverse chemical entities, their common mechanism of action is inhibition of prostaglandin-mediated amplification of chemical and mechanical irritants on the sensory pathways peripherally and centrally.
   2. **Acetaminophen (Paracetamol-APAP)** provides analgesic and antipyretic benefits but in overdose is associated with potentially fatal hepatic necrosis (a function of baseline glutathione levels and daily alcohol consumption [greater than three drinks daily]).
      a. Analgesic mechanisms of APAP are in part a function of COX inhibition.
      b. The half-life is 2 to 4 hours when used to treat postoperative pain.
      c. About 90% of APAP is hepatically metabolized to sulfate and glucuronide conjugates for renal excretion.
   3. **Clinical uses** of nonopioid analgesics are limited to treatment of events associated with sensitizing effects of prostaglandins (musculoskeletal, posttraumatic, and inflammatory pain).

TABLE 55-2

PHARMACOKINETIC PARAMETERS/MAXIMUM DOSAGE RECOMMENDATIONS FOR NONOPIOID ANALGESICS

	Route	Time to peak (hr)	Half-life (hr)	Analgesic onset (hr)	Analgesic duration (hr)	Maximum recommended daily dose (mg)
Salicylates						
Aspirin	Oral	0.5–2	2–3	0.5–1	2–4	3,600
Difunisal	Oral	0.2–3	>8–12	1–2	8–12	2,000
Propionic Acids						
Fenoprofen	Oral	1–2	2–3	1	4–6	3,200
Ibuprofen	Oral	1–2	1.8–2.5	0.5	4–6	3,200
Ketoprofen	Oral	0.5–2	2.4	4–6	300	
Naproxen	Oral	2–4	12–15	1	4–7	1,500
Acetic Acids						
Etodolac	Oral	1–2	7.3	0.5	4–12	200
Indomethacin	Oral	1–2	4.5	0.5	4–6	200
Sulindac	Oral	2–4	7.8			400
Ketorolac	Oral/im	1	2.4–6	0.5–1	4–6	120
Tomecin	Oral	0.5–1	1.1.5			2,000

(*continued*)

TABLE 55-2
CONTINUED

	Route	Time to peak (hr)	Half-life (hr)	Analgesic onset (hr)	Analgesic duration (hr)	Maximum recommended daily dose (mg)
Fenamates (anthranilic acids)						
Meclofenamate	Oral	0.5–1	2	0.5–1	4–6	400
Mefanamic acid	Oral	2–4	2–4	1	4–6	1,000
Oxicams						
Piroxicam	Oral	3–5	30–86	1	48–72	20
Phenylacetic acids						
Diclofenac	Oral	2–3	2	1	1.6	200
p-Aminophenols						
Acetaminophen	Oral	0.5–1	1.4	0.5	2–4	1,200
Phenacetin	Oral	1				2,400
Selective COX-2 Inhibitors						
Celecoxib	Oral	2–3		1	8–12	400
Rofecoxib	Oral	2–3		0.4	12–24	50

B. **Opioid analgesics** represented by morphine are used most often to treat severe postoperative pain (Table 55-3).

1. **Mechanism of analgesic effects** is most likely attributable to interaction with stereoselective opioid receptors (same sites of action as for endogenous neuromodulators represented by endorphins [Table 55-4]). Agonist-antagonist opioids may exhibit altered affinity for opioid receptors, accounting for the potential of these drugs to reverse the effects of an agonist (see Table 55-4).

2. **Absorption/biotransformation/elimination** is characterized by hepatic metabolism followed by renal elimination of conjugated metabolites (morphine-6-glucuronide is an active metabolite).
   a. Oral absorption may be extensive, but availability of the drug is limited by first-pass uptake into the liver and lungs.
   b. Distribution of drug depends on its lipid solubility.

3. **Adverse Effects** (Table 55-5)
   a. Physical dependence and analgesic tolerance are not generally a problem when opioids are used short term to treat acute pain.
   b. Respiratory depression is more likely when the opioid is administered in high doses and in the absence of pain.

4. **Clinical uses**
   a. Opioids remain the primary pharmacologic therapeutic drugs for management of moderate to severe pain.
   b. Agonist-antagonists can be effective analgesics in the postoperative period and have a ceiling effect for respiratory depression and often analgesia as well. Unlike NSAIDs, these drugs do not interfere with platelet function.
   c. As the patient's analgesic requirements decrease, the transition from parenteral to oral therapy is often empirical and generally involves replacing the opioid with an opioid-NSAID combination.
   d. Meperidine and propoxyphene use is decreasing because of recognition of the potential for neurotoxicity and cardiac/pulmonary toxicity respectively.

TABLE 55-3
PHARMACOKINETIC PARAMETERS/MAXIMUM DOSAGE RECOMMENDATIONS FOR ORAL AND PARENTERAL OPIOID ANALGESICS

	Dosage (mg)	Onset (hr)	Peak (hr)	Duration (hr)	Comment
Morphine	2.5–15 iv			0.125	Rapid onset, peak respiratory depression at 10 min
Meperidine	50–100 im	0.12–0.5	1	2–4	
Codeine	15–60 oral	0.25–1	0.5–2	3–4	Oral potency because of small first-pass effect
Methadone	2.5–10 oral	0.5–1	1.5–2	4–8	
Hydromorphone	1–4 oral	0.5–1	1	3–4	
	1–4 im	0.3–5	1	2–3	
	1–1.5 im	0.5		2–3	
Oxymorphone	5–7.5 oral				
Hydrocodone	5 oral	0.5	1–2	3–6	
Oxycodone	32–65 oral	0.25–1	1–2	3–6	
Propoxyphene	2–4 im	0.1–0.2	0.5–1	3–4	
Butorphanol	50 oral			4–7	Weak opioid
Pentazocine	30–60 im	0.12–0.5	1–3	3–6	

TABLE 55-4

PHARMACOLOGY OF OPIOIDS

	Receptor			
	μ-1	μ-2	δ	κ
Analgesia	Supraspinal		Spinal	Spinal
Affect	Euphoria			Sedation
Pupil	Miosis			Miosis
Ventilation		Depression	Depression	
Gastrointestinal	Nausea, vomiting	Constipation, vomiting	Nausea	
Genitourinary	Urinary retention		Urinary retention	Diuresis
Temperature	Increase			
Other	Pruritus		Pruritus	
Tolerance	Yes	Sedation	Yes	Little
Cross-tolerance	δ		μ	No

TABLE 55-5

ADVERSE EFFECTS OF SHORT-TERM AND MODERATE-DOSE OPIOID THERAPY

Central Nervous System (tolerance develops rapidly)
Sedation
Dizziness
Miosis

Gastrointestinal Effects
Nausea
Constipation
Spasm of the sphincter of Oddi (can persist for up to 24 hours after a single therapeutic dose)

Urinary Retention

      e. Alternative delivery techniques have evolved that may supplant the oral or intravenous delivery of opioids in certain clinical circumstances.

      f. Oxymorphone, sufentanil, fentanyl and morphine dosage preparations are being developed to provide greater long-acting analgesic postoperative opportunities. Oral slow release long-acting opioids (morphine, oxycodone, oxymoprphone) are finding a role in acute postoperative pain management.

IV. NEW METHODS OF OPIOID ADMINISTRATION

    A. Fentanyl patient-controlled transdermal analgesic (PCTA) can provide needleless analgesia for moderate to severe pain for ≥ 24 hours including the postoperative period.

    B. Sustained release morphine (15- to 25-mg epidural injection) provides analgesia for over 48 hours.

    C. Oxymorphone is a semisynthetic mu-specific opioid agonist for moderate to severe pain (oral sustained release and immediate release preparations available).

    D. During periods of acute postoperative pain scheduled administration of analgesics is typically more effective than use on a prn basis.

V. ADJUVANT ANALGESIA

    A. **Lidocaine topical patch** 5% provides relief for incision site pain and may provide an opioid sparing effect.

VI. METHODS OF ANALGESIA

    A. **Routes of Analgesic Delivery** (Table 55-6)

    B. **Patient-controlled analgesia (PCA)** provides excellent analgesia with a low total drug dose, minimal sedation, and prompt return to physical activity (Table 55-7). Use of PCA in pediatric and elderly patients may be difficult because the technique requires patient understanding and cooperation.

    C. **Central Neuraxial Analgesia** (Tables 55-8 and 55-9)

        1. **Intrathecal** administration of opioids (morphine 0.25 to 1 mg) produces long-lasting analgesia after a single injection.

            a. The onset of analgesic effect following the intrathecal administration of an opioid is directly proportional to the lipid solubility of the opioid (fentanyl has a rapid onset). The duration of the analgesic effect is longer with the more hydrophilic compounds (morphine).

TABLE 55-6

ROUTES OF ANALGESIC DELIVERY

Oral (unpredictable onset and duration; requires a functioning gastrointestinal tract)

Transepithelial (transdermal, transmucosal)

Intramuscular (administration of analgesics by this route on a 3- to 4-hour basis results in plasma concentrations that exceed the analgesic requirements for only about 35% of the dosing interval)

Intravenous (intermittent versus continuous versus patient controlled)

Central neuraxial analgesia
    Intrathecal
    Epidural

Peripheral nerve blocks (short duration limits usefulness)
    Local infiltration
    Intra-articular (bupivacaine up to 100 mg)
    Intercostal (bupivacaine with or without epinephrine; perform in the midaxillary line; risk is pneumothorax; cryoanalgesia lasts 1–3 months)
    Ilioinguinal (pain relief following inguinal or femoral herniorrhaphy, appendectomy, procedures on the scrotum)
    Penile
    Brachial plexus (continuous analgesia using bupivacaine 0.25% at 6–10 mL/hr)
    Intrapleural (bupivacaine 0.25–0.5%; 20 mL every 6 hours)

TABLE 55-7

GUIDELINES REGARDING THE BOLUS DOSES, LOCKOUT INTERVALS, AND CONTINUOUS INFUSIONS FOR PARENTERAL ANALGESICS WHEN USING A PATIENT-CONTROLLED ANALGESIA SYSTEM

Drug	Bolus dose (mg)	Lockout interval (min)	Continuous infusion (mg/hr)	Four hour limit (mg)
Agonists				
Fentanyl	0.015–0.05	3–10	0.02–0.1	0.2–0.4
Hydromorphone	0.10–0.5	5–15	0.2–0.5	
Oxymorphone	0.2–0.8	5–15	0.1–1	
Meperidine	5–15	5–15	5–40	200–300
Methadone	0.5–3.0	10–20		
Morphine	0.5–3.0	5–20	1–10	20–30
Sufentanil	0.003–0.015	3–10		
Agonist-Antagonists				
Buprenorphine	0.03–0.2	10–20		
Pentazocine	5–30	5–15	6–40	

TABLE 55-8

COMPLICATIONS OF THE USE OF NEURAXIAL OPIOIDS:
REPORTED INCIDENCE (%)

Complication	Spinal (%)	Epidural (%)	Treatment
Respiratory depression	5–7	0.1–2.0	Support ventilation, naloxone
Pruritus	60	1–100	Antihistamine, naloxone
Nausea and vomiting	20–30	20–30	Antiemetics, transdermal scopolamine, naloxone
Urinary retention	50	15–25	Catheterize, naloxone

    b. A disadvantage of this technique is the inability to titrate the drug effect.

    c. The use of combined spinal anesthesia followed by continuous epidural analgesia provides the advantages of spinal anesthesia (rapid onset, dense neural blockade) while facilitating the transition to an effective and titratable postoperative analgesia.

  2. **Epidural analgesia** by epidural administration of opioids reflects passage of the drug across the dura (2 to 10% of the injected dose) as well as systemic

TABLE 55-9

POSTOPERATIVE EPIDURAL ANALGESIA

Route	Group A (bupivacaine 25 mg/5 mL, 0.5%) Epidural bolus	Group B (morphine 5 mg) Epidural bolus	Group C (morphine 100 μg/hr) Epidural infusion
Urinary retention	30 (100%)	30 (100%)	2 (7%)
Hypotension	7 (23%)	0	0
Weakness of hands	12 (40%)	0	0
Pruritus	0	12 (40%)	1 (3%)
Decreased consciousness	0	8 (27%)	0

TABLE 55-10

COMPARISON OF TYPES OF EPIDURAL ADMINISTRATION

Advantages	Disadvantages
Continuous Epidural	
Less rostral spread	Need for sophisticated infusion device
Unchanging level of analgesia	
Permits concomitant use of a local anesthetic solution	
Permits use of short-acting opioids	
Less risk of catheter contamination	
Eliminates need for anesthesia personnel to perform injections	
Intermittent Epidural Bolus	
Simple	Limited number of suitable opioids
No need for infusion devices	High incidence of side effects
	Personnel needed to reinject catheter
	Excludes use of local anesthesia
	More difficult to titrate dose
Patient-Controlled Epidural Analgesia	
Manage dynamic changes in pain related to patient activity (coughing, chest physiotherapy)	

absorption of the opioid (morphine 10 mg iv or epidural produces peak plasma levels and decay curves that are similar).

a. Epidural opioids may be administered by a variety of techniques (Table 55-10).

b. The epidural catheter is often placed before the induction of anesthesia so that a test dose of local anesthetic can be administered to confirm the proper placement of the catheter. This practice also permits institution of the epidural analgesia intraoperatively (Table 55-11).

c. **Selection of analgesics** for epidural analgesia is influenced by the duration of action

TABLE 55-11
CONTINUOUS EPIDURAL INFUSION REGIMENS

Composition of Solution
Morphine (0.1 mg/mL) or fentanyl (100 μg/mL) with bupivacaine (1 mg/mL)

Rate of Infusion
Initiate intraoperatively at 4–6 mL/hr if operation is expected to exceed 3 hours
Precede infusion with 5- to 10-mL bolus of the solution if operation is expected to be of short duration

Placement of Epidural Catheter
Hydrophilic opioids (morphine) spread rostrally (lumbar epidural placement acceptable)
Lipophilic opioids (fentanyl) provide a segmental analgesic effect (epidural catheter placement at dermatome levels included in the surgical field)

(Table 55-12). Epidural coadministration of opioids with local anesthetics takes advantage of the desirable properties of each drug (potentiation of analgesia at lower opioid doses with a concentration of local anesthetic that does not produce significant motor blockade). The alpha-2 agonists such as clonidine produce antinociception with minimal ventilatory depression as compared with opioids.

    d. **Management of inadequate analgesia** (Fig. 55-1)

    e. **Safety considerations** (Table 55-13)

3. **Caudal** nerve blocks play a minor role in acute pain management in adults because they are technically more difficult to perform than a lumbar epidural block. In contrast, palpation of the sacral hiatus is easy in pediatric patients (use a short 22- or 23-gauge needle with the child in the lateral position to inject 0.75 to 1 mg/kg of bupivacaine, which produces analgesia to about T10).

4. Delayed depression of ventilation following neuraxial opioids is more likely in the presence of specific circumstances (Table 55-14).

D. **Other Modalities**

1. **Psychological interventions for postoperative analgesia** are more applicable to management of chronic pain but also have limited application in

TABLE 55-12

EPIDURAL OPIOIDS: LATENCY AND DURATION OF POSTOPERATIVE ANALGESIA

Drug	Bolus dose	Analgesic onset (min)	Analgesic peak (min)	Analgesic duration (hr)	Continuous infusion concentration (%)	Rate
Meperidine	30–100 mg	5–10	12–30	4–6		
Morphine	5 mg	23.5	30–60	12–24	0.01	1–6
Methadone	5 mg	12.5	17	7.2		
Fentanyl	100 µg	4–10	20	2.6	0.001	4–12
Sufentanil	30–50 mg	7.3	26.5	3.9	0.0001	10

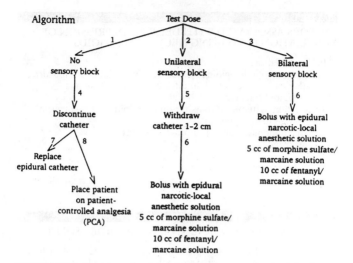

FIGURE 55-1. Test-dose algorithm for inadequate analgesia. A 5-mL test dose of 2% lidocaine in 1:200,000 epinephrine is injected into the lumbar epidural catheter.

TABLE 55-13

SAFETY CONSIDERATIONS IN THE MANAGEMENT OF A CONTINUOUS EPIDURAL TECHNIQUE

Subarachnoid migration of the catheter (add 0.1% bupivacaine to solution and monitor for onset of sensory blockade)

Infection-related problems (monitor patient's temperature and evaluate signs of infection; remove catheter and culture if signs of infection)

Epidural hematoma (epidural catheters should be placed at least 1 hour prior to intravenous heparinization using unfractionated heparin; placement and removal of epidural catheters are performed 10–12 hours after the last dose of low-molecular weight heparin and subsequent dosing with low-molecular weight heparin is not performed for at least 2 hours after removal of the catheter)

Respiratory depression (monitor respiratory rate and sedation every hour during the first 24 hours)

TABLE 55-14

FACTORS ASSOCIATED WITH DELAYED DEPRESSION OF VENTILATION FOLLOWING NEURAXIAL OPIOIDS

High opioid dose
Use of water-soluble opioid (lipid solubility of fentanyl limits drug available in cerebrospinal fluid for cephalad diffusion)
Lack of opioid tolerance
Concomitant systemic administration of opioids or other central nervous system depressants
Increased abdominal or intrathoracic pressure
Advanced age

TABLE 55-15

POSTOPERATIVE EPIDURAL ANALGESIA ORDER SHEET

(Please circle orders to be implemented and complete blanks where appropriate. Date and time for each procedure to be noted.)
1. Admit to postoperative pain service and institute routine vital signs (breathing rate every hour).
2. On ward (circle)
   a. Apnea monitor
   b. Telemetry
   c. Pulse oximetry
   d. Naloxone with syringe at bedside (administer 0.4 mg iv if breathing rate <8 and call anesthesiologist)
3. Epidural solution (circle one)[a]
   a. Morphine 7.5 mg with bupivacaine 150 mg in 150 mL saline (age >70 yr)
   b. Morphine 15 mg with bupivacaine 150 mg in 150 mL saline
   c. Fentanyl 750 μg with bupivacaine 150 mg in 150 mL saline (age >70 yr)
   d. Fentanyl 1500 μg with bupivacaine 150 mg in 150 mL saline
   e. Patient-assisted epidural mode _____ mL every _____ min with _____ mL/4-hour lockout
4. Supplemental medications (circle one)
   a. Morphine 2 mg iv or im every 2–4 hours as necessary for pain
   b. Metoclopramide 10 mg im every 4–6 hours as necessary for nausea
5. All other preoperative orders, medications, and diet per service with the exception of opioids and sedatives.
   Physician's signature _____ Date/Time _____

[a]Combined hourly rate not to exceed 10 mL.

TABLE 55-16

POSTOPERATIVE PATIENT-CONTROLLED ANALGESIA
ORDER SHEET

Medication: morphine 30 mg per 30-mL prefilled syringe
   Loading dose = 2 mg
   Maintenance dose = 1 mg
   Lockout interval = 6 minutes
   4-hour time limit at 20 mg[a]
Disregard all other opioid orders during patient-controlled
   analgesia use.
Physician's signature _____

[a]If analgesia is inadequate, 4-hour limit doses may be increased to 30 mg.

treatment of acute pain (relaxation techniques,
education, distraction).

VII. ORGANIZATION OF A POSTOPERATIVE
ANALGESIA SERVICE

- **A.** The basic goals of the postoperative analgesia service
  are (1) to administer and monitor postoperative
  analgesia and (2) to identify and manage complications
  or side effects of postoperative analgesic techniques.
- **B.** The delivery of central neuraxial opioid analgesia
  requires cooperation among the anesthesiology,
  nursing, surgery, and pharmacy staffs on a 24-hour
  basis.
- **C.** Written policy and procedure manuals for nursing staff
  as well as preprinted epidural analgesia orders are
  useful (Table 55-15).
- **D.** Protocols outlining the initial parameters for starting
  and maintaining PCA are useful (Table 55-16).
- **E.** An important aspect of the initiation of a postoperative
  analgesia service is the identification of patient
  populations that are most likely to benefit from
  improved postoperative pain management (Table
  55-17).

TABLE 55-17

PATIENTS MOST LIKELY TO BENEFIT FROM IMPROVED
POSTOPERATIVE PAIN MANAGEMENT

Thoracic surgery
Abdominal surgery
Orthopedic surgery
High-risk vascular surgery

TABLE 55-18

PHARMACOLOGIC CONSIDERATIONS FOR PEDIATRIC PATIENTS

	Dose (age >3 mo)	Interval (hr)	Route	Comments
Acetaminophen	5–15 mg/kg	4–6	Oral	Overdose may cause hepatotoxicity
	20 mg/kg	4–6	Rectal	
Ibuprofen	8 mg/kg	6	Oral	
Naproxen	5 mg/kg	8–12	Oral	Commonly combined with acetaminophen
Codeine	0.5–1 mg/kg	4–6	Oral	
Meperidine	1–1.5 mg/kg	3–4	im	Less constipation and urinary retention than morphine
	0.8–1 mg/kg	2–3	iv	
Morphine	0.1–0.15 mg/kg	3–4	im	
	0.08–0.1 mg/kg	2	iv	
	50–60 μg/kg/hr		iv	Continuous infusion
	50 μg/kg	12–24	Epidural	Abdominal surgery
	120–150 μg/kg	12–24	Epidural	Thoracic surgery
	50–100 μg/kg	12–24	Caudal	
Fentanyl	1–1.5 μg/kg	1–2	iv	
	2–3 μg/kg/hr		iv	Continuous infusion

1. Patients may be aware of the neuraxial opioid concept and request its use in their postoperative management.
2. Despite the absence of confirmation that neuraxial opioid analgesia improves outcome, there is sufficient evidence in the literature to support the increased use of sophisticated techniques to improve the quality of postoperative pain management.

VIII. SPECIAL CONSIDERATIONS IN PEDIATRIC ACUTE PAIN MANAGEMENT

A. A useful monitor of analgesic efficacy in children is **behavior observation**.
B. The selection and dosing of analgesics require special attention in the pediatric patient (Tables 55-18 and 55-19).
C. Oral Analgesics
   1. **Nonopioids** as represented by NSAIDs are useful for acute postoperative pain management in children (ibuprofen, acetaminophen, ketorolac).
   2. **Opioids** such as codeine in combination with acetaminophen are commonly used for management of moderate postoperative pain in children.
D. PCA, often using morphine (loading dose 0.1 to 0.2 mg/kg followed by 10 to 15 μg/kg/hr) may be beneficial.

TABLE 55-19

MAXIMUM LOCAL ANESTHETIC DOSES IN INFANTS AND CHILDREN

Drug	Infant dose (mg/kg): age	Child dose (mg/kg)
Lidocaine	5:from birth on	5
Lidocaine with epinephrine	7:from birth on	7
Mepivacaine	4:<6 months	5
Bupivacaine	2:<3 months	3
Bupivacaine with epinephrine	2:<3 months	4
Chloroprocaine	4:<6 months	8
Chloroprocaine with epinephrine	5:<6 months	10

IX. RELATIONSHIP BETWEEN ACUTE AND CHRONIC PAIN

A. It is generally agreed that pain lasting longer than 6 months can be viewed as chronic.

B. Differentiation between acute and chronic pain is important because therapy is generally vastly different (opioids used to treat chronic pain may lead to tolerance and dependence).

CHAPTER 56 ■ CHRONIC PAIN MANAGEMENT

Perhaps the most common factor associated with treatment failure of chronic pain is the assumption that treatment principles that apply to acute pain management are appropriate for chronic pain (Abram SE: Chronic pain management. In Barash PG, Cullen BF, Stoelting RK [eds]: *Clinical Anesthesia*, pp 1441–1472. Philadelphia, Lippincott Williams & Wilkins, 2006). Persistent pain, especially pain associated with nerve injury, produces significant and often permanent changes in the way the nervous system processes sensory information (Table 56-1). Each patient deserves assessment based on a careful medical, social, and psychological evaluation (rehabilitative therapies, close cooperation between multiple disciplines).

I. PAIN PATHWAYS AND MECHANISMS
(See Chapter 55)

II. MANAGEMENT OF COMMON CHRONIC PAIN SYNDROMES

A. Low Back Pain
1. Several low back structures (annulus of the intervertebral disk, vertebral bodies, facet joints, sacroiliac joint) are innervated by nociceptors and act as sources of pain under certain pathologic conditions.
2. Facet joints receive sensory innervation and, particularly if there are inflammatory changes in the joint, mechanical stimulation may result in pain that may be localized to the back or may radiate to the buttock, thigh, or leg (may account for 40% of patients with low back pain).
3. Mechanical compression of a chronically injured or inflamed nerve root, but not of a normal nerve root, produces sciatica or pain in the sensory distribution of that nerve root.

B. Lumbosacral Radiculopathy
1. Symptoms of lumbosacral radiculopathy consist of varying degrees of low back pain that may radiate to

TABLE 56-1

CHANGES THAT ACCOMPANY PERSISTENT PAIN

Changes in firing thresholds for neurons
Activation of glial cells (production of proinflammatory cytokines that enhance responses to stimulation)
Increased levels of excitatory amino acids in the central nervous system
Neuronal plasticity changes (sprouting of dendrites, ingrowth of sympathetic fibers into dorsal root ganglia)
Hyperalgesia accompanying chronic administration of opioids
Physical and mental changes (inactivity, muscle and tendon shortening, joint dysfunction, social withdrawal, depression)
Risk of opioid addiction (drug diversion may become a source of income)

the lower extremity and in severe cases may be associated with sensory and motor changes (Table 56-2).

2. **Epidural steroid injections** (often with a local anesthetic) may produce beneficial effects (especially with new onset pain), presumably by decreasing the inflammation initiated by either mechanical or chemical insult to the nerve root (Table 56-3). Nevertheless, the beneficial effects of epidural steroid injections are difficult to confirm using controlled randomized studies.

   a. **Methylprednisolone** (80 mg, consider smaller amounts in diabetic patients who may be at increased risk for formation of epidural abscess) is injected into the epidural space as close to the affected nerve root as possible. In occasional patients (especially those with S1 pathology), the drug will not spread adequately to the affected root and caudal injection may result in better drug access to the injured nerve.

   b. The addition of 3 to 4 mL of local anesthetic (lidocaine) to the injected solution produces analgesia, confirming proper drug placement.

   c. Fluoroscopic guidance with a small volume of nonionic radiographic dye is often used to facilitate proper placement of the needle (avoid intravascular or intrathecal placement) and to ensure that the drug reaches the target nerve root. Fluoroscopically controlled techniques are

TABLE 56-2

PAIN DISTRIBUTION AND PHYSICAL SIGNS ASSOCIATED WITH ACUTE DISK HERNIATION

Level of herniation	Pain distribution	Numbness	Weakness	Reflex changes
L3–4 disk (L4 root)	Low back, buttock, lateral thigh, anterior calf, ankle, and occasionally big toe	Lower anterior thigh and patella	Mild (quadriceps)	Diminished (knee jerk)
L4–5 disk (L5 root)	Low back, buttock, lateral thigh, calf, and big toe	Lateral calf, web space of first and second toe	Foot (dorsiflexion)	None
L5–S1 disk (S1 root)	Low back, buttock, posterior thigh, and calf	Posterior calf, lateral heel, and foot	Foot (plantar flexion)	Diminished or absent (ankle jerk)

TABLE 56-3

ALGORITHM FOR TREATMENT OF SCIATICA WITH EPIDURAL STEROID INJECTIONS

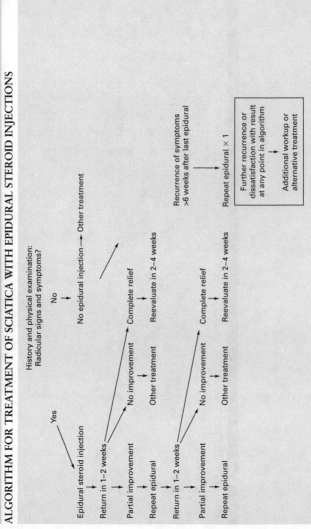

History and physical examination:
Radicular signs and symptoms?

Yes → Epidural steroid injection

No → No epidural injection → Other treatment

Epidural steroid injection

Return in 1–2 weeks
- No improvement → Other treatment
- Partial improvement → Repeat epidural
- Complete relief → Reevaluate in 2–4 weeks

Return in 1–2 weeks
- No improvement → Other treatment
- Partial improvement → Repeat epidural
- Complete relief → Reevaluate in 2–4 weeks

Recurrence of symptoms >6 weeks after last epidural → Repeat epidural × 1

Further recurrence or dissatisfaction with result at any point in algorithm → Additional workup or alternative treatment

especially indicated for patients who have had pervious surgery or who have anatomic conditions that are likely to make a blind epidural difficult.

d. Few patients obtain relief from repeated injections if the first epidural injection was of no help.

e. Patients with chronic radicular pain or previous back surgery may experience relief for several weeks to months (repeat injections every 3 to 4 months).

3. There appears to be little risk of serious complications associated with the use of epidural steroid injections.

a. Suppression of the hypothalamic-pituitary-adrenal axis (accentuated if midazolam is used in conjunction with the epidural steroids) may occur but usually recovers within 1 to 3 months.

b. Aseptic meningitis and bacterial meningitis are uncommon but real risks.

c. The polyethylene glycol vehicle for the epidural steroids does not cause neurologic damage in the doses used.

C. **Lumbosacral arthropathies** (degeneration and inflammation of the lumbar facet joints and sacroiliac joints) may produce low back pain that is difficult to distinguish from radicular pain.

1. Diagnosis is confirmed by injection of local anesthetic (1 mL) into the facet joint, often under fluoroscopic control. This injection may produce pain relief lasting 6 months.

2. Nonsteroidal anti-inflammatory drugs, radiofrequency coagulation, and cryoanalgesia may be of some benefit.

D. **Myofascial pain** is characterized by marked tenderness of discrete points (trigger points) within affected skeletal muscles and the appearance of tight, ropy bands of skeletal muscle. Acute skeletal muscle strain with disruption of sarcoplasmic reticulum and release of calcium and nociceptor-sensitizing substances (prostaglandins, bradykinin, serotonin) may play a role in the development of this pain.

1. **Scapulocostal Syndrome.** A trigger point is located just medial and superior to the upper portion of the scapula. Pain often radiates to the occipital region, shoulder, medial aspect of the arm, or anterior chest wall.

2. Myofascial pain involving gluteal muscles produces pain referred to the posterior thigh and calf, mimicking S1 radiculopathy. Myofascial pain involving the piriform muscle, which overlies the sciatic nerve, can produce sciatic irritation and resembles radiculopathy.

3. **Treatment**
   a. The most important aspect of treatment for myofascial pain is physical therapy designed to restore skeletal muscle strength and elasticity.
   b. Injection of local anesthetic solution directly into the trigger point (daily if necessary) provides analgesia that confirms the diagnosis and permits initiation of physical therapy. Injection of the trigger point with botulinum toxin produces long-lasting pain relief in myofascial syndrome.
   c. Ultrasound therapy, transcutaneous electrical nerve stimulation (TENS), or vapocoolant spray applied over the affected area may also produce periods of analgesia during physical therapy.

E. **Complex Regional Pain Syndromes (CRPS)**
   1. Although autonomic nervous system dysfunction (burning pain, dystrophic changes in skin, skin temperature changes) is evident in some cases of reflex sympathetic dystrophy (CRPS-I) and causalgia (CRPS-II), it is not a prominent feature in some cases and many patients with these conditions fail to respond to blockade or ablation of sympathetic fibers. For this reason, the term CRPS has been widely accepted.
   2. Pain that does not appear to be sympathetically mediated is termed sympathetically independent pain (SIP).
   3. **CRPS-I** (formerly termed reflex sympathetic dystrophy) is a syndrome of pain, autonomic nervous system dysfunction, and dystrophic changes that usually occurs after trauma (crush injuries, lacerations or surgery carpal tunnel release, palmar fasciectomy) (Table 56-4). CRPS-I occasionally occurs after a cerebrovascular accident or myocardial infarction.
      a. **Diagnosis and treatment.** Local anesthetic block of the sympathetic chain (stellate ganglion block or lumbar sympathetic block) is useful as a diagnostic test. Pain relief, however, does not guarantee that

TABLE 56-4

SYMPTOMS OF COMPLEX REGIONAL PAIN SYNDROME-I

Burning pain
Hyperalgesia
Warm and erythematous skin followed by vasoconstriction and
   edema
Bone demineralization
Joint stiffness

there is a sympathetically mediated component of
the patient's pain (placebo effect, spread of local
anesthetic to somatic afferent fibers). Similarly,
failure to achieve pain relief following sympathetic
block does not guarantee that the pain is not
sympathetically mediated (sympathetic efferent
fibers may not travel with the portion of the
sympathetic chain that has been interrupted).

b. Once the diagnosis is confirmed, treatment
consists of a series of sympathetic blocks (three to
seven are usually sufficient) until symptoms
become minimal. Physical therapy and often TENS
are carried out after each sympathetic block.

c. Patients whose condition is diagnosed and treated
early are more likely to respond to sympathetic
blocks (90% response reported). Nevertheless, the
high success rates associated with early
intervention may simply reflect the natural history
of the injury.

d. Surgical or neurolytic sympathectomy is reserved
for patients who do not respond to sympathetic
blocks. Success with sympathetic nerve ablation is
usually transient.

4. **CRPS-II** (formerly termed causalgia) refers to a
syndrome of burning pain and autonomic nervous
system dysfunction resulting from major nerve trunk
injury such as a gunshot wound, which causes a
violent deformation of the involved nerves (brachial
plexus, median nerve, sciatic nerve).

a. Pain often begins immediately after injury and is
commonly accompanied by deep shooting or
stabbing sensations. Movement or SNS activation
(noise, anxiety) often exacerbates pain. There is
usually evidence of decreased SNS activity in the
affected extremity (warm, dry, and venodilated).

Dystrophic changes resemble sympathetic dystrophy.

  b. Treatment with surgical sympathectomy (neurolytic lumbar sympathectomy is an alternative to surgical lumbar sympathectomy) seems to be more successful than local anesthetic-induced blockade.

F. Herpes Zoster

  1. Herpes zoster is caused by the varicella zoster virus, which is dormant in the dorsal root ganglia until immunity declines (advanced age, immunosuppression) and the virus becomes active again.

  2. As the latent virus in the sensory ganglion becomes active (most often thoracic and trigeminal dermatomes), it causes a vesicular skin eruption, inflammation in the dorsal root ganglion, and changes in the peripheral nerve. Patients with severe pain during the acute phase of the disease are more likely to develop persistent pain (postherpetic neuralgia).

  3. **Treatment** is intended to control pain associated with the acute eruption, and, if possible, prevent the occurrence of persistent pain (Table 56-5).

  4. Management of postherpetic neuralgia is often unsatisfactory because some patients respond poorly to nearly every therapy provided (Table 56-6).

TABLE 56-5

TREATMENT AND MANAGEMENT OF PATIENTS WITH ACUTE HERPES

Antiviral drugs

 Acyclovir modestly accelerates rate of cutaneous healing and decreases the severity of acute pain but there is little evidence it decreases the incidence of postherpetic neuralgia

Famcyclovir decreases the incidence of postherpetic neuralgia if initiated soon after the cutaneous eruption

Corticosteroids (systemic, epidural, local infiltration) may decrease the duration of acute pain but a decreased incidence of postherpetic neuralgia is unproven

Sympathetic block (paravertebral sympathetic block) produces dramatic decrease in pain, rapid drying of cutaneous lesions, and prevention of progression to postherpetic neuralgia (unproven if cause and effect or a reflection of the natural course of the disease in individual patients)

TABLE 56-6

TREATMENT AND MANAGEMENT OF PATIENTS WITH POSTHERPETIC NEURALGIA

Tricyclic antidepressants (onset of analgesia is slow often requiring 2–3 weeks)
Anticonvulsants (add to tricyclic antidepressants)
    Carbamazepine
    Valproic acid
    Phenytoin
    Gabapentin
Opioids (rarely of value)
Epidural stimulators (rarely of value)
TENS (may aggravate pain in some patients)

III. PHARMACOLOGIC TREATMENT OF CHRONIC PAIN

  A. **Opioids** prescribed to certain patients for treatment of chronic pain provide good pain control over long periods of time with minimal tolerance and few side effects (cognitive impairment, sedation, nausea, constipation, insomnia, sexual dysfunction).

    1. Predictors of a poor response to opioids are neuropathic pain and phasic pain. Patients with cognitive impairment or high levels of psychological distress are more likely to experience suboptimal pain control from opioids.

    2. A history of substance abuse is associated with a high risk of treatment failure and may be considered a contraindication to management of chronic pain with opioids.

    3. When opioids are prescribed over long intervals, there should be an agreement ("opioid contract") outlining the physician's obligation to continue treatment and the patient's obligation to meet behavioral expectations. Opioid withdrawal is commonly incorporated into chronic pain rehabilitation programs.

  B. **Adjuvant Drugs**

    1. **Tricyclic antidepressants** are useful in treatment of chronic pain presumably producing an analgesic effect via inhibition of the reuptake of serotonin and norepinephrine (increases the levels of these inhibitory neurotransmitters in the brain stem and

TABLE 56-7
SIDE EFFECTS OF ANTIDEPRESSANTS

Antimuscarinic Effects
Xerostomia
Impaired visual accommodation
Urinary retention
Constipation

Antihistaminic Effects
Sedation
Increase in gastric fluid pH

Cardiovascular Effects
Orthostatic hypotension
Cardiac conduction defects (overdose)

spinal cord). Nevertheless, serotonin-specific reuptake inhibitors (fluoxetine) are not predictably effective, suggesting that tricyclic antidepressants may exert their analgesic and antihyperalgesic effects by other mechanisms (binding at N-methyl-D-aspartate receptors).

    a. The clinically relevant benefits of these drugs in patients with chronic pain include normalization of sleep patterns (occurs promptly), reduction in anxiety and depression (delayed onset), and reduction in the perception of pain (delayed onset).

    b. Side effects (Table 56-7)

2. **Anticonvulsants** may have some efficacy in treatment of chronic pain syndromes.

    a. Side effects associated with anticonvulsants are variable and often specific for the specific drug (Table 56-8).

TABLE 56-8
SIDE EFFECTS OF ANTICONVULSANTS

Nausea
Ataxia
Folate deficiency and gingival hyperplasia (phenytoin)
Increased liver transaminase enzyme levels (valproic acid)
Pancytopenia (carbamazepine)
Emotional lability (clonazepam)
Somnolence, ataxia, peripheral edema (gabapentin)
Stevens-Johnson syndrome (lamotrigine)

   b. Gabapentin provides significant pain relief for
   patients with CRPS-I, diabetic neuropathy, and
   postherpetic neuralgia.
3. Sodium channel blocking drugs (systemic lidocaine,
   oral mexiletine) may produce analgesic properties in
   some patients with neuropathic pain.

IV. CANCER PAIN

   A. In assessing patients with malignant disease who seek
   treatment for pain, it is important to determine the
   specific site and mechanism of their pain as well as the
   state (prognosis) of their disease.
   B. Pharmacologic therapy (oral analgesics) is the mainstay
   of treatment of cancer pain, keeping in mind several
   guidelines (Table 56-9).
   1. Patients may experience diminishing analgesic effects
   from oral or parenteral opioids, reflecting either
   tolerance or more often increasing noxious
   stimulation related to tumor spread. When tolerance
   develops, there may be rationale for changing from
   morphine (low intrinsic activity) to fentanyl or
   sufentanil (high intrinsic activity means more
   receptors are occupied).
   2. When oral therapy is not possible or successful, a
   constant intravenous infusion technique is preferable
   to intermittent intramuscular injections.

TABLE 56-9
**GUIDELINES FOR THE TREATMENT OF CANCER PAIN
USING ORAL MEDICATIONS**

Use drugs appropriate for the nature and severity of the patient's
   pain (codeine versus morphine; repeated administration of
   meperidine can result in accumulation of normeperidine, which
   is a central nervous system stimulant)
Use adequate doses (varies tremendously)
Maintain steady blood and tissue medication levels (administering
   analgesics by the clock as treatment invariably results in periods
   of inadequate analgesia [better to administer analgesics as
   needed])
Consider the use of adjuvant drugs (tricyclic antidepressants,
   antiemetics, steroids)
Promptly treat side effects

TABLE 56-10

NONNEUROLYTIC NERVE BLOCKS FOR TREATMENT OF CANCER-RELATED PAIN

Local anesthetic injection or fluorimethane spray of trigger points (myofascial pain common in cancer patients perhaps reflecting bony infiltration, neural compression, or visceral pain)

Transcutaneous electrical nerve stimulation (TENS)

Perineural injection of steroids (tumor compression of nerve roots)

Epidural steroids (radicular pain caused by epidural tumor spread)

Local anesthetic blockade of sympathetic fibers (relieve pain of herpes zoster)

Continuous infusion of local anesthetic solution (monitor vital signs when using thoracic or cervical approaches)

3. **Transdermal fentanyl** offers an alternative to parenteral opioids for patients who are not able to take medication orally.

C. **Intraspinal Opioids**
   1. Morphine is the drug most often selected for epidural or intrathecal administration. The drug may be administered as a bolus, by infusion via an external pump and catheter, or by infusion via a totally implanted pump and catheter.
   2. Withdrawal symptoms may result if neuraxial opioid doses are abruptly decreased or discontinued.
   3. Intrathecal administration of baclofen may have analgesic effects in patients who are resistant or tolerant to opioids. Spasticity associated with multiple sclerosis and spinal cord injury may be decreased by intrathecal baclofen.

D. **Nonneurolytic Nerve Blocks** (Table 56-10)

E. **Neurolytic blocks** are usually reserved for patients with a terminal illness, in view of potential side effects such as loss of motor function and loss of voluntary control over the bowels or bladder.

TABLE 56-11

CHARACTERISTICS OF DRUGS USED FOR NEUROLYTIC BLOCK

Alcohol	Phenol
Pain on injection	No pain on injection
Prompt neurolysis	Neurolysis in about 15 minutes
Hypobaric	Hyperbaric

1. Drugs available for neurolysis are similar in efficacy but possess different characteristics (Table 56-11).
2. Intrathecal neurolysis requires precise positioning to place the affected sensory root uppermost (alcohol) or in the most dependent (phenol) position.

V. PAIN IN HIV/AIDS

A. The most common pain sources associated with human immunodeficiency virus (HIV) are abdominal pain, peripheral neuropathy, throat pain, headache, arthralgia, and herpes zoster-related pain.
B. Psychological sequelae of HIV pain are similar to cancer.
C. Pharmacologic treatment of HIV pain often begins with acetaminophen and nonsteroidal anti-inflammatory drugs (keep in mind the potential drug interaction with acetaminophen and AZT) progressing to use of opioids as necessary.
   1. Dementia may interfere with the ability to use drug therapy.
   2. Nerve blocks are not typically used for HIV-related pain.

VI. PSYCHOLOGICAL INTERVENTIONS FOR CHRONIC PAIN

A. Chronic pain is often accompanied by psychological changes that may with time become more disabling than the somatic pain (Table 56-12).

TABLE 56-12

PSYCHOLOGICAL FACTORS ASSOCIATED WITH CHRONIC PAIN

Mental depression
Loss of appetite
Insomnia
Avoidance of social and vocational obligations
Constant complaining
Dependence on analgesics
Physician shopping

TABLE 56-13

PSYCHOLOGICAL TREATMENTS FOR CHRONIC PAIN

Psychodynamic approaches
Cognitive therapies
Behavioral therapies
Biofeedback
Hypnosis

   B. Psychological treatment requires a knowledge of
   psychoanalytic and therapeutic principles that are also
   time consuming (Table 56-13).

VII. INTERVENTIONAL PAIN MANAGEMENT
   (Table 56-14)

TABLE 56-14

INTERVENTIONAL TECHNIQUES FOR MANAGEMENT OF CHRONIC PAIN

Intrathecal Drug Delivery Devices (external versus implantable)

Opioids (morphine most often selected) act preferentially on receptors in the dorsal horn of the substantia gelatinosa

Intrathecal baclofen used in treatment of spasticity but may provide persistent pain relief in patients who have failed intrathecal morphine treatment

Nociceptive pain is more responsive than neuropathic pain (cancer pain is often mixed and adjuvant therapy often needed)

Contraindications to placement of implantable infusion devices include limited life expectancy (<3 months), sepsis, anticoagulation, immune suppression, drug addiction

Efficacy trials are required prior to pump implantation

Complications following pump implantation include infection, bleeding, seroma formation, and CSF leakage

High dose spinal morphine or hydromorphone has been associated with formation of intrathecal mass lesions (granulomas)

Spinal Cord Stimulation

Efficacy limited to certain types of ischemic and neuropathic pain syndromes

Efficacy trials are required before implantation

Complications are lead migration and breakage with long-term stimulation

Radiofrequency Lesioning

Neurodestructive and more conservative techniques should be tried initially

Requires prior diagnosis with local anesthetic blocks

Lumbar spine often an area for this neurodestructive technique

Minimally Invasive Treatment for Disc Pathology

Discography is a diagnostic procedure to determine if a particular disc is a source of pain

Percutaneous annuloplasty (intradiscal electrothermal therapy)

Percutaneous disc decompression to reduce intradiscal pressure (nucleoplasty)

CHAPTER 57 ■ ANESTHESIA AND CRITICAL CARE MEDICINE

I. **INTRODUCTION: ANESTHESIOLOGISTS AND CRITICAL CARE MEDICINE.** In North America, anesthesiologists were integral to the development of critical care medicine as a specialty (Treggiari M, Deem S: Critical care medicine. In Barash PG, Cullen BF, Stoelting RK [eds]: *Clinical Anesthesia*, pp 1473–1498. Philadelphia, Lippincott Williams & Wilkins, 2006). However, in contrast to other countries, in the United States anesthesiologists have played an ever-diminishing role in the specialty and today comprise a small minority of the intensivist workforce. The driving forces behind intensive care unit (ICU) development included advances in surgical techniques, polio epidemics, which resulted in widespread respiratory failure, and later the recognition of the acute respiratory distress syndrome (ARDS). In the late 1960s, a group including Dr. Peter Safar and another anesthesiologist, Ake Grenvik, was instrumental in inaugurating the Society of Critical Care Medicine (SCCM). Anesthesiologists working through SCCM were instrumental in developing the board certification process for critical care medicine, and in 1986 the first Critical Care Medicine Certification examination was administered by the American Board of Anesthesiology.

II. **ANESTHESIOLOGY AND CRITICAL CARE MEDICINE: THE FUTURE.** Forces that will shape the evolution of the specialty of critical care medicine and the contribution that anesthesiologists will make to this evolution include (1) quality of care issues and the contribution of intensivists to improved ICU outcomes, (2) business/economic factors, and (3) the aging population and increasing demand for critical care services. Mortality and other intermediate end points such as ICU length of stay can be reduced when "high-intensity" physician staffing models that mandate management or co-management by intensivists are used.

A. **The Leapfrog Group** is a coalition of over 150 purchasers and providers of health care benefits with the stated goal to improve health care, in particular by reducing deaths as a result of medical error. To accomplish this aim, the group formulated the Leapfrog Initiative, which includes a series of "safety standards" that health care providers (largely hospitals) should strive for if they are to provide care for Leapfrog Group employees.

B. **Aging Population.** A final, important force driving the evolution of critical care medicine in the United States is the aging population. The predicted insufficient number of intensivists could be met by anesthesiologists who are hospital based and have sound fundamental training in physiology, pharmacology, and invasive procedures and monitoring.

III. CRITICAL CARE MEDICINE: A SYSTEM AND EVIDENCE BASED-APPROACH (Table 57-1)

IV. NEUROLOGICAL AND NEUROSURGICAL CRITICAL CARE

A. **Neuromonitoring** devices used in the ICU setting may help in assessing pathophysiologic processes and adjusting therapy.

TABLE 57-1
EVALUATING EVIDENCE FOR MEDICAL THERAPIES

Levels of Evidence

Large, randomized trials with clear-cut results; low risk of false-positive (alpha) error or false-negative (beta) error

Small, randomized trials with uncertain results; moderate to high risk of false-positive (alpha) and/or false-negative (beta) error

Nonrandomized, contemporaneous controls

Nonrandomized, historical controls and expert opinion

Case series, uncontrolled studies, and expert opinion

Grades of Recommendation Based on Expert Consensus

Supported by two or more Level I studies

Supported by only one Level I study

Supported by Level II studies

Supported by Level III studies

Supported by Level IV or V studies

1. **Transcranial Doppler (TCD) ultrasonography** measures mean, peak systolic and end-diastolic flow velocities and indirectly estimates cerebral blood flow. In patients with subarachnoid hemorrhage or traumatic brain injury (TBI), TCD can be used as a tool to identify vasospasm. In patients with TBI, flow velocities are depressed, and impaired autoregulation and vascular reactivity are common. In these patients, monitoring of TCD and jugular venous oxygen saturation (SjO_2) may be used to define the optimum cerebral perfusion pressure (CPP) level.

2. **Brain tissue oxygenation** ($PbrO_2$) measurements are performed by introducing a small, oxygen-sensitive catheter into the brain tissue (normal $PbrO_2$ values, 25 to 30 mm Hg). An increase in intracranial pressure (ICP) and a decrease in CPP or arterial oxygenation, and hyperventilation may result in decreased $PbrO_2$. CPP >60 mm Hg has been identified as the most important factor determining sufficient brain tissue oxygenation.

3. **Microdialysis** uses a probe as an interface to the brain to continuously monitor the chemistry of a small focal volume of the cerebral extracellular space (allows measurement of chemical substances such as lactate, pyruvate, glucose, glutamate, glycerol, metabolites of several biochemical pathways and electrolytes and thus provides insight into the bioenergetic status of the brain). Increased lactate, decreased glucose, and an elevated lactate/glucose ratio indicate accelerated anaerobic glycolysis. This metabolic pattern commonly occurs with cerebral ischemia or hypoxia, and increased glycolysis in this setting is associated with a poor outcome.

B. **Diagnosis and Clinical Management of the Most Common Types of Neurological Failure**

1. **Traumatic brain injury** is the leading cause of death from blunt trauma, and in patients between the age of 5 and 45 years, TBI represents the leading cause of death (Table 57-2).

   a. **Resuscitation.** The goal of resuscitation in traumatic and other types of brain injury is to prevent continuing cerebral insult after a primary injury has already occurred. A primary insult is often associated with intracranial hypertension

TABLE 57-2

**PREDICTORS OF POOR OUTCOME FOLLOWING
TRAUMATIC BRAIN INJURY**

Age >55 years
Poor pupillary reactivity (bilateral dilated and unreactive
 associated with poor neurological outcome and death as high
 as 90%)
Postresuscitation Glasgow Coma Scale score (most widely used
 measure of injury severity, may be unmeasurable initially,
 injury is severe when score is 8 or less)
Hypotension
Hypoxia
Unfavorable intracranial diagnosis based on radiologic features
 (CT scan, degree of diffuse injury and midline shift)
Hyperglycemia (>200 mg/dL)

and systemic hypotension, leading to decreased cerebral perfusion and brain ischemia. Concomitant hypoxemia aggravates brain hypoxia, especially in the presence of hyperthermia, which increases brain metabolic demand. The combined effect of these factors leads to secondary brain injury characterized by excitotoxicity, oxidative stress, and inflammation. The resulting cerebral ischemia may be the single most important secondary event affecting outcome following a cerebral insult.

 b. **Prevention of secondary injury** is the main goal of resuscitative efforts. Traumatized areas of the brain manifest impaired autoregulation, with increased dependency of flow on perfusion pressure, and disruption of the blood-brain barrier. The goals of neuroresuscitation are oriented at restoration of cerebral blood flow by maintenance of adequate CPP, reduction of ICP, evacuation of space occupying lesions, and initiation of therapies for cerebral protection, and avoidance of hypoxia (Table 57-3).

 c. **Drug-induced sedation.** A common practice is to provide sedation with propofol or benzodiazepines in patients following TBI. These agents have favorable effects on cerebral oxygen balance. Despite the induction of systemic hypotension, propofol decreases cerebral

TABLE 57-3

ICU MANAGEMENT OF PATIENTS WITH SEVERE
TRAUMATIC BRAIN INJURY (ASSUMING INITIAL SURGICAL
MANAGEMENT)

Head elevation 30–45°
CPP >70 mm Hg
Euvolemia, vasopressors as needed
ICP <20 mm Hg
   Mannitol, hypertonic saline
   CSF drainage
SaO_2 ≥95%; $PaCO_2$ 35–40 mm Hg
Temperature ≤37°C
Glucose < 180 mg/dL
Sedation and analgesia
Early enteral nutrition
Seizure, stress ulcer, and deep vein thrombosis prophylaxis
Refractory intracranial hypertension
   Optimized hyperventilation with SjO_2 and/or $PbrO_2$
      monitoring
   Barbiturate coma
   Mild therapeutic hypothermia (33°–35°C)
   Decompressive craniectomy

metabolism, resulting in a coupled decline in cerebral blood flow, with consequent decrease in ICP. Barbiturates should be considered if ICP is not controlled by moderate doses of propofol. Although neuromuscular blockade may result in a fall in ICP, the routine use of neuromuscular blockade is discouraged since its use has been associated with longer intensive care unit course, a higher incidence of pneumonia, and a trend toward more frequent sepsis without any improvement in outcome.

d. **Hyperventilation** effectively reduces ICP by reducing CBF but in small randomized trials, prophylactic hyperventilation has not proven to be beneficial in TBI. Prolonged or prophylactic hyperventilation should be avoided after severe TBI. Hyperventilation may be necessary for brief periods to reduce intracranial hypertension refractory to sedation, osmotic therapy, and CSF drainage, and should be guided by SjO_2 and/or

PbrO$_2$ (fall in either of these values suggests a harmful effect of hyperventilation).

   e. Hypothermia. There is insufficient evidence to provide recommendations for the use of moderate hypothermia in patients with TBI.

   f. Corticosteroids to reduce posttraumatic inflammatory injury should not be administered as therapy for acute TBI.

2. **Subarachnoid hemorrhage** (SAH) is most commonly caused by the rupture of an intracranial aneurysm with only one-third of the patients suffering from SAH being functional survivors. The leading causes of death and disability are the direct effect of the initial bleed, cerebral vasospasm, and rebleeding. At the time of aneurysm rupture, there is a critical reduction in CBF because of an increase in ICP toward arterial diastolic values. The persistence of a no-flow pattern is associated with acute vasospasm.

   In survivors of the initial bleed, emphasis has been placed on early aneurysm securing with either surgery or interventional neuroradiology (coiling). Early aneurysm occlusion substantially reduces the risk of this rebleeding.

   a. Cerebral vasospasm after SAH is correlated with the amount and location of subarachnoid blood. A reduction in cerebral blood flow is ultimately responsible for the appearance of *delayed ischemic neurological deficits (DINDs)*. Oral nimodipine (60 mg every 4 hours for 21 days) as prophylaxis for cerebral vasospasm is recognized as an effective treatment in improving neurological outcome (reduction of cerebral infarction and poor outcome) and mortality from cerebral vasospasm in patients suffering from SAH. The benefits of nimodipine have been attributed to a cytoprotective effect related to the reduced availability of intracellular calcium, and improved microvascular collateral flow.

   b. Hypervolemic/hypertensive and hemodilution ("triple-H") therapy is one of the mainstays of treatment for cerebral ischemia associated with SAH-induced vasospasm despite the lack of evidence for its effectiveness. The rationale for hypertension derives from the concept that a loss of cerebral autoregulation associated with vasospasm results in pressure-dependent blood flow. Hemodilution is a consequence of hypervolemic therapy and is thought to optimize the rheologic properties of the blood and thereby improve microcirculatory flow. Common complications of treatment are pulmonary edema and myocardial ischemia.

  c. **Interventional neuroradiology** with the use of balloon angioplasty (within 6 to 12 hours) can reverse or improve vasospasm-induced neurological deficits.

  d. **Hyponatremia** usually develops several days after the hemorrhage, and is attributed to a syndrome of inappropriate antidiuretic hormone secretion (SIADH) and an excess of free water.

3. **Acute Ischemic Stroke.** More than half of strokes can be attributed to a thrombotic mechanism. Transient ischemic attacks may precede stroke and thus should be considered a warning sign.

  a. **Thrombolysis.** Rapid clot lysis and restoration of circulation using alteplase (rt-PA) should be provided within 3 hours of stroke onset. Patients receiving systemic rt-PA should not receive aspirin, heparin, warfarin, clonidine, or other antithrombotic or antiplatelet aggregating drugs within 24 hours of treatment. Because hyperglycemia is associated with poor outcome in ischemic stroke, tight glucose control is recommended.

4. **Anoxic brain injury** most commonly occurs as a result of cardiac arrest. The pathophysiology of anoxic brain injury is multifactorial and includes excitatory neurotransmitter release, accumulation of intracellular calcium, and oxygen-free radical generation. A strong experimental literature supports a protective role for mild therapeutic hypothermia in anoxic brain injury (temperature 32°C to 34°C).

V. CARDIOVASCULAR AND HEMODYNAMIC ASPECTS OF CRITICAL CARE

  A. **Principles of Monitoring and Resuscitation.** Shock states are associated with impairment of adequate oxygen delivery, resulting in decreased tissue perfusion and tissue hypoxia (global hemodynamic monitoring may not reflect regional perfusion or the peripheral tissue energy status). Invasive monitoring in shock states provides insight into the circulatory status, organ perfusion, tissue microcirculation, and cellular metabolic status of the critically ill patient.

B. **Functional Hemodynamic Monitoring**

1. **Pulmonary Artery Catheter (PAC).** The information provided by the PAC may assist in the differentiation of cardiogenic and noncardiogenic circulatory and respiratory failure, and help guide fluid, inotropic, and vasopressor therapy. Despite the theoretical benefits of pulmonary artery catheterization, there are few data to support a positive effect of the PAC on mortality or other substantive outcome variables. There is increasing evidence that central venous and PA pressures do not predict the hemodynamic response to intravenous fluid administration in normal subjects or patients with shock. A consensus conference on the use of the PAC concluded that the catheter should only be used when noninvasive methods are not available to provide the information required.

2. **Fiberoptic Central Venous Catheter.** A less invasive and less costly alternative to placing a PAC for the measurement of SvO_2 is to measure central venous oxygen saturation $(ScvO_2)$ via a fiberoptic central venous catheter (target is an $ScvO_2 > 70\%$).

3. **Arterial Pressure Waveform Analysis.** The variation in systolic blood pressure and pulse pressure during positive-pressure ventilation is highly predictive (superior to static measures such as CVP and PaOP) of the response to intravascular fluid administration in both normal subjects and critically ill patients. Cardiac output derived using pulse contour analysis correlates well with thermodilution cardiac output in a variety of conditions, and has the advantage of providing continuous measurement without necessitating the placement of a PAC. The use of pulse contour analysis may potentially obviate the need for pulmonary artery catheterization to measure cardiac output, particularly if combined with the measurement of $ScvO_2$ as an indicator of the balance between oxygen delivery and consumption.

4. **Echocardiography.** Transthoracic and transesophageal echocardiography provide accurate noninvasive diagnostic information with regard to right and left ventricular function, valve function, pericardium anatomy, traumatic vascular injury, and pulmonary embolism (direct and indirect signs). Transesophageal echocardiography can also be used to assess volume status or preload via measurement of left-ventricular end-diastolic volume and/or area.

C. **Definition and Types of Circulatory Failure.** The common denominator of shock is circulatory instability characterized by severe hypotension and inadequate tissue perfusion. Shock states are classified according to the primary cause of circulatory failure. Distributive or vasodilatory shock results from a reduction in systemic vascular resistance, often associated with an increased cardiac output, whereas cardiogenic (left or right cardiac failure) and hypovolemic shock are low cardiac output states usually characterized by increased peripheral resistance. The most common forms of shock encountered in the ICU are cardiogenic, septic, and hypovolemic shock.

1. **Cardiogenic Shock.** The initiating event in cardiogenic shock is a primary pump failure (myocardial infarction, cardiomyopathy, arrhythmias, mechanical complications [mitral regurgitation, ventricular septal defect], tamponade). The onset of pump failure is associated with a compensatory reflex vasoconstriction in systemic vessels causing an increase in left ventricular workload and myocardial oxygen demand and a redistribution of blood volume toward the heart and the lungs. Consequently, therapy should minimize myocardial oxygen demand and raise oxygen delivery to the ischemic area; this goal is complicated by the fact that many resuscitative approaches to correct hypotension (preload augmentation, inotropes and vasopressors; see below) increase myocardial oxygen consumption. In patients without hypotension, pharmacological vasodilatation using nitrates or sodium nitroprusside may reduce myocardial oxygen consumption and improve ventricular ejection by reducing left ventricular afterload, and possibly produce a shift of blood from the lungs to

the periphery by reducing venous tone. When pharmacologic interventions are not sufficient to restore hemodynamic stability, the use of mechanical support with the insertion of intra-aortic balloon pump counterpulsation and ventricular assist devices can help unload the ventricles. In patients with myocardial infarction, coronary reperfusion can be achieved with thrombolysis or, preferably, primary percutaneous coronary intervention.

2. **Septic shock** is a form of distributive shock associated with the activation of the systemic inflammatory response and is usually characterized by a high cardiac output, low systemic vascular resistance, hypotension, and regional blood flow redistribution, resulting in tissue hypoperfusion. In patients with systemic infections, the physiologic response can be staged on a continuum from a systemic inflammatory response syndrome (SIRS) to sepsis, severe sepsis, and septic shock (Table 57-4). Multiple organ dysfunction syndrome (MODS) refers to the presence of altered organ function in an acutely ill patient such that homeostasis cannot be maintained without intervention. MODS accounts for most deaths in the intensive care unit.

D. **Clinical Management of Shock/Circulatory Failure Based on Hemodynamic Parameters.** The mainstay of treatment of hemodynamic instability is correction of hypotension and restoration of regional blood flow with intravascular volume expansion and vasopressors, and/or inotropes. Adequacy of regional perfusion is usually assessed by evaluating indices of organ function, including myocardial ischemia, renal dysfunction (urine output and renal function tests), arterial lactate levels as an indicator of anaerobic metabolism, central nervous system dysfunction as indicated by abnormal sensorium, and hepatic parenchymal injury by liver function tests. Additional end points of treatment consist of mean arterial pressure and oxygen delivery (DO_2), or some surrogate of the latter (SvO_2 or $ScvO_2$).

1. **Management of Hypotension with Fluid Replacement Therapy.** Intravascular volume expansion is the first line of therapy in all forms of shock. Clinical indicators of the response to a fluid challenge (bolus fluid therapy of 250 to 1,000 mL crystalloids over 5 to 15 minutes) are heart rate,

TABLE 57-4

DEFINITIONS OF SEPSIS AND ORGAN FAILURE

Clinical evidence of infection:
  Infection: Microbial phenomenon characterized by an
    inflammatory response to the presence of microorganisms or
    the invasion of normally sterile tissue by those organisms.
  Bacteremia: Presence of viable bacteria in the blood.

Systemic inflammatory response syndrome (SIRS): Systemic
  inflammatory response to a variety of severe clinical insults. The
  response is manifested by two or more of the following
  conditions:
  Core temperature <36°C or >38°C
  Tachycardia >90 beats/min
  Tachypnea >20 breaths/min while breathing spontaneously, or
    $PaCO_2$ <4.3 kPa
  White blood count > 12,000 cells/mm^3, <4,000 cells/mm^3, or
    >10% immature forms

Sepsis: The systemic response to infection. This systemic response is
  manifested by three or more of the conditions described above
  (SIRS) and clinical or microbiological evidence of infection.

Severe sepsis: Sepsis associated with organ dysfunction,
  hypoperfusion, or hypotension. Hypoperfusion and perfusion
  abnormalities may include, but are not limited to, lactic acidosis,
  oliguria, or an acute alteration in mental status.

Septic shock: Sepsis with hypotension, despite adequate fluid
  resuscitation, along with the presence of perfusion abnormalities
  that may include, but are not limited to: lactic acidosis, oliguria,
  or an acute alteration in mental status. Patients who are on
  inotropic or vasopressor agents may not be hypotensive at the
  time that perfusion abnormalities are measured.

Sepsis-induced hypotension: A systolic BP of <90 mm Hg or a
  reduction of >40 mm Hg from baseline in the absence of other
  causes for hypotension.

Multiple organ dysfunction syndrome: Presence of several altered
  organ function in an acutely ill patient such that homeostasis
  cannot be maintained without intervention.

blood pressure, and urine output as well as
invasively acquired measures including CVP,
pulmonary artery occlusion pressure, systolic and
pulse pressure variation, and cardiac output.
2. **Management of Shock with Vasopressors/Inotropes.**
   If patients remain persistently hypotensive despite

volume expansion and markers of adequate preload, the use of vasopressors is indicated.

a. **Norepinephrine** (NE) increases systemic arterial pressure, with variable effects on cardiac output and heart rate. A concern that NE may compromise renal perfusion has led to some hesitancy to use this drug; however, the majority of available evidence suggests that NE improves renal function in volume-resuscitated, hypotensive patients with septic shock. NE is the drug of first choice in the management of septic shock.

b. **Dopamine** raises mean arterial pressure by increasing cardiac index and less so systemic vascular resistance. Comparing low-dose dopamine to placebo in critically ill patients shows no differences in either renal function tests or survival, and the use of low-dose dopamine is therefore not recommended. In addition, dopamine may have detrimental effects on the splanchnic circulation and gastric mucosal perfusion.

c. **Dobutamine** demonstrates potent inotropic and chronotropic effects, and mild peripheral vasodilatation, with the ultimate effect of increasing oxygen delivery and consumption. Dobutamine is the drug of choice in patients with circulatory failure primarily because of cardiac pump failure (cardiogenic shock). However, dobutamine should not be used as first-line single therapy when hypotension is present.

d. **Epinephrine** increases cardiac index by increasing contractility and heart rate, and also increases systemic vascular resistance. In patients with septic shock, epinephrine may reduce splanchnic perfusion despite an increase in global hemodynamic and oxygen transport. In addition, epinephrine therapy consistently increases plasma lactate levels in septic shock. Epinephrine treatment brings no additional benefit to other catecholamine therapy in the management of patients with septic shock.

e. **Vasopressin** is a potent vasoconstrictor when administered in low doses to patients in shock, particularly those with distributive shock as a result of sepsis or hepatic failure, or with circulatory failure following cardiopulmonary bypass. Vasopressin may also be useful in resuscitation from cardiac arrest, particularly asystole. Vasopressin administration during shock typically results in dramatically increased systemic blood pressure, with either no effect or a mild decrease in cardiac output, little change in heart rate, and no effect on pulmonary vascular resistance. The use of vasopressin is currently reserved for cases of catecholamine-refractory shock.

3. **Additional Treatment Considerations for Critically Ill Patients with Septic Shock.**
   a. **Activated Protein C.** Clinical or subclinical manifestations of intravascular disseminated coagulation and consumption coagulopathy (increase in D-dimers, decreased protein C, thrombocytopenia, and increased prothrombin time) are present in essentially all patients with septic shock. The activation of protein C is thought to be an important mechanism for modulating sepsis-induced consumption coagulopathy. Activated protein C works as an antithrombotic agent by inactivating factors Va and VIIIa. The rationale for replacing activated protein C relates to its anticoagulant and profibrinolytic properties, which interrupt the consumption coagulopathy and are particularly effective at preventing microvascular thrombosis.
   b. **Corticosteroids** are of no benefit for the treatment of septic shock but low doses (hydrocortisone 200 to 300 mg per day) can reduce dependency on vasopressors.
   c. **Treatment of Infection.** Identifying the source of the infection, source control, and early initiation of appropriate antibiotic therapy are critical priorities in addition to hemodynamic support. Empiric antibiotic therapy should be started as soon as possible after appropriate culture collection.

VI. **ACUTE RESPIRATORY FAILURE** is a generic term that encompasses the need for mechanical ventilation and/or airway intubation, independent of cause.

A. **Principles of Mechanical Ventilation.** Mechanical ventilation in the ICU is provided through the application of positive pressure to the airway; commonly a preset tidal volume and rate are provided, and any breathing that the patient does above this set minute ventilation is either supported (assist-control; AC) or not (intermittent mandatory ventilation; IMV). There is little evidence to suggest that the mode of mechanical ventilation contributes significantly to any major outcome measure. Mechanical ventilation utilizing tidal volumes of 10 to 15 mL/kg may be injurious in certain settings.

  1. **Air-trapping** and auto-PEEP (positive end-expiratory pressure) leads to significant morbidity and mortality in patients with obstructive lung disease. Ventilatory strategy in these patients should focus on prolongation of expiratory time by limiting minute ventilation by using low tidal volumes (6 to 8 mL/kg or less) and a low breathing rate (8 to 12 breaths per minute), and by reducing the inspiratory time of the respiratory cycle. In order to accomplish these goals, deep sedation is often required, and rarely neuromuscular blockade must be used. Separation from mechanical ventilation is expedited when respiratory therapy–driven protocols are used that focus on daily assessment of the ability to breath without assistance, assuming improvement of the inciting process, adequate oxygenation, and hemodynamic stability (Grade A recommendation). Once the patient can breathe comfortably for 30 to 120 minutes without support, the trachea can be extubated, assuming that there are not other precluding factors such as airway abnormalities and coma.

B. **Acute Lung Injury (ALI) and Acute Respiratory Distress Syndrome (ARDS)** are characterized by acute hypoxemic respiratory failure and diffuse alveolar damage, with resulting increased lung permeability and diffuse alveolar edema. and mortality in ARDS and ALI appear to be similar. The treatment of ALI/ARDS is largely supportive and includes aggressive treatment of inciting events, avoidance of complications, and mechanical ventilation. It is critical that tidal volumes (6 mL/kg or less) and static ventilatory pressures

($\leq$30 cm H_2O) are minimized in order to avoid further injury to the remaining relatively uninjured lung. Since ARDS is marked by high intrapulmonary shunt, hypoxemia is relatively unresponsive to oxygen therapy. Thus, strategies to recruit collapsed lung are necessary. This is most commonly achieved by using PEEP. Long-term outcome benefits of inhaled nitric oxide have not been demonstrated, although inhaled nitric oxide may still be useful as "rescue" therapy in selected patients with severe, refractory hypoxemia.

VII. **ACUTE RENAL FAILURE** (ARF) is reported to occur in as many as 25% of critically ill patients. Mortality associated with ARF requiring dialysis has remained approximately 60% for nearly five decades. In the ICU, ARF occurs because of pre-renal causes and tubular injury (acute tubular necrosis; ATN) in the vast majority of cases. Urine sodium concentration and fractional excretion of sodium can help identify pre-renal azotemia (Table 57-5).

   A. **Treatment.** In incipient and established ARF, supportive care is the rule, with the focus on maintenance of euvolemia, avoidance of renal toxins, adjustment of medication doses, and monitoring of electrolytes and acid base status. Pharmacologic approaches to the prevention and treatment of ARF have been uniformly disappointing including low-dose dopamine. Diuretics may in fact be harmful in early ARF, and their use should probably be restricted to the treatment of hypervolemia prior to the institution of dialysis or ultrafiltration. The weight of evidence supports an increased intensity of dialysis.

VIII. **ENDOCRINE ASPECTS OF CRITICAL CARE MEDICINE**

   A. **Glucose Management in Critical Illness.** Hyperglycemia is associated with increased risk of postoperative infection (wound and otherwise), and poor outcome in patients with stroke or TBI. Strict glycemic control in critically ill patients is likely to confer substantial outcome benefits. Data clearly favor an aggressive approach to blood glucose control in the ICU.

TABLE 57-5

URINALYSIS, URINE CHEMISTRIES, AND OSMOLALITY IN ACUTE RENAL FAILURE

	Hypovolemia	Acute tubular necrosis	Acute interstitial nephritis	Glomerulonephritis	Obstruction
Sediment	Bland	Broad, brownish granular casts	WBCs, eosinophils, cellular casts	RBCs, RBC casts	Blood or bloody
Protein	None or low	None or low	Minimal but may be ↑ with NSAIDs	Increased, >100 mg/dL	Low
Urine Na +, mEq/L[a]	<20 <40 (days)	>30	>30	<20	<20 (Acute)
Urine osmolality, mOsm/kg	>400	<350	<350	>400	<350
FENa+, %[b]	<1	>1	Varies	<1	<1 (Acute) >1 (days)

WBCs, white blood cells; RBCs, red blood cells; NSAIDs, nonsteroidal anti-inflammatory drugs.

[a] The sensitivity and specificity of urine sodium of less than 20 in differentiating pre-renal azotemia from acute tubular necrosis are 90% and 82%, respectively.

[b] FENa+, Fractional excretion of sodium is the urine to plasma (U/P) of sodium divided by U/P of creatinine × 100. The sensitivity and specificity of fractional excretion of sodium is the urine to plasma (U/P) of sodium divided by U/P of creatinine × 100. The sensitivity and specificity of fractional excretion of sodium of less than 1% in differentiating pre-renal azotemia from acute tubular necrosis are 96% and 95%, respectively.

B. **Adrenal Function in Critical Illness.** The stress response to injury includes an increase in serum cortisol levels in most critically ill patients. Adrenal insufficiency may also occur in critically ill patients reflecting inhibition of adrenal stimulation or corticosteroid synthesis by drugs or cytokines and direct injury to or infection of the pituitary or adrenal glands. Until free cortisol assays are more widely available, the diagnosis of adrenal insufficiency in critical illness must be based on clinical suspicion and total cortisol levels. Adrenal insufficiency should be considered in all critically ill patients with pressor-dependent shock.

C. **Thyroid function in Critical Illness.** Depression of T3 occurs within hours of injury or illness and can persist for weeks. Low thyroid hormone levels, particularly for T3, correlate with the severity of illness and are associated with an increased risk of death. Hypothyroidism elevation of TSH in the presence of a low T4 level may be present in the critically ill, particularly in the geriatric population, and should be considered in the face of refractory shock, adrenal insufficiency, unexplained coma, and prolonged, unexplained respiratory failure.

D. **Somatotropic Function in Critical Illness.** Growth hormone levels are low in prolonged critical illness.

IX. **ANEMIA AND TRANSFUSION THERAPY IN CRITICAL ILLNESS.** The vast majority of patients admitted to the ICU are anemic at some point in their hospital stay, and more than one-third of them will receive transfused blood. The cause of anemia in critical illness is multifactorial and related to blood loss from the primary injury or illness, iatrogenic blood loss because of daily blood sampling, and nutritional deficiencies (folate). It is assumed that critically ill patients have less efficient compensatory mechanisms and reduced physiologic reserve, and thereby require a higher hemoglobin (Hb) concentration than unstressed individuals. Data collected from ICUs at multiple centers in the United States suggest that the transfusion trigger is nearer 8.6 g/dL than the previously recommended 7 g/dL. Hb is an important DO_2, and transfusion is an integral component of goal-directed therapeutic strategies that aim to optimize DO_2 in early shock states.

X. **NUTRITION IN THE CRITICALLY ILL PATIENT.** Poor nutritional status is associated with increased mortality and morbidity among critically ill patients (adequate nutritional support should be considered a standard of care). Enteral nutrition is preferred over parenteral nutrition whenever possible because of its lower cost and less frequent complications.

A. **Complications** associated with enteral feedings include aspiration of gastric feeding, diarrhea, and fluid and electrolyte imbalance. To prevent aspiration with gastric feeding, the head of the patient's bed should be raised 30° to 45° during feeding; jejunal access can be considered in patients with recurrent tube-feeding aspiration. To prevent or reduce diarrhea, all potential etiologies should be considered and corrected.

XI. **SEDATION OF THE CRITICALLY ILL PATIENT.** Critically ill patients are often deeply sedated because of potential benefits afforded by a reduction in the sympathoadrenal response to injury. Additionally, complications associated with undersedation include ventilator dysynchrony, patient injury, agitation, anxiety, stress disorders, and, possibly, unplanned extubation. Recent studies have tempered the enthusiasm for deep sedation in the ICU (daily interruption of continuous sedative and analgesic drug infusions was effective in reducing the length of mechanical ventilation and length of ICU stay). It is important to titrate medications according to established therapeutic goals and reevaluate the sedation requirements frequently (Ramsay sedation scale).

A. **Confusion and agitation** are common in ICU patients and could have unfavorable consequences on patient outcome. Agitation needs to be distinguished from delirium, which is relatively common in ICU patients and equally associated with increased length of stay, morbidity, and mortality. The distinguishing characteristics of delirium include acute onset and fluctuating course, inattention, disorganized thinking, and altered level of consciousness.

B. **Nonpharmacological and pharmacological** means can be used to provide comfort and safety to ICU patients. The former include communication and frequent

reorientation, maintenance of a day-night cycle, noise
reduction, and ensuring ventilation synchrony.
Pharmacological agents include hypnotics-anxiolytics,
opioids, and antipsychotics.
1. **Hypnotics** most commonly used are propofol,
   midazolam, and lorazepam (despite the observation
   that oversedation occurred twice as often with
   lorazepam than with propofol or midazolam).
2. **Dexmedetomidine** has been effectively used as a
   single agent or in combination with other drugs in
   postsurgical and medical ICU patients.
3. **Opioids.** Morphine and fentanyl are the most
   commonly used opioids to provide analgesia in the
   ICU. Morphine should be avoided in patients with
   renal failure as a result of active metabolites that
   accumulate in the presence of impaired renal
   elimination.
4. **Neuromuscular blockade** may be occasionally
   indicated in ICU patients with severe TBI or
   respiratory failure, but routine use is discouraged
   because of concerns that this practice may
   predispose to critical illness polyneuropathy and
   myopathy and because of an increased risk of
   nosocomial pneumonia in patients receiving these
   agents.

XII. COMPLICATIONS IN THE ICU: DETECTION, PREVENTION, AND THERAPY

A. **Nosocomial infections** are a major source of morbidity
   and mortality in the critically ill. At some level,
   nosocomial infections are unavoidable and occur
   because of the nature of intensive care: patients are
   critically ill with altered host defenses, they require
   invasive devices (endotracheal tubes, intravascular
   catheters) for support, they receive monitoring and
   therapy that provide portals of entry for infectious
   organisms, and they receive therapies that increase the
   risk of infection (glucocorticoids, parenteral nutrition).
   On the other hand, many nosocomial infections are
   preventable with relatively simple interventions.
   1. **Sinusitis** is common in critically ill patients with
      indwelling oral and nasal tubes. Prevention of
      sinusitis should focus on efforts to improve sinus
      drainage, including semirecumbent positioning and

avoidance of nasal tubes. Bacterial sinusitis should be considered in patients with unexplained fever and leukocytosis in the ICU.

2. **Ventilator-Associated Pneumonia (VAP).** Endotracheal intubation and mechanical ventilation increase the risk of VAP. Interventions that can reduce the incidence of VAP include strict hand washing between patients and semirecumbent positioning of the patient (head height at 30° or greater from horizontal) (Level II evidence). These practices should be rigorously applied in all ICUs (granted that semirecumbent positioning is not possible in all patients). Acid-suppression therapies as prophylaxis against gastrointestinal bleeding have been associated with an increased risk of VAP because they allow bacterial overgrowth in the stomach (sucralfate should be considered as an alternative agent to acid-suppressive regimens). An important approach to reduce the overall mortality from VAP involves refinement of the diagnostic process and limitation of antibiotic therapy to avoid the development of antibiotic resistance. Antibiotics can be narrowed in spectrum or discontinued depending on the results from quantitative cultures after 48 to 72 hours.

3. **Intravascular catheter–associated bacteremia** is strictly defined as clinical suspicion of catheter-related infection plus positive culture of blood drawn from the catheter or of a segment of catheter and matching positive blood culture drawn from another site. Catheter infection is more likely when placement occurs under emergency conditions, and is reduced by the use of strict aseptic technique with full barrier precautions. Catheter-related infection and bacteremia increase with the duration of catheterization, particularly for durations of greater than 2 days. However, routine catheter replacement at 3 or 7 days does not reduce the incidence of infection, and results in increased mechanical complications. Thus, routine guidewire change of catheters is not recommended. Catheters coated with either antiseptics (chlorhexidine and silver sulfadiazine) or antibiotics (rifampin and minocycline) reduce catheter-related infection and bacteremia (consider use of these catheters if

placement longer than 2 days is anticipated). Based on incidence of infection at the insertion site, the subclavian route should be used when possible if the duration of catheterization is predicted to be longer than 2 days. Catheter-related venous thrombosis occurs commonly, and is associated with an increased risk of infection. Routine flushing of catheter ports with heparin reduces both the incidence of thrombosis and infection. When catheter-related bacteremia is confirmed, the offending catheter should be removed and appropriate antibiotics continued for a minimum of 7 days.

4. **Urinary tract infection** is the second most common source of infection in the ICU and the incidence increases with the duration of bladder catheterization.

5. **Invasive fungal infections** in nonneutropenic patients as caused by *Candida* species in the vast majority of cases, is increasingly common in the ICU population, and accounts for 5 to 10% of all blood stream infections in the ICU. A high level of suspicion for invasive *Candida* infection in critically ill patients is necessary, and "preemptive" therapy should be considered in patients with a high likelihood of invasive *Candida* infection while awaiting blood culture results. An ophthalmologic exam is warranted in patients with documented or suspected blood stream infection, as patients with endopthalmitis may require longer courses of therapy. Intravascular catheters that are potential sources of blood stream infection should be removed. Organisms sensitive to the azole derivative fluconazole cause the majority of invasive *Candida* infections in the ICU, and fluconazole is the first-line treatment given its reasonable efficacy and limited toxicity.

B. **Stress Ulceration and Gastrointestinal Hemorrhage.** Gastric mucosal breakdown with resulting gastritis and ulceration ("stress ulceration") can lead to gastrointestinal (GI) bleeding in the ICU. The major risk factors for stress-related GI bleeding are mechanical ventilation and coagulopathy; secondary risk factors among mechanically ventilated patients include renal failure, thermal injury, and possibly head injury. Enteral nutrition may protect against significant GI bleeding.

1. **Prevention.** Agents used to prevent stress ulceration and GI bleeding include methods to suppress acid production (H2 blockers and proton pump inhibitors) and cytoprotective agents (sucralfate). The agent of choice—and whether any prophylaxis is beneficial or indicated—is somewhat controversial. It appears that stress ulcer prophylaxis is more widely used than necessary. Thus, although stress ulcer prophylaxis, predominantly with ranitidine, is commonly used in critically ill patients, the utility of this intervention is unclear.

C. **Venous thromboembolism** (VTE) occurs frequently in critically ill patients, with incidences of deep venous thrombosis (DVT) of 10 to 30% and of pulmonary embolism (PE) of 1.5 to 5%. In addition to classic lower extremity DVT, upper extremity DVT occurs with increased frequency in the ICU population. This is directly associated with the use of central venous catheters in the subclavian and internal jugular sites. Upper extremity DVT can result in pulmonary embolism in up to two thirds of cases, with occasional fatalities.

1. **Prophylaxis.** The risks of VTE prophylaxis, including heparin-induced thrombocytopenia and bleeding, must be weighed when considering prophylaxis in the ICU population. Nonetheless, it is generally agreed that high-risk patients without contraindications should receive prophylaxis with low-molecular weight heparin (LMWH), and that patients with low-to-moderate risk should receive low dose unfractionated heparin (UFH) (Table 57-6). To reduce central venous catheter–associated thrombosis and infection, catheter tips should be positioned in the superior vena cava and catheters should be flushed with a dilute heparin solution. Heparin bonding of catheters may also reduce local thrombosis.

2. **Diagnosis.** Despite the high incidence of DVT, routine screening studies for DVT do not appear to improve clinical outcomes in the ICU. VTE should be considered in critically ill patients in the face of relatively nonspecific findings, such as unexplained tachycardia, tachypnea, fever, asymmetric extremity

TABLE 57-6
RISK FACTORS FOR VENOUS THROMBOEMBOLISM

Strong Risk Factors
Fracture (hip or leg)
Hip or knee replacement
Major trauma
Spinal cord injury

Moderate Risk Factors
Arthroscopic knee surgery
Central venous lines
Chemotherapy
Congestive heart or respiratory failure
Hormone replacement therapy
Malignancy
Oral contraceptive therapy
Paralytic stroke
Pregnancy/postpartum
Previous venous thromboembolism
Thrombophilia

Weak Risk Factors
Bed rest >3 days
Immobility as a result of sitting (prolonged car or air travel)
Increasing age
Laparoscopic surgery (cholecystectomy)
Obesity
Pregnancy/antepartum
Varicose veins

edema, and gas exchange abnormalities, including high dead space ventilation. Compression Doppler ultrasonography is the most commonly utilized test for diagnosis of DVT. Ventilation-perfusion scanning and/or pulmonary angiography may have utility in specific circumstances, including in the presence of renal insufficiency (concerns about contrast-induced nephrotoxicity) or equivocal results on CT scan. Pulmonary angiography may be the test of choice when the likelihood of PE is high and anticoagulation is contraindicated, necessitating immediate placement of a vena cava filter.

3. **Treatment.** The mainstay of treatment for VTE is heparin, which should be started prior to confirmatory studies if clinical suspicion is high. LMWH may be superior to UFH in efficacy with

comparable rates of bleeding. The advantage of UFH in the ICU population is its titratability and rapid reversibility, which may be desirable in patients at high risk for bleeding. For patients who have contraindications to anticoagulation or who have recurrent PE despite anticoagulation, vena cava filters can be placed in the SVC or IVC, depending on DVT location.

D. **Acquired Neuromuscular Disorders in Critical Illness.** Neuromuscular abnormalities developing as a consequence of critical illness can be found in the majority of patients hospitalized in the ICU for a week or more (ranges from isolated nerve entrapment with focal pain or weakness to disuse muscle atrophy with mild weakness, to severe myopathy or neuropathy with associated severe, prolonged weakness). Critical illness polyneuropathy and myopathy (CIPNM) and a similar and likely related disorder, acute quadraplegic myopathy (AQM), produce significant morbidity and are associated with increased mortality in critically ill patients.

1. **Critical illness polyneuropathy and myopathy** is the most common form of myopathy in ICU patients. In addition to sepsis, factors associated with the development of CIPNM include duration of illness, hyperglycemia, and corticosteroid and neuromuscular blocking drug administration.

2. **Acute quadraplegic myopathy** was initially described in asthmatics with respiratory failure that were receiving high-dose corticosteroids and neuromuscular blocking drugs, but has since been described in other patients receiving similar therapeutic regimens. It is likely that the combination of these two drugs, in addition to as yet undefined patient factors, results in toxic injury to muscle that can range from a mild myopathy to rhabdomyolysis. It is also likely that CIPNM and AQM overlap, and it is often difficult to differentiate one from the other. It is likely that CIPNM and AQM prolong the duration of mechanical ventilation, ICU stay, and hospitalization; provide a significant impediment to long-term functional recovery from critical illness; and are a significant contributor to ICU and hospital mortality.

3. **Prevention** of acquired neuromuscular disorders in the ICU centers on avoidance or minimization of

contributory risk factors, including high-dose
steroids, prolonged administration of
neuromuscular blockade, and hyperglycemia.

4. **Diagnosis** of CIPNM and/or AQM should be
   entertained in all critically ill patients with
   unexplained weakness; electrodiagnostic studies can
   help confirm the diagnosis and rule out other,
   potentially treatable causes of weakness such as
   Gullain-Barrè syndrome.

5. **Treatment.** No treatment for either CIPNM or
   AQM has been identified; avoidance of potentially
   contributing agents and aggressive physical therapy
   are warranted.

CHAPTER 58 ■
CARDIOPULMONARY
RESUSCITATION

The cardiopulmonary physiology and pharmacology that form the basis of anesthesia practice are applicable to treating the victim of cardiac arrest (Otto CW: Cardiopulmonary resuscitation. In Barash PG, Cullen BF, Stoelting RK [eds]: *Clinical Anesthesia*, pp 1499–1520. Philadelphia, Lippincott Williams & Wilkins, 2006).

I. HISTORY (Table 58-1)

II. SCOPE OF THE PROBLEM

A. Cardiopulmonary resuscitation (CPR) is symptomatic therapy, aimed at sustaining vital organ function until natural cardiac function can be restored.

B. In clinical practice, the severity of underlying cardiac disease is the major determining factor in the success or failure of CPR.

1. Factors associated with poor outcomes are long arrest time before CPR is begun, prolonged ventricular fibrillation without definitive therapy, and inadequate coronary and cerebral perfusion during cardiac massage.

   a. Optimum outcome from ventricular fibrillation is obtained only if basic life support is begun within 4 minutes of arrest and defibrillation applied within 8 minutes.

   b. Blood flow falls rapidly with interruptions of chest compressions (checking pulse, intubation, defibrillation attempts, starting intravenous lines) and resumes slowly with reinstitution of compressions emphasizing the importance of continued chest compressions in overall outcome.

2. Overall initial resuscitation rates (40%) and survival to discharge (10%) are similar for out-of-hospital and in-hospital arrests (intercurrent illness of hospitalized patients decreases the likelihood of survival, and the arrest victim is likely to be elderly).

TABLE 58-1
HISTORY OF CARDIOPULMONARY RESUSCITATION
Bible story of Elisha breathing life back into the son of a Shunammite woman
Andreas Versalius described tracheostomy and artificial ventilation in 1543
Teaching of resuscitation by the Society for the Recovery of Persons Apparently Drowned founded in London in 1774
Establishment of mouth-to-mouth ventilation as the only effective means of artificial ventilation in the 1950s by Elam, Safar, and Gordon
Successful use of the internal defibrillator in 1947
External defibrillation introduced in late 1950s
Description by Kouwenhoven, Jude, and Knickerbocker of closed chest compression
Description by Redding and Pearson of the value of epinephrine

  a. Within the hospital, the operating room (OR) is where CPR has the highest rate of success (resuscitation is successful in about 90% of anesthesia-related cardiac arrests).

  b. Outside the operating suite, the best initial resuscitation rates are found in the intensive care unit (ICU), whereas the best survival rates are for patients arresting in the emergency department.

III. ORGANIZING A SOLUTION

 A. A standardized protocol is used for teaching CPR to numerous individuals with varying levels of expertise (lay public, emergency personnel, nurses, physicians) (Table 58-2).

 B. The two levels of CPR are referred to as basic life support (BLS) for ventilation and chest compressions (appropriate for lay public) and advanced cardiac life support (**ACLS**) using all modalities available for resuscitation.

 C. **Algorithms** for approaching the patient with cardiac arrest have been developed by the American Heart Association in conjunction with the International Liaison Committee on Resuscitation (Fig. 58-1).

TABLE 58-2

STANDARD APPROACH TO THE UNCONSCIOUS PATIENT

Determine unresponsiveness
Activate emergency medical services or code team
Position victim supine on a firm surface
Open airway
Determine absence of breathing
Deliver two breaths
Determine absence of pulse
Initiate external chest compressions
Alternate 15 compressions with 2 breaths (when there are two
  rescuers, a 1.5- to 2-second pause after every 5 chest
  compressions will allow a breath to be given)

IV. ETHICAL ISSUES: DO NOT RESUSCITATE ORDERS IN THE OPERATING ROOM

A. The patient's right to limit medical treatment including refusing CPR (do not resuscitate [DNR]) is firmly established in modern medical practice based on the ethical principle of respect for patient autonomy.

B. There are ethically sound arguments on both sides of the issue of whether DNR orders should be upheld in the operating room (OR).

   1. A desire by the anesthesiologist and/or surgeon to suspend DNR orders during surgery is often based on the knowledge that nearly 75% of the cardiac arrests in the operating room are related to a surgical or anesthetic complication and resuscitation attempts are highly successful.

   2. A mutual decision to suspend or limit a DNR order in the perioperative period may be achieved by communication among the patient, family, and caregivers.

     a. Many interventions used commonly in the OR (mechanical ventilation, vasopressors, cardiac antidysrhythmics, blood products) may be considered forms of resuscitation in other situations. The only modalities that are not routine anesthetic care are cardiac massage and defibrillation.

     b. Specific interventions included in a DNR status must be clarified with specific allowance made for methods necessary to perform anesthesia and surgery.

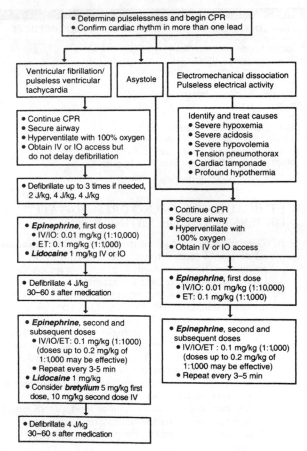

FIGURE 58-1. Algorithm for adult emergency cardiopulmonary resuscitation in the presence of ventricular fibrillation, asystole, or pulseless electrical activity.

V. BASIC LIFE SUPPORT

A. Airway Management

1. The techniques used for airway maintenance during anesthesia are applicable to the cardiac arrest victim (Table 58-3).

TABLE 58-3

TECHNIQUES USED FOR AIRWAY MAINTENANCE DURING CARDIOPULMONARY RESUSCITATION

Head tilt-chin lift (head is extended by pressure applied to the brow while the mandible is pulled forward by pressure on the front of the jaw, lifting the tongue away from the posterior pharynx)
Jaw thrust (applying pressure behind the rami of the mandible)
Oropharyngeal or nasopharyngeal airway (danger of inducing vomiting or laryngospasm in a semiconscious victim)
Tracheal intubation (do not perform until adequate ventilation and chest compressions have been established)
Alternatives to tracheal intubation
    Laryngotracheal mask airway
    Esophageal obturator airway
    Translaryngeal ventilation
    Tracheostomy

2. **Foreign body airway obstruction** must be considered in any victim who suddenly stops breathing and becomes cyanotic and unconscious (occurs most commonly during eating and is usually because of food [especially meat] impacting in the laryngeal inlet, at the epiglottis, or in the vallecula).
   a. The signs of total airway obstruction are the lack of air movement despite respiratory efforts and the inability of the victim to speak or cough.
   b. Treatment is the abdominal thrust maneuver (chest thrusts an alternative for the parturient and massively obese) and the finger sweep.
   c. In an awake victim, the rescuer reaches around the victim from behind, placing the fist of one hand in the epigastrium between the xiphoid and umbilicus. The fist is grasped with the other hand and pressed into the victim's epigastrium with a quick upward thrust. If the first attempt is unsuccessful, repeated attempts should be made because hypoxia-related muscular relaxation may eventually allow success.
B. **Ventilation**
   1. Currently airway management and ventilation (mouth to mouth is the most immediately available, providing an inspired gas containing about 4% carbon dioxide and 17% oxygen) remain the standard first steps of CPR.

TABLE 58-4

TECHNIQUES OF RESCUE BREATHING

Mouth-to-mouth ventilation (rescuer delivers exhaled air to victim and exhalation by victim is passive)
Mouth-to-nose ventilation
Oropharyngeal airway with an external extension mouthpiece (often difficult to obtain a good mouth seal)
Mouth-to-mask ventilation (mask may include one-way valve to direct victim's exhaled gases away from the rescuer and a side port for delivery of supplemental oxygen)
Self-inflating resuscitation bag
Tracheal intubation (following placement of the tracheal tube no pause should be made for ventilation as blood flow during CPR decreases rapidly when chest compressions are stopped)

2. Closed chest compressions alone may be as efficacious as compressions and mouth-to-mouth ventilation especially when the arrest is witnessed, likely to be a cardiac rather than respiratory cause, the upper airway is patent, and tracheal intubation will be available in a short time.
3. **Physiology of Ventilation During CPR**
   a. Avoiding gastric insufflation requires that peak inspiratory airway pressures remain below esophageal opening pressure (about 20 cm H_2O). Partial airway obstruction by the tongue and pharyngeal tissues is a major cause of increased airway pressure contributing to gastric insufflation during CPR. Properly applied pressure to the anterior arch of the cricoid (Sellick maneuver) causes the cricoid lamina to seal the esophagus and can prevent air from entering the stomach at airway pressures up to 100 cm H_2O.
   b. Achievement of an acceptable tidal volume during low inspiratory pressures characteristic of rescue breathing requires a slow inspiratory flow rate and long inspiratory time (breaths over 1.5 to 2 seconds during a pause in chest compressions).
4. **Techniques of Rescue Breathing** (Table 58-4)
C. **Circulation**
   1. **Physiology of Circulation During Closed Chest Compression.** Two theories of the mechanism of blood flow during closed chest compression have been suggested. Which mechanism predominates

varies from victim to victim and even during the resuscitation of the same victim.

   a. The **cardiac pump mechanism** proposes that pressure on the chest compresses the heart between the sternum and spine. Compressions raise the pressure in the ventricular chambers (closing the atrioventricular valves) and ejects blood into the lungs and aorta. During the relaxation phase of closed chest compression, expansion of the thoracic cage causes a subatmospheric intrathoracic pressure facilitating blood return.

   b. The **thoracic pump mechanism** proposes that the increase in intrathoracic pressure caused by sternal compressions forces blood out of the chest (backward flow into veins is prevented by valves) with the heart acting as a passive conduit.

2. **Distribution of Blood Flow During CPR.** Cardiac output is decreased to 10 to 33% of normal during CPR, and nearly all the blood flow is directed to organs above the diaphragm (abdominal viscera and lower extremity blood flow decreased to <5% of normal).

   a. Myocardial perfusion is 20 to 50% of normal; cerebral perfusion is maintained at 50 to 90% of normal.

   b. Total flow tends to decrease with time during CPR, but the relative distribution is not altered. **Epinephrine** may help sustain cardiac output over time during CPR.

3. **Gas Transport During CPR**

   a. During the low flow state of CPR, excretion of carbon dioxide is decreased to the same extent that cardiac output is reduced.

   b. Exhaled carbon dioxide concentrations reflects only the metabolism of the part of the body that is being perfused

   c. When normal circulation is restored, carbon dioxide that has accumulated in nonperfused tissues is washed out and a temporary increase in carbon dioxide excretion is seen.

   d. Although carbon dioxide excretion is decreased during CPR, measurement of blood gases reveals an arterial respiratory alkalosis and a venous respiratory acidosis reflecting the severely reduced cardiac output.

TABLE 58-5

TECHNIQUES OF CLOSED CHEST COMPRESSION

Rescuer should stand or kneel next to victim's side
Heel of one hand is placed on the lower sternum and the other
 hand is placed on top of the hand on the victim (avoid pressing
 on the xiphoid, which can lead to liver laceration; even with
 proper technique costochondral separation and rib fractures are
 common)
Apply pressure only with heel of hand (fingers free of contact with
 chest) straight down on sternum with the arms straight and
 elbows locked into position so entire weight of the upper body is
 used to apply force
During relaxation all pressure is removed but hands should not
 lose contact with the chest wall
Sternum must be depressed 3.5–5.0 cm in the average adult
 (palpable pulse when systolic pressure >50 mm Hg)
Duration of compression should equal that of relaxation
Compression rate should be 80–100/min

4. **Technique of Closed Chest Compression**
   a. Some circulation may be present in a "pulseless"
      patient (systolic blood pressure of about
      50 mm Hg is necessary to palpate a peripheral
      pulse) with primary respiratory arrest. In such a
      patient, opening the airway and ventilation of the
      lungs may be sufficient for resuscitation. For this
      reason, a further search for a pulse should be
      made following artificial ventilation before
      beginning sternal compressions.
   b. Important considerations in performing closed
      chest compressions are the position of the rescuer
      relative to the victim, the position of the rescuer's
      hands, and the rate and force of compression
      (Table 58-5).
5. **Alternative Methods of Circulatory Support**
   a. Standard CPR will sustain most patients for only
      15 to 30 minutes.
   b. Alternatives to standard techniques for CPR
      (simultaneous ventilation-compression CPR and
      abdominal binding, interposed abdominal comp-
      ression CPR, pneumatic vest CPR, active
      compression–decompression CPR) are intended
      to provide better hemodynamics usually by taking
      advantage of the thoracic pump mechanism.

TABLE 58-6

CRITICAL VARIABLES ASSOCIATED WITH SUCCESSFUL RESUSCITATION

Myocardial blood flow	15–20 mL/min/100 g
Aortic diastolic pressure	40 mm Hg
Coronary perfusion pressure	15–25 mm Hg
End-tidal carbon dioxide	>10 mm Hg

None of these alternatives has proved reliably superior to the standard technique.

   c. **Invasive Techniques.** Open chest cardiac massage or cardiopulmonary bypass must be instituted early to improve survival. If open chest massage is begun after 30 minutes of ineffective closed chest compressions, there is no better survival even though hemodynamics are improved.

6. **Assessing the Adequacy of Circulation During CPR** (Table 58-6)

   a. The adequacy of closed chest compressions is usually judged by palpation of a pulse in the carotid or femoral artery (palpable pulse primarily reflects systolic blood pressure).

   b. The return of spontaneous circulation is greatly dependent on restoring oxygenated blood flow to the myocardium. Obtaining such flow depends on closed chest compressions developing adequate cardiac output and coronary perfusion pressure (diastolic blood pressure minus central venous pressure) (see Table 58-6). Damage to the myocardium from underlying disease may preclude survival no matter how effective the CPR efforts.

   c. During CPR with a tracheal tube in place, exhalation of carbon dioxide is dependent on pulmonary blood flow (cardiac output) rather than alveolar ventilation. End-tidal carbon dioxide concentrations can be used to judge the effectiveness of chest compressions. Attempts should be made to maximize the end-tidal carbon dioxide concentration by alterations in technique or drug therapy (epinephrine). It should be remembered that sodium bicarbonate produces a transient (3 to 5 minutes) increase in end-tidal carbon dioxide concentration.

VI. ADVANCED CARDIAC LIFE SUPPORT (see Fig. 58-1)

A. Defibrillation

1. **Electrical Pattern and Duration of Ventricular Fibrillation.** Ventricular fibrillation is the most common electrocardiographic pattern found during cardiac arrest in adults and the only effective treatment is electrical defibrillation. **Defibrillation should be performed as soon as the fibrillation is diagnosed and equipment is available.** Immediate defibrillation is only effective when applied within 4 to 5 minutes of collapse. Otherwise, a brief period of 2 to 3 minutes of chest compressions before defibrillation is necessary.

   a. The most important controllable determinant of failure to resuscitate a patient with ventricular fibrillation is the duration of fibrillation (fibrillating heart has a high oxygen consumption).

   b. If defibrillation occurs within 1 minute of fibrillation, CPR is not necessary.

   c. Defibrillation should not be delayed for epinephrine administration (no evidence that epinephrine improves the success of defibrillation or decreases the energy setting needed for defibrillation).

   d. Fibrillation amplitude on an electrocardiogram lead varies with the orientation of that lead to the vector of the fibrillatory wave (flat line can be present if lead is oriented at right angles to the fibrillatory wave).

   e. A nonfibrillatory rhythm will not respond to defibrillation

2. **Defibrillators: Energy, Current, and Voltage**

   a. The typical defibrillator consists of a variable transformer that allows selection of a variable voltage potential, an AC to DC converter to provide a direct current that is stored in a capacitor, a switch to charge the capacitor, and discharge switches to complete the circuit from the capacitor to the paddle electrodes.

   b. Defibrillation is accomplished by direct current passing through a critical mass of myocardium resulting in simultaneous depolarization of the myofibrils.

TABLE 58-7
DETERMINANTS OF TRANSTHORACIC IMPEDANCE

Diameter of electrode paddles (most common diameter is 8–10 cm)
Impedance between metal electrode and skin (decreased with gel
 designed to conduct electricity in the defibrillation setting)
Successive shocks (may decrease impedance and partially explain
 why an additional shock of the same energy can cause
 defibrillation when previous shocks failed)
Lung volume (air is a poor electrical conductor so impedance is
 slightly higher during inspiration)
Paddle pressure (pressure of at least 11 kg decreases resistance by
 improving paddle-skin contact and by expelling air from the
 lungs)

   c. Even at a constant delivered energy, the delivered
      current (critical determinant of defibrillation) will
      be decreased as impedance (resistance) increases.
3. **Transthoracic impedance** (Table 58-7)
4. Adverse effects and energy requirements
   a. Repeated defibrillation with high-energy shocks,
      especially if repeated at short intervals, may
      result in myocardial damage.
   b. Current recommendations for adults are to use
      200 J for the initial shock followed by a second
      shock at 200 to 300 J if the first is unsuccessful. If
      both fail to defibrillate the patient's heart,
      additional shocks should be given at 300 to 360 J.

VII. PHARMACOLOGIC THERAPY (Table 58-8)

A. Establishing intravenous access and pharmacologic
   therapy should come after other interventions are
   established.
   1. Of the drugs given during CPR, only epinephrine is
      acknowledged as being useful in helping restore
      spontaneous circulation.
   2. Asystole and pulseless electrical activity
      (electromechanical dissociation) are circumstances
      in which drugs are most frequently given.
B. **Routes of Administration**
   1. The preferred route of administration of all drugs
      during CPR is intravenous (central injection
      produces a higher drug level and more rapid onset
      than peripheral injection). Because of poor blood

TABLE 58-8

ADULT ADVANCED CARDIAC LIFE SUPPORT DRUGS
AND DOSES

	Dose (iv)	Dosing interval (min)	Maximum dose (mg/kg)
Epinephrine	1 mg 3–8 mg[a]	3–5	None
Lidocaine	1–5 mg/kg	3–5	3.0
Amiodarine	150 mg over 10 min		
Sodium bicarbonate	1 mEq/kg	As needed	check *p*H

[a]Consider if no response to lower doses of epinephrine.

flow below the diaphragm during CPR, drugs
administered into the lower extremity may not reach
sites of action.
2. If venous access cannot be established, the
endotracheal tube is an alternative route of
administration for epinephrine, lidocaine, and
atropine (not sodium bicarbonate). Doses 2 to
2.5 times the established intravenous dose
administered in 5- to 10-mL volumes are
recommended when using the tracheal route of
administration.
C. Catecholamines and Vasopressors
1. **Mechanism of Action.** The efficacy of **epinephrine**
lies entirely in its α adrenergic actions (peripheral
vasoconstriction leads to an increase in aortic
diastolic pressure causing an increase in coronary
perfusion pressure and myocardial blood
flow).
a. It is commonly believed that the ability of
epinephrine to increase the amplitude of
ventricular fibrillation (alpha-adrenergic effect)
makes defibrillation easier. There is no proof,
however, that epinephrine improves the success
or decreases the energy necessary for successful
defibrillation.
b. Epinephrine when added to chest compressions
helps develop the critical coronary perfusion
pressure necessary to provide myocardial blood
flow for restoration of spontaneous circulation.

2. **Epinephrine dose** is 1 mg iv every 3 to 5 minutes in the adult. If this dose remains ineffective, higher doses (3 to 8 mg iv) should be considered.

D. **Vasopressin** is recommended as an alternative to epinephrine in a dose of 40 units iv as a one time injection. If additional vasopressor doses are needed, epinephrine should be administered.

E. **Amiodarone and Lidocaine**

1. These drugs are used during cardiac arrest to aid in defibrillation when ventricular fibrillation is refractory to electrical countershock or when ventricular fibrillation recurs. Amiodarone may be considered the first drug for treatment of ventricular fibrillation that is resistant to electrical countershock.

   a. Lidocaine has few hemodynamic effects when given intravenously.

   b. Amiodarone can cause hypotension and tachycardia especially with rapid intravenous administration.

2. Ventricular fibrillation threshold is decreased by acute myocardial ischemia or infarction, and this effect is partially reversed by lidocaine and amiodarone.

3. To rapidly achieve and maintain therapeutic blood levels during CPR, relatively large doses of lidocaine or amiodarone are necessary (Table 58-8).

F. **Sodium Bicarbonate**

1. The use of sodium bicarbonate during CPR is based on theoretical considerations that acidosis lowers ventricular fibrillation threshold and respiratory acidosis impairs the physiologic response to catecholamines.

2. Little to no evidence supports the efficacy of sodium bicarbonate treatment during CPR. The lack of effect of buffer therapy may be explained by the slow onset of metabolic acidosis during cardiac arrest (acidosis as measured by blood lactate concentrations does not become severe for 15 to 20 minutes of cardiac arrest).

3. In contrast to the lack of evidence that buffer therapy during CPR improves survival, the adverse effects of excessive sodium bicarbonate administration are well documented: metabolic alkalosis, hypernatremia, and hyperosmolarity.

   a. Intravenous sodium bicarbonate combines with hydrogen ions to produce carbonic acid that dissociates into carbon dioxide and water ($PaCO_2$ is temporarily increased until ventilation eliminates the excess carbon dioxide).

   b. Tissue acidosis during CPR is caused primarily by low tissue blood flow and accumulation of carbon dioxide in the tissues (theoretically there is concern that carbon dioxide liberated from sodium bicarbonate could worsen existing tissue acidosis).

   4. Current practice restricts the use of sodium bicarbonate (1 mEq/kg iv initially with additional doses of 0.5 mEq/kg every 10 minutes [better if guided by blood gas determinations]) primarily to cardiac arrests that are associated with hyperkalemia, severe preexisting metabolic acidosis, and tricyclic antidepressant overdose.

G. Atropine

   1. Atropine (1 mg iv repeated every 3 to 5 minutes up to a total dose of 0.04 mg/kg, which is totally vagolytic) is commonly administered during cardiac arrest associated with a pattern of asystole or slow pulseless electrical activity on the electrocardiogram. Atropine enhances sinus node automatically and atrioventricular conduction *via* its vagolytic effects.

   a. Excessive parasympathetic tone probably contributes little to asystole or pulseless electrical activity in adults (most often a result of myocardial ischemia).

   b. Even in children, it is doubtful that parasympathetic tone plays a significant role during most cardiac arrests.

   2. Full vagolytic doses of atropine may be associated with fixed mydriasis following successful resuscitation confounding neurologic evaluation.

H. Calcium

   1. The only indications for administration of calcium during CPR is hyperkalemia, hypocalcemia, or calcium blocker toxicity.

   2. When calcium is administered, the chloride salt (2 to 4 mg/kg of the 10% solution iv) is recommended because it produces higher and more consistent levels of ionized calcium than other salts (calcium gluconate contains one-third as much molecular calcium as the chloride salt).

VIII. PEDIATRIC CARDIOPULMONARY RESUSCITATION

A. The basic approach to the pediatric cardiac arrest victim is the same as in the adult (see Table 58-2 and Fig. 58-1).
   1. Cardiac arrest is less likely to be a sudden event and more likely related to progressive deterioration of ventilation and cardiac function in the pediatric age group.
   2. Effective ventilation of the lungs is critical since ventilatory problems are frequently the cause of cardiac arrest in this age group.
B. Cardiac compression in the infant is provided with two fingers on the midsternum or by encircling the chest with the hands and using the thumbs to provide compression.
C. Defibrillation is less frequently necessary in children, but the same principles apply as in the adult (recommended starting energy is 2 J/kg, which is doubled if defibrillation is unsuccessful).
D. Drug therapy is similar to the adult but plays a larger role because electrical therapy is less often needed.

IX. POSTRESUSCITATION CARE

A. The major factors contributing to mortality following successful resuscitation are progression of the primary disease and cerebral damage suffered as a result of the cardiac arrest. Furthermore, even brief cardiac arrest causes generalized decreases in myocardial function (global myocardial stunning) and may require treatment with inotropic drugs.
   1. When cerebral blood flow is restored after a period of global cerebral ischemia there are initially multifocal areas of the brain with no reflow (may reflect effects of epinephrine administered during CPR) followed within an hour by global hyperemia, which is followed quickly by global hypoperfusion.
   2. Support after resuscitation is focused on providing stable oxygenation (PaO_2 >100 mm Hg), ventilation

(PaCO$_2$ 25 to 35 mm Hg), neuromuscular blockers to prevent coughing or restlessness, and optimal hemodynamics (hematocrit 30 to 35%).

   a. A brief 5-minute period of hypertension (mean arterial pressure 120 to 140 mm Hg) may help overcome the initial cerebral no reflow.

   b. Hyperglycemia during cerebral ischemia results in increased neurologic damage. Although it is unknown if hyperglycemia in the postresuscitation period influences outcome, it seems prudent to maintain the blood glucose level between 100 and 250 mg/dL.

   c. Increased intracranial pressure is unusual following resuscitation from cardiac arrest (ischemic injury can lead to cerebral edema and increased intracranial pressure in the ensuing days).

   d. In contrast to general supportive care, specific pharmacologic therapy directed at brain preservation has not been shown to have further benefit.

3. Most severely damaged victims die of multisystem organ failure within 1 to 2 weeks.

4. It is recommended that unconscious patients with spontaneous circulation following out-of-hospital cardiac arrest should be cooled to 32° to 34°C for 12 to 24 hours when the initial rhythm was ventricular fibrillation. Such cooling may also be beneficial for other rhythms or in-hospital cardiac arrest.

B. **Prognosis.** Most patients who completely recover show rapid improvement in the first 48 hours.

CHAPTER 59 ■ DISASTER PREPAREDNESS AND WEAPONS OF MASS DESTRUCTION

I. INTRODUCTION (Murray MJ: Disaster preparedness and weapons of mass destruction. In Barash PG, Cullen BF, Stoelting RK [eds]: *Clinical Anesthesia*, pp 1521–1537. Philadelphia, Lippincott Williams & Wilkins, 2006).

   A. After September 11, 2001, physicians have been faced with a prospect that challenges their scientific training.

   B. We must confront the possibility that terrorists can attack our cities with conventional, nuclear, biologic, and chemical weapons.

   C. As anesthesiologists, we must now be prepared at any time to care for the victims of such assaults.

II. JOINT COMMISSION ON ACCREDITATION OF HEALTHCARE ORGANIZATIONS (JCAHO)

   A. Following the events of September 11, 2001, and subsequent anthrax attacks, the Joint Commission on Accreditation of Healthcare Organizations (JCAHO) published a "white paper" to help hospitals develop systems to create and sustain community-wide emergency preparedness. It is incumbent on physicians to be familiar with what their hospital has done to comply with the JCAHO standards, in anticipation of what their roles may be.

   B. The JCAHO white paper focuses on three major areas:

   1. Enlisting the Community to Develop the Local Response

   a. Central to the JCAHO disaster preparedness standards and their requirements is the recognition that the initial response needs to be a local response.

   b. There has traditionally been poor communication between law enforcement agencies, fire and rescue services, and emergency medical services. There is a fundamental need to formalize an organization of community resources of which hospitals and physicians are but one component.

c. Community planning needs to occur and the results of that planning need to be widely disseminated to as many potential partners in implementing the plan as possible.

2. **Focusing on the Key Aspects of the System That Prepares the Community Health Care Resources to Mobilize to Care for Patients, Protect Its Staff, and Serve the Public**

   a. In order to respond to a mass casualty event, an emergency medical system must be able to assess and expand its surge capacity—the ability to provide care for and transport countless numbers of patients to facilities with appropriate capacity, resources, and staff.

   b. In order to maintain surge capacity, it is imperative that every health care provider recognize the importance of protecting herself or himself.

   c. After having established the basics, the most important aspect of managing a mass casualty event, again whether it is natural, unintentional, or intentional, is having a command and control structure with which everyone is familiar.

   d. The public must be mobilized to participate in the response. As part of this response, the health care system and its leaders must identify communication and information needs.

   e. JCAHO requires two drills annually (provides health care providers an opportunity to hone their skills and anticipate problems they might confront in the future in dealing with natural disasters and terrorist attacks).

3. **Establishing the Accountabilities, Oversight, Leadership, and Sustainment of a Community-Preparedness System.** Most of the responsibility for preparedness is with local, state, and federal governments and with hospitals and hospital organizations.

III. DISASTER PREPAREDNESS

A. While we recognize the critical importance for planning and preparing to deal with the use of weapons of mass

TABLE 59-1
DISASTERS THAT RESULT IN MASS CASUALTIES

Natural
Hurricanes
Tornados
Floods
Earthquakes
Fires

Unintentional
Airplane/train/bus crash
Boat sinking

Fire
Nuclear accident
Industrial accident
Building collapse/sports stadium disaster

Intentional
Bombing
Nuclear
Biologic
Chemical

destruction, the reality is that we are far more likely to
have to manage patients and health care facilities that are
victims of natural and unintentional disasters
(Table 59-1).

B. Role of Government
1. The initial response to any disaster, whether natural,
unintended, or terrorist initiated, begins at the local
level and would involve law enforcement agencies,
especially if there was criminal activity suspected,
firefighters, and paramedics.
2. If the event supersedes the state's ability to respond,
the federal government would become involved. The
anesthesiologist needs to know there are a number of
local, state, and federal agencies that are mobilizing to
help her or him handle the situation depending on the
gravity and number of casualties.
3. The CDC has established a National Pharmaceutical
Stockpile program as a national repository of
antibiotics, chemical antidotes, life-support
medications, intravenous administration and
airway maintenance supplies, and medical/surgical
items.

C. **Role of Anesthesiologist in Managing Mass Casualties**
   1. It is difficult to anticipate every measure in which anesthesiologists could be asked to assist in managing mass casualty situations.
   2. However, their basic understanding of physiology and pharmacology; their airway skills; and their fluid resuscitation expertise; and their ability to manage ventilators and to provide anesthesia in the field environment, in the emergency department, in the operating room, and in intensive care units (ICUs) will be invaluable.

IV. **NUCLEAR ACCIDENTS** (Table 59-2)
   A. The experience from Chernobyl should indicate the kind of injuries and results that anesthesiologists can anticipate from nuclear accidents including radiation burns, bone marrow suppression, the destruction of the lining of the gastrointestinal (GI) tract, and GI bleeding with translocation of bacteria, infection, sepsis, septic shock, and death.
      1. Potassium iodide is indicated to protect the thyroid gland from taking up 131_I and other drugs are being considered such as 5-androstenediol.
      2. Because of the possibility of exposure to ionizing radiation from nuclear power plants the American Academy of Pediatrics has recommended that at least two tablets of potassium iodide be available for all inhabitants within 10 miles of any nuclear power plant.
   B. **Potential Sources of Ionizing Radiation Exposure**
      1. The greatest concern is the exposure to ionizing radiation that is unintentional, as occurred at the Chernobyl nuclear power plants, or is intentional.

TABLE 59-2

NUCLEAR ACCIDENTS IN DECREASING ORDER OF PROBABILITY

Accidents (nuclear power plants, reactors)
Terrorist action
Single nuclear bomb detonation
Theater nuclear war
Strategic nuclear war

TABLE 59-3

TYPES OF RADIATION

Ionizing radiation (a high-frequency, low-amplitude form of radiation that interacts significantly with biologic systems)

Alpha particle (alpha particles have poor penetration, pose little hazard after external exposure, but can produce tissue injury when inhaled or ingested)

Beta particle (a high-speed particle, identical to an electron, emitted from the nucleus of an atom)

Neutrons (emitted only after a nuclear detonation, neutrons are highly destructive, producing 10 times more tissue damage than gamma-rays)

Gamma-rays (significant penetrance and are the most important external radiation hazard after a radiation disaster)

X rays (their energy is emitted from electrons)

2. Exposure to ionizing radiation may be as a result of terrorism (radiologic dispersion device remains the most likely event).
3. Individuals should be familiar with types of ionizing radiation (Table 59-3).
4. The most likely injury from ionizing radiation is to those tissues that have the greatest turnover rate (greatest for lymphoid tissues).
   a. Thrombocytopenia, granulocytopenia, and GI injury lead to bleeding and bacterial translocation across the GI epithelium, the net result of which is sepsis, bleeding, and the hallmarks of acute radiation syndrome, which lead to death.
   b. Because ionizing radiation is invisible, individuals may appear normal or may present with nausea, vomiting, diarrhea, fever, hypotension, erythema, and central nervous system (CNS) dysfunction.
   c. Patients who present with nausea, vomiting, diarrhea, and fever are likely to have severe acute radiation syndrome. Hypotension, erythema, and CNS dysfunction will manifest later.
   d. Long-term effects include thyroid cancer and psychologic injury as has been documented many times in the past.
C. Management
   1. Depending on the type of radiation event, the first step is immediate evacuation of the area.

2. The principle of disaster management always involves containment (avoid bringing patients with material emitting ionizing radiation to the hospital). To the extent possible, patients should be decontaminated at the site.
3. Potassium iodide can prevent radiation-induced thyroid effects (give within 24 hours).
4. Acute radiation syndrome manifests as bleeding and sepsis.

V. BIOLOGIC DISASTERS

A. Anesthesiologists need to be familiar with contagious diseases that are not initiated by terrorist groups (influenza, SARS, and West Nile virus). Anesthesiologists, because of their airway and ventilator management skills, will be involved in providing care for many of these patients.
B. Biologic Terrorism
   1. The ideal biologic agent is one that has the greatest potential for adverse public health impact, generating mass casualties and with potential for easy large-scale dissemination that could cause mass hysteria and civil disruption.
   2. There are three categories of biologic weapons (Table 59-4). Category A are those weapons which are highly contagious and fit all the characteristics of a relatively ideal biologic agent.

TABLE 59-4
BIOLOGIC AGENTS USED FOR WARFARE

Category A	Category B	Category C
Anthrax	Q fever	Various equine encephalitic viruses
Smallpox	Cholera	
Plague	Glanders	
Botulism	Enteric pathogens (salmonella, shigella)	
Tularemia	Cholera,	
Viral hemorrhagic fever		
Various encephalitic viruses (Ebola, Lassa, Marburg, Argentine)	Various biologic toxins	

3. **Smallpox.** In 1972, routine vaccination for smallpox was discontinued in the United States. It is precisely because of this that we are at most risk for terrorists using smallpox as a biologic weapon.
4. **Anthrax** has appeal as a bioterrorism agent because it can be "weaponized" (aerosolized).
    a. There are three primary types of anthrax infection: cutaneous, inhalation, and GI. Ninety-five percent of cases are cutaneous. Inhalation anthrax is hard to detect and manifests as an influenza-like disease with fever, myalgias, malaise, and a nonproductive cough with or without chest pain.
    b. The most notable finding on physical examination and laboratory testing is a widened mediastinum. Usually when a patient develops profound dyspnea, death ensues within 1 to 2 days.
    c. In the past, penicillin G was the treatment of choice, but because weaponized anthrax has been engineered to be resistant to penicillin G, ciprofloxacin or doxycycline is more commonly used.
5. **Plague** (bubonic and pneumonic). With bubonic plague, there is a 2- to 6-day incubation period at which time there is the sudden onset of fever, chills, weakness, and headache. Without treatment, patients become septic and develop septic shock with cyanosis and gangrene in peripheral tissues, leading to the "black death" descriptor that was used during the epidemics in Europe.
    a. The treatment of choice is streptomycin, but chloramphenicol and tetracycline are acceptable alternatives.
    b. Patients with pneumonic plague should be managed as one would manage a patient with drug resistance to tuberculosis as the respiratory secretions are highly infectious.
6. **Tularemia.** Normally, humans acquire *tularenis* with direct contact of an infected animal or from the bite of an infected tick or deerfly.
    a. There is a 3- to 5-day incubation period, and then the onset of disease is marked with fever, pharyngitis, bronchitis, pneumonia, pleuritis, and hilar lymphadenopathy.
    b. Prophylaxis with streptomycin, ciprofloxacin, or doxycycline has been recommended.

966 Postanesthesia and Consultant Practice

7. **Botulism** is a neuroparalytic disease caused by the toxin (most potent poison known) from *botulinum*.
   a. Victims develop progressive weakness, a flaccid paralysis that begins in the extremities and progresses until the respiratory muscles are paralyzed.
   b. Patients with profound respiratory embarrassment should have their tracheas protected and mechanical ventilation initiated.
8. **Hemorrhagic Fevers.** There are at least 18 viruses that cause human hemorrhagic fevers, which form a special group of viruses characterized by viral replication in lymphoid cells, after which patients develop fever and myalgia, evidence of capillary leak (peripheral or pulmonary edema), disseminated intravascular coagulation (DIC), and thrombocytopenia. There are no specific antiviral therapies for this class of viruses.

C. **Role of the Anesthesiologist in Bioterrorism**
   1. Airway management and ventilator management may be critical, as would the establishment of intravascular access and volume resuscitation.
   2. Anesthesiologists must protect themselves by using 100% effective respiratory protection going so far as to consider an oxygen-rebreathing system.

VI. **CHEMICAL** (Table 59-5)

A. **Nerve agents** are chemicals that affect nerve transmission by inhibiting acetylcholinesterase so that acetylcholine accumulates at muscarinic and nicotinic acetylcholine receptors and within the CNS.
   1. Nicotinic stimulation leads to tachycardia and hypertension at preganglionic sites, and at nicotinic acetylcholine receptors on the neuromuscular junction, to fasciculations, twitching, fatigue, and flaccid paralysis.

TABLE 59-5

CHEMICAL AGENTS

Nerve (tabun, sarin, soman)
Pulmonary (chlorine, phosgene)
Blood (hydrogen cyanide, cyanogen chloride)
Vesicants (sulfur mustard, nitrogen mustard)

2. Excess parasympathetic activity leads to miosis and loss of accommodation so that patients complain of blurred vision.
    a. Within the respiratory system, the increased parasympathetic activity leads to bronchospasm, dyspnea, and rhinorrhea.
    b. Within the cardiovascular system, activity within the muscarinic system leads to bradycardia, and at the nicotinic site, an increase in heart rate.
3. Treatment for nerve agent poisoning is with atropine and/or pralidoxime chloride.
    a. The U.S. military travels with automatic injectors containing 2 mg of atropine and 600 mg of 2-PAM CL (pyridostigmine) or pralidoxime chloride.
    b. For situations in which one is anticipating nerve agent exposure, pyridostigmine is a long-acting agent that binds with acetylcholinesterase, allowing the enzyme to spontaneously regenerate. It does not cross the blood-brain barrier and, if used, must be taken more than 30 minutes prior to exposure.
    c. Patients are decontaminated by removing their clothing and with copious amounts of water in 5% hypochlorite (household bleach).
B. Pulmonary Agents
1. There are primarily four pulmonary agents: chloropicrine, chlorine, phosgene, and diphosgene.
2. Phosgene is a prototypical agent because it is deadlier than any of the other compounds. It is a colorless gas and has an odor of recently cut hay at 22° to 28° celsius and normal pressure conditions.
    a. It is highly soluble in lipids and, therefore, can easily penetrate pulmonary epithelium and the cells lining the alveoli.
    b. Though it is very lipid soluble, it reacts rapidly with water forming hydrochloric acid (extremely toxic to tissues causing ARDS) and carbon dioxide.
    c. For individuals who are exposed, gas masks provide the best protection.
3. **Blood agents** (cyanogens) are inhaled and release hydrogen cyanide, which impairs cytochrome oxidase and aerobic metabolism at the level of the mitochondria (metabolic acidosis).
    a. The blood agents are hydrogen cyanide, hydrocyanic acid, cyanogen chloride, and arsine.

      b. Hydrogen cyanide is a colorless liquid and can be taken up through the skin as a liquid or inhaled.

      c. Treatment for cyanide toxicity (nitroprusside a medical cause of cyanide toxicity) involves the administration of sodium thiosulfate, with supportive care in terms of tracheal intubation, ventilation, 100% oxygen, and cardiac support with inotropes and vasopressors.

C. Vesicants

  1. Sodium mustard and related compounds such as nitrogen mustard, phosgene oxime, and lewisite, also known as "blister agents," get their names by the fact that on contact with skin, these compounds produce burns and blisters. Though these are the most readily apparent manifestations, these compounds can also be inhaled and can inflict severe damage to the respiratory system and the eyes, as well as produce multiple organ dysfunction syndrome.

  2. Blister agents are colorless and almost odorless. If the ambient temperature is high enough, odor is present, which smells like rotten onions or mustard.

      a. Individuals lose their sight while nausea, vomiting, and diarrhea develop along with severe respiratory difficulty (same thing that happens to the skin can happen in the pulmonary epithelium).

      b. A nuclear-biologic-chemical protective suit and gas mask provide the best protection against sulfur mustard. Individuals who are exposed should be decontaminated as they would if they were exposed to a nerve agent (clothing is removed and they are washed with warm soapy water with or without 0.5% hypochlorite).

A ■ FORMULAS
    Hemodynamic Formulas
    Respiratory Formulas
    Lung Volumes and Capacities
B ■ ELECTROCARDIOGRAPHY ATLAS
C ■ AMERICAN HEART ASSOCIATION (AHA)
    RESUSCITATION PROTOCOLS
    Adult
        Comprehensive ECC Algorithm
        Ventricular Fibrillation/Pulseless VT Algorithm
        Pulseless Electrical Activity Algorithm
        Asystole: The Silent Heart Algorithm
        Bradycardia Algorithm
        The Tachycardia Overview Algorithm
        Narrow-Complex Supraventricular Tachycardia
          Algorithm
        Stable Ventricular Tachycardia (Monomorphic or
          Polymorphic) Algorithm
        Synchronized Cardioversion Algorithm
        The Acute Pulmonary Edema, Hypotension, and
          Shock Algorithm
        Algorithm for Suspected Stroke
    Pediatric
        PALS (Pediatric Advanced Life Support) Bradycardia
          Algorithm
        PALS Pulseless Arrest Algorithm
        PALS Tachycardia Algorithm for Infants and Children
          with Rapid Rhythm and Adequate Perfusion
        PALS Tachycardia Algorithm for Infants and Children
          with Rapid Rhythm and Evidence of Poor Perfusion
        PALS Medications for Cardiac Arrest and Sympomatic
          Arrhythmias
        PALS Medications to Maintain Cardiac Output and
          for Postresuscitation Stabilization
    Neonatal
        Algorithm for Resuscitation of the Newly Born Infant
        Therapeutic Guidelines
    Conveying News of a Sudden Death to Family Members
    Recommendations for Critical Incident Debriefing
D ■ AMERICAN SOCIETY OF ANESTHESIOLOGISTS
    STANDARDS
    Standards for Basic Anesthetic Monitoring
    Continuum of Depth of Sedation: Definition of General
        Anesthesia and Level of Sedation/Analgesia

Basic Standards for Pre-Anesthesia Care
Standards for Postanesthesia Care
E ■ THE AIRWAY APPROACH ALGORITHM AND
DIFFICULT AIRWAY ALGORITHMS
F ■ MALIGNANT HYPERTHERMIA PROTOCOL
G ■ DRUG LIST
H ■ HERBAL MEDICATIONS

APPENDIX A ■ FORMULAS

Hemodynamic Formulas
Respiratory Formulas
Lung Volumes and Capacities

HEMODYNAMIC FORMULAS

HEMODYNAMIC VARIABLES: CALCULATIONS AND NORMAL VALUES

Variable	Calculation	Normal values
Cardiac index (CI)	CO/BSA	$2.5-4.0$ L/min/m^2
Stroke volume (SV)	CO $\times$ 1000/HR	$60-90$ mL/beat
Stroke index (SI)	SV/BSA	$40-60$ mL/beat/m^2
Mean arterial pressure (MAP)	Diastolic pressure + $\frac{1}{3}$ pulse pressure	$80-120$ mm Hg
Systemic vascular resistance (SVR)	$\frac{MAP - \overline{CVP}}{CO} \times 79.9$	$1200-1500$ dyne-cm-sec^{-5}
Pulmonary vascular resistance (PVR)	$\frac{\overline{PAP} - \overline{PCWP}}{CO} \times 79.9$	$100-300$ dyne-cm-sec^{-5}
Right ventricular stroke work index (RVSWI)	0.0136 ($\overline{PAP}$ − CVP) $\times$ SI	$5-9$ g-m/beat/m^2
Left ventricular stroke work index (LVSWI)	0.0136 (MAP − PCWP) $\times$ SI	$45-60$ g-m/beat/m^2

HR = heart rate; $\overline{CVP}$ = mean central venous pressure; BSA = body surface area; CO = cardiac output; $\overline{PAP}$ = mean pulmonary artery pressure; PCWP = pulmonary capillary wedge pressure; MAP = mean arterial blood pressure.

RESPIRATORY FORMULAS

	Normal values (70 kg)
Alveolar oxygen tension	110 mm Hg
$P_{AO_2} = (P_B - 47)\,F_{IO_2} - P_{ACO_2}$	$(F_{IO_2} = 0.21)$
Alveolar–arterial oxygen gradient	<10 mm Hg
$A_{aO_2} = P_{AO_2} - P_{aO_2}$	$(F_{IO_2} = 0.21)$
Arterial-to-alveolar oxygen ratio, a/A ratio	>0.75
Arterial oxygen content	21 mL/100 mL
$Ca_{O_2} = (Sa_{O_2})(Hb \times 1.34) + Pa_{O_2}(0.0031)$	
Mixed venous oxygen content	15 mL/100 mL
$C\bar{v}_{O_2} = (S\bar{v}_{O_2})(Hb \times 1.34) + P\bar{v}_{O_2}\,(0.0031)$	
Arterial–venous oxygen content difference	
$av\,O_2 = Ca_{O_2} - C\bar{v}_{O_2}$	4–6 mL/100 mL
Intrapulmonary shunt	<5%
$\dot{Q}s/\dot{Q}T = (Cc_{O_2} - Ca_{O_2})/(Cc_{O_2} - C\bar{v}_{O_2})$	
$Cc_{O_2} = (Hb \times 1.34) + (P_{AO_2} \times 0.0031)$	
Physiologic dead space	0.33
$V_D/V_T = (Pa_{CO_2} - Pe_{CO_2})/Pa_{CO_2}$	
Oxygen consumption	240 mL/min
$\dot{V}_{O_2} = CO\,(Ca_{O_2} - C\bar{v}_{O_2})$	
Oxygen transport	
$O_2T = CO\,(Ca_{O_2})$	1000 mL/min

Ca_{O_2} = arterial oxygen content; $C\bar{v}_{O_2}$ = mixed venous oxygen content; Cc_{O_2} = pulmonary capillary oxygen content; CO = cardiac output; F_{IO_2} = fraction inspired oxygen; O_2T = oxygen transport; P_B = barometric pressure; $\dot{Q}S/\dot{Q}T$ = intrapulmonary shunt; Pa_{CO_2} = alveolar carbon dioxide tension; Pa_{CO_2} = arterial carbon dioxide tension; P_{AO_2} = alveolar oxygen tension; Pa_{O_2} = arterial oxygen tension; Pe_{CO_2} = expired carbon dioxide tension; V_D = dead space gas volume; V_T = tidal volume; $\dot{V}_{O_2}$ = oxygen consumption (minute).

LUNG VOLUMES AND CAPACITIES

	Lung Volume (% TLC)
IRV	45–50%
TV	10–15%
ERV	15–20%
RV	20–25%

		Normal values (70 kg)
Vital capacity	VC	4,800 mL
Inspiratory capacity	IC	3,800 mL
Functional residual capacity	FRC	2,400 mL
Inspiratory reserve volume	IRV	3,500 mL
Tidal volume	TV	1,500 mL
Expiratory reserve volume	ERV	1,200 mL
Residual volume	RV	1,200 mL
Total lung capacity	TLC	6,000 mL

APPENDIX B ■
ELECTROCARDIOGRAPHY ATLAS

ELECTROCARDIOGRAM

LEAD PLACEMENT

| | Electrode | |
	Positive	Negative
BIPOLAR LEADS		
I	LA	RA
II	LL	RA
III	LL	LA
AUGMENTED UNIPOLAR		
aVR	RA	LA, LL
aVL	LA	RA, LL
aVF	LL	RA, LA
	Position	
PRECORDIAL		
V_1	4 ICS–RSB	
V_2	4 ICS–LSB	
V_3	Midway between V_2 and V_4	
V_4	5 ICS–MCL	
V_5	5 ICS–AAL	
V_6	5 ICS–MAL	

We wish to thank Dr. Malcom S. Thaler for graciously permitting re-production of electrocardiographic tracings from his book. The Only EKG Book You'll Ever Need *(Philadelphia, JB Lippincott, 1988).*

THREE-LEAD SYSTEMS

Bipolar lead system	Electrode placement	ECG lead[a]	Advantage
II	RA R–clavicle LA L–10th rib (midclavicular line) LL Ground	II (II)	Dysrhythmias
MCL 1	RA Ground LA L–clavicle LL V_1	III (V_1)	Dysrhythmias and conduction defects
CS 5	RA R–clavicle LA V_5 LL Ground	I (V_5)	Precordial ischemia
CB 5	RA R–scapula LA V_5 LA Ground	I (V_5)	Precordial ischemia and dysrhythmias

MCL = modified central lead; CB = central back; CS = central subclavian.
[a] Selected lead on monitor; () = simulated ECG lead.

THE NORMAL ELECTROCARDIOGRAM—
CARDIAC CYCLE

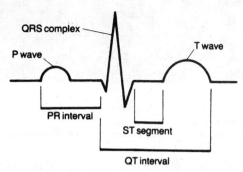

In this section the ECG complex is divided into the atrial (PR interval) and ventricular (QT interval) components.

ASHMAN BEATS

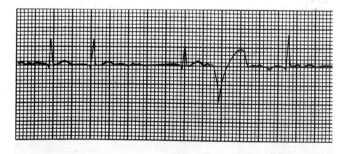

Rate: Variable.

Rhythm: Irregular.

PR interval: P wave may be present if supraventricular premature beat.

QT interval: QRS prolonged (>0.12 s) and altered, revealing bundle-branch pattern, most commonly right bundle. ST segment abnormal.

Note: Ashman beats are often confused with ventricular premature contractions. Ashman beats, usually seen with atrial fibrillation, have no compensatory pause and are a benign ECG finding requiring no treatment.

ATRIAL FIBRILLATION

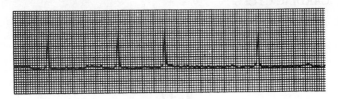

Rate: Variable (~150–200 beats/min).
Rhythm: Irregular.
PR interval: No P wave, and PR interval not discernible.
QT interval: QRS normal.

Note: Must be differentiated from atrial flutter: (1) absence of flutter waves and presence of fibrillatory line; (2) flutter usually associated with higher ventricular rates (>150 beats/min). Loss of atrial contraction reduces cardiac output (10–20%). Mural atrial thrombi may develop. Considered controlled if ventricular rate <100 beats/min.

ATRIAL FLUTTER

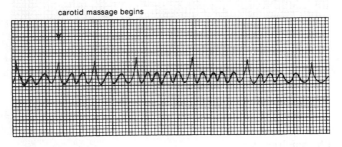

carotid massage begins

Rate: Rapid, atrial usually regular (250–350 beats/min); ventricular usually regular (<100 beats/min).
Rhythm: Atrial and ventricular regular.
PR interval: Flutter (F) waves are saw-toothed. PR interval cannot be measured.
QT interval: QRS usually normal; ST segment and T waves are not identifiable.

Note: Carotid massage will slow ventricular response, simplifying recognition of the F waves.

ATRIOVENTRICULAR BLOCK
(First Degree)

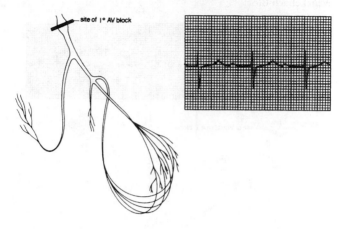

Rate: 60–100 beats/min.
Rhythm: Regular.
PR interval: Prolonged (>0.20 s) and constant.
QT interval: Normal.

Note: Usually clinically insignificant; may be early harbinger of drug toxicity.

ATRIOVENTRICULAR BLOCK
(Second Degree), Mobitz Type I/
Wenckebach Block

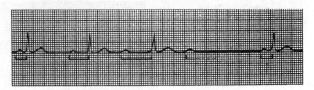

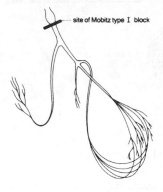

site of Mobitz type I block

Rate: 60–100 beats/min.

Rhythm: Atrial regular; ventricular irregular.

PR interval: P wave normal; PR interval progressively lengthens with each cycle until QRS complex is dropped (dropped beat). PR interval following dropped beat is shorter than normal.

QT interval: QRS complex normal but dropped periodically.

Note: Commonly seen (1) in trained athletes and (2) with drug toxicity.

ATRIOVENTRICULAR BLOCK
(Second Degree), Mobitz Type II

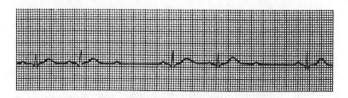

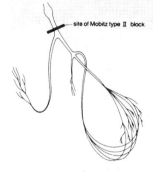

site of Mobitz type II block

Rate: <100 beats/min.

Rhythm: Atrial regular; ventricular regular or irregular.

PR interval: P waves normal, but some are not followed by QRS complex.

QT interval: Normal but may have widened QRS complex if block is at level of bundle branch. ST segment and T wave may be abnormal, depending on location of block.

Note: In contrast to Mobitz type I block, the PR and RR intervals are constant and the dropped QRS occurs without warning. The wider the QRS complex (block lower in the conduction system), the greater the amount of myocardial damage.

ATRIOVENTRICULAR BLOCK
(Third Degree), Complete Heart Block

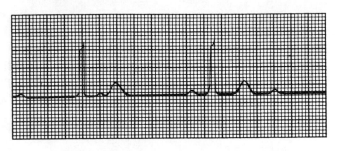

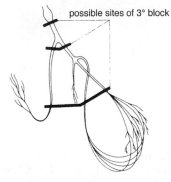

possible sites of 3° block

Rate: <45 beats/min.

Rhythm: Atrial regular; ventricular regular; no relationship between P wave and QRS complex.

PR interval: Variable because atria and ventricles beat independently.

QT interval: QRS morphology variable, depending on the origin of the ventricular beat in the intrinsic pacemaker system (atrioventricular junctional versus ventricular pacemaker). ST segment and T wave normal.

Note: Immediate treatment with atropine or isoproterenol is required if cardiac output is reduced. Consideration should be given to insertion of a pacemaker. Seen as a complication of mitral valve replacement.

ATRIOVENTRICULAR DISSOCIATION

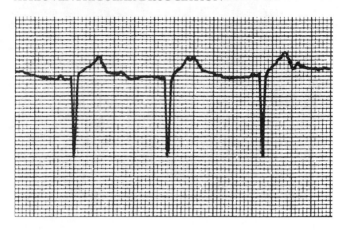

Rate: Variable.

Rhythm: Atrial regular; ventricular regular; ventricular rate faster than atrial rate; no relationship between P wave and QRS complex.

PR interval: Variable because atria and ventricles beat independently.

QT interval: QRS morphology depends on location of ventricular pacemaker. ST segment and T wave abnormal.

Note: Digitalis toxicity can present as atrioventricular dissociation.

BUNDLE-BRANCH BLOCK—LEFT (LBBB)

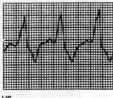

V6

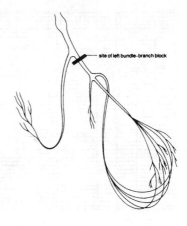

site of left bundle-branch block

Rate: <100 beats/min.
Rhythm: Regular.
PR interval: Normal.
QT interval: Complete LBBB (QRS >0.12 s); incomplete LBBB
  (QRS = 0.10–0.12 s). Lead V_1 negative rS complex; I, aVL, V_6
  wide R wave without Q or S component. ST segment and T
  wave defection opposite direction of the R wave.

Note: LBBB does not occur in healthy patients and usually indicates serious heart disease with a poorer prognosis. In patients
with LBBB, insertion of a pulmonary artery catheter may lead to
complete heart block.

BUNDLE-BRANCH BLOCK—RIGHT (RBBB)

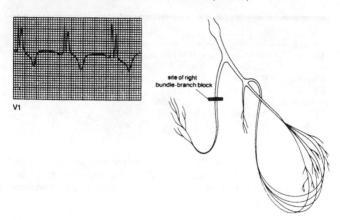

Rate: <100 beats/min.
Rhythm: Regular.
PR interval: Normal.
QT interval: Complete RBBB (QRS >0.12 s); incomplete RBBB (QRS = 0.10–0.12 s). Varying patterns of QRS complex; rSR (V_1); RS, wide R with M pattern. ST segment and T wave opposite direction of the R wave.

Note: In the presence of RBBB, Q waves may be seen with a myocardial infarction.

ELECTROLYTE DISTURBANCES

	$\downarrow Ca^{2+}$	$\uparrow Ca^{2+}$	$\downarrow K^{+}$	$\uparrow K^{+}$
Rate	<100 beats/min	<100 beats/min	<100 beats/min	<100 beats/min
Rhythm	Regular	Regular	Regular	Regular
PR interval	Normal	Normal/increased	Normal	Normal
QT interval	Increased	Decreased	T flat U wave	T peaked QT decreased

Note: ECG changes usually do not correlate with serum calcium. Hypocalcemia rarely causes dysrhythmias in the absence of hypokalemia. In contrast, abnormalities in serum potassium concentration can be diagnosed by ECG.

DIGITALIS EFFECT

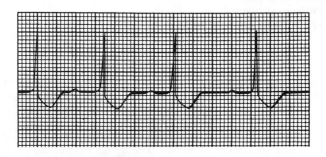

Rate: <100 beats/min.
Rhythm: Regular.
PR interval: Normal or prolonged.
QT interval: ST segment sloping ("digitalis effect").

Note: Digitalis toxicity can be the cause of many common dysrhythmias (e.g., premature ventricular contractions, second-degree heart block). Verapamil, quinidine, and amiodarone cause an increase in serum digitalis concentration.

CORONARY ARTERY DISEASE—Ischemia

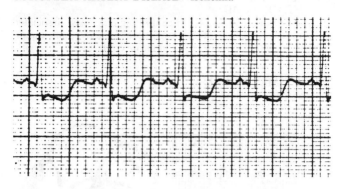

Rate: Variable.

Rhythm: Usually regular, but may show atrial and/or ventricular dysrhythmias.

PR interval: Normal.

QT interval: ST segment depressed; J point depression; T-wave inversion: conduction disturbances. Coronary vasospasm (Prinzmetal) ST segment elevation.

Note: Intraoperative ischemia is usually seen in the presence of "normal" vital signs (e.g., ± 20% of preinduction values).

CORONARY ARTERY DISEASE—
Myocardial Infarction

Anatomic site	Leads	ECG changes	Coronary artery
Inferior	II, III, aVF	Q, ST, T	Right
Lateral	I, aVL, V_5–V_6	Q, ST, T	Left circumflex
Anterior	I, aVL, V_1–V_4	Q, ST, T	Left
Anteroseptal	V_1–V_4	Q, ST, T	Left anterior descending

SUBENDOCARDIAL MYOCARDIAL INFARCTION (SEMI)

Persistent ST segment depression and/or T-wave inversion in the absence of Q wave. Usually requires additional laboratory data (e.g., isoenzymes) to confirm diagnosis.

TRANSMURAL MYOCARDIAL INFARCTION (TMI)

Q waves seen on ECG useful in confirming diagnosis. Associated with poorer prognosis and more significant hemodynamic impairment; dysrhythmias frequently complicate course.

PAROXYSMAL ATRIAL TACHYCARDIA (PAT)

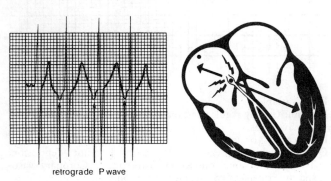

retrograde P wave

Rate: 150–250 beats/min.

Rhythm: Regular.

PR interval: Difficult to distinguish because of tachycardia obscuring P wave. P wave may precede, be included in, or follow QRS complex.

QT interval: Normal, but ST segment and T wave may be difficult to distinguish.

Note: Therapy depends on degree of hemodynamic compromise. In contrast to management of PAT in awake patients, synchronized cardoversion rather than pharmacologic treatment is preferred in hemodynamically unstable anesthetized patients.

PREMATURE ATRIAL CONTRACTION (PAC)

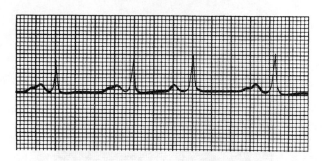

Rate: < 100 beats/min.

Rhythm: Irregular.

PR interval: P waves may be lost in preceding T waves. PR interval is variable.

QT interval: QRS normal configuration; ST segment and T wave normal.

Note: Nonconducted PAC appearnace similar to that of sinus arrest; T waves with PAC may be distorted by inclusion of P wave in the T wave.

PREMATURE VENTRICULAR CONTRACTION (PVC)

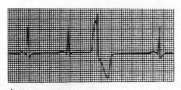

A

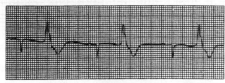

B

Rate: Usually <100 beats/min.
Rhythm: Irregular.
PR interval: P wave and PR interval absent; retrograde conduction of P wave can be seen.
QT interval: Wide QRS (>0.12 s); ST segment cannot be evaluated (e.g., ischemia); T wave opposite direction of QRS with compensatory pause (*A*). Bigeminy: every other beat a PVC (*B*); trigeminy: every third beat a PVC. R-on-T occurs when PVC falls in the T wave and can lead to ventricular tachycardia or fibrillation.

Note: If compensatory pause is not seen following an ectopic beat, the complex is most likely supraventricular in origin.

SINUS TACHYCARDIA

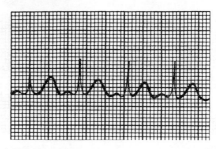

Rate: 100–160 beats/min.
Rhythm: Regular.
PR interval: Normal; P wave may be difficult to see.
QT interval: Normal.

Note: Should be differentiated from paroxysmal atrial tachycardia (PAT). With PAT, carotid massage terminates dysrhythmia. Sinus tachycardia may respond to vagal maneuvers but reappears as soon as vagal stimulus is removed.

TORSADES DE POINTES

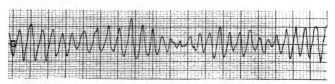

Rate: 150–250 beats/min.
Rhythm: No atrial component seen; ventricular rhythm regular or irregular.
PR interval: P wave buried in QRS complex.
QT interval: QRS complexes usually wide and with phasic variation twisting around a central axis (a few complexes point upward then a few point downward). ST segments and T waves difficult to discern.

Note: Type of ventricular tachycardia associated with prolonged QT interval. Seen with electrolyte disturbances (e.g., hypokalemia, hypocalcemia, and hypomagnesemia) and bradycardia. Administering standard antidysrhythmics (lidocaine, procainamide, etc.) may worsen Torsades de Pointes. Treatment includes increasing heart rate pharmacologically or by pacing.

VENTRICULAR FIBRILLATION

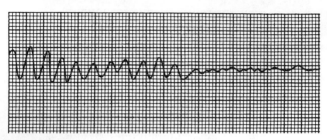

Rate: Absent.
Rhythm: None.
PR interval: Absent.
QT interval: Absent.

Note: "Pseudoventricular fibrillation" may be the result of a monitor malfunction (e.g., ECG lead disconnect). Always check for carotid pulse before instituting therapy.

VENTRICULAR TACHYCARDIA

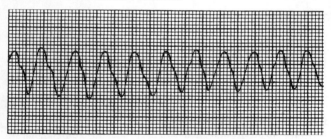

Rate: 100–250 beats/min.
Rhythm: No atrial component seen; ventricular rhythm irregular or regular.
PR interval: Absent; retrograde P wave may be seen in QRS complex.
QT interval: Wide, bizarre QRS complex. ST segment and T wave difficult to determine.

Note: In the presence of hemodynamic compromise, immediate DC synchronized cardioversion is required. If the patient is stable, with short bursts of ventricular tachycardia, pharmacologic management is preferred. Should be differentiated from supraventricular tachycardia with aberrancy (SVT-A). Compensatory pause and atrioventricular dissociation suggest a PVC. P waves and SR' (V_1) and slowing to vagal stimulus suggest SVT-A.

WOLFF-PARKINSON-WHITE SYNDROME (WPW)

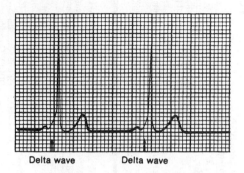

Delta wave   Delta wave

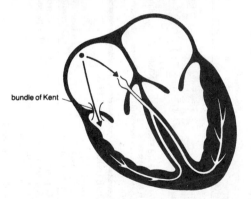

bundle of Kent

Rate: <100 beats/min.
Rhythm: Regular.
PR interval: P wave normal; PR interval short (<0.12 s).
QT interval: Duration (>0.10 s) with slurred QRS complex.
  Type A has delta wave, RBBB, with upright QRS complex V_1.
  Type B has delta wave and downward QRS-V_1. ST segment and
  T wave usually normal.

Note: Digoxin should be avoided in the presence of WPW because
it increases conduction through the accessory bypass tract (bundle
of Kent) and decreases atrioventricular node conduction; consequently, ventricular fibrillation can occur.

PACEMAKER

GENERIC PACEMAKER CODE (NBG*): NASPE/BPEG REVISED (2002)

Position I, pacing chamber(s)	Position II, sensing chamber(s)	Position III, response(s) to sensing	Position IV, programmability	Position V, multisite pacing
O = none	O = none	O = none	O = none	O = none
A = atrium	A = atrium	I = Inhibited	R = rate modulation	A = atrium
V = ventricle	V = ventricle	T = triggered		V = ventricle
D = dual (A+V)	D = dual (A+V)	D = dual (T+I)		D = dual (A+V)

ICD, implanted cardioverter defibrillator.

*NBG: N refers to North American Society of Pacing and Electrophysiology (NASPE), now called the Heart Rhythm Society (HRS), B refers to British Pacing and Electrophysiology Group (BPEG), and G refers to generic.

From Practice Advisory for Perioperative Management of Patients with Cardiac Rrhythm Management Devices: Pacemakers and Implantable Cardioventer Defibrillators. Anesthesiology, 103:186, 2005.

GENERIC DEFIBRILLATOR CODE (NBD): NASPE/BPEG

Position I, shock chamber(s)	Position II, antitachycardia pacing chamber(s)	Position III, tachycardia detection	Position IV,* antibradycardia pacing chamber(s)
O = none	O = none	E = electrogram	O = none
A = atrium	A = atrium	H = hemodynamic	A = atrium
V = ventricle	V = ventricle		V = ventricle
D = dual (A+V)	D = dual (A+V)		D = dual (A+V)

*For robust identification, position IV is expanded into its complete NBG code. For example, a biventricular pacing–defibrillator with ventricular shock and antitachycardia pacing functionality would be identified as VVE-DDDRV, assuming that the pacing section was programmed DDDRV. Currently, no hemodynamic sensors have been approved for tachycardia detection (position III).

From Practice Advisory for Perioperative Management of Patients with Cardiac Rrhythm Management Devices: Pacemakers and Implantable Cardioventer Defibrillators. Anesthesiology, 103:186, 2005.

EXAMPLE OF A STEPWISE APPROACH TO THE PERIOPERATIVE TREATMENT OF THE PATIENT WITH A CARDIAC RHYTHM MANAGEMENT DEVICE (CRMD)

Perioperative period	Patient/CRMD condition	Intervention
Preoperative evaluation	Patient has CRMD	• Focused history • Focused physical examination
	Determine CRMD type (pacemaker, ICD, CRT)	• Manufacture's CRMD identification card • Chest x-ray studies (no data available) • Supplemental resources*
	Determine whether patient is CRMD-dependent for pacing function	• Verbal history • Bradyarrhythmia symptoms • Atrioventricular node ablation • No spontaneous ventricular activity†
	Determine CRMD function	• Comprehensive CRMD evaluation‡ • Determine whether pacing pulses are present and create paced beats
Preoperative preparation	EMI unlikely during procedure	• If EMI unlikely, special precautions are not needed
	EMI likely: CRMD is pacemaker	• Reprogram to asynchronous mode when indicated • Suspend rate-adaptive functions§
	EMI likely: CRMD is ICD	• Suspend antitachyarrhythmia functions • If patient is dependent on pacing function, after pacing functions as above
	EMI likely: all CRMD	• Use bipolar cautery; ultrasonic scalpel • Temporary pacing and external cardioversion–defibrillation available
	Intraoperative physiologic changes likely (e.g., bradycardia, ischemia)	• Plan for possible adverse CRMD–patient interaction

EXAMPLE OF A STEPWISE APPROACH TO THE PERIOPERATIVE TREATMENT OF THE PATIENT WITH A CRMD (CONTINUED)

Perioperative period	Patient/CRMD condition	Intervention
Intraoperative management	Monitoring	• Electrocardiographic monitoring per ASA standard • Peripheral pulse monitoring
	Electrocautery interference	• CT/CRP—no current through PG/leads • Avoid proximity of CT to PG/leads • Short bursts at lowest possible energy • Use bipolar cautery; ultrasonic scalpel
	Radiofrequency catheter ablation	• Avoid contact of radiofrequency catheter with PG/leads • Radiofrequency current path far away from PG/leads • Discuss these concerns with operator
	Lithotripsy	• Do not focus lithotripsy beam near PG • R wave triggers lithotripsy? Disable atrial pacing||
	MRI	• Generally contraindicated • If required, consult ordering physician, cardiologist, radiologists, and manufacturer
	RT	• PG/leads must be outside of RT field • Possible surgical relocation of PG • Verify PG function during/after RT course
	ECT	• Consult with ordering physician, patient's cardiologist, a CRMD service, or CRMD manufacturer

Emergency defibrillation–cardioversion	
ICD: magnet disabled	• Terminate all EMI sources • Remove magnet to reenable therapies • Observe for appropriate therapies
ICD: programming disabled	• Programming to reenable therapies or proceed directly with external cardioversion–defibrillation
ICD: either of above	• Minimize current flow through PG/leads • PP as far as possible from PG. • PP perpendicular to major axis PG/leads • To extent possible, PP in anterior–posterior location
Regardless of CRMD type	• Use clinically appropriate cardioversion/defibrillation energy
Immediate postoperative period	• Monitor cardiac R&R continuously • Backup pacing and cardioversion/defibrillation capability
Postoperative management	
Postoperative interrogation and restoration of CRMD function	• Interrogation to assess function • Setting appropriate?# • Is CRMD an ICD?** • Use cardiology/pacemaker–ICD service if needed

*Manufacturer's databases, pacemaker clinic records, cardiology consultation. †With cardiac rhythm management device (CRMD) programmed WI at lowest programmable rate. ‡Ideally CRMD function assessed by interrogation, with function altered by reprogramming if required. §Most times this will be necessary; when in doubt, assume so. ||Atrial pacing spikes may be interpreted by the lithotriptor as R waves, possibly inciting the lithotriptor to deliver a shock during a vulnerable period in the heart. #If necessary, reprogram appropriate setting. **restore all antitachycardia therapies.
CRP, current return pad; CRT, cardiac resynchronization therapy; CT, cautery tool; ECT, electroconvulsive therapy; EMI, electromagnetic interference; ICD, internal cardioverter–defibrillator; MRI, magnetic resonance imaging; PG, pulse generator; PP, external cardioversion–defibrillation pads or paddles; R&R, rhythm and rate; RT, radiation therapy.
From Practice Advisory for Perioperative Management of Patients with Cardiac Rhythm Management Devices: Pacemakers and Implantable Cardioventer Defibrillators. Anesthesiology, 103:186, 2005.

TREATMENT OF PACEMAKER FAILURE

Rate	Possible treatment
Adequate to maintain blood pressure	1. Observe, oxygen
	2. Atropine
	3. Try magnet
Severe bradycardia hypotension	1. Oxygen, airway control
	2. Atropine
	3. Isoproterenol
	4. Try magnet
	5. Transcutaneous pacing
No escape rhythm	1. CPR
	2. Isoproterenol
	3. Try magnet
	4. Transcutaneous pacing

Reprinted with permission from Zaldan JR: Pacemakers. In Youngberg JA, Lake CL, Roizeu MF, Wilson KS (eds): Cardiac, Vascular and Thoracic Anesthesia. New York, Churchill Livingsteon, 2000.

ATRIAL PACING

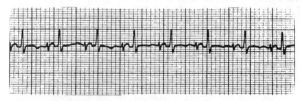

Atrial pacing as demonstrated in this figure is used when the atrial impulse can proceed through the AV node. Examples are sinus bradycardia and junctional rhythms associated with clinically significant decreases in blood pressure.

VENTRICULAR PACING

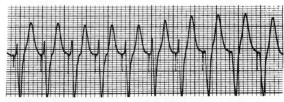

In this tracing ventricular pacing is evident by absence of atrial wave (*P wave*) and pacemaker spike preceding QRS complex. Ventricular pacing is used in the presence of bradycardia secondary to AV block or atrial fibrillation.

DDD PACING

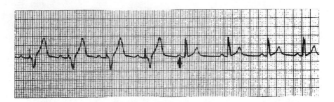

The DDD pacemaker (generator), one of the most commonly used, paces and senses both atrium and ventricle. In the first four beats, the P waves were not followed by a QRS complex within the programmed PR interval. Therefore, a ventricular pacing spike and a ventricular paced beat occurred. In the last four beats (*after the arrow*), atrial activity proceeded through the AV node in the allotted amount of time; therefore, ventricular pacing was inhibited.

ATRIAL ELECTROGRAM (AEG)

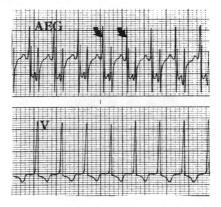

The AEG is useful in differentiating various atrial dysrhythmias. The AEG is obtained from an intracardiac or esophageal lead, if P waves are not clearly seen on the surface ECG. In this trace the V lead does not have obvious P waves; however, the AEG reveals large P waves (*arrows*) that precede each QRS complex. Locate the QRS on the AEG by matching the R wave on the surface ECG to the AEG. The surface and AEG must be simultaneously recorded.

GUIDELINES FOR USING THE ELECTROCAUTERY

1. Electromagnet interference created by an electrocautery can cause a number of problems with pacemaker or ICD function including, but not limited to, reprogramming, inhibition, noise reversion mode, electrical reset, myocardial burns, increase in threshold, rate increment changes in rate adaptive pacemakers, and inappropriate sensing and charging in ICDs.[2,3]
2. When positioning the return plate of the electrocautery,
   a. Ensure it is located so the pacemaker or ICD is not between this return plate and the active electrode.
   b. Ensure the plane described by the return plate and the active electrode of the electrocautery is perpendicular to a plane described by the pacemaker or ICD and the pacemaker's electrodes.
3. Use the smallest current required to cut or coagulate.
4. Use the electrocautery in short bursts.
5. Avoid using the electrocautery within 6 in. of the device or leads.
6. Consider using the bipolar electrocautery or the ultrasonic scalpel[4,5] to minimize interference with pacemaker or ICD function.
7. Activating the electrocautery in the area of the pacemaker or ICD, even if the active electrode is not touching the patient, will cause interference.
8. Do not use the electrocautery when an ICD is programmed to sense and deliver therapy.
9. Convert the ICD to no response either by programming or by using the magnet, depending on the manufacturer of the ICD so the device will not deliver therapy secondary to misinterpretation of signals from the electrocautery as a dysrhythmia. These maneuvers will not change the program of a pacemaker that is incorporated into an ICD.
10. If desired, convert a pacemaker that does not have an ICD to the asynchronous mode so it is not inhibited by the electrocautery.
11. A magnet will not change bradycardia-related pacing parameters in the ICD.
12. ICDs must be programmed to respond to a magnet.

ICD, implanted cardioverter defibrillator.

ADDITIONAL ISSUES FOR PATIENTS WITH IMPLANTED CARDIOVERTER DEFIBRILLATORS

1. All ICDs have pacemakers incorporated into the circuitry.
2. Preoperative assessments should include those procedures that are standard for patients with heart disease.
3. Obtain a cardiology consult to help assess the patient, interrogate the ICD, program the device to no response, and program the device to respond to the magnet.
4. There is no particular anesthetic technique that is clearly right or wrong for a patient who has an ICD.
5. Apply patches for external defibrillation when the ICD is programmed to no response. Ensure these external patches are as far away as possible from the device and, if possible, not in the same plane as the device and electrodes.
6. Monitor as required for patient care. If monitoring with a pulmonary arterial catheter, discuss the issues of dislodgment of the ICD's electrodes with the patient and cardiologist. Document in the chart your discussions and the logic supporting the necessity for a pulmonary arterial catheter. Maintain sterile technique, and consider administering antibiotics just before inserting central lines.
7. Continue antidysrhythmic agents until the time of surgery. Discuss with the cardiologist the necessity of administering an additional dose of an antidysrhythmic agent if the patient experiences an intraoperative dysrhythmia.
8. Intraoperative dysrhythmias:
   a. If the patient has a dysrhythmia, rule out and treat the usual intraoperative causes to prevent a recurrence.
   b. If the dysrhythmia continues and a magnet has been used to create the no response mode, remove the magnet from the ICD and allow the ICD to charge and deliver a response.
   c. If the ICD has been programmed to the no response mode, then either quickly reprogram the ICD to deliver a response or proceed directly to external defibrillation.
   d. If external defibrillation or cardioversion is required, apply the defibrillator paddles in an anterior-posterior position if possible and deliver the shock at a level sufficient to terminate the dysrhythmia.
   e. External pacing might be required if the pacemaker/ICD is damaged with the shock.
9. Monitor the patient's ECG and be prepared to deliver an external defibrillation when transporting the patient to and from the operating room.
10. Interrogate and reprogram the ICD when the patient has entered the postoperative care unit.

ECG, electrocardiogram; ICD, implanted cardioverter defibrillator.

1. Practice advisory for perioperative management of patients with cardiac rhythm management devices: Pacemakers and implantable cardioverter-defibrillators. A Report by the American Society of Anesthesiologists Task Force on Perioperative Management of Patients with Cardiac Rhythm Management Devices. Anesthesiology, 103:186, 2005
2. Hayes DL, Strathmore NF: Electromagnetic interference with implantable devices. In Ellenbogen KA, Kay GN, Wilkoff BL (eds): Clinical Cardiac Pacing and Defibrillation, 2nd ed, p 939. Philadelphia, WB Saunders, 2000
3. Atlee JL, Bernstein AD: Cardiac rhythm management devices (part II): Perioperative management. Anesthesiology 95:1492, 2001
4. Epstein MR, Mayer JE Jr, Duncan BW: Use of an ultrasonic scalpel as an alternative to electrocautery in patients with pacemakers. Ann Thorac Surg 65:1802, 1998
5. Ozeren M, Dogan OV, Duzgun C, Yucel E: Use of an ultrasonic scalpel in the open-heart reoperation of a patient with pacemaker. Eur J Cardiothorac Surg 21:761, 2002

APPENDIX C ■ AMERICAN HEART ASSOCIATION (AHA) RESUSCITATION PROTOCOLS

Adult
  Comprehensive ECC Algorithm
  Ventricular Fibrillation/Pulseless VT Algorithm
  Pulseless Electrical Activity Algorithm
  Asystole: The Silent Heart Algorithm
  Bradycardia Algorithm
  The Tachycardia Overview Algorithm
  Narrow-Complex Supraventricular Tachycardia Algorithm
  Stable Ventricular Tachycardia (Monomorphic or Polymorphic) Algorithm
  Synchronized Cardioversion Algorithm
  The Acute Pulmonary Edema, Hypotension, and Shock Algorithm
  Algorithm for Suspected Stroke
Pediatric
  PALS (Pediatric Advanced Life Support) Bradycardia Algorithm
  PALS Pulseless Arrest Algorithm
  PALS Tachycardia Algorithm for Infants and Children with Rapid Rhythm and Adequate Perfusion
  PALS Tachycardia Algorithm for Infants and Children with Rapid Rhythm and Evidence of Poor Perfusion
  PALS Medications for Cardiac Arrest and Symptomatic Arrhythmias
  PALS Medications to Maintain Cardiac Output and for Postresuscitation Stabilization
Neonatal
  Algorithm for Resuscitation of the Newly Born Infant
  Therapeutic Guidelines
Conveying News of a Sudden Death to Family Members
Recommendations for Critical Incident Debriefing

For more detailed information, the reader is referred to the American Heart Association: Guidelines 2000 for Cardiopulmonary Resuscitation and Emergency Cardiovascular Care: International Consensus on Science. Circulation 102(8), 2000.

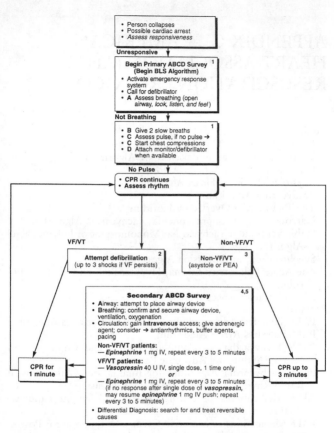

FIGURE 1. Comprehensive emergency cardiac care (ECC) algorithm.

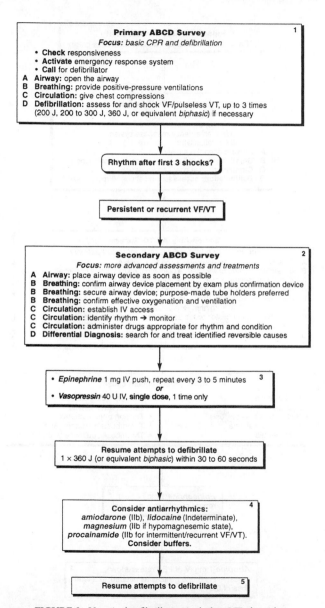

FIGURE 2. Ventricular fibrillation/pulseless VT algorithm.

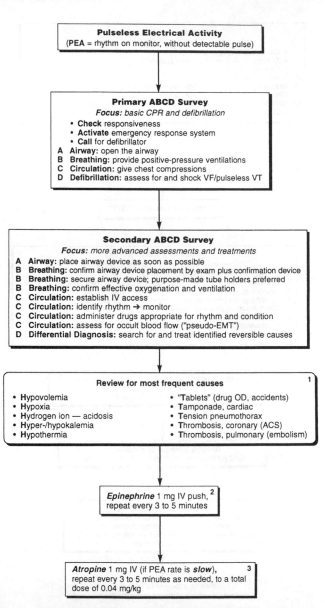

FIGURE 3. Pulseless electrical activity algorithm.

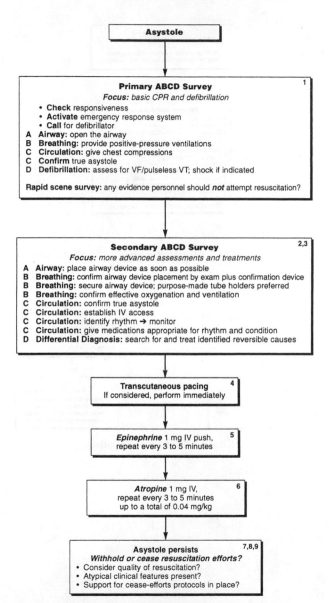

FIGURE 4. Asystole: The silent heart algorithm.

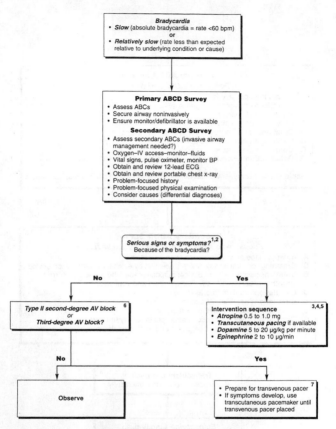

FIGURE 5. Bradycardia algorithm.

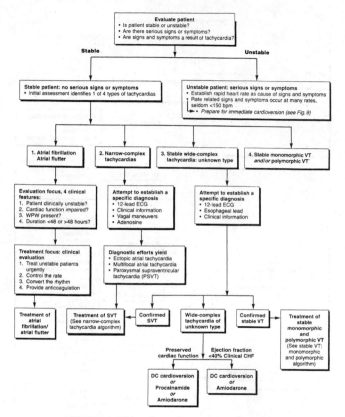

FIGURE 6. The tachycardia overview algorithm.

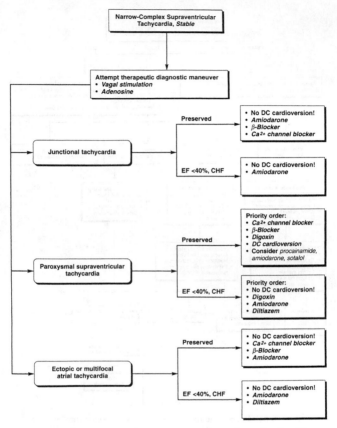

FIGURE 7. Narrow-complex supraventricular tachycardia algorithm.

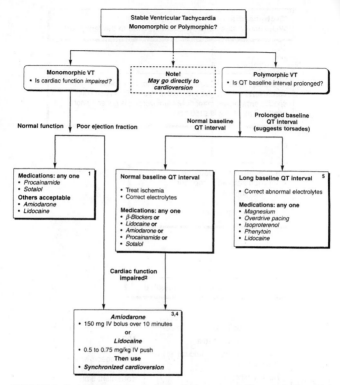

FIGURE 8. Stable ventricular tachycardia (monomorphic or polymorphic) algorithm.

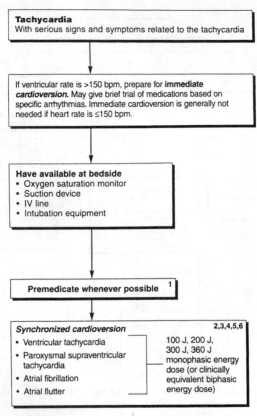

Tachycardia
With serious signs and symptoms related to the tachycardia

If ventricular rate is >150 bpm, prepare for **immediate cardioversion.** May give brief trial of medications based on specific arrhythmias. Immediate cardioversion is generally not needed if heart rate is ≤150 bpm.

Have available at bedside
- Oxygen saturation monitor
- Suction device
- IV line
- Intubation equipment

Premedicate whenever possible [1]

Synchronized cardioversion [2,3,4,5,6]
- Ventricular tachycardia
- Paroxysmal supraventricular tachycardia
- Atrial fibrillation
- Atrial flutter

100 J, 200 J, 300 J, 360 J monophasic energy dose (or clinically equivalent biphasic energy dose)

FIGURE 9. Synchronized cardioversion algorithm.

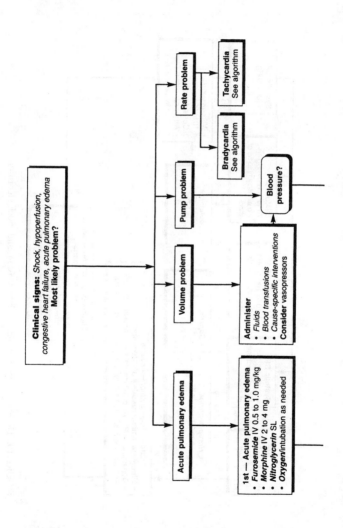

Clinical signs: *Shock, hypoperfusion, congestive heart failure, acute pulmonary edema*
Most likely problem?

Acute pulmonary edema

Volume problem

Pump problem

Rate problem

1st — Acute pulmonary edema
- *Furosemide* IV 0.5 to 1.0 mg/kg
- *Morphine* IV 2 to 4 mg
- *Nitroglycerin* SL
- *Oxygen*/intubation as needed

Administer
- *Fluids*
- *Blood transfusions*
- *Cause-specific interventions*
- **Consider vasopressors**

Blood pressure?

Bradycardia
See algorithm

Tachycardia
See algorithm

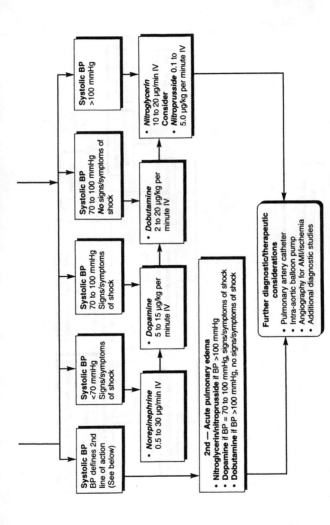

FIGURE 10. The acute pulmonary edema, hypotension, and shock algorithm.

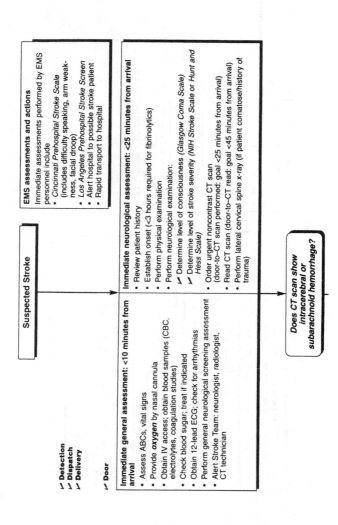

Suspected Stroke

✓ **Detection**
✓ **Dispatch**
✓ **Delivery**

✓ **Door**

EMS assessments and actions

Immediate assessments performed by EMS personnel include
- *Cincinnati Prehospital Stroke Scale* (includes difficulty speaking, arm weakness, facial droop)
- *Los Angeles Prehospital Stroke Screen*
- Alert hospital to possible stroke patient
- Rapid transport to hospital

Immediate general assessment: <10 minutes from arrival
- Assess ABCs, vital signs
- Provide **oxygen** by nasal cannula
- Obtain IV access; obtain blood samples (CBC, electrolytes, coagulation studies)
- Check blood sugar; treat if indicated
- Obtain 12-lead ECG; check for arrhythmias
- Perform general neurological screening assessment
- Alert Stroke Team: neurologist, radiologist, CT technician

Immediate neurological assessment: <25 minutes from arrival
- Review patient history
- Establish onset (<3 hours required for fibrinolytics)
- Perform physical examination
- Perform neurological examination:
  ✓ Determine level of consciousness (*Glasgow Coma Scale*)
  ✓ Determine level of stroke severity (*NIH Stroke Scale or Hunt and Hess Scale*)
- Order urgent noncontrast CT scan (door-to-CT scan performed): goal <25 minutes from arrival)
- Read CT scan (door-to-CT read: goal <45 minutes from arrival)
- Perform lateral cervical spine x-ray (if patient comatose/history of trauma)

Does CT scan show intracerebral or subarachnoid hemorrhage?

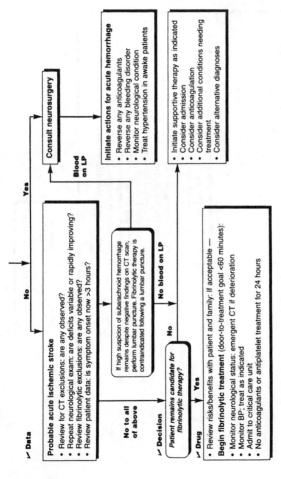

FIGURE 11. Algorithm for suspected stroke.

Data

Probable acute ischemic stroke
- Review for CT exclusions: are any observed?
- Repeat neurological exam: are deficits variable or rapidly improving?
- Review fibrinolytic exclusions: are any observed?
- Review patient data: is symptom onset now >3 hours?

No to all of above

If high suspicion of subarachnoid hemorrhage remains despite negative findings on CT scan, perform lumbar puncture. Fibrinolytic therapy is contraindicated following a lumbar puncture.

Consult neurosurgery

Blood on LP

No blood on LP

Initiate actions for acute hemorrhage
- Reverse any anticoaguants
- Reverse any bleeding disorder
- Monitor neurological condition
- Treat hypertension in awake patients

Decision

Patient remains candidate for fibrinolytic therapy?

Drug

No

Yes

Begin fibrinolytic treatment (door-to-treatment goal <60 minutes):
- Monitor neurological status: emergent CT if deterioration
- Monitor BP; treat as indicated
- Admit to critical care unit
- No anticoagulants or antiplatelet treatment for 24 hours

- Review risks/benefits with patient and family: If acceptable —

- Initiate supportive therapy as indicated
- Consider admission
- Consider anticoagulation
- Consider additional conditions needing treatment
- Consider alternative diagnoses

1016

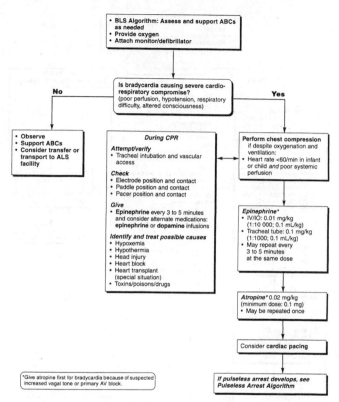

FIGURE 12. PALS (Pediatric Advanced Life Support) bradycardia algorithm.

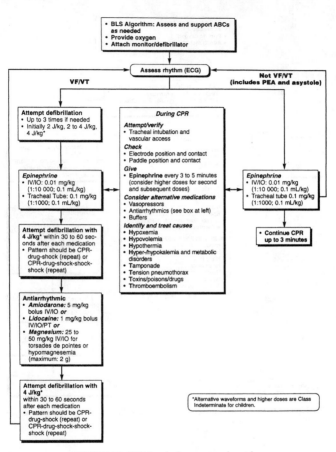

FIGURE 13. PALS pulseless arrest algorithm.

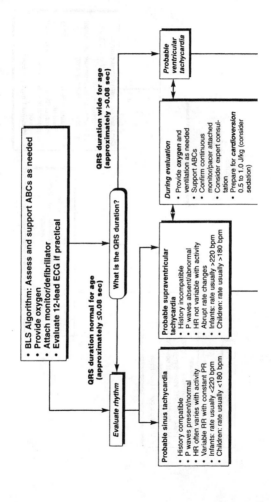

- BLS Algorithm: Assess and support ABCs as needed
- Provide oxygen
- Attach monitor/defibrillator
- Evaluate 12-lead ECG if practical

Evaluate rhythm

What is the QRS duration?

QRS duration normal for age (approximately ≤0.08 sec)

QRS duration wide for age (approximately >0.08 sec)

Probable sinus tachycardia
- History compatible
- P waves present/normal
- HR often varies with activity
- Variable RR with constant PR
- Infants: rate usually <220 bpm
- Children: rate usually <180 bpm

Probable supraventricular tachycardia
- History incompatible
- P waves absent/abnormal
- HR not variable with activity
- Abrupt rate changes
- Infants: rate usually >220 bpm
- Children: rate usually >180 bpm

Probable ventricular tachycardia

During evaluation
- Provide *oxygen* and ventilation as needed
- Support ABCs
- Confirm continuous monitor/pacer attached
- Consider expert consultation
- Prepare for *cardioversion* 0.5 to 1.0 J/kg (consider sedation)

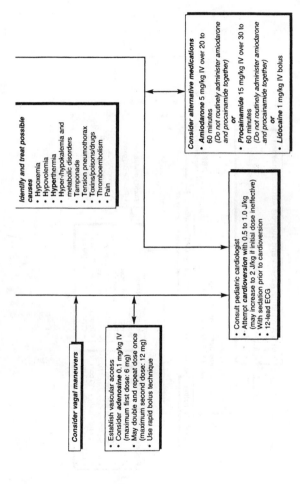

Identify and treat possible causes
- Hypoxemia
- Hypovolemia
- Hyperthermia
- Hyper-/hypokalemia and metabolic disorders
- Tamponade
- Tension pneumothorax
- Toxins/poisons/drugs
- Thromboembolism
- Pain

Consider alternative medications
- **Amiodarone** 5 mg/kg IV over 20 to 60 minutes
  (Do not routinely administer amiodarone and procainamide together)
  or
- **Procainamide** 15 mg/kg IV over 30 to 60 minutes
  (Do not routinely administer amiodarone and procainamide together)
  or
- **Lidocaine** 1 mg/kg IV bolus

Consider vagal maneuvers

- Establish vascular access
- Consider **adenosine** 0.1 mg/kg IV (maximum first dose: 6 mg)
- May double and repeat dose once (maximum second dose: 12 mg)
- Use rapid bolus technique

- Consult pediatric cardiologist
- Attempt **cardioversion** with 0.5 to 1.0 J/kg (may increase to 2 J/kg if initial dose ineffective)
- With sedation prior to cardioversion
- 12-lead ECG

FIGURE 14. PALS tachycardia algorithm for infants and children with rapid rhythm and adequate perfusion.

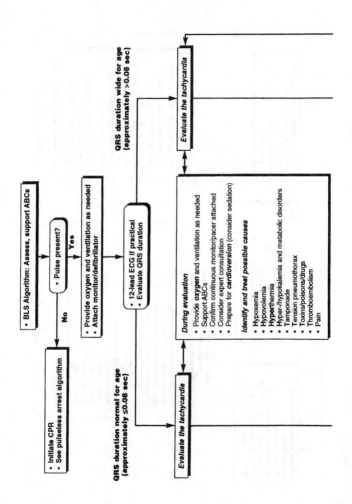

- **BLS Algorithm: Assess, support ABCs**

- **Pulse present?**

  No →
  - Initiate CPR
  - See pulseless arrest algorithm

  Yes →
  - Provide oxygen and ventilation as needed
  - Attach monitor/defibrillator

- 12-lead ECG if practical
- Evaluate QRS duration

QRS duration normal for age (approximately ≤0.08 sec)

Evaluate the tachycardia

QRS duration wide for age (approximately >0.08 sec)

Evaluate the tachycardia

During evaluation
- Provide **oxygen** and ventilation as needed
- Support ABCs
- Confirm continuous monitor/pacer attached
- Consider expert consultation
- Prepare for **cardioversion** (consider sedation)

Identify and treat possible causes
- Hypoxemia
- Hypovolemia
- Hyperthermia
- Hyper-/hypokalemia and metabolic disorders
- Tamponade
- Tension pneumothorax
- Toxins/poisons/drugs
- Thromboembolism
- Pain

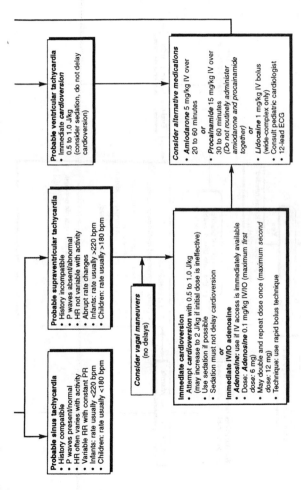

Probable sinus tachycardia
- History compatible
- P waves present/normal
- HR often varies with activity
- Variable RR with constant PR
- Infants: rate usually <220 bpm
- Children: rate usually <180 bpm

Probable supraventricular tachycardia
- History incompatible
- P waves absent/abnormal
- HR not variable with activity
- Abrupt rate changes
- Infants: rate usually >220 bpm
- Children: rate usually >180 bpm

Probable ventricular tachycardia
- Immediate *cardioversion* 0.5 to 1.0 J/kg
  (consider sedation, do not delay cardioversion)

Consider vagal maneuvers
(no delays)

Immediate cardioversion
- Attempt *cardioversion* with 0.5 to 1.0 J/kg
  (may increase to 2 J/kg if initial dose is ineffective)
- Use sedation if possible
- Sedation must not delay cardioversion
  or
Immediate IV/IO adenosine
- *Adenosine*: use if IV access is immediately available
- Dose: *Adenosine* 0.1 mg/kg IV/IO (maximum *first dose*: 6 mg)
- May double and repeat dose once (maximum *second dose*: 12 mg)
- Technique: use rapid bolus technique

Consider alternative medications
- *Amiodarone* 5 mg/kg IV over 20 to 60 minutes
  or
- *Procainamide* 15 mg/kg IV over 30 to 60 minutes
  (Do not routinely administer amiodarone and procainamide together)
  or
- *Lidocaine* 1 mg/kg IV bolus (wide-complex only)
- Consult pediatric cardiologist
- 12-lead ECG

FIGURE 15. PALS tachycardia algorithm for infants and children with rapid rhythm and evidence of poor perfusion.

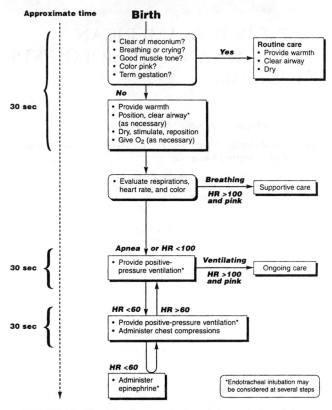

FIGURE 16. Algorithm for resuscitation of the newly born infant.

APPENDIX D ■ AMERICAN SOCIETY OF ANESTHESIOLOGISTS STANDARDS

Standards for Basic Anesthetic Monitoring

Continuum of Depth of Sedation: Definition of General Anesthesia and Level of Sedation/Analgesia

Basic Standards for Pre-Anesthesia Care

Standards for Postanesthesia Care

STANDARDS FOR BASIC ANESTHETIC MONITORING

(Approved by ASA House of Delegates on October 21, 1986 and last amended on October 27, 2004)

These standards apply to all anesthesia care, although, in emergency circumstances, appropriate life-support measures take precedence. These standards may be exceeded at any time based on the judgment of the responsible anesthesiologist. They are intended to encourage quality patient care, but observing them cannot guarantee any specific patient outcome. They are subject to revision from time to time, as warranted by the evolution of technology and practice. They apply to all general anesthetics, regional anesthetics, and monitored anesthesia care. This set of standards addresses only the issue of basic anesthetic monitoring, which is one component of anesthesia care. In certain rare or unusual circumstances, (1) some of these methods of monitoring may be clinically impractical, and (2) appropriate use of the described monitoring methods may fail to detect untoward clinical developments. Brief interruptions of continual[a] monitoring may be unavoidable. *Under extenuating circumstances, the responsible anesthesiologist may waive the requirements marked with an asterisk (*); it is recommended that when this is done, it should be so stated (including the reasons) in a note in the patient's medical record.* These standards are not intended for application to the care of the obstetrical patient in labor or in the conduct of pain management.

Standard I

Qualified anesthesia personnel shall be present in the room throughout the conduct of all general anesthetics, regional anesthetics, and monitored anesthesia care.

Objective

Because of the rapid changes in patient status during anesthesia, qualified anesthesia personnel shall be continuously present to monitor the patient and provide anesthesia care. In the event there is a direct known hazard, for example, radiation, to the anesthesia personnel that might require intermittent remote observation of the patient, some provision for monitoring the patient must be made. In the event that an emergency requires the temporary absence of the person primarily responsible for the anesthetic, the best judgment of the anesthesiologist will be exercised in comparing the emergency with the anesthetized patient's condition and in

---

[a] Note that "continual" is defined as "repeated regularly and frequently in steady rapid succession" whereas "continuous" means "prolonged without any interruption at any time."

the selection of the person left responsible for the anesthetic during the temporary absence.

Standard II
During all anesthetics, the patient's oxygenation, ventilation, circulation, and temperature shall be continually evaluated.

Oxygenation
Objective
To ensure adequate oxygen concentration in the inspired gas and the blood during all anesthetics.
Methods
1. Inspired gas: During every administration of general anesthesia using an anesthesia machine, the concentration of oxygen in the patient breathing system shall be measured by an oxygen analyzer with a low oxygen concentration limit alarm in use.*
2. Blood oxygenation: During all anesthetics, a quantitative method of assessing oxygenation such as pulse oximetry shall be employed.* Adequate illumination and exposure of the patient are necessary to assess color.*

Ventilation
Objective
To ensure adequate ventilation of the patient during all anesthetics.
Methods
1. Every patient receiving general anesthesia shall have the adequacy of ventilation continually evaluated. Qualitative clinical signs such as chest excursion, observation of the reservoir breathing bag, and auscultation of breath sounds are useful. Continual monitoring for the presence of expired carbon dioxide shall be performed unless invalidated by the nature of the patient, procedure, or equipment. Quantitative monitoring of the volume of expired gas is strongly encouraged.*
2. When an endotracheal tube or laryngeal mask is inserted, its correct positioning must be verified by clinical assessment and by identification of carbon dioxide in the expired gas. Continual end-tidal carbon dioxide analysis, in use from the time of endotracheal tube/laryngeal mask placement until extubation/removal or initiating transfer to a postoperative care location, shall be performed using a quantitative method such as capnography, capnometry, or mass spectroscopy.*
3. When ventilation is controlled by a mechanical ventilator, there shall be in continuous use a device that is capable of detecting disconnection of components of the breathing system. The device must give an audible signal when its alarm threshold is exceeded.

4. During regional anesthesia and monitored anesthesia care, the adequacy of ventilation shall be evaluated by continual observation of qualitative clinical signs and/or monitoring for the presence of exhaled carbon dioxide.

Circulation
Objective
To ensure the adequacy of the patient's circulatory function during all anesthetics.
Methods
1. Every patient receiving anesthesia shall have the electrocardiogram continuously displayed from the beginning of anesthesia until preparing to leave the anesthetizing location.*
2. Every patient receiving anesthesia shall have arterial blood pressure and heart rate determined and evaluated at least every 5 minutes.*
3. Every patient receiving general anesthesia shall have, in addition to the above, circulatory function continually evaluated by at least one of the following: palpation of a pulse, auscultation of heart sounds, monitoring of a tracing of intra-arterial pressure, ultrasound peripheral pulse monitoring, or pulse plethysmography or oximetry.

Body Temperature
Objective
To aid in the maintenance of appropriate body temperature during all anesthetics.
Methods
Every patient receiving anesthesia shall have temperature monitored when clinically significant changes in body temperature are intended, anticipated, or suspected.

CONTINUUM OF DEPTH OF SEDATION DEFINITION OF GENERAL ANESTHESIA AND LEVELS OF SEDATION ANALGESIA[a]

(Approved by ASA House of Delegates on October 13, 1999, and amended on October 27, 2004)

	Minimal sedation (anxiolysis)	Moderate sedation/ analgesia ("conscious sedation")	Deep sedation/ analgesia	General anesthesia
Responsiveness	Normal response to verbal stimulation	Purposeful[b] response to verbal or tactile stimulation	Purposeful[b] response following repeated or painful stimulation	Unarousable even with painful stimulus
Airway	Unaffected	No intervention required	Intervention may be required	Intervention often required
Spontaneous Ventilation	Unaffected	Adequate	May be inadequate	Frequently inadequate
Cardiovascular Function	Unaffected	Usually maintained	Usually maintained	May be impaired

Minimal Sedation (Anxiolysis) is a drug-induced state during which patients respond normally to verbal commands. Although cognitive function and coordination may be impaired, ventilatory and cardiovascular functions are unaffected.

Moderate Sedation/Analgesia ("Conscious Sedation") is a drug-induced depression of consciousness during which patients respond purposefully[b] to verbal commands, either alone or accompanied by light tactile stimulation. No interventions are required to maintain a patent airway, and spontaneous ventilation is adequate. Cardiovascular function is usually maintained.

Deep Sedation/Analgesia is a drug-induced depression of consciousness during which patients cannot be easily aroused but respond purposefully[b] following repeated or painful stimulation. The ability to independently maintain ventilatory function may be

---

[a] Monitored Anesthesia Care does not describe the continuum of depth of sedation, rather it describes "a specific anesthesia service in which an anesthesiologist has been requested to participate in the care of a patient undergoing a diagnostic or therapeutic procedure."

[b] Reflex withdrawal from a painful stimulus is NOT considered a purposeful response.

impaired. Patients may require assistance in maintaining a patent airway, and spontaneous ventilation may be inadequate. Cardiovascular function is usually maintained.

General Anesthesia is a drug-induced loss of consciousness during which patients are not arousable, even by painful stimulation. The ability to independently maintain ventilatory function is often impaired. Patients often require assistance in maintaining a patent airway, and positive-pressure ventilation may be required because of depressed spontaneous ventilation or drug-induced depression of neuromuscular function. Cardiovascular function may be impaired.

Because sedation is a continuum, it is not always possible to predict how an individual patient will respond. Hence, practitioners intending to produce a given level of sedation should be able to rescue[c] patients whose level of sedation becomes deeper than initially intended. Individuals administering Moderate Sedation/Analgesia ("Conscious Sedation") should be able to rescue[c] patients who enter a state of Deep Sedation/Analgesia, while those administering Deep Sedation/Analgesia should be able to rescue[c] patients who enter a state of General Anesthesia.

---

[c]Rescue of a patient from a deeper level of sedation than intended is an intervention by a practitioner proficient in airway management and advanced life support. The qualified practitioner corrects adverse physiologic consequences of the deeper-than-intended level of sedation (such as hypoventilation, hypoxia, and hypotension) and returns the patient to the originally intended level of sedation.

BASIC STANDARDS FOR PRE-ANESTHESIA CARE
(Approved by House of Delegates on October 14, 1987,
and affirmed on October 18, 1998)

These standards apply to all patients who receive anesthesia or monitored anesthesia care. Under unusual circumstances, for example, extreme emergencies, these standards may be modified. When this is the case, the circumstances shall be documented in the patient's record.

Standard I: An anesthesiologist shall be responsible for determining the medical status of the patient, developing a plan of anesthesia care, and acquainting the patient or the responsible adult with the proposed plan.

The development of an appropriate plan of anesthesia care is based on:

1. Reviewing the medical record.
2. Interviewing and examining the patient to:
   a. Discuss the medical history, previous anesthetic experiences, and drug therapy.
   b. Assess those aspects of the physical condition that might affect decisions regarding perioperative risk and management.
3. Obtaining and/or reviewing tests and consultations necessary to the conduct of anesthesia.
4. Determining the appropriate prescription of preoperative medications as necessary to the conduct of anesthesia.

The responsible anesthesiologist shall verify that the above has been properly performed and documented in the patient's record.

STANDARDS FOR POSTANESTHESIA CARE
*(Approved by House of Delegates on October 12, 1988,
and last amended on October 27, 2004)*
These standards apply to postanesthesia care in all locations. These standards may be exceeded based on the judgment of the responsible anesthesiologist. They are intended to encourage quality patient care, but cannot guarantee any specific patient outcome. They are subject to revision from time to time as warranted by the evolution of technology and practice. *Under extenuating circumstances, the responsible anesthesiologist may waive the requirements marked with an asterisk (*); it is recommended that when this is done, it should be so stated (including the reasons) in a note in the patient's medical record.*

Standard I
All patients who have received general anesthesia, regional anesthesia, or monitored anesthesia care shall receive appropriate postanesthesia management.[a]

1. A Postanesthesia Care Unit (PACU) or an area that provides equivalent postanesthesia care (for example, a Surgical Intensive Care Unit) shall be available to receive patients after anesthesia care. All patients who receive anesthesia care shall be admitted to the PACU or its equivalent **except** by specific order of the anesthesiologist responsible for the patient's care.
2. The medical aspects of care in the PACU (or equivalent area) shall be governed by policies and procedures that have been reviewed and approved by the Department of Anesthesiology.
3. The design, equipment, and staffing of the PACU shall meet requirements of the facility's accrediting and licensing bodies.

Standard II
A patient transported to the PACU shall be accompanied by a member of the anesthesia care team who is knowledgeable about the patient's condition. The patient shall be continually evaluated and treated during transport with monitoring and support appropriate to the patient's condition.

Standard III
Upon arrival in the PACU, the patients shall be reevaluated and a verbal report provided to the responsible PACU nurse by the member of the anesthesia care team who accompanies the patient.

---

[a] Refer to *Standards of Post Anesthesia Nursing Practice 1992* published by ASPAN for issues of nursing care.

1. The patient's status on arrival in the PACU shall be documented.
2. Information concerning the preoperative condition and the surgical/anesthetic course shall be transmitted to the PACU nurse.
3. The member of the Anesthesia Care Team shall remain in the PACU until the PACU nurse accepts responsibility for the nursing care of the patient.

Standard IV
The patient's condition shall be evaluated continually in the PACU.

1. The patient shall be observed and monitored by methods appropriate to the patient's medical condition. Particular attention should be given to monitoring oxygenation, ventilation, circulation, level of consciousness, and temperature. During recovery from all anesthetics, a quantitative method of assessing oxygenation such as pulse oximetry shall be employed in the initial phase of recovery.* This is not intended for application during the recovery of the obstetrical patient in whom regional anesthesia was used for labor and vaginal delivery.
2. An accurate written report of the PACU period shall be maintained. Use of an appropriate PACU scoring system is encouraged for each patient on admission, at appropriate intervals prior to discharge and at the time of discharge.
3. General medical supervision and coordination of patient care in the PACU should be the responsibility of an anesthesiologist.
4. There shall be a policy to assure the availability in the facility of a physician capable of managing complications and providing cardiopulmonary resuscitation for patients in the PACU.

Standard V
A Physician is responsible for the discharge of the patient from the postanesthesia care unit.

1. When discharge criteria are used, they must be approved by the Department of Anesthesiology and the medical staff. They may vary depending on whether the patient is discharged to a hospital room, to the Intensive Care Unit, to a short-stay unit, or to home.
2. In the absence of the physician responsible for the discharge, the PACU nurse shall determine that the patient meets the discharge criteria. The name of the physician accepting responsibility for discharge shall be noted on the record.

APPENDIX E ■ THE AIRWAY APPROACH ALGORITHM AND DIFFICULT AIRWAY ALGORITHM

AIRWAY APPROACH ALGORITHM

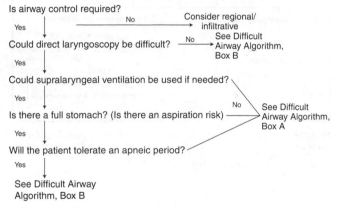

FIGURE 1. Airway Approach Algorithm. From: Rosenblatt W: The airway approach algorithm. J Clin Anes 16:312, 2004.

DIFFICULT AIRWAY ALOGRITHM

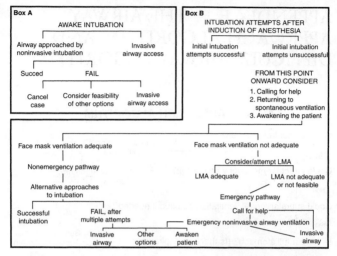

FIGURE 2. Difficult Airway Algorithm. From: Practice guidelines for the management of the difficult airway: An updated report by the American Society of Anesthesiologists Task Force on Management of the Difficult Airway. Anesthesiology 98:1269, 2003.

APPENDIX F ■ MALIGNANT HYPERTHERMIA PROTOCOL

DIAGNOSIS
Signs of Malignant Hyperthermia (MH)
 A. Increased $ETCO_2$
 B. Trunk or limb rigidity
 C. Masseter spasm or trismus
 D. Tachycardia/tachypnea
 E. Acidosis
 F. Increased temperature (late sign)
Sudden/Unexpected Cardiac Arrest in Young Patients
 A. Presume hyperkalemia and initiate treatment (see #6).
 B. Measure CK, myoglobin, ABGs, until normalized.
 C. Consider dantrolene.
 D. Realize it is usually secondary to occult myopathy
    (e.g., muscular dystrophy).
 E. Understand resuscitation may be difficult and prolonged
Trismus or Masseter Spasm with Succinylcholine
 A. Early sign of MH in many patients.
 B. If limb muscle rigidity, begin treatment with dantrolene.
 C. For emergent procedures, continue with nontriggering
    agents, consider dantrolene.
 D. Follow CK and urine myoglobin for 36 hours at least.
 E. Observe in ICU for at least 12 hours.

ACUTE PHASE TREATMENT

1. **GET HELP. GET DANTROLENE—Notify surgeon.**
 A. Discontinue volatile agents and succinylcholine (SCh).
 B. Hyperventilate with 100% oxygen at flows of
    10 L/min or more.
 C. Halt the procedure as soon as possible; if emergent, use
    nontriggers.
2. **Dantrolene 2.5 mg/kg rapidly iv**
 A. Repeat until there is control of the signs of MH.
 B. Sometimes more than 10 mg/kg is necessary.
 C. Dissolve the 20 mg in each vial with at least 60 mL **sterile
    distilled water** for injection.
 D. The crystals also contain NaOH for a pH of 9, mannitol
    3 g.

3. **Bicarbonate for metabolic acidosis**
   A. 1 to 2 mEq/kg if blood gas values are not yet available.
4. **Cool** the patient with core temperature >39°C, via cold saline iv, surface, open body cavities, stomach, bladder, or rectum. Stop cooling if temp <38°C and falling. Avoid excess cooling to prevent drift <36°.
5. **Dysrhythmias** usually respond to treatment of acidosis and hyperkalemia.
   A. Use standard drug therapy **except calcium channel blockers, which may cause hyperkalemia or cardiac arrest in the presence of dantrolene sodium.**
6. **Hyperkalemia**— Treat with hyperventilation, bicarbonate, glucose/insulin, calcium
   A. 10 units regular insulin and 50 mL 50% glucose (adult)
      OR
   B. 0.15 units insulin/kg and 1 mL/kg 50% glucose (pediatric)
   C. Calcium chloride 10 mg/kg or calcium gluconate 10 to 50 mg/kg for life-threatening hyperkalemia
7. **Follow** $ETCO_2$, electrolytes, blood gases, CK, core temperature, urine output and color, coagulation factors.
   A. Venous blood gas (e.g., femoral vein) values may document hypermetabolism better than arterial values.
   B. Central venous or PA monitoring as needed.

POST ACUTE PHASE

   A. Observe the patient in an ICU for a minimum of 36 hours.
   B. Dantrolene 1 mg/kg q4 to 6 hours for 24 to 48 hours, depending on recovery phase.
   C. Follow vitals and labs as above (see #7)
      ■ Frequent ABG
      ■ CK every 6 to 8 hours
   D. Counsel the patient and family regarding MH and further precautions. Refer them to MHAUS, fill and send in the Adverse Metabolic Reaction to Anesthesia (AMRA) form, and send a letter to the patient and his or her physician.
   E. Refer patient to the nearest biopsy center for follow up.

CAUTION: This protocol may not apply to every patient and may require alteration according to specific patient needs.

APPENDIX G ■ DRUG LIST

The authors and publisher have exerted every effort to ensure that the drug selection and dosage set forth in this appendix are in accord with current recommendations and practice at the time of publication. However, in view of ongoing research, changes in government regulations, and the constant flow of information relating to drug therapy and drug reactions, the reader is urged to check the package insert for each drug for any change in indications and dosage and for added warnings and precautions. This is particularly important when the recommended agent is a new or infrequently used drug. Unless specified otherwise, all doses are for adults.

The editors acknowledge the contribution of Stella A. Haddadin, BSc, PharmD, Yale–New Haven Hospital, Department of Pharmacy Services, in the preparation of this appendix.

ABBREVIATIONS

BBW: black box warning **BBW**
CrCl: creatinine clearance
ESRD: end-stage renal disease
HTN: hypertension
IV: intravenous
IM: intramuscular
MR: may repeat
N/A: not available
NTE: not to exceed
PO: orally
SC: subcutaneous
t$_{1/2}$: half-life

ACETAMINOPHEN (VARIOUS)

■ **Uses:** analgesic, antipyretic
■ **Dose:** Adults: (PO) 325–650 mg q4h, max daily dose 4 g. Children >12 yr: (PO) 10–15 mg/kg q4h, NTE 5 doses. Children 6–12 yr: (rectal) 325 mg q4–6h, max daily dose 2.6 g. Children 3–6 yr: (rectal) 120 mg q4h, max daily dose 720 mg. Children 1–3 yr: (rectal) 80 mg q4–6h.
■ **Site of clearance:** hepatic

- $t^{1}/_{2}$: 1–3 h
- **Interaction/toxicity:** Has no significant anti-inflammatory effect. Causes severe liver toxicity when combined with alcohol. Use with caution in patients with alcoholic-related liver disease. Therapeutic doses can cause liver failure in alcoholics. Potentiates toxicity of barbiturates, carbamazepine, and hydantoins. Beta-blockers and anticholinergics intensify effect.

ACETAZOLAMIDE (VARIOUS)

- **Uses:** reduce intraocular pressure, acute altitude sickness, diuretic
- **Dose:** *Glaucoma:* Adults: (IV) 250 mg q6h; (PO) 250–1,000 mg/day qid, max 1.0 g/24 h. Children: (IV, IM) 5–10 mg/kg q6h; (PO) 10–15 mg/kg/day q6–8h.
  Acute altitude sickness: (PO) 250 mg q8–12h; begin Rx 24–48 h before and continue for 24–48 h after arrival at altitude.
- **Site of clearance:** renal
- $t^{1}/_{2}$: 2.4–5.8 h
- **Interaction/toxicity:** Contraindicated in sulfonamide allergy, hepatic disease, decreased serum sodium or potassium levels, adrenocortical insufficiency, hyperchloremic acidosis, renal disease, long-term use in glaucoma. Use with caution in respiratory acidosis, diabetes mellitus (may cause significant blood glucose increase). Paresthesias and myalgias may be experienced. Decreased effects of lithium. Increases toxicity of cyclosporine and digitalis toxicity (hypokalemia present). Salicylates may cause accumulation.

ADENOSINE (ADENOCARD)

- **Uses:** antidysrhythmic (paroxysmal supraventricular tachycardia)
- **Dose:** Adults: (IV) 6 mg, if not effective within 1–2 min give 12 mg, MR 12 mg bolus prn, max single dose 12 mg. Infants and children: (IV) 0.1 mg/kg, if not effective give 0.2 mg/kg, medium dose 0.15 mg/kg, max single dose 12 mg.
- **Site of clearance:** enzymatic
- $t^{1}/_{2}$: <10 sec
- **Interaction/toxicity:** Transient dysrhythmias seen before conversion to sinus rhythm. Excessive doses may cause significant hypotension, shortness of breath, and flushing. Adenosine does not convert atrial flutter/atrial fibrillation/ventricular tachycardia to sinus rhythm but may be used to distinguish paroxysmal supraventricular tachycardia and other tachycardias.

ALBUTEROL (VARIOUS)

- Uses: bronchodilator
- Dose: Adults: (PO) 4–8 mg/kg bid, NTE 16 mg q12h; (inhalation) 90 mcg/spray, 1–2 inhalations q4–6h, NTE 12 inhalations/day. Children 6–12 yr: (PO) 4 mg bid, NTE 24 mg/day; (inhalation) 90 mcg/spray, 1–2 inhalations q6–8h, NTE 12 inhalations/day.
- Site of clearance: hepatic
- t$^1/_2$: 1.5–2.5 h
- Interaction/toxicity: Use with spacer for inhalations. Use with caution in patients with hypothyroidism, diabetes mellitus, CAD, and HTN, and those using MAOIs, tricyclic antidepressants. Decreased effect with beta-blockers. Enhanced effect with sympathomimetics. Excessive use leads to tolerance. May contain sulfites.

ALFENTANIL (ALFENTA)

- Uses: analgesia
- Dose: (IV) induction 130–245 mcg/kg, maintenance 0.5–1.5 mcg/kg/min.
- Site of clearance: hepatic
- t$^1/_2$: 83–97 min
- Interaction/toxicity: Diazepam potentiates hypotensive action; truncal muscle rigidity may be seen during induction and emergence. Erythromycin delays clearance.

AMINOCAPROIC ACID (VARIOUS)

- Uses: antifibrinolytic
- Dose: (IV, PO) loading 5 g, then 1.25 g/h, max daily dose 30 g.
- Site of clearance: renal
- t$^1/_2$: 1–2 h
- Interaction/toxicity: Adjust dose in renal dysfunction. Rapid IV administration may cause hypotension, bradycardia, or dysrhythmias. Do not administer if DIC is present. Use with caution in presence of upper urinary tract bleeding (may cause intrarenal thrombosis).

AMIODARONE (CORDARONE)   BBW

- Uses: antidysrhythmic
- Dose: *Cardiac arrest:* Pulseless VF or VT: (IV) Initial: 300 mg in 20–30 ml NS or D$_5$W; if VF or VT recurrs, supplemental

dose of 150 mg followed by infusion of 1 mg/min for 6 h, then 0.5 mg/min × 18 hr (max daily dose 2.2 gm)

Break through VF or VT: (IV) 150 mg supplemental dose in 100 ml D_5W over 10 min (PO) loading 800–1,000 mg divided bid–tid, then 400 mg/day.

- Site of clearance: hepatic
- $t^1/_2$: 13–37 days
- Interaction/toxicity: Contraindicated in cardiogenic shock, severe sinus node dysfunction, second- and third-degree heart arteriovenous block and bradycardia-induced syncope in absence of pacemaker. Pulmonary toxicity (hypersensitivity pneumonitis) and optic neuropathy can occur. Inhibits peripheral conversion of T_4 to T_3. Potentiates anticoagulants, beta-blockers, calcium channel blockers, digoxin, fentanyl, hydantoins, lidocaine, procainamide, quinidine, and theophylline.

AMINOPHYLLINE (VARIOUS)

- Uses: bronchodilator
- Dose: *Acute bronchospasm:* Adults and children >1 yr: (IV) loading 6 mg/kg (diluted in 100 mL D_5W or NS), NTE 25 mg/min use ideal body weight for obese patients (each 0.6 mg/kg increases serum theophylline level 1.0 mcg/mL); maintenance 0.5–1.0 mg/kg/h (adjust dose based on serum level). Infants 6–52 wk: (IV) 0.008 [age in wk] + 0.21 mg/kg/h theophylline.
- Site of clearance: hepatic
- $t^1/_2$: infants (4–52 wk) 4–30 h, children/adolescents 2–16 h, adults 4–16 h
- Interaction/toxicity: Increases effects on sympathomimetics, digitalis, oral anticoagulants; decreases effects of phenytoin, lithium, nondepolarizing muscle relaxants. Phenobarbital increases aminophylline metabolism. Antagonizes beta-blockers; toxicity with halothane (dysrhythmias) and ketamine (seizures).

AMITRIPTYLINE (VARIOUS)

- Uses: antidepressant, chronic pain, migraine headaches
- Dose: *Antidepressant:* (IM) 20–30 mg qid; (PO) 10–25 mg tid. *Pain management:* (PO) initial 25 mg qhs, may increase to 100 mg/day.
- Site of clearance: hepatic
- $t^1/_2$: 16–26 h
- Interaction/toxicity: Contraindicated in patients with narrow-angle glaucoma, Rx with MAOIs within previous 14 days. Use with caution in patients receiving electroshock Rx, and those with cardiac dysrhythmias, hyperthyroidism, renal or

hepatic dysfunction. Blocks antihypertensive effect of guanethidine. Barbiturates increase metabolism. Increases amount of inhalation anesthesia required. Potentiates sympathomimetics, CNS depressants, and anticoagulants. Cimetidine decreases metabolism. Do not discontinue abruptly. Cardiovascular toxicity leading cause of death.

AMOBARBITAL (VARIOUS)

- **Uses:** hypnotic, sedative, anticonvulsant, premedicant
- **Dose:** (IV, IM) 60–500 mg; (PO) 30–50 mg tid, 60–200 mg qhs.
- **Site of clearance:** hepatic
- **$t^1/_2$:** 8–42 h
- **Interaction/toxicity:** Contraindicated in patients with severe liver dysfunction or porphyria. Potentiates sedatives, hypnotics tranquilizers, and other CNS depressants. Decreases effects of beta-blockers, theophylline, and corticosteroids. MAOIs increase actions. Increases metabolism of methadone and can result in withdrawal. Tolerance can develop.

AMOXICILLIN (VARIOUS)

- **Uses:** antibiotic
- **Dose:** Adults: (PO) 250–500 mg q8h. Children: (PO) 20–40 mg/kg q8h.
     Prophylaxis for bacterial endocarditis (dental, respiratory, oral procedures): Adults: (PO) 2 g 1 h before procedure. Children: (PO) 50 mg/kg 1 h before procedure.
- **Site of clearance:** renal
- **$t^1/_2$:** infants and children 1–2 h, adults 0.7–1.4 h
- **Interaction/toxicity:** Adjust dose with renal dysfunction. Potentiates anticoagulants.

AMPICILLIN (VARIOUS)

- **Uses:** antibiotic
- **Dose:** Adults: (IV) 500 mg to 2 g q4–6h, max daily dose 12 g; (IM) 0.5–1.5 g q4–6h; (PO) 250–500 mg q6h. Children: (IV, IM) 100–400 mg/kg/day divided q4–6h; (PO) 50–100 mg/kg/day divided q6h, max daily dose 2–3 g.
     Sepsis/meningitis: Adults: (IV) 150–250 mg/kg/day divided q4h, max 2 g q4h. Children: (IV) 200 mg/kg/day divided q4–6h, max daily dose 12 g.
- **Site of clearance:** renal
- **$t^1/_2$:** 1–1.8 h

■ **Interaction/toxicity:** Adjust dose with renal dysfunction. Potentiates anticoagulants. Rapid infusion >100 mg/min may cause
rigors.

ANTITHROMBIN III (THROMBATE III)

■ **Uses:** antithrombin III replacement
■ **Dose:** (IV) International units required = [(desired − baseline AT
III level)/(1.4)](weight in kg); administer over 10–20 min.
■ **Site of clearance:** N/A
■ **t$\frac{1}{2}$:** 2.6–3.8 days
■ **Interaction/toxicity:** Derived from human plasma; risk of HIV
and infectious viruses. Potentiates action of heparin.

APROTININ (TRASYLOL)   BBW

■ **Uses:** protease inhibitor of plasmin and kallikrein
■ **Dose:** (IV) (administer all IV doses via central catheter) test dose
1.0 mL; observe 10 min for allergic reaction.
    Regimen A: loading 200 mL (2 million KIU) over
20 min, infusion 50 mL/h (500,000 KIU/h). If administered
during procedures requiring cardiopulmonary bypass, "pump
prime" is 200 mL.
    Regimen B: loading 100 mL (1 million KIU) over 20–30
min, infusion 25 mL/h (250,000 KIU/h). If administered during
procedures requiring cardiopulmonary bypass, "pump prime"
is 100 mL.
■ **Site of clearance:** renal
■ **t$\frac{1}{2}$:** 2.5 h
■ **Interaction/toxicity:** Prolongs ACT as determined by celite ACT.
Consequently, celite ACT >450 s may lead to inadequate anticoagulation; Kaolin ACT much less affected. Use Kaolin ACT
or another method of determining coagulation status, or use
fixed-dose heparin regimen. Anaphylactic reactions including
first time and reexposures.

ARDEPARIN (NORMIFLO) (DISCONTINUED BY MANUFACTURER IN FEBRUARY 2002)   BBW

■ **Uses:** anticoagulant (low-molecular weight [LMW] heparin)
■ **Dose:** (SQ) 50 anti-Xa units/kg q12h up to 14 days.
■ **Site of clearance:** N/A
■ **t$\frac{1}{2}$:** 1.2–3.3 h
■ **Interaction/toxicity:** Administer as deep SQ (not IM) injection. Contraindicated in patients with pork allergy, active
hemorrhage, severe HTN and thrombocytopenia (ardeparin

induced antiplatelet antibodies). Use with caution in patients with heparin-induced thrombocytopenia (HIT) or recent lumbar puncture. Concomitant use with other anticoagulants, antiplatelet drugs, aspirin or NSAIDs may cause bleeding. May cause epidural or spinal hematoma in presence of spinal or epidural anesthetic. Single-dose spinal anesthetic may be safest technique. Needle placement should occur 10–12 h after last dose of LMW heparin; 24-h delay is required with higher doses of LMW heparin. For neuraxial catheter techniques LMW heparin should not be administered for 24 h postoperatively. Preferable to remove catheters before initiating LMW heparin Rx. Catheter removal should be delayed for 10–12 h after last dose of LMW heparin. Subsequent dosing should not occur for at least 2 h after catheter removal. Presence of blood during spinal, epidural needle, or catheter placement should delay administration of LMW heparin for 24 h. Overdose treated with protamine.

ARGATROBAN (ARGATROBAN)

- **Uses:** anticoagulant, thrombin inhibitor
- **Dose:** *Prophylaxis of thrombosis (heparin-induced thrombocytopenia):* (IV) initial 2 mcg/kg/min, NTE 10 mcg/kg/min.
  Myocardial infarction: 100 mcg/kg bolus followed by 1–3 mcg/kg/min for 6–72 h. *Percutaneous coronary interventions:* 350 mcg/kg IV over 3–5 min and 25 mcg/kg/min IV continuous infusion.
- **Site of clearance:** liver
- **$t^1/_2$:** 30–51 min
- **Interaction/toxicity:** Use with caution in patients with increased risk of hemorrhage: severe HTN, lumbar puncture, spinal anesthesia, major surgery, bleeding disorders, GI ulcers hepatic impairment.

ATENOLOL (TENORMIN) `BBW`

- **Uses:** antianginal, antihypertensive, antidysrhythmic
- **Dose:** Adults: (IV) 5 mg over 5 min, MR after 10 min; (PO) 25–50 mg/day.
- **Site of clearance:** renal
- **$t^1/_2$:** 6–9 h, ESRD 15–35 h
- **Interaction/toxicity:** Adjust dose in renal dysfunction. Administer with caution to patients with diabetes mellitus, bronchospastic disorders, CHF, second- and third-degree heart block, and myasthenia gravis. Increases effects of calcium channel blockers,

H_2 antagonists, MAOIs, IV anesthetic agents, and local anesthetics. Avoid abrupt withdrawal. Clonidine may cause life-threatening HTN.

ATRACURIUM (TRACRIUM) `BBW`

- **Uses:** nondepolarizing neuromuscular blocker
- **Dose:** Dose to effect; doses will vary due to interpatient variability; use ideal body weight for obese patients. Adults and children >2 yr: (IV) 0.4–0.5 mg/kg, then 0.08–0.1 mg/kg 20–45 min after initial dose to maintain neuromuscular block, followed by repeat doses of 0.08–0.1 mg/kg at 15–25 min intervals.

  Initial dose after succinylcholine for intubation: Adults and Children >2 yr: 0.2–0.4 mg/kg.

  Neuromuscular blockade: Children 1 mo to 2 yr: (IV) 0.3–0.5 mg/kg followed by 0.25 mg/kg maintenance doses.

  Continuous infusion: Adults and Children > 2 yr: surgery initial 9–10 mcg/kg/min at initial signs of recovery from bolus dose, block usually maintained by a rate of 5–9 mcg/kg/min under balanced anesthesia.

  ICU: Adults and Children >2 yr: neuromuscular blockade usually maintained by rate of 11–13 mcg/kg/min.
- **Site of clearance:** plasma (Hofmann elimination) and ester hydrolysis; hepatic
- **t$\frac{1}{2}$:** 16–20 min
- **Interaction/toxicity:** Potentiated by volatile anesthetics, hypokalemia, antibiotics (aminoglycosides), lithium, verapamil, trimethaphan, and procainamide. Antagonized by theophylline and phenytoin (decrease action). Releases histamine at high doses.

ATROPINE (VARIOUS)

- **Uses:** antisialagogue; vagolysis
- **Dose:** *Paradoxical bradycardia has been associated with the following doses:* Adults: <0.5 mg. Neonates, infants, and children: <0.1 mg.

  Asystole or pulseless electrical activity: (IV) 1.0 mg, MR in 3–5 min if asystole persists to a total dose of 0.04 mg/kg; (intratracheal) 2–2.5 times the IV dose in 10 mL NS.

  Pre-anesthetic: Adults: (IV, IM, SC) 0.4–0.6 mg 30–60 min preop then q4–6h prn. Children >5 kg: (IV, IM, SC, PO) 0.01–0.02 mg/kg to a max 0.4 mg/dose 30–60 min preop, min dose 0.1 mg. Children <5 kg: (IV, IM, SC, PO) 0.02 mg/kg 30–60 min preop then q4–6h prn. Use of a minimum dosage of

0.1 mg in neonates <5 kg will result in dosages >0.02 mg/kg. There is no documented minimum dosage in this age group.

Bradycardia: Adults: (IV) 0.5–1.0 mg q5min, NTE total 3 mg or 0.04 mg/kg; may give intratracheally in 10 mL NS. Children: (IV, intratracheal) 0.02 mg/kg, min dose 0.1 mg, max single dose 0.5 mg in children and 1 mg in adolescents; MR in 5-min intervals to max total dose 1.0 mg in children and 2 mg in adolescents (for intratracheal administration, dilute in NS to total volume of 1–2 mL). When treating bradycardia in neonates, reserve use for patients unresponsive to improved oxygenation and epinephrine.

Neuromuscular blockade reversal: (IV) 25–30 mcg/kg 60 sec before neostigmine or 7–10 mcg/kg in combination with edrophonium.
- **Site of clearance:** renal
- **$t^1/_2$:** 2–3 h
- **Interaction/toxicity:** Potentiated by antihistamines, procainamide, tricyclic antidepressants, and monoamine oxidase inhibitors. Antagonizes effects of cholinesterase inhibitors and metoclopramide.

BENZOCAINE (AMERICAINE, HURRICAINE)

- **Uses:** topical anesthesia
- **Dose:** (topical) Spray applied for ≤1 sec. A spray >2 sec is contraindicated. The average expulsion rate of residue from the spray is 200 mg/sec.
- **Site of clearance:** plasma cholinesterase
- **$t^1/_2$:** N/A
- **Interaction/toxicity:** methemoglobinemia

BISOPROLOL (ZEBETA)

- **Uses:** antianginal, antihypertensive, antidysrhythmic
- **Dose:** Adults: (PO) 5 mg/day, may be increased to 10 mg and then up to 20 mg/day if necessary. Elderly: (PO) initial 2.5 mg/day, may be increased by 2.5–5 mg/day, max daily dose 20 mg.
- **Site of clearance:** renal
- **$t^1/_2$:** 9–12 h
- **Interaction/toxicity:** Adjust dose in renal dysfunction. Administer with caution to patients with diabetes mellitus, bronchospastic disorders, CHF, second- and third-degree heart block, and myasthenia gravis. Increases effects of calcium channel blockers, H_2 antagonists, MAOIs, IV anesthetic agents, and local anesthetics. Avoid abrupt withdrawal. Clonidine may cause life-threatening HTN.

BIVALRUDIN (ANGIOMAX)

- Uses: anticoagulant, thrombin inhibitor
- Dose: *Anticoagulant, patients with unstable angina undergoing PTCA:* (IV) 1.0 mg/kg bolus followed by 2.5 mg/kg/h infusion for 4 h, additional 0.2 mg/kg/h for 20 h prn.

  Renal impairment: for CrCl 30–59 mL/min reduce dose by 20%, for CrCl 10–29 mL/min reduce dose by 60%, for CrCl <10 mL/min reduce dose by 90%.
- Site of clearance: renal and proteolysis
- $t^{1}/_{2}$: 25 min
- Interaction/toxicity: Contraindicated in patients with active bleeding. Use with caution in patients for brachytherapy procedures (increased risk of thrombus formation with possible fatal outcomes), cerebral aneurysm, renal impairment, gastrointestinal ulceration (risk of hemorrhage). There is limited data to support use in patients with heparin induced thrombocytopenia-thrombosis syndromes (HIT/HITTS) undergoing PTCA. However, in vitro studies exhibited no platelet aggregation response against sera from patients with a history of HIT/HITTS.

BRETYLIUM (BRETYLOL)

- Uses: prophylaxis; treatment of ventricular fibrillation
- Dose: *Immediate life-threatening ventricular dysrhythmias:* (IV) initial 5 mg/kg (undiluted) over 1 min; if dysrhythmia persists 10 mg/kg (undiluted) over 1 min and prn (usually at 15–30 mg intervals) up to total dose of 30–35 mg/kg.

  Other life-threatening ventricular dysrhythmias: (IV) loading 5–10 mg/kg, maintenance 1–2 mg/min (dilute 500 mg in 100 mL D_5W or NS).
- Site of clearance: renal
- $t^{1}/_{2}$: 7–11 h, ESRD 16–32 h
- Interaction/toxicity: Digitalis toxicity may follow initial release of norepinephrine; transient HTN and increased frequency of dysrhythmias follow initial release of norepinephrine from postganglionic nerve terminals.

BUPIVACAINE (MARCAINE, SENSORCAINE) BBW

- Uses: local/regional anesthesia
- Dose: Doses vary; max daily dose 3 mg/kg.

  Local anesthesia: infiltration 0.25% infiltrated locally, max dose 175 mg.

Caudal block (with or without epinephrine, preservative free): Adults: 15–30 mL of 0.25% or 0.5%. Children: 1.0–3.7 mg/kg.

Epidural block (other than caudal block with or without epinephrine, preservative free): Adults: 10–20 mL of 0.25% or 0.5%. Children: 1.25 mg/kg/dose. Always administer in 3–5 mL increments, allowing sufficient time to detect toxic manifestations of inadvertent IV or IT administration.

Surgical procedures requiring a high degree of muscle relaxation and prolonged effects only: 10–20 mL of 0.75% (do not use in obstetrical cases).

Maxillary and mandibular infiltration and nerve block: 9 mg (1.8 mL) of 0.5% (with epinephrine) per injection site, MR after 10 min to produce adequate anesthesia, max 90 mg per dental appointment.

Obstetrical anesthesia: incremental 3–5 mL of 0.5%, NTE 50–100 mg in any dosing interval; allow sufficient time to detect toxic manifestations or inadvertent IV or IT injection.

Peripheral nerve block: 5 mL of 0.25 or 0.5%, max daily dose 400 mg

Sympathetic nerve block: 20–50 mL of 0.25%

Retrobulbar anesthesia: 2–4 mL of 0.75%

Spinal anesthesia: solution of 0.75% bupivacaine in 8.25% dextrose (a hyperbaric solution); lower extremity and perineal procedures 1.0 mL, lower abdominal procedures 1.6 mL.

Obstetrical: normal vaginal delivery 0.8 mL (higher doses may be required); C section 1.0–1.4 mL

- **Site of clearance:** hepatic
- **t$^1/_2$:** 3–5 h
- **Interaction/toxicity:** Bupivacaine 0.75% not recommended for obstetrics or IV regional anesthesia. Diazepam increases bioavailability. Acute CV collapse following accidental injection; cardiac toxicity greater than CNS toxicity.

BUPRENORPHINE (BUPRENEX)

- **Uses:** analgesia, opioid agonist-antagonist
- **Dose:** *Acute pain (moderate to severe):* Adults and children ≥13 yr: (IM, slow IV) opiate-naïve initial 0.3 mg q6–8h prn, MR once 30–60 min after initial dose, usual range 0.15–0.6 mg q4–6h prn. Children 2–12 yr: 2–6 mcg/kg q4–6h. Elderly: 0.15 mg q6h. Doses should be titrated to pain relief and control.
- **Site of clearance:** hepatic
- **t$^1/_2$:** 2.2–3 h

■ **Interaction/toxicity:** Potentiates barbiturates and CNS depressants. Potentiated in patients with hepatic disease. May precipitate withdrawal in opioid-dependent patient. Increases intracholedochal pressure.

BUTORPHANOL (STADOL)

■ **Uses:** analgesia; opioid agonist-antagonist
■ **Dose:** *Acute pain (moderate to severe):* Adults: (IM) initial 2 mg, MR q3–4h prn, usual range 1–4 mg q3–4h prn; (IV) initial 1.0 mg, MR q3–4h prn, usual range 0.5–2 mg q3–4h prn.
   Preoperative medication: (IM) 2 mg 60–90 min before surgery.
   Supplement to balanced anesthesia: (IV) 2 mg shortly before induction and/or incremental dose of 0.5–1.0 mg (up to 0.06 mg/kg).
   Pain during labor (fetus >37 wk gestation and no signs of fetal distress): (IM, IV) 1–2 mg, MR in 4 h.
■ **Site of clearance:** hepatic, renal
■ **t$^{1}/_{2}$:** 3–6 h
■ **Interaction/toxicity:** May precipitate withdrawal in opioid-dependent patients.

CALCIUM CHLORIDE (VARIOUS)

■ **Uses:** electrolyte replacement; inotropic
■ **Dose:** 1.0 g = 13.6 mEq calcium. Calcium chloride is 3 times as potent as calcium gluconate.
   Cardiac arrest in the presence of hyperkalemia or hypocalcemia, magnesium toxicity, or calcium antagonist toxicity: Adults: (IV) 2–4 mg/kg (10% solution), MR q10min if necessary. Infants and children: (IV) 20 mg/kg, MR in 10 min.
   Hypocalcemia: Children: (IV) 2.7–5 mg/kg q4–6h. Alternate dosing for infants and children: (IV) 10–20 mg/kg (infants <1.0 mEq, children 1.0–7.0 mEq), repeat q4–6h prn.
   Hypocalcemic tetany: Adults: (IV) 1.0 g over 10–30 min, MR after 6 h. Infants and children: (IV) 10 mg/kg (0.5–0.7 mEq/kg) over 5–10 min, MR after 6–8 h or follow with an infusion, max daily dose 200 mg/kg.
   Hypocalcemia secondary to citrated blood transfusion: Adults: (IV) 1.35 mEq calcium for each 100 mL of citrated blood infused. Neonates, infants, and children: (IV) 0.45 mEq elemental calcium for each 100 mL citrated blood infused.
■ **Site of clearance:** GI, renal
■ **t$^{1}/_{2}$:** N/A

■ **Interaction/toxicity:** Increases risk of dysrhythmias in digitalized patients; antagonizes verapamil; skin slough (necrosis) seen with extravasation.

CALCIUM GLUCONATE (VARIOUS)

■ **Uses:** electrolyte replacement; inotropic
■ **Dose:** (IV) 500–2,000 mg (1.0 g = 4.5 mEq calcium).
■ **Site of clearance:** GI, renal
■ **t$^{1}/_{2}$:** N/A
■ **Interaction/toxicity:** Increases risk of dysrhythmias in digitalized patients; antagonizes verapamil; risk of skin slough (necrosis) seen with extravasation.

CAPSAICIN (VARIOUS)

■ **Uses:** chronic pain Rx
■ **Dose:** (topical) apply tid–qid.
■ **Site of clearance:** N/A
■ **t$^{1}/_{2}$:** N/A
■ **Interaction/toxicity:** Burning diminishes with repeated use. Do not bandage area tightly.

CAPTOPRIL (CAPOTEN) `BBW`

■ **Uses:** antihypertensive; CHF
■ **Dose:** *Acute HTN (urgency/emergency):* (PO) 12.5–25 mg, MR prn.
　　HTN: (PO) initial 12.5–25 mg bid–tid, may increase by 12.5–25 mg/dose at 1–2-wk intervals up to 50 mg tid, add diuretic before further dosage increase, max dose 150 mg tid.
　　CHF: (PO) initial 6.25–12.5 mg tid, max dose 150 mg tid.
　　LVD after MI: (PO) initial 6.25 mg followed by 12.5 mg tid, increase to 25 mg tid during next several days to weeks to target dose 50 mg tid.
　　Diabetic nephropathy: Adults: (PO) 25 mg tid; other antihypertensives given concurrently. Adolescents: (PO) initial 12.5–25 mg given q8–12h, increase by 25 mg/dose to max daily dose 450 mg. Older children: (PO) initial 6.25–12.5 mg q12–24h, titrate up to max daily dose 6 mg/kg. Children: (PO) initial 0.5 mg/kg, titrate up to max 6 daily dose mg/kg in 2–4 divided doses. Infants: (PO) initial 0.15–0.3 mg/kg, titrate up to max daily dose 6 mg/kg in 1–4 divided doses; usual dose 2.5–6 mg/kg/day.
　　Renal dosing: (PO) for CrCl 10–50 mL/min reduce to 75% of normal dose; for CrCl <10 mL/min reduce to 50% of normal dose.

- **Site of clearance:** renal
- **$t^{1}/_{2}$:** adults 1.9 h, CHF 2 h, anuria 20–40 h; renal and cardiac function dependent
- **Interaction/toxicity:** Potentiates hypotensive effects of anesthetics; elevates serum digoxin level; enhances hemodynamic effects of vasodilators, calcium channel blockers, and beta-blockers.

CARBAMAZEPINE (VARIOUS) **BBW**

- **Uses:** anticonvulsant, chronic pain
- **Dose:** *Anticonvulsant:* Adults and children >12 yr: (PO) initial 200 mg bid, increase by 200 mg/day at weekly intervals until therapeutic levels achieved, usual dose 400–1,200 mg/day divided bid–qid, max daily dose 12–15 yr 1,000 mg. Children >15 yr: (PO) 1,200 mg; some patients require up to 1.6 to 2 g/day. Children 6–12 yr: (PO) initial 100 mg bid or 10 mg/kg/ day divided bid; increase by 100 mg/day at weekly intervals depending on response, usual maintenance 20–30 mg/kg/day divided bid–qid, max daily dose 1,000 mg. Children <6 yr: (PO) initial 5 mg/kg/day; may be increased q5–7days to 10 mg/kg/day, up to 20 mg/kg/day if necessary divided bid to qid.

  Trigeminal or glossopharyngeal neuralgia: Adults: (PO) initial 100 mg q12h, gradually increase in increments of 100 mg bid prn, maintenance 400–600 mg bid, max daily dose 1,200 mg. Elderly: (PO) 100 mg qd–bid, increase in increments of 100 mg/ day at weekly intervals until therapeutic levels are achieved, usual dose 400–1,000 mg/day.

  Renal impairment: for CrCl <10 mL/min reduce dose to 75%.
- **Site of clearance:** hepatic
- **$t^{1}/_{2}$:** 10–20 h
- **Interaction/toxicity:** Contraindicated in patients with bone-marrow suppression and liver dysfunction, and those using MAOIs. Discontinue MAOIs for 14 days before starting carbamazepine Rx. Induces its own metabolism as well as that of other drugs (e.g., benzodiazepines, corticosteroids, tricyclic antidepressants). Potentiated by cimetidine, verapamil, and barbiturates. Enhances the toxicity of acetaminophen. Risk of aplastic anemia.

CEFAZOLIN (VARIOUS)

- **Uses:** antibiotic
- **Dose:** Adults: (IV, IM) 250 mg to 2 g q6–12h (usually q8h) depending on severity of infection, max daily dose 12 g. Children

and infants >1 mo: (IV, IM) 25–100 mg/kg/day divided q6–8h, max daily dose 6 g.

Prophylaxis against bacterial endocarditis: Adults: (IV) 1.0 g 30 min before procedure. Infants/children: 25 mg/kg 30 min before procedure, max 1.0 g.

Renal adjustment: for CrCl 10–30 mL/min dose q12h, for CrCl <10 mL/min dose q24h.
- **Site of clearance:** renal
- **t^1/$_2$:** 1.5–2.5 h
- **Interaction/toxicity:** Adjust dose with renal dysfunction. May increase toxicity of nephrotoxic drugs such as aminoglycosides. Large doses in patients with renal failure may cause seizures. Potentiates anticoagulants. Ingestion of alcohol may cause a disulfiram-like reaction.

CEFOTAXIME (CLAFORAN)

- **Uses:** antibiotic
- **Dose:** *Bacterial infections:* Adults and children >12 yr: (IV, IM) 1–2 g q6–8h. Infants and children 1 mo to 12 yr <50 kg: (IV, IM) 50–180 mg/kg/day divided q4–6h. *Meningitis/other serious infections:* Adults and children >12 yr: 2 g q4–6h, max daily dose 12 g. Infants and children 1 mo to 12 yr <50 kg: 200 mg/kg/day divided q6h.

  Preoperative: (IM, IV) 1.0 g 30–90 min before surgery.

  C section: 1.0 g when umbilical cord clamped, then 1.0 g q6–12h.

  Renal adjustment: for CrCl 10–50 mL/min dose q8–12 h, for CrCl <10 mL/min dose q24h.
- **Site of clearance:** renal
- **t^1/$_2$:** adults 1–1.5 h; prolonged with renal or hepatic impairment
- **Interaction/toxicity:** Adjust dose in renal dysfunction. Potentiates aminoglycoside nephrotoxicity. Alcohol ingestion causes disulfiram-like reaction. Potentiates anticoagulants.

CEFOTETAN (CEFOTAN)

- **Uses:** antibiotic
- **Dose:** Adults: (IV, IM) 1–2 g q12h, max daily dose 6 g. Children: (IV, IM) 20–40 mg/kg q12h.

  Perioperative prophylaxis: Adults: (IV) 1.0–2 g 30–60 min before procedure. Children: (IV) 20–40 mg/kg 30–60 min before procedure.

  Renal adjustment: for CrCl 10–30 mL/min dose q24h, for CrCl <10 mL/min dose q48h.

- Site of clearance: renal
- $t^{1}/_{2}$: 3–5 h
- Interaction/toxicity: Adjust dose in renal dysfunction. Potentiates aminoglycoside nephrotoxicity. Alcohol ingestion causes disulfiram-like reaction. Potentiates anticoagulants.

CELECOXIB (CELEBREX) ▪BBW▪

- Uses: nonsteroidal analgesic (selective COX-2 inhibitor)
- Dose: (PO) 100–200 mg/day
- Site of clearance: hepatic
- $t^{1}/_{2}$: 11 h
- Interaction/toxicity: GI bleeding (including ulceration and perforation), liver dysfunction, renal impairment, and worsening of aspirin-sensitive asthma have been reported. Aspirin potentiates GI ulceration. Reduces natriuretic effect of furosemide. Diminish antihypertensive effect of ACE inhibitors. Increased INR and PTT in patients receiving warfarin. Fluconazole and lithium increase plasma levels. Contraindicated in patients with sulfa allergy. Use increases the risk of cardiovascular events such as heart attack and stroke.

CHLORAL HYDRATE (VARIOUS)

- Uses: sedative
- Dose: Adults: (PO) 250 mg tid, 500–1,000 mg qhs, max daily dose 2 g. Children: (PO/rectal) 25 mg/kg.
  Preoperative: Adults: (PO) 500–1,000 mg 30–60 min before procedure, NTE 2 g in 24 h. Children (PO/rectal): 50–75 mg/kg 30–60 min before procedure, NTE 1.0 g in single dose.
- Site of clearance: renal
- $t^{1}/_{2}$: 8–11 h
- Interaction/toxicity: Contraindicated in patients with severe hepatic or renal dysfunction. Use with caution in patients with porphyria. Potentiates CNS depressants and warfarin.

CHLORAMPHENICOL (VARIOUS) ▪BBW▪

- Uses: antibiotic
- Dose: Adults: (IV) 50 mg/kg/day q6h, max daily dose 4 g. Children: (IV) 50–75 mg/kg/day q6h. Neonates: (IV) 25 mg/kg/day.
- Site of clearance: renal
- $t^{1}/_{2}$: 1.6–3.3 h
- Interaction/toxicity: Adjust dose with renal or hepatic dysfunction. Use with caution in patients with porphyria or G6PD

deficiency. Barbiturates antagonize effect. Potentiates barbiturates, anticoagulants, hydantoins. Severe blood dyscrasias seen. Causes gray syndrome in neonates.

CHLORDIAZEPOXIDE (LIBRIUM)

- **Uses:** antianxiety
- **Dose:** *Anxiety:* Adults: (IM, IV) initial 50–100 mg followed by 25–50 mg tid–qid prn; up to 300 mg may be given IM or IV during a 6-h period but not more than this in any 24-h period; (PO) 15–100 mg divided tid–qid. Children >6 yr: (PO, IM) 0.5 mg/kg/24 h divided q6–8h. Children <6 yr: not recommended.
  Preoperative anxiety: (IM) 50–100 mg.
  Ethanol withdrawal symptoms: (PO, IV) initial 50–100 mg, MR in 2–4 h prn to max 300 mg/24 h.
  Renal adjustment: for CrCl <10 mL/min reduce dose to 50%.
  Hepatic impairment: avoid use
- **Site of clearance:** hepatic
- **t$^1/_2$:** 10–48 h
- **Interaction/toxicity:** Cimetidine, metoprolol, propranolol decrease elimination. Increases effect of digoxin.

CHLOROPROCAINE (NESACAINE)

- **Uses:** regional anesthesia
- **Dose:** Dosage varies with anesthetic procedure; range 1.5–25 mL of 2–3% solution, max 800 mg.
  Infiltration and peripheral nerve block: 1–2%.
  Infiltration, peripheral and central nerve block, including caudal and epidural block: 2–3%, without preservative.
- **Site of clearance:** plasma cholinesterase
- **t$^1/_2$:** 1.5–4.7 min
- **Interaction/toxicity:** Rapid inadvertent IT injection of low pH and bisulfite-containing solution may be associated with residual motor/sensory deficit.

CHLORPROMAZINE (THORAZINE)

- **Uses:** psychiatric disorders; premedication; vasodilator
- **Dose:** *Nausea/vomiting:* Adults: (IV, IM) 25–50 mg q4–6h; (PO) 10–25 mg q4–6h; (rectal) 50–100 mg q6–8h. Children: (IV, IM) 0.5–1.0 mg/kg q6–8h, max daily dose 40 mg for ≤5 yr (22.7 kg), max daily dose 75 mg for 5–12 yr (22.7–45.5 kg). Infants

>6 mo: (PO) 0.5–1.0 mg/kg q6h prn; (rectal) 1.0 mg/kg q6–8h prn.

Hepatic impairment: avoid use if severe.
- **Site of clearance:** hepatic
- **t^1/$_2$:** 2 h
- **Interaction/toxicity:** Potentiates sedative–hypnotics. Lithium reduces bioavailability. Mephentermine and epinephrine potentiate chlorpromazine-induced hypotension.

CIMETIDINE (TAGAMET)

- **Uses:** histamine antagonist (H$_2$)
- **Dose:** *Premedication:* (IV) 300 mg (dilute in 20–100 mL NS); (PO) 300 mg.

  Children: (PO, IM, IV) 20–40 mg/kg/day divided q4h

  Adults: Short-term treatment of active ulcers: (PO) 300 mg qid or 800 mg at bedtime or 400 mg bid for up to 8 weeks

  (IM, IV) 300 mg q6h or 37.5 mg/hr by continuous infusion; IV dosage should be adjusted to maintain intragastric pH$\geq$5.

  Renal adjustment: for CrCl 20–40 mL/min dose q8h or reduce dose to 75%, for CrCl 0–20 mL/min dose q12h or reduce dose to 50%.

  Hepatic impairment: caution and reduce dose in severe liver disease; increased risk of CNS toxicity in cirrhosis.
- **Site of clearance:** renal
- **t^1/$_2$:** children 1.4 h, adults 2 h
- **Interaction/toxicity:** Rapid IV administration may cause hypotension and dysrhythmias. Potentiates respiratory depressant effects of morphine. High serum level associated with confusional states in the elderly. Reduces hepatic metabolism of drugs requiring cytochrome P-450 (beta-blockers, calcium channel blockers, theophylline, tranquilizers).

CIPROFLOXACIN (CIPRO)

- **Uses:** antibiotic
- **Dose:** (IV) 200–400 mg q12h; (PO) 250–500 mg q12h.
- **Site of clearance:** renal and hepatic
- **t^1/$_2$:** 3–5 h
- **Interaction/toxicity:** Adjust dose in renal or hepatic failure. May cause CNS stimulation (e.g., tremor, confusion, and seizures). Potentiates anticoagulants and theophylline. Cimetidine potentiates. Antagonizes hydantoins. Not recommended in children <18yr.

CISATRACURIUM BESYLATE (NIMBEX)

■ **Uses:** nondepolarizing neuromuscular blocker
■ **Dose:** Children 2–12 yr: (IV) intubating 0.1 mg over 5–15 sec.
   Adults: (IV) intubating 0.15–0.2 mg/kg; maintenance 0.03 mg/kg 40–60 min after initial dose, then at ~20-min intervals based on clinical criteria.
   Continuous infusion: Adults and children ≥2 yr: (IV) initial rate of 3 mcg/kg/min may be required to rapidly counteract spontaneous recovery of neuromuscular function; thereafter a rate of 1–2 mcg/kg/min should be adequate to maintain continuous neuromuscular block in the 89 to 99% range in most pediatric and adult patients. Consider reduction of infusion rate by 30–40% when administering during stable level of anesthesia.
■ **Site of clearance:** plasma (Hofmann elimination)
■ **t$^1/_2$:** 22–29 min
■ **Interaction/toxicity:** Potentiated by volatile anesthetics, hypokalemia, antibiotics (aminoglycosides), lithium, magnesium, verapamil, local anesthetics, quinidine, and procainamide. Antagonized by phenytoin and carbamazepine. Does not release histamine at high doses.

CLINDAMYCIN (VARIOUS)   **BBW**

■ **Uses:** antibiotic
■ **Dose:** Adults: (IM, IV) 1.2–1.8 g/day q6–12h, max daily dose 4,800 mg; (PO) 150–450 mg q6–8h. Children >1 mo: (IM, IV) 20–40 mg/kg/day q6–8h; (PO) 8–16 mg/kg/day q6–8h.
■ **Site of clearance:** hepatic
■ **t$^1/_2$:** 1.6–5.3 h
■ **Interaction/toxicity:** Adjust dose in renal or hepatic dysfunction. Rapid injection may cause cardiac arrest. Potentiates effects of nondepolarizing neuromuscular blockers and digoxin. Theophylline antagonizes effects. May cause fatal colitis.

CLONAZEPAM (VARIOUS)

■ **Uses:** anticonvulsant, chronic pain
■ **Dose:** *Seizure disorders:* Adults: (PO) initial NTE 1.5 mg in 3 divided doses, may increase by 0.5–1.0 mg every third day until seizures are controlled or adverse effects seen, maintenance 0.05–0.2 mg/kg, max daily dose 20 mg. Children: (PO) initial 0.01–0.03 mg/kg/day in 2–3 divided doses (max 0.05 mg/kg/day), increase by no more than 0.5 mg every third day until

seizures controlled or adverse effects seen, maintenance 0.1–0.2 mg/kg/day divided TID, NTE 0.2 mg/kg/day.

Panic disorder: (PO) 0.25 mg bid; increase in increments of 0.125–0.25 mg bid q3days; target dose 1.0 mg/day, max daily dose 4 mg.

- Site of clearance: renal
- $t^{1}/_{2}$: children 22–33 h, adults 19–50 h
- Interaction/toxicity: Use with caution in patients with chronic respiratory or renal dysfunction. Abrupt withdrawal may cause seizures. Potentiated by general anesthetics, cimetidine, CNS depressants, and verapamil.

CLONIDINE (CATAPRES) BBW

- Uses: antihypertensive
- Dose: *HTN:* Adults: (PO) initial 0.1 mg bid, usual maintenance 0.2–1.2 mg/day in 2–4 divided doses, max daily dose 2.4 mg; (transdermal) apply once q7days; for initial therapy start with 0.1 mg and increase by 0.1 mg at 1–2 week intervals; dosages >0.6 mg do not improve efficacy. Children: (PO) initial 5–10 mcg/kg/day divided q8–12h, increase gradually at 5–7 day intervals to 25 mcg/kg/day divided q6h, max daily dose 0.9 mg.

  Acute HTN (urgency): (PO) initial 0.1–0.2 mg, may be followed by additional doses of 0.1 mg q1h prn to max total 0.6 mg.

  Pain management: Adults: (epidural infusion) initial 30 mcg/h, titrate for relief of pain or presence of side effects. Minimal experience with doses >40 mcg/h; should be considered an adjunct to intraspinal opiate therapy. Children (reserved for patients with severe intractable pain, unresponsive to other analgesics or epidural or spinal opiates): (epidural infusion) initial 0.5 mcg/kg/h; adjust with caution, based on clinical effect.
- Site of clearance: renal, hepatic
- $t^{1}/_{2}$: adults 6–20 h, renal impairment 18–41 h
- Interaction/toxicity: Rebound HTN follows abrupt withdrawal. Enhances effects of anesthetics, tranquilizers, sedatives, and hypnotics. Tolazoline and tricyclic antidepressants can block antihypertensive effects.

COCAINE (VARIOUS)

- Uses: topical anesthesia
- Dose: (topical) 1–4% solution to mucous membranes, max 1–3 mg/kg (or 400 mg); generally 1.0 mg/kg sufficient
  Doses reduced for children, elderly or debilitated patients.
- Site of clearance: plasma cholinesterase

- t$^{1}/_{2}$: 75 min
- **Interaction/toxicity:** Potentiates vasopressors; cardiac dysrhythmias and seizures at high doses.

CODEINE (VARIOUS)

- **Uses:** analgesic
- **Dose:** Adults: (IV, IM, SC, PO) 15–60 mg q4–6h, max daily dose 360 mg. Children: (IV, IM, SC, PO) 0.5–1.0 mg/kg q4–6h, max dose 60 mg.
- **Site of clearance:** hepatic
- t$^{1}/_{2}$: 2.5–3.5 h
- **Interaction/toxicity:** Use with caution with other CNS depressants and MAOIs, and in patients with respiratory diseases. May contain sulfites.

DALTEPARIN (FRAGMIN) **BBW**

- **Uses:** anticoagulant (LMW heparin)
- **Dose:** *Abdominal surgery:* Low to moderate risk: (SQ) 2,500 IU 1–2 h before surgery, then 2,500 IU, then once daily 5–10 days postoperatively. High-risk: (SQ) 5,000 IU 1–2 h before surgery, then 5,000 IU qd for 5–10 days.

  Hip replacement surgery: (SQ) 2,500 IU 1–2 h before surgery, then 2,500 IU on evening of surgery (>6 h after last dose), then 5,000 IU qd for 5–10 days.

  Unstable angina: 120 IU/kg (max 10,000 IU) q12h concurrently with aspirin.
- **Site of clearance:** renal
- t$^{1}/_{2}$: 2–5 h
- **Interaction/toxicity:** Adjust dose with renal dysfunction. Administer as deep SQ (not IM) injection. Contraindicated in patients with pork allergy, active hemorrhage, severe HTN, and thrombocytopenia (ardeparin induced antiplatelet antibodies). Use with caution in patients with HIT. Concomitant use with other anticoagulants, antiplatelet drugs, aspirin, or NSAIDs may cause bleeding. May cause epidural or spinal hematoma in presence of spinal or epidural anesthetic. Single-dose spinal anesthetic may be safest technique. Needle placement should occur 10–12 h after last dose of LMW heparin; 24-h delay is required with higher doses of LMW heparin. For neuraxial catheter techniques, do not administer LMW heparin for 24 h postoperatively. Remove catheters before initiating LMW heparin Rx. Delay catheter removal 10–12 h after last dose of LMW heparin. Subsequent dosing should not occur for <2 h after catheter removal. Presence of blood during spinal, epidural needle, or

catheter placement should delay administration of LMW heparin for 24 h. Overdose treated with protamine.

DANAPAROID (ORGARAN) (DISCONTINUED BY MANUFACTURER IN AUGUST 2002)

■ **Uses:** anticoagulant (LMW heparin)
■ **Dose:** (SQ) 750 anti-Xa units bid not sooner than 1–4 h before surgery, then 750 anti-Xa units bid not sooner than 2 h postoperatively for 7–10 days.
■ **Site of clearance:** renal
■ $t^1/_2$: 24 h
■ **Interaction/toxicity:** Adjust dose with renal dysfunction. Cannot be used interchangeably with heparin or LMW heparins. Administer as deep SQ (not IM) injection. Contraindicated in patients with pork allergy, active hemorrhage, severe HTN, and thrombocytopenia (ardeparin induced antiplatelet antibodies). Concomitant use with other anticoagulants, antiplatelet drugs, aspirin, or NSAIDs may cause bleeding. May cause epidural or spinal hematoma in presence of spinal or epidural anesthetic. Single-dose spinal anesthetic may be safest technique. Needle placement should occur 10–12 h after last dose of LMW heparin; 24-h delay required with higher doses of LMW heparin. For neuraxial catheter techniques, do not administer LMW heparin for 24 h postoperatively. Remove catheters before initiating LMW heparin Rx. Delay catheter removal for 10–12 h after last dose of LMW heparin. Subsequent dosing should not occur for at least 2 h after catheter removal. Presence of blood during spinal, epidural needle, or catheter placement should delay administration of LMW heparin for 24 h. Monitor effect by use anti-Factor Xa assays (ACT, PT, PTT relatively insensitive). Overdose treated with protamine may be ineffective. May contain sulfites.

DANTROLENE (DANTRIUM)   **BBW**

■ **Uses:** malignant hyperthermia
■ **Dose:** *Preoperative prophylaxis:* Adults and children: (IV) 2.5 mg/kg about 75 min prior to anesthesia and infused over 1 h with additional doses prn (dilute 20 g in 60 mL sterile distilled H_2O); (PO) 4–8 mg/kg/day in 4 divided doses 1–2 days prior to surgery with last dose 3–4 h before surgery.

    Crisis: Adults and children: (IV) 2.5 mg/kg, MR to cumulative dose of 10 mg/kg; if physiologic and metabolic abnormalities reappear, repeat regimen.

Postcrisis follow-up: Adults and children: (PO) 4–8 mg/kg/day in 4 divided doses for 1–3 days. IV used when PO not practical. Individualize dosage beginning with 1.0 mg/kg, then switch to PO dosage.
- **Site of clearance:** hepatic
- **t½:** 8.7 h
- **Interaction/toxicity:** Skeletal muscle weakness.

DESIPRAMINE (VARIOUS)

- **Uses:** antidepressant, chronic pain
- **Dose:** (PO) 100–200 mg/day tid.
- **Site of clearance:** hepatic
- **t½:** 7–60 h
- **Interaction/toxicity:** Contraindicated in patients with narrow-angle glaucoma, Rx with MAOIs within previous 14 days. Use with caution in patients with cardiac dysrhythmias and conduction defects, seizure disorders, hyperthyroidism, renal or hepatic dysfunction. Phenobarbital increases metabolism. Increases amount of inhalation anesthesia required. Potentiates sympathomimetics, CNS depressants, and anticoagulants. Cimetidine decreases metabolism. Do not discontinue abruptly. Cardiovascular toxicity leading cause of death.

DESMOPRESSIN ACETATE (DDAVP, STIMATE)

- **Uses:** antidiuretic hormone, coagulation (von Willebrand disease type I)
- **Dose:** *Diabetes insipidus:* Adults and children >12 yr: (IV, SC) 2–4 mcg/day (0.5–1.0 mL) in 2 divided doses; (intranasal) 100 mcg/mL nasal solution at 10–40 mcg/day (0.1–0.4 mL) divided 1–3 times/day; adjust morning and evening doses for an adequate diurnal rhythm of water turnover; (PO) initial 0.05 mg bid, total daily dose increased or decreased prn to obtain adequate antidiuresis, range 0.1–1.2 mg divided 2–3 times/day.
  Hemophilia A and mild to moderate von Willebrand disease (type 1): Adults and children >12 yr: (IV) 0.3 mcg/kg by slow infusion begun 30 min before procedure (dilute in 50–100 mL NS).
- **Site of clearance:** renal
- **t½:** IV 75 min, PO 1.5–2.5 h.
- **Interaction/toxicity:** Chlorpropamide, clofibrate, and carbamazepine potentiate antidiuretic effects.

DEXMEDETOMIDINE (PRECEDEX)

■ **Uses:** sedative
■ **Dose:** (IV) loading 1 mcg/kg over 10 min, infusion 0.2–0.7 mcg/kg/h, not indicated for infusions >24 h; (IM) 0.5–1.5 mcg/kg.
■ **Site of clearance:** hepatic
■ **t$^1/_2$:** 6 min
■ **Interaction/toxicity:** HTN and bradycardia following rapid IV injection. Hypotension and bradycardia can be seen with sedation. Potentiates sedative, hypnotics, and inhalation anesthetics. May impair recognition of signs of light anesthesia (tearing, movement, or sweating). Renal and hepatic impairment prolong actions.

DEXAMETHASONE (HEXADROL, DECADRON)

■ **Uses:** cerebral edema; allergic reactions; replacement Rx
■ **Dose:** *Cerebral edema:* Adults: (IV) 10 mg, then 4 mg IV or IM q6h. Children: (IV) loading 1–2 mg/kg as single dose, maintenance 1–1.5 mg/kg/day to max daily dose 16 mg, divided q4–6h for 5 days then taper for 5 days.

   Extubation or airway edema: Children: (IV, IM, PO) 0.5–2 mg/kg/day divided q6h beginning 24 h before extubation and continuing for 4–6 doses afterward.

   Physiologic replacement: Adults and children: (IV, IM, PO) 0.03–0.15 mg/kg/day divided q6–12h.
■ **Site of clearance:** hepatic
■ **t$^1/_2$:** 1.8–3.5 h
■ **Interaction/toxicity:** Increases insulin requirements; phenytoin, phenobarbital, and ephedrine may increase metabolic clearance of steroid.

DIAZEPAM (VALIUM)

■ **Uses:** antianxiety
■ **Dose:** *Anxiety/sedation/skeletal muscle relaxant:* Adults: (IV, IM) 2–10 mg, MR in 3–4 h prn; (PO) 2–10 mg tid–qid. Children: (PO) 0.12–0.8 mg/kg/day divided q6–8h; (IM, IV): 0.04–0.3 mg/kg q2–4h to max 0.6 mg/kg in 8-h period.

   Sedation in the ICU: (IV) 0.03–0.1 mg/kg q30min to q6h.

   Conscious sedation for procedures: Children: (PO) 0.2–0.3 mg/kg to max 10 mg 45–60 min prior to procedure.
■ **Site of clearance:** hepatic, renal
■ **t$^1/_2$:** 20–50 h
■ **Interaction/toxicity:** Elimination reduced by cimetidine, metoprolol, propranolol. Increases effect of digoxin.

DICLOFENAC (VARIOUS)

- **Uses:** anti-inflammatory, analgesic, antipyretic
- **Dose:** *Analgesia:* (PO) initial 50 mg tid.
  Rheumatoid arthritis: 150–200 mg/day in 2–4 divided doses (100 mg/day of sustained-release product).
  Osteoarthritis: 100–150 mg/day in 2–3 divided doses (100–200 mg/day of sustained-release product).
- **Site of clearance:** hepatic
- **t$^1/_2$:** 2 h
- **Interaction/toxicity:** Adjust dose in renal failure. Use with caution in patients with CHF, hepatic or renal dysfunction, HTN, history of GI bleed. Higher doses are associated with adverse CNS effects, especially in the elderly (agitation, confusion, and hallucination). Aspirin decreases effect. Potentiates digoxin, lithium, and anticoagulants. Inhibits loop diuretics, ACE inhibitors, and beta-blockers.

DIGOXIN (LANOXIN)

- **Uses:** heart failure; antidysrhythmic
- **Dose:** Loading (IV) 0.5–1.0 mg, (PO) 0.75–1.5 mg; give half total digitalizing dose initially, then one-fourth in two subsequent doses at 8–12-h intervals; maintenance (IV, PO) 0.125–0.5 mg once daily.
- **Site of clearance:** renal, hepatic
- **t$^1/_2$:** 38–48 h
- **Interaction/toxicity:** Potentiated by hypokalemia; synergistic with catecholamines, calcium.

DILTIAZEM (CARDIZEM)

- **Uses:** antidysrhythmic (atrial fibrillation/flutter paroxysmal supraventricular tachycardia), HTN
- **Dose:** *Antidysrhythmic:* (IV) 0.25 mg/kg (bolus over 2 min), wait 15 min; if inadequate response 0.35 mg/kg (bolus over 2 min); infusion 2 mcg/kg/min or 10 mg/h.
  HTN: (PO) usual starting dose 30 mg tid; sustained release 120–180 mg/day; increase gradually at 14 day intervals until optimal dose obtained.
- **Site of clearance:** hepatic, renal
- **t$^1/_2$:** 4–6 h
- **Interaction/toxicity:** Potentiated by hepatic and renal disease. Potentiates theophylline and CV depressant effects of volatile anesthetics. Cimetidine and ranitidine may increase

bioavailability. Intensifies sick sinus syndrome, second- and third-degree arteriovenous block, hypotension, and cardiogenic shock. Should not be used in patients with Wolf-Parkinson-White syndrome or short PR interval.

DIPHENHYDRAMINE (BENADRYL)

- **Uses:** histamine blocker (H_1); allergic reaction
- **Dose:** Adults: (IV, IM) 25–50 mg; (PO) 25–50 mg q6–8h. Children >10 kg: (IV) 5 mg/kg/day divided q6–8h; (PO)12.5–25 mg tid–qid.
- **Site of clearance:** hepatic
- $t^{1}/_{2}$: 2–8 h, elderly 13.5 h
- **Interaction/toxicity:** MAOIs intensify effects; may antagonize effect of heparin.

DIPYRIDAMOLE (VARIOUS)

- **Uses:** antiplatelet agent, coronary vasodilator
- **Dose:** Adults: (PO) 75–400 mg divided tid–qid. Children: (PO) 3–6 mg/kg/day divided tid–qid.
- **Site of clearance:** hepatic
- $t^{1}/_{2}$: 10 h
- **Interaction/toxicity:** Use with caution in patients receiving other anticoagulants, aspirin, and NSAIDs. May cause hypotension and "coronary steal." Theophylline inhibits effects.

DOBUTAMINE (DOBUTREX)

- **Uses:** inotropic support
- **Dose:** Adults and children: (IV) 2.5–20 mcg/kg/min, max 20 mcg/kg/min; titrate to desired response
- **Site of clearance:** hepatic
- $t^{1}/_{2}$: 2 min
- **Interaction/toxicity:** Halogenated anesthetics (especially halothane) sensitize myocardium to sympathomimetic effects (dysrhythmias).

DOPAMINE (INTROPIN)

- **Uses:** inotropic support
- **Dose:** (IV) 2–20 mcg/kg/min (dilute 200 mg in 250 mL D_5W or NS).
- **Site of clearance:** enzymatic transformation (COMT and MAOI)
- $t^{1}/_{2}$: 2 min

■ **Interaction/toxicity:** Reduce dose in patients receiving MAOIs; combined with phenytoin, causes seizures, hypotension, and bradycardia; halogenated anesthetics (especially halothane) sensitize myocardium to sympathomimetic effects (dysrhythmias).

DOXACURIUM (NUROMAX) BBW

■ **Uses:** Nondepolarizing neuromuscular blocker
■ **Dose:** Adults: (IV) 0.05–0.08 mg/kg with thiopental/narcotic or 0.025 mg/kg after initial dose of succinylcholine for intubation, initial maintenance 0.005–0.01 mg/kg after 100–160 min followed by repeat doses every 30–45 min.
  Children >2 yr: (IV) initial 0.03–0.05 mg/kg followed by maintenance 0.005–0.01 mg/kg after 30–45 min.
■ **Site of clearance:** renal
■ **t$\frac{1}{2}$:** 1.2–2 h
■ **Interaction/toxicity:** Potentiated by volatile anesthetics, hypokalemia, antibiotics (aminoglycosides), lithium, magnesium, local anesthetics, procainamide, quinidine. Anticonvulsants (phenytoin and carbamazepine) lengthen onset and shorten duration of neuromuscular blockade. Contains benzyl alcohol, which may be associated with increased incidence of neurologic complications in neonates. Due to long duration of action, not recommended for patients undergoing cesarean section.

DOXAPRAM (DOPRAM)

■ **Uses:** respiratory and CNS stimulant
■ **Dose:** (IV) 0.5–1.0 mg/kg, repeat q5min prn, max 2 mg/kg; infusion 5 mg/min then 1–3 mg/min then taper, max daily dose 300 mg.
■ **Site of clearance:** hepatic
■ **t$\frac{1}{2}$:** 2.4–9.9 h
■ **Interaction/toxicity:** Contraindicated in patients with epilepsy, cerebral edema, cerebral vascular accident, severe cardiopulmonary disease, HTN, mechanical obstruction to ventilation, pheochromocytoma, and hyperthyroidism. Associated with cholestatic hepatitis. Continuous infusion in neonates can deliver large amounts of benzyl alcohol.

DROPERIDOL (INAPSINE) BBW

■ **Uses:** antianxiety; antiemetic

- **Dose:** *Nausea and vomiting:* Adults: (IV, IM) 0.625–2.5 mg. Children 2–12 yr: (IV, IM) 0.05–0.06 mg/kg, max initial dose 0.1 mg/kg.
- **Site of clearance:** hepatic
- $t^1/_2$: 2.3 h
- **Interaction/toxicity:** Intensifies hypotension of vasodilators; produces extrapyramidal signs. Contraindicated in patients with known or suspected QT-interval prolongation (QTc interval above 440 msec for males and above 450 msec for females) and congenital long QT syndrome.

DROTRECOGIN ALFA (XIGRIS)

- **Uses:** anti-inflammatory, blood modifier, coagulation inhibitor, profibrinolytic
- **Dose:** *Severe sepsis:* (IV) 24 mcg/kg/h for 96 h.
- **Site of clearance:** endogenous plasma protease inhibitors
- $t^1/_2$: 13 min
- **Interaction/toxicity:** Hypersensitivity to drotrecogin alfa, active internal bleeding, recent hemorrhagic stroke (within 3 months), recent intracranial, intraspinal surgery; severe head trauma (within 2 months), intracranial neoplasm or mass lesion or evidence of cerebral herniation, existing epidural catheter, trauma with an increased risk of life-threatening bleeding. May prolong activated partial thromboplastin time (aPTT) but has minimal effect of the prothrombin time (PT); the PT should be used to monitor the status of the coagulopathy in these patients, should be discontinued 2 hours prior to procedures with an inherent risk of bleeding.

EDROPHONIUM (TENSILON)

- **Uses:** anticholinesterase; antidysrhythmic
- **Dose:** *Titration of oral anticholinesterase therapy:* Adults: (IV) 1–2 mg given 1 h after oral dose of anticholinesterase. If strength improves an increase in neostigmine or pyridostigmine dose is indicated. Children: (IV) 0.04 mg/kg given 1 h after oral intake of the drug being used in treatment.
- **Site of clearance:** hepatic, renal
- $t^1/_2$: 1.8 h
- **Interaction/toxicity:** Bradycardia, salivation. Overdosage can cause cholinergic crisis which may be fatal. IV atropine should be readily available for treatment of cholinergic reactions.

ENOXAPARIN (LOVENOX) `BBW`

- **Uses:** anticoagulant (LMW heparin)
- **Dose:** *Abdominal surgery:* (SQ) 40 mg 2 h before surgery, then 40 mg qd for 7–10 days.

    Hip or knee replacement: (SQ) 40 mg 9–15 h before surgery and 40 mg qd for 3 wk; alternatively 30 mg q12h with first dose given 12–24 h postoperatively in presence of adequate hemostasis; continue for 7–14 days.

    Treatment of DVT with or without PE: 1.0 mg/kg q12h or 1.5 mg/kg qd.

    Anticoagulant prophylaxis: Infants >2 mo and children ≤18 yr: (SQ) 0.5 mg/kg q12h.

    Anticoagulant treatment: Infants >2 mo and children ≤18 yr: (SQ) 1.0 mg/kg q12h.
- **Site of clearance:** renal
- **t$\frac{1}{2}$:** 4.5–7 h
- **Interaction/toxicity:** Adjust dose with renal dysfunction. Administer as deep SQ (not IM) injection. Contraindicated in patients with pork allergy, active hemorrhage, severe HTN, and thrombocytopenia (ardeparin induced antiplatelet antibodies). Contraindicated in patients with heparin induced thrombocytopenia. Concomitant use with other anticoagulants, antiplatelet drugs, aspirin, or NSAIDs may cause bleeding. May cause epidural or spinal hematoma in presence of spinal or epidural anesthetic. Single-dose spinal anesthetic may be safest technique. Needle placement should occur 10–12 h after last dose of LMW heparin; 24-h delay is required with higher doses of LMWH. For neuraxial catheter techniques, do not administer LMW heparin for 24 h postoperatively. Remove catheters before initiating of LMW heparin Rx. Delay catheter for 10–12 h after last dose of LMW heparin. Subsequent dosing should not occur for <2 h after catheter removal. Presence of blood during spinal, epidural needle, or catheter placement should delay administration of LMW heparin for 24 h. In elderly there is increased incidence of bleeding with therapeutic doses. Careful attention should be paid to elderly patients <45kg. Overdose treated with protamine.

EPHEDRINE (VARIOUS)

- **Uses:** sympathomimetic
- **Dose:** (IV) 5–10 mg.
- **Site of clearance:** hepatic
- **t$\frac{1}{2}$:** 3–6 h

■ **Interaction/toxicity:** Potentiated by tricyclic antidepressants and MAOIs; halogenated anesthetics sensitize myocardium to sympathomimetic effects (dysrhythmias).

EPINEPHRINE (VARIOUS)

■ **Uses:** sympathomimetic; allergic reaction
■ **Dose:** (IV) 2–8 mcg; infusion 0.01–0.02 mcg/kg/min.
■ **Site of clearance:** enzymatic transformation (COMT and MAOI)
■ **t$\frac{1}{2}$:** 2 min
■ **Interaction/toxicity:** Halogenated anesthetics (especially halothane) sensitize myocardium to sympathomimetic effects (dysrhythmias); potentiated by tricyclic antidepressants, MAOIs, and antihistamines.

EPINEPHRINE, RACEMIC (VAPONEFRIN, MICRONEFRIN)

■ **Uses:** bronchodilator, croup (laryngotracheobronchitis)
■ **Dose:** (inhalation) q4h (dilute 1:6 with NS).
■ **Site of clearance:** enzymatic transformation (COMT and MAOI)
■ **t$\frac{1}{2}$:** 2 min
■ **Interaction/toxicity:** Halogenated anesthetics (especially halothane) sensitize myocardium to sympathomimetic effects (dysrhythmias).

ERGONOVINE (ERGOTRATE)

■ **Uses:** increases uterine contractions
■ **Dose:** (IM) 0.2 mg q2–4h for uterine bleeding.
■ **Site of clearance:** hepatic
■ **t$\frac{1}{2}$:** 0.5–3.5 h
■ **Interaction/toxicity:** Can induce coronary artery spasm.

ERYTHROMYCIN (VARIOUS)

■ **Uses:** antibiotic
■ **Dose:** Adults: (IV) 15–20 mg/kg/day q4–6h, max daily dose 4 g; (PO) base 250–500 mg q6h; preop bowel prep 1.0 g erythromycin base at 1:00, 2:00, and 11:00 PM on the day before surgery combined with mechanical cleansing of the large intestine and oral neomycin. Children: (IV) lactobionate 20–40 mg/kg/day q6h; (PO) 30–50 mg/kg/day q6–8h, max daily dose

1–2 g; preop bowel prep 20 mg/kg erythromycin base at 1:00, 2:00, and 11:00 PM on the day before surgery combined with mechanical cleansing of the large intestine and oral neomycin.
- **Site of clearance:** hepatic
- **t^1/$_2$:** 1.5–2 h, ESRD 5–6 h
- **Interaction/toxicity:** Modify dose in hepatic dysfunction. Ventricular dysrhythmias including ventricular tachycardia and abnormal prolongation of the QT interval (Torsades de Pointes) have been reported. Potentiates effects of warfarin, benzodiazepines, alfentanil, carbamazepine, corticosteroids, cyclosporine, digoxin, ergot alkaloids, and theophylline. May potentiate effects of myasthenia gravis.

ESMOLOL (BREVIBLOC)

- **Uses:** supraventricular tachycardia, HTN
- **Dose:** (IV) bolus 0.25–0.5 mg/kg,; continuous infusion loading dose 500 mcg/kg/min over 1–2 min; maintenance 50–200 mcg/kg/min (dilute 5 g in 500 mL D$_5$W or NS).
- **Site of clearance:** red blood cell esterase
- **t^1/$_2$:** 9 min
- **Interaction/toxicity:** Increases digoxin and serum morphine levels.

ETHACRYNIC ACID (EDECRIN)

- **Uses:** diuretic
- **Dose:** Adults: (IV) 0.5–1.0 mg/kg, max 100 mg/dose; repeat doses not routinely recommended but if indicated repeat doses q8–12h; (PO) 50–200 mg/day in 1–2 divided doses, may increase up to max 200 mg bid. Children: (PO) 1.0 mg/kg/dose qd, increase to max of 3 mg/kg/day.
- **Site of clearance:** renal
- **t^1/$_2$:** 2–4 h
- **Interaction/toxicity:** Administration with aminoglycoside antibiotics can cause ototoxicity. Reduces renal clearance of lithium. Reduce warfarin dose.

ETIDOCAINE (DURANEST)

- **Uses:** regional anesthesia
- **Dose:** *Neural blockade:* 300 mg (with epinephrine 1: 200,000).
- **Site of clearance:** hepatic
- **t^1/$_2$:** 2.5 h

- **Interaction/toxicity:** Not recommended for obstetric anesthesia because of profound motor blockade.

ETOMIDATE (AMIDATE)

- **Uses:** induction agent
- **Dose:** Adults and children >10 yr: (IV) initial 0.2–0.6 mg/kg over 30–60 sec, maintenance 5–20 mcg/kg/min.
- **Site of clearance:** hepatic
- **t^1/$_2$:** 2.6–3.5 h
- **Interaction/toxicity:** Interferes with adrenal function (reduced release of cortisol). Myoclonus and pain with rapid IV injection.

FACTOR VIIa RECOMBINANT (NOVOSEVEN)

- **Uses:** factor replacement for hemophiliacs
- **Dose:** (IV) 90 mcg/kg q2h until adequate coagulation occurs.
- **Site of clearance:** N/A
- **t^1/$_2$:** 2.3 h
- **Interaction/toxicity:** Contraindicated in patients with known allergies to mouse, hamster, or bovine proteins. Increase in thrombotic events in DIC, advanced arteriosclerotic disease, and crush injury.

FACTOR VIII (ANTIHEMOPHILIAC FACTOR [AHF]; VARIOUS)

- **Uses:** factor VIII replacement
- **Dose:** (IV) 10–25 AHF IU/kg q12–24h to increase level to 80%–100% of normal.
- **Site of clearance:** N/A
- **t^1/$_2$:** 12–17 h
- **Interaction/toxicity:** Ineffective for von Willebrand's disease. Risk of HIV and infectious viral agents (hepatitis). Patients with factor VIII inhibitor may not respond appropriately. Hemolysis may occur due to AHF solution containing anti-A and anti-B isoagglutinins.

FACTOR IX CONCENTRATE (VARIOUS)

- **Uses:** factor IX deficiency (hemophilia B, Christmas disease)
- **Dose:** (IV) IU (recombinant) = (1.2 IU/kg)(kg)(desired increase % of normal); IU (human derived factor) = (1.0 IU/kg)(kg)(desired increase % of normal) (titrate to >20 % normal). 1.0 IU/kg will increase level by 1%.

- Site of clearance: N/A
- t^1/$_2$: 18–36 h
- Interaction/toxicity: Contraindicated in patients with known allergy to mouse protein. Risk of HIV, infectious viruses (human-derived factor). May cause thromboembolic complications including MI, pulmonary embolism, venous thrombosis, and DIC. Rapid infusion can cause hemodynamic instability.

FAMOTIDINE (PEPCID)

- Uses: histamine blocker (H$_2$)
- Dose: Adults: (PO, IV) 20 mg q12h (dilute in 10 mg D$_5$W or NS). Children 1–16 yr: (PO) 0.5 mg/kg/day qhs or divided q12h; (IV) 0.25 mg/kg q12h.
- Site of clearance: renal
- t^1/$_2$: 2.5–3.5 h
- Interaction/toxicity: Antacids decrease oral absorption.

FENOLDOPAM (CORLOPAM)

- Uses: HTN
- Dose: (IV) infusion 0.1 mcg/kg/min, increase 0.05–0.2 mcg/kg/min until target blood pressure is achieved; average rate 0.25–0.5 mcg/kg/min; usual length of treatment 1–6 h with tapering of 12% q15–30min.
- Site of clearance: hepatic
- t^1/$_2$: 9.8 min
- Interaction/toxicity: Use with caution in patients with cirrhosis, glaucoma, unstable angina. Causes dose-related tachycardia. Hypokalemia may occur. Contains sulfites.

FENTANYL (SUBLIMAZE)

- Uses: analgesia
- Dose: *Sedation for minor procedures/analgesia:* Adults and children >12 yr: (IM, IV) 0.5–1.0 mcg/kg/dose; higher doses are used for major procedures. Children 1–12 yr: (IM, IV): 1.0–2 mcg/kg/dose, MR at 30–60 min intervals. Note: Children 18–38 mo may require 2–3 mcg/kg/dose.
  General anesthesia without additional anesthetic agents: Adults and children >12 yr: (slow IV) 50–100 mcg/kg.
  Mechanically ventilated adults and children >12 yr: (IV) 0.35–1.5 mcg/kg every 30–60 min prn, infusion 0.7–10 mcg/kg/h.

Continuous sedation: Children 1–12 yr: (IV) initial bolus 1–2 mcg/kg then 1.0 mcg/kg/h, titrate upward, usual 1–3 mcg/kg/h.
- **Site of clearance:** hepatic
- **t^1/$_2$:** 2–4 h
- **Interaction/toxicity:** Diazepam potentiates hypotensive action; truncal muscle rigidity may be seen during induction and emergence.

FENTANYL (DURAGESIC)   `BBW`

- **Uses:** analgesia
- **Dose:** (transdermal) 2.5 mg patch (therapeutically equivalent to 15 mg morphine IM or 90 mg morphine PO).
- **Site of clearance:** hepatic
- **t^1/$_2$:** 17 h
- **Interaction/toxicity:** Potentiates opioid analgesics, tranquilizers, and sedatives.

FENTANYL ORALET (ACTIQ)   `BBW`

- **Uses:** analgesia
- **Dose:** 5 mcg/kg, suck on lozenge vigorously for approximately 20–40 min before start of procedure; drug effect begins in 10 min. Available in 200 mcg, 300 mcg, 400 mcg.
- **Site of clearance:** hepatic
- **t^1/$_2$:** 6.6 h
- **Interaction/toxicity:** Potentiates opioid analgesics, tranquilizers, and sedatives.

FLUMAZENIL (MAZICON)   `BBW`

- **Uses:** benzodiazepine receptor antagonist
- **Dose:** *Reversal of conscious sedation:* Adults: (IV) 0.1–0.2 mg over 30 sec, MR 0.2 mg at 1 min intervals if desired level of consciousness not obtained, max cumulative dose 3 mg. Children: (IV) initial 0.01 mg/kg (max 0.2 mg) over 15 sec, MR 0.005–0.01 mg/kg (max 0.2 mg) at 1 min intervals, max cumulative dose 1.0 mg.
- **Site of clearance:** hepatic
- **t^1/$_2$:** 7–15 min
- **Interaction/toxicity:** Benzodiazepine reversal may be associated with seizures in high-risk populations: major hypnotic drug withdrawal, previous seizure activity, and cyclic antidepressant poisoning. May precipitate withdrawal syndrome in benzodiazepine dependent patients.

FLURAZEPAM (DALMANE)

- **Uses:** antianxiety
- **Dose:** (PO) 15–30 mg
- **Site of clearance:** hepatic
- **t$^1/_2$:** single dose 74–90 h, multiple doses 111–113 h; elderly (61–85 yr) single dose 120–160 h, multiple doses 126–158 h
- **Interaction/toxicity:** Significantly longer elimination half-time in the elderly. Caution in patients with chronic pulmonary insufficiency.

FUROSEMIDE (LASIX)

- **Uses:** diuretic
- **Dose:** Adults: (IM, IV) 20–40 mg, MR in 1–2 h prn and increase by 20 mg/dose until desired effect; (PO) 20–80 mg initially increased in increments of 20–40 mg/dose at intervals of 6–8 h; usual maintenance dosing interval is q12h or q24h. Infants and children: (IM, IV) initial 1.0 mg/kg, increasing each succeeding dose by 1.0 mg/kg at intervals of 6–12 h up to 6 mg/kg/dose; (PO) initial 1–2 mg/kg, increasing by 1.0 mg/kg/dose no more frequently than q6h until desired effect up to 6 mg/kg/dose.
- **Site of clearance:** renal
- **t$^1/_2$:** 0.5–1.1 h, ESRD 9 h
- **Interaction/toxicity:** Stimulates release of renal prostaglandin E_2 (increases incidence of patent ductus arteriosus in premature infants). Administration with aminoglycoside antibiotics can cause ototoxicity.

GABAPENTIN (NEURONTIN)

- **Uses:** epilepsy
- **Dose:** Adults and children >12 yr: (PO) 300–600 mg tid.
- **Site of clearance:** renal
- **t$^1/_2$:** 5–6 h
- **Interaction/toxicity:** Antacids reduce bioavailability; cimetidine and oral contraceptives increase bioavailability.

GALLAMINE (FLAXEDIL)

- **Uses:** nondepolarizing neuromuscular blocker
- **Dose:** (IV): initial 1.0 mg/kg up to 100 mg, maintenance 0.5 to 1.0 mg/kg q30–40min prn, max 100 mg.
- **Site of clearance:** renal
- **t$^1/_2$:** 134 minutes

- **Interaction/toxicity:** Tachycardia. Do not administer to patients with iodide allergy.

GENTAMICIN (VARIOUS) BBW

- **Uses:** antibiotic
- **Dose:** Adults: (IV, IM) (use ideal body weight) 1–1.7 mg/kg q8h. Children >5 yr: (IV, IM): 1.5–2.5 mg/kg q8h. Infants and children <5 yr: (IV, IM) 2.5 mg/kg q8h.
  Renal impairment: extend dosing interval.
- **Site of clearance:** renal
- $t^{1}/_{2}$: 1.5–4 h
- **Interaction/toxicity:** Adjust dose with renal dysfunction. Associated with significant nephrotoxicity and ototoxicity. In burn patients, reduced serum concentration of gentamicin may be observed. Potentiates nondepolarizing neuromuscular blockers and effects of myasthenia gravis. Antibiotics, loop diuretics, cyclosporine, and enflurane increase risk of nephrotoxicity and/or ototoxicity.

GLUCAGON (GLUCAGON)

- **Uses:** treatment of hypoglycemia; relaxes sphincter of Oddi
- **Dose:** *Hypoglycemia or insulin shock therapy:* Adults: (IV, IM, SQ) 0.5–1.0 mg, MR in 20 min prn. Children: (IV, IM, SQ) 0.025–0.1 mg/kg, NTE 1.0 g/dose, MR in 20 min prn.
- **Site of clearance:** renal
- $t^{1}/_{2}$: 3–10 min
- **Interaction/toxicity:** Intensifies action of anticoagulants; causes significant increase in BP.

GLYCOPYRROLATE (ROBINUL)

- **Uses:** anticholinergic
- **Dose:** *Preoperative:* Adult: (IM) 0.004 mg/kg 30–60 min before procedure. Children <2 yr: (IM) 0.004–0.008 mg/kg 30–60 in before procedure. Children >2 yr: (IM) 0.004 mg/kg 30–60 min before procedure.
  Intraoperative: Adult: (IV) 0.1 mg repeated prn at 2–3-min intervals. Children: (IV) 0.004 mg/kg, NTE 0.1 mg, MR at 2–3-min intervals prn.
  Control of secretions: Children: (PO) 0.04–0.1 mg/kg q3–4h; (IM, IV) 0.004–0.01 mg/kg q3–4h, max 0.2 mg/dose or 0.8 mg/24 h.
- **Site of clearance:** renal

- **t$^1/_2$:** 20–40 min
- **Interaction/toxicity:** Contraindicated in patients with myasthenia gravis; paralytic ileus, obstructive diseases of GI tract; obstructive uropathy; tachycardia; acute hemorrhage; ulcerative colitis; narrow-angle glaucoma. Incompatible with secobarbital, sodium bicarbonate, thiopental.

GRANISETRON (KYTRIL)

- **Uses:** antiemetic
- **Dose:** *PONV prevention:* 1.0 mg undiluted over 30 sec, administered before induction of anesthesia or before reversal of anesthesia.

    PONV treatment: 1 mg undiluted over 30 sec.

    Chemotherapy-related emesis: Adults and children >2 yr: (IV) 10 mcg/kg or 1.0 mg/dose infused over 5 min; (PO) 1.0 mg bid.
- **Site of clearance:** hepatic
- **t$^1/_2$:** 9 h
- **Interaction/toxicity:** Use with caution in patients with liver disease. Has minimal sedative properties.

HALOPERIDOL (HALDOL)

- **Uses:** tranquilizer
- **Dose:** *Psychosis:* (IM) (as lactate) 2–5 mg q4–8h prn; (PO) 0.5–5 mg bid–tid, max daily dose 30 mg.

    ICU delirium: (IV, IM): 2–10 mg; MR bolus doses q20–30 min until calm achieved then administer 25% of max dose q6h; monitor ECG and QT$_c$ interval.

    Sedation/psychotic disorders: Children 6–12 yr: (IM, as lactate) 1–3 mg q4–8h to max daily dose 0.15 mg/kg; change to PO as soon as possible. Children 3–12 yr (15–40 kg): (PO) initial 0.05 mg/kg/day or 0.25–0.5 mg/day in 2–3 divided doses; increase by 0.25–0.5 mg q5–7days, max daily dose 0.15 mg/kg.
- **Site of clearance:** hepatic
- **t$^1/_2$:** 20 h
- **Interaction/toxicity:** Coadministration with lithium may produce neurotoxicity.

HEPARIN (VARIOUS) **BBW**

- **Uses:** anticoagulant
- **Dose:** *Cardiopulmonary bypass:* (IV) 350–400 units/kg, using ACT as therapeutic guide.

Deep vein thrombosis and pulmonary embolism: (IV) 80 units/kg IV bolus then 18 units/kg/h.

Low-dose prophylaxis: (SC) 5,000 units q8–12h.

- **Site of clearance:** hepatic
- **$t^1/_2$:** 1.5 h
- **Interaction/toxicity:** Increases diazepam plasma levels; digitalis and antihistamines interfere with anticoagulant properties; nitroglycerin may antagonize heparin.

HETASTARCH (HESPAN)

- **Uses:** volume expander
- **Dose:** (IV) 500–1,000 mL with total dosage NTE 1,500 mL/day (or ~20 mL/kg/day).
- **Site of clearance:** enzymatic
- **$t^1/_2$:** 12 h
- **Interaction/toxicity:** Anaphylactoid reaction. Large volumes may cause coagulopathy.

HYDRALAZINE (APRESOLINE)

- **Uses:** antihypertensive
- **Dose:** *HTN:* Adults: (IM, IV) 5–10 mg q4–6h prn, may increase to 40 mg/dose; change to PO as soon as possible. Children: (IM, IV) 0.1–0.2 mg/kg (max 20 mg) q4–6h prn, up to 1.7–3.5 mg/kg/day in 4–6 divided doses.

Pre-eclampsia/eclampsia: 5 mg then 5–10 mg q20–30 min prn.

- **Site of clearance:** hepatic
- **$t^1/_2$:** 3–5 h
- **Interaction/toxicity:** Increases bioavailability of beta-blockers; may require coadministration of beta-blockers to blunt cardiac stimulation.

HYDROCORTISONE (SOLU-CORTEF)

- **Uses:** anti-inflammatory; steroid replacement; allergic reaction
- **Dose:** *Acute adrenal insufficiency:* Adults: (IV, IM) 100 mg q8h. Older children: (IV, IM) 1–2 mg/kg bolus then 150–250 mg/day divided q6–8h. Infants and young children: (IV, IM) 1–2 mg/kg bolus, then 25–150 mg/day divided q6–8h.
- **Site of clearance:** hepatic
- **$t^1/_2$:** 8–12 h
- **Interaction/toxicity:** Increases insulin requirements; phenytoin, phenobarbital, and ephedrine may increase metabolic clearance.

HYDROMORPHONE (DILAUDID)

- **Uses:** analgesia
- **Dose:** Adults and older children >50 kg: (PO) start at 2–4 mg q3–4h in opiate-naïve patients, usual range 2–8 mg q3–4h; (IV) start at 0.2–0.6 mg q2–3h or (IM, SC) 0.8–1 mg q4–6h in opiate-naïve patients, usual range 1–4 mg (IV, IM, SC) q4–6h; (epidural) bolus 0.5–1.0 mg, continuous infusion 0.10–0.15 mg/h. Young children ≥6 mo and <50 kg: (PO) 0.03–0.08 mg/kg q3–4h prn; (IV) 0.015 mg/kg q3–6h prn.
- **Site of clearance:** liver
- **$t^{1}/_{2}$:** 1–3 h
- **Interaction/toxicity:** Hypotension, respiratory depression, nausea, and pruritus. Potentiated by sedatives, hypnotics, tranquilizers; decreases effects of diuretics in CHF.

IBUPROFEN (VARIOUS)

- **Uses:** analgesia, antipyretic, anti-inflammatory drug
- **Dose:** Adults: (PO) 200–800 mg q4–8h, max daily dose 3.2 g. Children: (PO) 30–70 mg/kg/day divided q6–8h.
- **Site of clearance:** hepatic
- **$t^{1}/_{2}$:** 2–4 h
- **Interaction/toxicity:** Use with caution in patients with CHF, hepatic or renal dysfunction, HTN, history of GI bleed. May inhibit platelet aggregation. Higher doses are associated with adverse CNS effects, especially in the elderly (agitation, confusion, and hallucination). Aspirin decreases effect. Potentiates digoxin, lithium, and warfarin. Inhibits loop diuretics, beta-blockers, ACE inhibitors, anticoagulants, lithium, and dipyridamole.

IMIPENEM AND CILASTIN (PRIMAXIN)

- **Uses:** antibiotic
- **Dose:** Adults: (IV) 125–500 mg over 30 min q6–8h. Children: (IV) 15–25 mg/kg q6h, max daily dose 2 g.
- **Site of clearance:** renal
- **$t^{1}/_{2}$:** 60 min
- **Interaction/toxicity:** Adjust dose in renal dysfunction. May cause allergic reaction in patients with penicillin allergy. Benzyl alcohol preservative associated with toxicity in neonates.

IMIPRAMINE (VARIOUS)

- **Uses:** antidepressant, chronic pain management

- **Dose:** Adults: (PO) 25 mg q6–8h, max daily dose 300 mg. Children: (PO) 25 mg/day, max daily dose 2.5 mg/kg.
- **Site of clearance:** hepatic
- **$t^1/_2$:** 6–18 h
- **Interaction/toxicity:** Contraindicated in patients with narrow-angle glaucoma, Rx with MAOIs within previous 14 days. Use with caution in patients with cardiac dysrhythmias, hyperthyroidism, renal or hepatic dysfunction. Barbiturates increase metabolism. Increases amount of inhalation anesthesia required. Potentiates sympathomimetics, CNS depressants, and anticoagulants. Cimetidine decreases metabolism. Do not abruptly discontinue. Intermediate metabolite has tricyclic activity. May contain sulfites. Cardiovascular toxicity leading cause of death.

INAMRINONE (INOCOR)

- **Uses:** inotropic support
- **Dose:** (IV) loading 0.75 mg/kg, maintenance 5–10 mcg/kg/min.
- **Site of clearance:** renal
- **$t^1/_2$:** 3.6 h; CHF 5.8 h
- **Interaction/toxicity:** Marked vasodilator action seen in hypovolemic patients. Thrombocytopenia following long-term therapy. Should not be diluted with D_5W or given in same IV tubing with furosemide. Contains sodium metabisulfate, which may cause allergic and/or anaphylactic reactions in patients allergic to sulfites.

INDOMETHACIN (VARIOUS)

- **Uses:** analgesia, antipyretic, anti-inflammatory drug, closure PDA in neonates
- **Dose:** (PO) 25–50 mg q8–12h, max daily dose 200 mg.
  Closure of PDA: Neonates: (IV) initial 0.2 mg/kg, followed by 2 doses depending on postnatal age. (Withhold with anuria or oliguria.)
- **Site of clearance:** hepatic
- **$t^1/_2$:** 4.5 h
- **Interaction/toxicity:** Contraindicated in patients with active GI bleed, neonates with necrotizing enterocolitis, and active bleeding. Use with caution in patients with CHF, hepatic or renal dysfunction, HTN, history of GI bleed. Higher doses are associated with adverse CNS effects, especially in the elderly (agitation, confusion, and hallucination). Aspirin decreases effect. Potentiates digoxin, lithium, and anticoagulants. Inhibits loop diuretics. Inhibits effect of antihypertensives, beta-blockers, and furosemide.

ISOPROTERENOL (ISUPREL)

- **Uses:** inotropic/chronotropic; bronchodilator
- **Dose:** Adults: (IV) initial 2 mcg/min, titrate to patient response, usual effective dose 2–10 mcg/min (dilute 2–4 mg/500 mL D_5W). Children: (IV) initial 0.1 mcg/kg/min, usual effective dose 0.2–2 mcg/kg/min.
- **Site of clearance:** hepatic
- **$t^1/_2$:** 2.5–5 min
- **Interaction/toxicity:** Halogenated anesthetics (especially halothane) sensitize myocardium to sympathomimetic effects (dysrhythmias); effects of MAOIs and tricyclic antidepressants are potentiated.

KANAMYCIN (KANTREX) BBW

- **Uses:** antibiotic
- **Dose:** *Infection:* Adults: (IV, IM) 5–7.5 mg/kg q8–12h, max daily dose 1.5 g. Children: (IV, IM) 15 mg/kg/day divided q8–12h.
  Preoperative intestinal antisepsis: (PO) 1 g q1h for 4 h, then q4–6h for 36–72 h.
  Intraperitoneal irrigation: (PO) 500 mg diluted in 20 mL distilled water.
- **Site of clearance:** renal
- **$t^1/_2$:** 2.2–2.4 h
- **Interaction/toxicity:** Use with caution in patients with renal dysfunction, otologic impairment, and myasthenia gravis. Potentiates nondepolarizing neuromuscular blockers. Antibiotics, loop diuretics, cyclosporins, and enflurane increase risk of nephrotoxicity and ototoxicity. Antagonizes digoxin.

KETAMINE (KETALAR) BBW

- **Uses:** induction agent; anesthesia
- **Dose:** Adults: (IV) 1–2 mg/kg; (IM) 5–10 mg/kg. Children: (IM) 3–7 mg/kg. (IV) 0.5–2 mg/kg, with smaller doses (0.5–1.0 mg/kg) for sedation for minor procedures; usual induction dosage 1–2 mg/kg.
- **Site of clearance:** hepatic
- **$t^1/_2$:** 11–17 min
- **Interaction/toxicity:** Potentiates action of sedatives, hypnotics, and opioids; dysphoric reactions; increases cerebral blood flow and IOP. Increases upper airway secretions and heightens laryngeal reflexes.

KETOROLAC (TORADOL) **BBW**

- Uses: analgesic
- Dose: (IV, IM) 60 mg as single dose or 30 mg q6h.
- Site of clearance: renal
- $t^1/_2$: 2–8 h, prolonged in elderly
- Interaction/toxicity: Potentiates NSAIDs. Reversibly inhibits platelet aggregation and is contraindicated before major surgery or intraoperatively where hemostasis is critical. May cause renal toxicity and is potentiated by acute renal failure; contraindicated in patients with advanced renal impairment or those at risk for renal failure due to hypovolemia. May cause peptic ulcers, GI bleeding, and/or perforation. Anaphylactic allergic reaction may be seen with first dose. Contraindicated in patients with previously demonstrated hypersensitivity to ketorolac, aspirin, or other NSAIDs. Contraindicated for spinal or epidural anesthesia. Contraindicated in labor and delivery due to adverse effects on fetal circulation and inhibition of fetal contractions. Contraindicated for patients receiving other NSAIDs or aspirin (cumulative risk of serious adverse effects). Duration of oral Ketorolac not to be >5 days, and oral dose is significantly lower than IV or IM routes. For patients aged >65, those who weigh <110 lbs, and those with elevated serum creatinine, IV/IM dose is not to be >60 mg/day.

LABETALOL (NORMODYNE, TRANDATE)

- Uses: Alpha- and beta-adrenergic blockade; antihypertensive
- Dose: (IV) 5–20 mg (0.25 mg/kg for an 80 kg patient) over 2 min, may administer 40–80 mg at 10 min intervals, up to 300 mg total; infusion 2 mg/min, titrate to response up to 300 mg total dose prn.
- Site of clearance: hepatic
- $t^1/_2$: 2.5–8 h
- Interaction/toxicity: Cimetidine increases bioavailability; halothane or diazepam prolongs effects.

LEPIRUDIN (REFLUDAN)

- Uses: anticoagulant for heparin-induced thrombocytopenia
- Dose: (IV) bolus 0.4 mg/kg over 15–20 sec, continuous infusion 0.15 mg/kg/h. Bolus and infusion must be reduced in renal insufficiency.
- Site of clearance: renal
- $t^1/_2$: 0.8–2 h

- **Interaction/toxicity:** Adjust dose in renal dysfunction. Contraindicated in patient with renal failure, intracranial bleeding, concomitant thrombolytic Rx, active bleeding, recent puncture of large blood vessels, recent surgery, neuraxial anesthesia, and bacterial endocarditis. Should not be administered to patients receiving other anticoagulant drugs.

LEVOBUPIVACAINE (CHIROCAINE)

- **Uses:** local anesthetic
- **Dose:** infiltration 5–200 mg; epidural 50–150 mg; peripheral nerve block 75–150 mg.
- **Site of clearance:** renal
- **t$^{1}/_{2}$:** 1.3 h
- **Interaction/toxicity:** CV toxicity less than that of bupivacaine, otherwise similar.

LIDOCAINE (XYLOCAINE)

- **Uses:** local anesthetic; antidysrhythmic
- **Dose:** *Antidysrhythmic:* (IV) 1.0 mg/kg over 2–3 min, then infusion 2–4 mg/min (20–50 mcg/kg/min).
  Anesthetic: (topical) <4 mg/kg, do not repeat within 2 h; (infiltration) 4 mg/kg, with epinephrine (1:200,000), max dose 7 mg/kg.
- **Site of clearance:** hepatic
- **t$^{1}/_{2}$:** 1.5–2 h
- **Interaction/toxicity:** Beta-blockers decrease hepatic clearance; cimetidine increases serum level. Plasma concentration >8 mcg/mL may cause seizures, respiratory/cardiac depression.

LIDOCAINE/PRILOCAINE (EMLA)

- **Uses:** anesthetic, local, topical
- **Dose:** *Anesthesia for major dermal procedure:* Adult: (topical) apply 2 g of cream per 10 cm^2 of skin, allow to remain in contact with skin for at least 2 h. Children 0–3 mo or <5 kg: (topical) max dose 1.0 g, max application area 10 cm^2, max application time 1 h. Children 3–12 mo or >5 kg: (topical) max dose 2 g, max application area 20 cm^2, max application time 4 h. Children 1–6 yr or >10 kg: (topical) max dose 10 g, max application area 100 cm^2, max application time 4 h. Children 7–12 yr or >20 kg: (topical) max dose 20 g, max application area 200 cm^2, max application time 4 h.
- **Site of clearance:** hepatic

■ $t^1/_2$: lidocaine 65–150 min; prilocaine 10–150 min
■ **Interactions/toxicity:** Neonates and infants up to 3 months of age should be monitored for Met-hemoglobin levels before, during, and after the application of EMLA, provided the test results can be obtained quickly. Patients taking drugs associated with drug-induced methemoglobinemia such as sulfonamides, acetaminophen, acetanilid, aniline dyes, benzocaine, chloroquine, dapsone, naphthalene, nitrates and nitrites, nitrofurantoin, nitroglycerin, nitroprusside, pamaquine, para-aminosalicylic acid, phenacetin, phenobarbital, phenytoin, primaquine, quinine, are also at greater risk for developing methemoglobinemia. EMLA should be used with caution in patients receiving Class I antiarrhythmic drugs (such as tocainide and mexiletine) since the toxic effects are additive and potentially synergistic.

Repeated doses of EMLA may increase blood levels of lidocaine and prilocaine. EMLA should be used with caution in patients who may be more sensitive to the systemic effects of lidocaine and prilocaine including acutely ill, debilitated, or elderly patients.

Lidocaine and prilocaine have been shown to inhibit viral and bacterial growth. The effect of EMLA on intradermal injections of live vaccines has not been determined.

LORAZEPAM (ATIVAN)

■ **Uses:** antianxiety agent
■ **Dose:** *Preoperative:* (IM) 0.05 mg/kg administered 2 h before surgery, max 4 mg/dose; (IV) 0.44 mg/kg 15–20 min before surgery, max 2 mg/dose.
   Operative amnesia: (IV) up to 0.05 mg/kg, max 4 mg/dose.
   Agitation in ICU: (IV) 0.02–0.06 mg/kg q2–6h; infusion 0.01–0.1 mg/kg/h.
   Sedation/anxiety: Adults: (PO) usual 2–6 mg/day in 2–3 divided doses. Infants and children: (PO, IM, IV) 0.05 mg/kg (range 0.02–0.09 mg/kg) q4–6h prn.
■ **Site of clearance:** hepatic, renal
■ $t^1/_2$: 12 h
■ **Interaction/toxicity:** Cimetidine, metoprolol, propranolol decrease elimination. Increases effect of digoxin.

MAGNESIUM (VARIOUS)

■ **Uses:** toxemia, preeclampsia, hypomagnesemia
■ **Dose:** *Hypomagnesemia:* Adults: (IV) 1–4 g; infusion <2 mL/min (4 g in 250 mL). Children: (IM, IV) 25–50 mg/kg q4–6h

for 3–4 doses, max single dose 2g. Neonates: (IV) 25–50 mg/kg q4–6h for 2–3 doses.
- **Site of clearance:** renal
- **t^1/$_2$:** N/A
- **Interaction/toxicity:** Potentiates neuromuscular blockade (non-depolarizing/depolarizing), potentiates CNS effects of anesthetics, hypnotics, and opioids. Toxicity seen with serum levels >7–10 mEq/L.

MANNITOL (OSMITROL)

- **Uses:** osmotic diuretic
- **Dose:** *Osmotic diuretic:* Adults: Test dose to produce urine flow of at least 30–50 mL/h over next 2–3 h: (IV) 12.5 g (200 mg/kg) over 3–5 min; initial 0.5–1 g/kg, maintenance 0.25–0.5 g/kg q4–6h, usual dose 20–200g/24h. Children: Test dose to produce urine flow of at least 1.0 mL/kg for 1–3 h: (IV) 200 mg/kg over 3–5 min; initial 0.5–1 g/kg, maintenance 0.25–0.5 g/kg q4–6h.
  Neurosurgery: Adults (IV) 0.5–2 g/kg (10–20% solution over 30–60 min) 1–1.5 h before surgery.
- **Site of clearance:** renal
- **t^1/$_2$:** 1–2 h
- **Interaction/toxicity:** Abrupt increases in intravascular volume.

MEPERIDINE (DEMEROL)

- **Uses:** analgesia, antishivering
- **Dose:** Adults: (IM, SC) 50–75mg q3–4h prn. Children: (IV, IM, SC) 1–1.5 mg/kg q3–4h prn.
  Preoperative: Adults: (IM, SC) 50–100 mg 30–90 min before beginning of anesthesia; (slow IV) initial 5–10 mg q5min prn. Children: (IV, IM, SC) 1–2 mg/kg as single dose, max 100 mg/dose.
- **Site of clearance:** hepatic
- **t^1/$_2$:** adults 2.5–4 h, liver disease 7–11 h; normeperidine (active metabolite) 15–30 h; accumulates with high doses or decreased renal function.
- **Interaction/toxicity:** Combined with MAOIs can cause hyperthermia and death. High doses may cause seizures.

MEPHENTERMINE (WYAMINE)

- **Uses:** sympathomimetic
- **Dose:** (IV) 15–30 mg.
- **Site of clearance:** hepatic

■ t^1/$_2$: 17–18 h
■ **Interaction/toxicity:** Pressor effect exaggerated in patients treated with MAOIs; halogenated anesthetics (especially halothane) sensitize myocardium to sympathomimetic effects (dysrhythmias).

MEPIVACAINE (CARBOCAINE)

■ **Uses:** regional; local anesthesia
■ **Dose:** nerve blockade 400 mg; epidural 400 mg, with epinephrine (1:200,000), max dose 500 mg.
■ **Site of clearance:** hepatic
■ t^1/$_2$: 1.9 h
■ **Interaction/toxicity:** Beta-blockers decrease hepatic clearance; cimetidine increases serum level. High plasma concentration causes seizures, respiratory/cardiac depression.

MEROPENEM (MERREM)

■ **Uses:** antibiotic
■ **Dose:** Adults and children >50 kg: (IV) 1 g q8h infused over 5–30 min. Children >3 mo and <50 kg: (IV) 20–40 mg/kg q8h, max dose 2g q8h.
■ **Site of clearance:** renal
■ t^1/$_2$: 1–1.5h
■ **Interaction/toxicity:** Adjust dose in renal dysfunction. Use with caution in seizure disorders. May cause allergic reaction in patients with penicillin allergy.

METAPROTERENOL (VARIOUS)

■ **Uses:** bronchodilator
■ **Dose:** Adults: (PO) 20 mg q6–8h. Children >9 yr: (PO) 10 mg q6–8h. Children 6–9 yr: (PO) 10 mg q6h. Children 2–6 yr: (PO) 1.3–2.6 mg/kg/day q6h. Children <2 yr: (PO) 0.4 mg/kg tid–qid. Infants: (PO) 0.4 mg/kg q8–12h. Adults and children: (inhalation) 2–3 inhalations q3–4h, not >12 inhalations/day.
■ **Site of clearance:** N/A
■ t^1/$_2$: N/A
■ **Interaction/toxicity:** Use with spacer for inhalations. Use with caution in patients with hypothyroidism, diabetes mellitus, CAD, and HTN, and those using MAOIs, tricyclic antidepressants. Decreased effect with beta-blockers. Enhanced effect with sympathomimetics. Excessive use leads to tolerance.

METARAMINOL BITARTRATE (ARAMINE)

- **Uses:** vasoconstrictor
- **Dose:** Adult: (IV, IM, SC) bolus 0.5–10 mg. Children: (IV) bolus 0.01 mg/kg; infusion 5 mcg/kg/min. May be given via ETT.
- **Site of clearance:** N/A
- **t$^1/_2$:** N/A
- **Interaction/toxicity:** Contraindicated in patients receiving MAOIs. May sensitize myocardium to halogenated anesthetics. Use with caution in patients with hyperthyroidism. Extravasation may cause sloughing of skin. Prolonged action associated with cumulative effect. May contain sulfites.

METHADONE (DOLOPHINE) `BBW`

- **Uses:** analgesia, opioid addiction
- **Dose:** *Analgesia:* Adults: (IM, IV, SQ) 2.5–10 mg q6–8h; (PO) 2.5–5 mg q6–8h prn; patients with prior opiate exposure may require higher initial doses. Children: (PO, IM, SC) 0.7 mg/kg/day divided q4–6h prn or 0.1–0.2 mg/kg q4–12h prn, max 10 mg/dose; (IV) 0.1 mg/kg q4h initially for 2–3 doses, then q6–12h prn, max 10 mg/dose.
- **Site of clearance:** hepatic
- **t$^1/_2$:** 15–29 h; prolonged with alkaline pH
- **Interaction/toxicity:** Phenytoin reduces bioavailability by increasing hepatic clearance.

METHOHEXITAL (BREVITAL)

- **Uses:** induction agent; cardioversion; electroconvulsive shock Rx
- **Dose:** Adults: (IV) induction 50–120 mg to start, 20–40 mg q4–7min. Children and infants ≥1 mo: (IM) induction 6.6–10 mg/kg of a 5% solution; (rectal) induction usually 25 mg/kg of a 1% solution.
- **Site of clearance:** hepatic
- **t$^1/_2$:** 3.9 h
- **Interaction/toxicity:** Infrequent allergic reactions; myoclonus, hiccups, and seizures.

METHOXAMINE (VASOXYL)

- **Uses:** vasoconstrictor
- **Dose:** (IV) 3–5 mg administered slowly; (IM, SQ) 10–15 mg may be used to supplement IV administration to provide more prolonged effect. May be given via ETT.
- **Site of clearance:** N/A

■ t^1/$_2$: N/A
■ **Interaction/toxicity:** Potentiated by bretylium, guanethidine, oxytocics, and tricyclic anti-depressants. May contain sulfites. Sloughing may be seen with extravasation.

METHYLDOPA (ALDOMET, METHYLDOPATE) BBW

■ **Uses:** antihypertensive
■ **Dose:** Adults: (IV) 250–500 mg q6–8h, max dose 1 g q6h. Children (IV): 5–10 mg/kg q6–8h up to total dose of 65 mg/kg/24 h or 3 g/24 h.
■ **Site of clearance:** hepatic, renal
■ t^1/$_2$: 75–80 min, ESRD 6–16 h
■ **Interaction/toxicity:** Reduces anesthetic requirements, potentiates sympathomimetics and levodopa. Concomitant Rx with propranolol may cause paradoxical HTN.

METHYLENE BLUE (VARIOUS)

■ **Uses:** antidote cyanide poisoning, methemoglobinemia.
■ **Dose:** *Methemoglobinemia:* Adults and children: (IV) 1–2 mg/kg over several minutes, MR in 1 h prn.
    Genitourinary antiseptic: Adults: (PO) 65–130 mg TID with full glass of water.
■ **Site of clearance:** renal
■ t^1/$_2$: 5–6.5 h
■ **Interaction/toxicity:** Contraindicated in patients with renal insufficiency. May cause hemolysis in patients with G6PD deficiency. Rapid injection may cause increased levels of methemoglobinemia. Turns urine and stool blue-green.

METHYLERGONOVINE (METHERGINE)

■ **Uses:** increases uterine contractions
■ **Dose:** (IM) 0.2 mg after delivery of anterior shoulder or placenta or during puerperium, MR q2–4h; (PO) 0.2 mg 3–4 times/day for 2–7 days.
■ **Site of clearance:** hepatic
■ t^1/$_2$: 1–5 min
■ **Interaction/toxicity:** Acute HTN; additive effects with sympathomimetics.

METHYLPREDNISOLONE (SOLU-MEDROL)

■ **Uses:** anti-inflammatory, allergic reaction, steroid replacement

- **Dose:** *Anti-inflammatory or immunosuppressive:* Adults: (PO) 2–60 mg/day in 1–4 divided doses, followed by gradual reduction to the lowest possible level to maintain adequate clinical response; (IM) 10–80 mg/day; (IV) 10–40 mg over several minutes and repeated IV or IM depending on clinical response; when high dosages needed, give 30 mg/kg over ≥30 min and MR q4–6h for 48 h. Children: (PO, IM, IV) 0.5–1.7 mg/kg/day in divided q6–12h; "pulse" therapy 15–30 mg/kg/dose over ≥30 min given once daily for 3 days.

  Status asthmaticus: Adults and children: (IV) loading 2 mg/kg, then 0.5–1.0 mg/kg q6h for up to 5 days.

  Acute spinal cord injury: Adults and children: (IV) 30 mg/kg over 15 min, followed in 45 min by continuous infusion of 5.4 mg/kg/h for 23 h.
- **Site of clearance:** hepatic
- **t$^1/_2$:** 3–3.5 h
- **Interaction/toxicity:** Increases insulin requirements; phenytoin, phenobarbital, and ephedrine may increase metabolic clearance of steroid.

METOCLOPRAMIDE (REGLAN)

- **Uses:** stimulates gastric emptying; antiemetic
- **Dose:** *Reduce risk of aspiration:* Adults: (IV) 10 mg. Children <6 yr: (IV) 0.1 mg/kg. Children 6–14 yr: (IV) 2.5–5 mg.

  Postoperative nausea and vomiting: (IM) 10 mg near end of surgery.

  Gastroesophageal reflux: Adults: (PO) 10–15 mg qid. Children: (PO): 0.1–0.2 mg/kg qid.
- **Site of clearance:** renal
- **t$^1/_2$:** 4–7 h
- **Interaction/toxicity:** Antagonized by anticholinergics and opioids; potentiated by sedatives, hypnotics, opioids, and tranquilizers. Potentiates extrapyramidal effects of phenothiazines.

METOCURINE (METUBINE)

- **Uses:** nondepolarizing neuromuscular blocker
- **Dose:** (IV) 0.2–0.4 mg/kg.
- **Site of clearance:** renal
- **t$^1/_2$:** 6 h
- **Interaction/toxicity:** Histamine release. Cross-sensitivity in patients allergic to other muscle relaxants. Do not administer to patients with iodide allergy.

METOPROLOL (LOPRESSOR) BBW

- Uses: cardioselective beta-blocker; antidysrhythmic
- Dose: Adults: *HTN/ventricular rate control:* (IV) initial 1.25–5 mg q6–12h.

    Myocardial infarction: (IV) 2–5 mg q2min for 3 doses then 50 mg PO q6h starting 15 min after last IV dose and continuing for 48 h; maintenance max 100 mg q12h.

    Children: (PO) 1–5 mg/kg/24 h divided q12h.
- Site of clearance: hepatic
- $t^{1}/_{2}$: 3–4 h
- Interaction/toxicity: Increases digoxin and morphine serum levels.

METRONIDAZOLE (VARIOUS) BBW

- Uses: amebicide and antibiotic
- Dose: *Anaerobic infections:* Adults: (PO, IV) 250–500 mg q6–8h. Infants and children: (PO) 15–35 mg/kg/day divided q8h for 10 days; (IV) 30 mg/kg/day divided q6h.
- Site of clearance: hepatic
- $t^{1}/_{2}$: 6–8 h
- Interaction/toxicity: Reduce dose in hepatic or renal dysfunction. High sodium content. Disulfiram-like reaction seen with alcohol ingestion. Potentiates anticoagulants, lithium, phenytoin. Cimetidine potentiates effect. Antagonizes barbiturates. Barbiturates interfere with therapeutic effects.

MIDAZOLAM (VERSED) BBW

- Uses: premedicant, induction agent
- Dose: Depends on patient physical status and/or concomitant administration of opioids or other CNS depressants.

    Adults: Preoperative sedation: (IM) 0.07–0.08 mg/kg 30–60 min prior to surgery/procedure; usual dose: 5 mg; (IV) 1–2 mg MR q5min prn to desired effect (max dose <5 mg).

    Conscious sedation: (IV) 0.5–1 mg over at least 2 min; usual dose 2–4 mg

    Anesthesia Induction: Unpremedicated patients: (IV) 0.3–0.35 mg/kg (in resistant cases total dose <0.6 mg/kg)

    Premedicated patients: (IV) 0.15–0.35 mg/kg

    Continuous infusion: Loading dose: (IV) 0.01–0.05 mg/kg, MR at 10–15 min intervals until sedation achieved. Maintenance: (IV): 0.02–0.1 mg/kg/hr

Infants and Children: Conscious sedation for procedures or preoperative sedation: (PO): 0.25–1 mg/kg as a single dose pre-procedural dose or anxiolysis (max < 20 mg); Children <6 years, or less cooperative patients may require as much as 1 mg/kg as a single dose; 0.25 mg/kg may suffice for children 6–16 yrs of age. (IM): 0.01–0.15 mg/kg; range 0.05–0.15 mg/kg; doses up to 0.5 mg/kg have been used in more anxious patients; max dose <10 mg

(IV): Infants <6 months: Limited information is available therefore dosing recommendations unclear.

Infants 6 mos to Children 5 yrs: Initial: 0.05–0.1 mg/kg; total dose <0.6 mg/kg may be required; max dose <6 mg.

Children 6–12 yrs: Initial: 0.025–0.05 mg/kg; total doses of 0.4 mg/kg may be required; max <10 mg.

Children 12–16 yrs: Dose as adults; max dose <10 mg

- Site of clearance: renal
- $t^{1}/_{2}$: 1–4 h; prolonged with cirrhosis, CHF, obesity, and in elderly
- Interaction/toxicity: Intensifies effects of CNS depressants, sedatives, hypnotics, opioids, and tranquilizers. Potentiated by antimycotics and erythromycin.

MILRINONE (PRIMACOR)

- Uses: inotropic support
- Dose: (IV) loading 50 mcg/kg over 10 min; infusion rate 0.375–0.75 mcg/kg/min (dilute in sodium chloride or D_5W).
- Site of clearance: renal
- $t^{1}/_{2}$: 1–3 h
- Interaction/toxicity: Marked vasodilator effect seen in hypovolemic patients. Use with caution in patients with atrial fibrillation/flutter (milrinone may decrease AV nodal conduction and increase ventricular rate), electrolyte abnormalities, hypotension, recent myocardial infarction, renal disease, severe aortic or pulmonic valvular disease (may aggravate outflow tract obstruction in hypertrophic subaortic stenosis).

MIVACURIUM (MIVACRON)

- Uses: nondepolarizing neuromuscular blocker
- Dose: Adults: (IV) initial 0.15–0.25 mg/kg bolus, then 0.1 mg/kg at 15 min intervals; for prolonged neuromuscular block, initial infusion 9–10 mcg/kg/min used on evidence of spontaneous recovery from initial dose, usual infusion rate 6–7 mcg/kg/min (1–15 mcg/kg/min) under balanced anesthesia. Children 2–12 yr: (IV) (duration of action is shorter and disease requirements are

higher) 0.2 mg/kg bolus, then 14 mcg/kg/min (5–31 mcg/kg/min) on evidence of spontaneous recovery from initial dose.
- **Site of clearance:** plasma cholinesterase
- **t^1/$_2$:** 2 min
- **Interaction/toxicity:** Potentiated by volatile anesthetics, hypokalemia, antibiotics (aminoglycosides), lithium, magnesium local anesthetics, procainamide, quinidine. Chronic administration of oral contraceptives, glucocorticoids, MAOIs, or echothiophate enhances neuromuscular block by decreasing plasma cholinesterase activity. Releases histamine at high doses.

MORPHINE (VARIOUS) BBW

- **Uses:** analgesia
- **Dose:** *Acute pain:* Adults: (PO) initial for opiate naïve 10 mg q3–4h prn; initial for prior opiate exposure 10–30 mg q3–4h prn; (IV) opiate naïve 2.5–5 mg q3–4h; patients with prior opiate exposure may require higher initial doses; (IM, SC) initial for opiate naïve 5–10 mg q3–4h prn; initial for prior opiate exposure 5–20 mg q3–4h prn. Children >6 mo and <50 kg: (PO) 0.15–0.3 mg/kg q3–4h prn; (IM):0.1 mg/kg q3–4h prn; (IV) 0.05–0.1 mg/kg q3–4h prn.
    Patient-controlled analgesia (PCA): usual concentration 1.0 mg/mL, usual demand dose 1.0 mg (range 0.5–2.5 mg), lockout interval 5–10 min.
    Epidural: bolus 1–6 mg, infusion rate 0.1–1.0 mg/h, max dose 10 mg/24 h.
    Intrathecal: opiate naïve 0.2 mg/dose.
- **Site of clearance:** hepatic
- **t^1/$_2$:** 2–4 h
- **Interaction/toxicity:** Hypotension and respiratory depression. Potentiates cimetidine; increases anticoagulation with warfarin. Releases histamine in high doses.

MORPHINE, CONTROLLED RELEASE
(MS CONTIN) BBW

- **Uses:** opioid analgesic
- **Dose:** (PO) 15 mg q12h.
- **Site of clearance:** hepatic
- **t^1/$_2$:** 15 h
- **Interaction/toxicity:** Hypotension and respiratory depression. Potentiates sedatives, hypnotics, general anesthetics, and cimetidine (increases anticoagulation with warfarin). Causes nausea and pruritus and can release histamine in high doses. Higher plasma concentrations seen in hepatic and renal failure.

NAFCILLIN (VARIOUS)

- Uses: antibiotic
- Dose: Adults: (IV, IM) 500 mg q4–6h, max daily dose 18 g; (PO) 250–500 mg q4–6h.
     Children: (IV) 25 mg/kg bid; (PO) 25–50 mg/kg/day q6h.
- Site of clearance: renal
- $t^{1}/_{2}$: Children (3 mo to 14 yr) 0.75–2 h, adults 30 min to 2 h
- Interaction/toxicity: Antagonizes effect of warfarin ("warfarin resistance").

NALBUPHINE (NUBAIN)

- Uses: analgesia, opioid agonist-antagonist
- Dose: Adults: (IV) 10 mg/70 kg q3–6h, max single dose 20 mg, max daily dose 160 mg.
     Premedication: Children 10 mo to 14 yr: (IV) 0.2 mg/kg; max 20 mg/dose.
- Site of clearance: hepatic
- $t^{1}/_{2}$: 3–3.5 h
- Interaction/toxicity: Does not antagonize effects of opioids in nondependent patient.

NALMEFENE HYDROCHLORIDE (REVEX)

- Uses: opioid antagonist
- Dose: (IV) 0.25 mcg/kg, cumulative total dose NTE 1.0 mcg/kg.
- Site of clearance: hepatic
- $t^{1}/_{2}$: 11 h
- Interaction/toxicity: Can cause abrupt CV stimulation and pulmonary edema; withdrawal in opioid-dependent patients.

NALOXONE (NARCAN)

- Uses: opioid antagonist
- Dose: Adults: (IV) 40–100 mcg prn. Children: (IV) 10 mcg/kg.
- Site of clearance: hepatic
- $t^{1}/_{2}$: 1–1.5h
- Interaction/toxicity: Can cause abrupt CV stimulation and pulmonary edema; causes withdrawal in opioid-dependent patients.

NAPROXEN (VARIOUS)

- Uses: analgesia, antipyretic, anti-inflammatory
- Dose: Adults: (PO) 250–500 mg bid, max daily dose 1.25 g. Children: (PO) 5–10 mg/kg/day divided bid.

- Site of clearance: hepatic
- $t^1/_2$: 12–15 h
- Interaction/toxicity: Use with caution in patients with CHF, hepatic or renal dysfunction, HTN, history of GI bleed. Higher doses are associated with adverse CNS effects, especially in the elderly (agitation, confusion, and hallucination). Aspirin decreases effect. Potentiates digoxin, lithium, and anticoagulant. Inhibits loop diuretics. Antagonizes ACE inhibitors and beta-blockers.

NEOSTIGMINE (PROSTIGMIN)

- Uses: anticholinesterase
- Dose: Adults: (IV) 0.5–2.5 mg, total dose NTE 5 mg. Children: (IV) 0.025–0.08 mg/kg. Infants: (IV) 0.025–0.1 mg/kg.
- Site of clearance: hepatic
- $t^1/_2$: 0.5–2 h, prolonged in ESRD
- Interaction/toxicity: Bradycardia, salivation.

NESIRITIDE (NATRECOR)

- Uses: natriuretic peptide, B-type, human, vasodilator
- Dose: *Congestive heart failure:* (IV) loading 2 mcg/kg IV bolus over 60 sec, followed by 0.01 mcg/kg/min continuous IV infusion; titration may increase by 0.005 mcg/kg/min (after a bolus of 1.0 mcg/kg IV) no more frequently than q3h up to a max dose of 0.03 mcg/kg/min. If hypotension occurs, discontinue drug; restart at 70% of dose (without bolus).
- Site of clearance: renal
- $t^1/_2$: 18 min, biologic effects persist longer than expected half-life.
- Interaction/toxicity: cardiogenic shock (not as primary therapy), hypersensitivity to nesiritide or any of its components, systolic blood pressure less than 90 mm Hg.

NICARDIPINE (CARDENE IV)

- Uses: antihypertensive, antidysrhythmic, and antianginal
- Dose: (IV) 1–2 mcg/kg/min or 5 mg/h (dilute in 250 mL NS or D_5W; incompatible with LR solution).
- Site of clearance: hepatic
- $t^1/_2$: 2–4 h
- Interaction/toxicity: Cimetidine and ranitidine may increase bioavailability. Potentiated in patient with liver disease may increase hepatic portal pressure in cirrhotic patients.

NIFEDIPINE (PROCARDIA, ADALAT)

- **Uses:** coronary vasospasm; angina; antihypertensive
- **Dose:** (PO) 10–20 mg tid.
- **Site of clearance:** hepatic, renal
- **$t^1/_2$:** 2–5 h, cirrhosis 7 h, elderly 6–7 h
- **Interaction/toxicity:** Decreases platelet aggregation. Cimetidine and ranitidine may increase bioavailability. Potentiates theophylline.

NIMODIPINE (NIMOTOP)

- **Uses:** prevent cerebral arterial spasm (subarachnoid hemorrhage)
- **Dose:** (PO) 60 mg q4h for 21 days.
- **Site of clearance:** hepatic
- **$t^1/_2$:** 3 h
- **Interaction/toxicity:** Potentiated in patients with hepatic disease. Potentiates effects of antihypertensive drugs.

NITRIC OXIDE (INOMAX)

- **Uses:** selective pulmonary vasodilator
- **Dose:** (inhalation) 10–20 ppm.
- **Site of clearance:** enzymatic and renal
- **$t^1/_2$:** 3–6 sec
- **Interaction/toxicity:** Abrupt withdrawal can result in hypoxemia and pulmonary HTN. Inspiratory N_2O, NO_2, and blood methemoglobin concentrations should be monitored. May cause thrombocytopenia and decrease in platelet aggregation.

NITROGLYCERIN (TRIDIL, NITROL IV, NITROSTAT IV)

- **Uses:** vasodilator, antianginal; controlled hypotension
- **Dose:** (IV) 1–3 mcg/kg/min (dilute 50 mg in 250 mL D_5W or NS).
- **Site of clearance:** hepatic, renal
- **$t^1/_2$:** 1–4 min
- **Interaction/toxicity:** Increases bioavailability of dihydroergotamine. Methemoglobinemia seen with high doses, especially in individuals with methemoglobin reductase deficiency. Treat with O_2 and methylene blue (0.2 mL/kg IV). Dose may be increased to 1–2 mg/kg.

NITROPRUSSIDE (NIPRIDE, NITROPRESS) **BBW**

- Uses: antihypertensive; vasodilator; controlled hypotension
- Dose: *Antihypertensive, vasodilator, controlled hypotension:*
  Adults: (IV) initial 0.3–0.5 mcg/kg/min, increase in increments
  of 0.5 mcg/kg/min, titrating to the desired hemodynamic effect
  or the appearance of headache or nausea; usual dose 3 mcg/
  kg/min, rarely need >4 mcg/kg/min, max 10 mcg/kg/min.
  Pulmonary HTN: Children: (IV) initial 0.5–1.0 mcg/kg/min
  by continuous IV infusion, increase in increments of 1 mcg/
  kg/min at intervals of 20–60 min, titrating to the desired response; usual dose 3 mcg/kg/min, rarely need >4 mcg/kg/min,
  max 5 mcg/kg/min.
- Site of clearance: hepatic
- $t^1/_2$: <10 min
- Interaction/toxicity: Cyanide toxicity may occur at doses
  >10 mcg/kg/min. Tachyphylaxis, elevated mixed venous O_2 tension (saturation), and acidosis suggest diagnosis of cyanide toxicity. Hydroxocobalamin may reduce risk of cyanide toxicity.
  Treatment of cyanide toxicity is IV administration of sodium
  thiosulfate, 150 mg/kg over 15 min. Thiocyanate ion can be
  removed by hemodialysis.

NOREPINEPHRINE (LEVOPHED)

- Uses: vasoconstrictor
- Dose: Adults: (IV) initial 0.5–1 mcg/min and titrate to desired
  response (dilute 4 mg in 250 mL D_5W). Children: (IV) initial
  0.03–0.1 mcg/kg/min, max dose 1–2 mcg/kg/min.
- Site of clearance: enzymatic
- $t^1/_2$: 2–3 min
- Interaction/toxicity: MAOIs and tricyclic antidepressants
  may cause severe HTN. Halogenated anesthetics (especially
  halothane) may sensitize myocardium to sympathomimetic effects (dysrhythmias). Furosemide may decrease arterial vasoconstrictor properties. Extravasation may cause skin slough.

NORTRIPTYLINE (VARIOUS)

- Uses: antidepressant, chronic pain management, migraine
  headaches
- Dose: (PO) 25 mg tid.
- Site of clearance: hepatic
- $t^1/_2$: 28–31 h
- Interaction/toxicity: Contraindicated in patients with narrow-
  angle glaucoma, Rx treated with MAOIs within previous

14 days. Use with caution in patients with cardiac dysrhythmias, hyperthyroidism, renal or hepatic dysfunction. Phenobarbital increases metabolism. Increases amount of inhalation anesthesia required. Potentiates sympathomimetics, CNS depressants, and anticoagulants. Cimetidine decreases metabolism. Should not be abruptly discontinued. May contain sulfites.

ONDANSETRON (ZOFRAN)

- **Uses:** antiemetic
- **Dose:** *Postoperative nausea and vomiting:* Adults: (IV) 4 mg as a single dose 30 min before the end of anesthesia. Children 2–12 yr and ≤40 kg: (IV) 0.1 mg/kg. Children >40 kg: (IV) 4 mg.
- **Site of clearance:** hepatic
- **t^1/$_2$:** children (<15 yr) 2–3 h, adults 3–6 h
- **Interaction/toxicity:** Potentiated by hepatic disease. ECG abnormalities with rapid injection.

OXACILLIN (VARIOUS)

- **Uses:** antibiotic
- **Dose:** Adults: (IV, IM) 250–500 mg q4–6h; (PO) 500 mg q4–6h. Children: (IV) 50 mg/day q6h; (PO) 50 mg/kg/day q6h.
- **Site of clearance:** hepatic
- **t^1/$_2$:** Children (1 wk to 2 yr) 1–2 h, adults 23–60 min
- **Interaction/toxicity:** Potentiates anticoagulants.

OXYCODONE, CONTROLLED RELEASE (OXYCONTIN) BBW

- **Uses:** opioid analgesic
- **Dose:** Adults: (PO) 10 mg q12h.
- **Site of clearance:** renal
- **t^1/$_2$:** 4.5–8 h
- **Interaction/toxicity:** Hypotension and respiratory depression. Potentiates sedatives, hypnotics, general anesthetics and cimetidine (increases anticoagulation with warfarin). Causes nausea and pruritus and can release histamine in high doses. Higher plasma concentrations in hepatic and renal failure.

OXYTOCIN (PITOCIN) BBW

- **Uses:** increases uterine contraction
- **Dose:** (IV) 10 units, infusion 0.002 units/min.
- **Site of clearance:** hepatic

■ $t^{1}/_{2}$: 1–5 min
■ **Interaction/toxicity:** Potentiates sympathomimetics.

PANCURONIUM (PAVULON) `BBW`

■ **Uses:** nondepolarizing neuromuscular blocker
■ **Dose:** Adults, children, and infants >1 mo: (IV) initial 0.05–0.10 mg/kg prn.
■ **Site of clearance:** renal, hepatic
■ $t^{1}/_{2}$: 110 min
■ **Interaction/toxicity:** Potentiated by volatile anesthetics, hypokalemia, antibiotics (aminoglycosides), magnesium local anesthetics, procainamide, quinidine. Conditions associated with increased volume of distribution (e.g., slower circulation time, edematous states, and old age) may be associated with delay in onset. Prolongation of neuromuscular blockade may occur in patients with renal and/or hepatic disease. Patients receiving tricyclic antidepressants who are anesthetized with halothane and receive pancuronium may develop dysrhythmias.

PENICILLIN G (VARIOUS)

■ **Uses:** antibiotic
■ **Dose:** Adults: (IV) 10,000,000–20,000,000 units/day divided q4–6h. Children: (IV) 100,000–250,000 units/kg/day divided q6h.
■ **Site of clearance:** renal
■ $t^{1}/_{2}$: 20–50 min
■ **Interaction/toxicity:** Reduce dose with renal dysfunction. May exacerbate seizure disorders. Large doses may prolong bleeding time and potentiates anticoagulants. Electrolyte abnormalities (sodium and potassium) may be seen with large IV doses.

PENTAZOCINE (TALWIN)

■ **Uses:** analgesia; opioid agonist–antagonist
■ **Dose:** Adults: (IV, IM) 30 mg q4h. Adults and children >12 yr: (PO) 50 mg q4h.
■ **Site of clearance:** hepatic, renal
■ $t^{1}/_{2}$: 2–3 h
■ **Interaction/toxicity:** Potentiates barbiturates and CNS depressants. Potentiated in patients with hepatic and/or renal disease. May precipitate withdrawal in opioid-dependent patients.

PENTOBARBITAL (NEMBUTAL)

- **Uses:** hypnotic; premedication
- **Dose:** *Hypnotic, preoperative sedation:* Adults: (IM) 150–200 mg; (IV) initial 100 mg, MR q1–3min up to 200–500 mg total dose. Children ≥6 mo: (IM) 2–6 mg/kg, max 100 mg/dose; (IV) 1–3 mg/kg to max of 100 mg until asleep.

  Conscious sedation prior to a procedure: Adolescents: (IV) 100 mg before procedure. Children 5–12 yr: (IV) 2 mg/kg 5–10 min before procedure, MR once.

  Barbiturate coma in head injury patients: Adults and children: (IV) loading 5–10 mg/kg over 1–2 h while monitoring blood pressure and respiratory rate; maintenance initial 1.0 mg/kg/h, may increase to 2–3 mg/kg/h; maintain burst suppression on EEG.
- **Site of clearance:** hepatic, renal
- **t$\frac{1}{2}$:** adults 22 h, children 25 h (range 15–50 h)
- **Interaction/toxicity:** Barbiturates decrease effects of theophylline, β-adrenergic blockers, corticosteroids, and tricyclic antidepressants. MAOIs increase action.

PHENOBARBITAL (VARIOUS)

- **Uses:** sedative, hypnotic, anticonvulsant
- **Dose:** *Sedation:* Adults (IV, IM): 30–120 mg in 2–3 divided doses; (PO) 30–120 mg/day q8–12h. Children: 2 mg/kg tid.

  Premedication: Adults: (IM) 100–200 mg. Children: 1–3 mg/kg 1–1.5 h before procedure.

  Anticonvulsant, status epilepticus, loading: Adults (IV): 300–800 mg followed by 120–240 mg/dose at 20 min intervals until seizures controlled or total dose of 1–2 g in 24 h. Infants and children: (IV) loading 10–20 mg/kg in single or divided doses q15–30min until seizures controlled or total dose of 40 mg/kg in 24 h.

  Anticonvulsant, maintenance: Adults and children >12 yr: (PO, IV) 1–3 mg/kg/day in divided doses or 50–100 mg 2–3 times/day. Children 5–12 yr: (PO, IV) 4–6 mg/kg/day in 1–2 divided doses. Children 1–5 yr (PO, IV) 6–8 mg/kg/day in 1–2 divided doses. Infants (PO, IV) 5–8 mg/kg/day in 1–2 divided doses.
- **Site of clearance:** hepatic
- **t$\frac{1}{2}$:** adults 53–140 h, children 37–73 h
- **Interaction/toxicity:** Contraindicated in patients with severe liver or renal dysfunction or porphyria. Rapid IV injection may laryngospasm, respiratory depression, and hypotension.

Potentiates sedatives, hypnotics, tranquilizers, and other CNS depressants. Decreases the effects of beta-adrenergic blockers, theophylline, verapamil, corticosteroids, tricyclic antidepressants. MAOIs increase actions. Increases metabolism of methadone and can result in withdrawal. Tolerance may develop. Avoid abrupt withdrawal.

PHENOXYBENZAMINE (DIBENZYLINE)

- Uses: antihypertensive, vasodilator, pheochromocytoma
- Dose: (PO) 10 mg bid, increase by 10 mg every other day, usual range 20–40 mg bid–tid.
- Site of clearance: renal
- $t^1/_2$: 24 h
- Interaction/toxicity: Use with caution in patients with coronary, cerebral, renal dysfunction. Exaggerated response (hypotension and tachycardia) may be seen with catecholamine administration such as epinephrine.

PHENTOLAMINE (REGITINE)

- Uses: arterial dilator
- Dose: *Diagnosis of pheochromocytoma:* Adults: (IM, IV) 5 mg. Children: (IM, IV) 0.05–0.1 mg/kg, max single dose 5 mg.
      Surgery for pheochromocytoma, HTN: Adults: (IM, IV) 2.5–5.0 mg 1–2 h before procedure and MR prn q2–4h. Children: (IM, IV) 0.05–0.1 mg/kg given 1–2 h before procedure, MR prn q2–4h until controlled, max single dose of 5 mg.
- Site of clearance: unknown
- $t^1/_2$: 19 min
- Interaction/toxicity: Vasoconstrictor effects of epinephrine and ephedrine are blocked by phentolamine.

PHENYLEPHRINE (NEO-SYNEPHRINE)

- Uses: vasoconstrictor
- Dose: *Hypotension/shock:* Adults: (IV) bolus 50–100 mcg; infusion 0.5–1.0 mcg/kg/min (dilute 4 mg in 250 mL D_5W or NS). Children: (IV) bolus 5–20 mcg/kg q10–15min prn; infusion 0.1–0.5 mcg/kg/min.
- Site of clearance: hepatic
- $t^1/_2$: 2.5 h, prolonged after long-term infusion
- Interaction/toxicity: Effects potentiated by oxytocic drugs, MAOIs, and tricyclic antidepressants.

PHENYTOIN (DILANTIN)

- **Uses:** anticonvulsant; antidysrhythmic
- **Dose:** *Status epilepticus:* Adults: (IV, PO) loading 10–20 mg/kg in single or divided dose, maintenance 5–6 mg/kg/day in 3 divided doses. Infants and children: (IV, PO) loading 15–20 mg/kg in a single or divided dose, maintenance initial 5 mg/kg/day in 2 divided doses.
- **Site of clearance:** hepatic
- **$t^1/_2$:** 22 h
- **Interaction/toxicity:** Increased effects seen with cimetidine and diazepam; decreased effects seen with barbiturates, theophylline, and antacids. Decreases effectiveness of corticosteroids, dicumarol, haloperidol, quinidine, furosemide, dopamine, and nondepolarizing muscle relaxants. Increases toxicity of lithium.

PHYSOSTIGMINE (ANTILIRIUM)

- **Uses:** anticholinesterase; nonspecific reversal of CNS side effects of benzodiazepines, scopolamine, and ketamine
- **Dose:** Adults: (IV) initial 0.5–1.0 mg, MR q20min until response or adverse effect occurs. Children (reserve for life-threatening situations): (IV) 0.02 mg/kg/dose (max 0.5 mg/min), MR after 5–10 min to max total dose of 2 mg or until response or adverse cholinergic effects occur.
- **Site of clearance:** cholinesterase enzyme
- **$t^1/_2$:** 15–40 min
- **Interaction/toxicity:** Rapid administration can cause bradycardia, salivation, and seizures.

PHYTONADIONE (AQUAMEPHYTON, KONAKION) BBW

- **Uses:** hepatic synthesis of prothrombin (II); proconvertin (VII); plasma thromboplastin (IX); and Stuart factor (X)
- **Dose:** Adults: (slow IV) 2.5–10.0 mg. Children: (slow IV) 0.5–2.0 mg.
- **Site of clearance:** hepatic
- **$t^1/_2$:** 26–193 h
- **Interaction/toxicity:** Severe reaction resembling anaphylaxis has been seen even with administration of dilute phytonadione.

PIPECURONIUM (ARDUAN) `BBW`

- **Uses:** nondepolarizing neuromuscular blocker
- **Dose:** (IV) 0.07 mg/kg.
- **Site of clearance:** renal
- **$t^{1}/_{2}$:** 137–161 min
- **Interaction/toxicity:** Potentiated by volatile anesthetics, hypokalemia, antibiotics (aminoglycosides), lithium, magnesium, local anesthetics, procainamide, quinidine. Conditions associated with increased volume of distribution (e.g., slower circulation time, edematous states, and old age) may be associated with delay in onset. Contains benzyl alcohol, which may be associated with increased incidence of neurologic complications in neonates. Due to long duration of action not recommended for patient undergoing cesarean section.

PREDNISOLONE (VARIOUS)

- **Uses:** anti-inflammatory, steroid replacement, allergic reaction
- **Dose:** Adults: (PO) 5–60 mg/day. Children: (PO) 0.5–1.0 mg/kg q12–24h.
- **Site of clearance:** hepatic
- **$t^{1}/_{2}$:** 3.6 h
- **Interaction/toxicity:** Contraindicated in patients with serious infections or varicella. Use with caution in patients with hypothyroidism, CHF, peptic ulcer disease. Increases insulin requirements. Hydantoins, barbiturates, and ephedrine increase metabolic clearance of steroid. Withdraw drug gradually if used for chronic Rx. Must be metabolized by liver to active form.

PRILOCAINE (CITANEST)

- **Uses:** regional anesthesia
- **Dose:** nerve block 600 mg.
- **Site of clearance:** hepatic
- **$t^{1}/_{2}$:** 10–150 min
- **Interaction/toxicity:** Methemoglobinemia may be associated with doses >500 mg; treat with methylene blue (IV), 1–2 mg/kg over 5 min.

PROCAINAMIDE (PRONESTYL) `BBW`

- **Uses:** antidysrhythmic
- **Dose:** Adults: (IV) 100–200 mg, MR q5min prn to a total dose of 1.0 g, maintenance 1.0–4 mg/min by continuous infusion (dilute 1,000 mg in 500 mL D_5W). Children: (IV) 3–6 mg/kg/dose over

5 min NTE 100 mg/dose, MR q5–10min to max 15 mg/kg/load, maintenance as continuous infusion 20–80 mcg/kg/min, max 2 g/24 h.
- **Site of clearance:** hepatic
- **t$^1/_2$:** children 1.7 h, adults 2.5–4.7 h, anephric 11 h; NAPA (dependent on renal function): children 6 h, adults 6–8 h, anephric 42 h.
- **Interaction/toxicity:** Enhances anticholinergic drugs, potentiates neuromuscular blockers.

PROCAINE (NOVOCAIN)

- **Uses:** regional anesthesia
- **Dose:** nerve block 1,000 mg; epidural 1,000 mg; spinal 50–200 mg.
- **Site of clearance:** plasma cholinesterase
- **t$^1/_2$:** 7.7 min
- **Interaction/toxicity:** Potential for allergic reaction with repeated use.

PROCHLORPERAZINE (COMPAZINE)

- **Uses:** antiemetic, antipsychotic
- **Dose:** *Antiemetic:* Adults: (PO) tablet 5–10 mg tid–qid, max 40 mg/day; (rectal) 25 mg bid; (IV, IM) 5–10 mg, max 10 mg/dose and 40 mg/day.
  Surgical nausea and vomiting: Adults: (IV) 5–10 mg 15–30 min before induction. Children >10 kg: (PO, rectal) 0.4 mg/kg/24 h divided tid–qid; (IM) 0.1–0.15 mg/kg/dose.
- **Site of clearance:** hepatic
- **t$^1/_2$:** PO 3–5 h, IV ~7 h
- **Interaction/toxicity:** Hypersensitivity reaction may manifest as jaundice, extrapyramidal symptoms.

PROMETHAZINE (PHENERGAN)

- **Uses:** antiemetic
- **Dose:** *Allergic conditions (including allergic reactions to blood or plasma):* Adults: (IM, IV, PO, rectal) 12.5–25.0 mg, MR in 2 h. Children ≥2 yr: (PO, rectal) 0.1 mg/kg q6h max 12.5 mg/dose.
  Antiemetic: Adults: (IV, IM, PO, rectal) 12.5–25 mg q4–6h prn. Children: (IV, IM, PO, rectal) 0.25–1.0 mg/kg 4–6 times/day prn, max 25 mg/dose.
- **Site of clearance:** hepatic

- $t^1/_2$: 9–16 h
- **Interaction/toxicity:** Hypersensitivity reaction may manifest as jaundice.

PROPOFOL (DIPRIVAN)

- **Uses:** induction agent
- **Dose:** Adults: (IV) induction 1.5–2.5 mg/kg approximately 40 mg q10sec until induction onset; (IV infusion) maintenance initial 150–200 mcg/kg/min, usual infusion rate 100–200 mcg/kg/min. Children: (IV) induction 2.5–3.5 mg/kg over 20–30 sec; (IV infusion) maintenance initial 200–300 mcg/kg/min, titrate 50–100 mcg/kg/min, usual infusion rate 125–150 mcg/kg/min.
- **Site of clearance:** hepatic
- $t^1/_2$: 40 min
- **Interaction/toxicity:** Hypotension, respiratory depression, and pain with injection. Prepared in lipid emulsion; infection potential, allergic reaction.

PROPRANOLOL (INDERAL) BBW

- **Uses:** Beta blockade, antidysrhythmic, antihypertensive
- **Dose:** *Tachyarrhythmias:* Adults: (IV) 0.5–1.0 mg, repeat q5min up to total of 5 mg, titrate initial dose to desired response. Children and infants: (IV) 0.01–0.1 mg/kg over 10 min; max 1.0 mg for infants, 3 mg for children.
- **Site of clearance:** hepatic
- $t^1/_2$: children 3.9–6.4 h, adults 4–6 h
- **Interaction/toxicity:** Increases digoxin, local anesthesia, and morphine serum levels. Bradycardia, hypotension, and bronchospasm can be seen.

PROSTAGLANDIN E$_1$, ALPROSTADIL (PROSTIN VR)

- **Uses:** maintain patency of ductus arteriosus; vasodilator
- **Dose:** (IV) continuous infusion into large vein, or alternatively through umbilical artery catheter placed at ductal opening at 0.05–0.1 mcg/kg/min with therapeutic response, rate reduced to lowest effective dosage; with unsatisfactory response, rate is increased gradually; maintenance 0.01–0.4 mcg/kg/min (dilute 500 mcg in 250 mL D$_5$W or sodium chloride).
- **Site of clearance:** lungs
- $t^1/_2$: 5–10 min

■ **Interaction/toxicity:** In premature newborns produces apnea; inhibits platelet aggregation.

PROTAMINE (VARIOUS)

■ **Uses:** heparin antagonist
■ **Dose:** titrated on basis of coagulation test (e.g., ACT); protamine 1.0 mg neutralizes 90 units heparin (lung) or 115 units heparin (intestinal mucosa).
■ **Site of clearance:** N/A
■ $t^1/_2$: 7.4 min
■ **Interaction/toxicity:** Potentiates vasodilators; anaphylactic reactions especially in patients with fish allergy or diabetics treated with protamine-containing insulin solutions; complement-mediated pulmonary vasoconstriction.

PYRIDOSTIGMINE (REGONOL, MESTINON)

■ **Uses:** anticholinesterase; myasthenia gravis
■ **Dose:** (IV) 0.2 mg/kg. Note: Atropine sulfate 0.6–1.2 mg IV immediately prior to pyridostigmine minimizes dose effects.
■ **Site of clearance:** renal, hepatic
■ $t^1/_2$: 1–2 h
■ **Interaction/toxicity:** Bradycardia, salivation.

QUINIDINE GLUCONATE (VARIOUS) `BBW`

■ **Uses:** antidysrhythmic
■ **Dose:** (IV) 100–300 mg administer at rate <1 mL/min (16 mg/min) (dilute 10 mL [880 mg] in 50 mL D_5W).
■ **Site of clearance:** hepatic
■ $t^1/_2$: adults 6–8 h, prolonged in elderly or with cirrhosis or CHF
■ **Interaction/toxicity:** Reduced by hypokalemia (also increases risk of Torsades de Pointes). Verapamil, cimetidine, antacids enhance activity by increasing quinidine plasma concentration. Potentiates nondepolarizer neuromuscular blockers and succinyl-choline.

RANITIDINE (ZANTAC)

■ **Uses:** histamine antagonist (H_2)
■ **Dose:** Adults: (PO) 150 mg q12h; (IV) 50 mg q6–8h (dilute in 100 mL NS or D_5W). Children 1 mo to 16 yr: (PO) 2–4 mg/kg/day divided q12h, max 300 mg/day; (IV) 2–4 mg/kg/day divided q6–8h, max 150 mg/day.

- **Site of clearance:** hepatic, renal
- **t$^{1}/_{2}$:** PO 2.5–3h, IV 2–2.5 h
- **Interaction/toxicity:** Bradycardia with IV administration.

REMIFENTANIL (ULTIVA)

- **Uses:** analgesia
- **Dose:** (IV) induction 0.5–1.0 mcg/kg/min (through intubation) over 30–60 sec, continuous infusion 0.1–2.0 mcg/kg/min.
  Monitored anesthesia care: (IV) 1.0 mcg/kg, continuous infusion 0.025–0.2 mcg/kg/min.
- **Site of clearance:** plasma and tissue esterases
- **t$^{1}/_{2}$:** 10 min
- **Interaction/toxicity:** Hypotension, respiratory depression, and nausea and pruritus. Potentiated by sedatives, hypnotics, tranquilizers. Decreases effects of diuretics in congestive heart failure. Contraindicated for use in epidural or intrathecal administration due to glycine in formulation.

RITODRINE (YUTOPAR)

- **Uses:** uterine relaxation
- **Dose:** (IV) 0.1–0.3 mg/min.
- **Site of clearance:** renal
- **t$^{1}/_{2}$:** 60–156 min
- **Interaction/toxicity:** CV effects (dysrhythmias and hypotension) seen with meperidine and general anesthetics. Concomitant use of corticosteroids may lead to pulmonary edema.

ROFECOXIB (VIOXX) (CURRENTLY NOT AVAILABLE IN THE US) BBW

- **Uses:** nonsteroidal analgesic (selective COX-2 inhibitor)
- **Dose:** (PO) 12.5–25 mg/day.
- **Site of clearance:** hepatic
- **t$^{1}/_{2}$:** 17 h
- **Interaction/toxicity:** GI bleeding (including ulceration and perforation), liver dysfunction, renal impairment and worsening of aspirin-sensitive asthma have been reported. Aspirin potentiates GI ulceration. Reduces natruretic effect of furosemide. Diminish antihypertensive effect of ACE inhibitors. Increased INR and PTT in patients receiving warfarin. Fluconazole and lithium increase plasma levels. Use increases the risk of cardiovascular events such as heart attack and stroke.

ROPIVACAINE (NAROPIN)

- **Uses:** local anesthetic
- **Dose:** infiltration 5–200 mg; peripheral nerve block 175–250 mg; lumbar epidural 75–150 mg; thoracic epidural 25–75 mg.
- **Site of clearance:** renal
- **t$^1/_2$:** epidural 5–7 h, IV 2–4 h
- **Interaction/toxicity:** Increased plasma ropivacaine levels seen with theophylline, imipramine, fluvoxamine, and verapamil. CV toxicity less than that of bupivacaine, otherwise similar.

SCOPOLAMINE (VARIOUS)

- **Uses:** anticholinergic; amnesia
- **Dose:** *Preoperative:* Adults: (IV, IM, SC) 0.2–0.4 mg, MR q4–6h. Children: (IM, SC) 6 mcg/kg, max 0.3 mg/dose.
- **Site of clearance:** renal
- **t$^1/_2$:** 9.5 h
- **Interaction/toxicity:** CNS excitation or sedation (central anticholinergic syndrome). Antihistamines, procainamide, sedatives, hypnotics, and opioids intensify effect. Amnesia, vertigo, and dry mouth.

SECOBARBITAL (SECONAL)

- **Uses:** hypnotic; premedication
- **Dose:** *Preoperative sedation:* Adults: (IV) 100–300 mg 1–2 h before procedure. Children: (IV) 2–6 mg/kg (max dose 100 mg) 1–2 h before procedure.
- **Site of clearance:** hepatic
- **t$^1/_2$:** 19–34 h
- **Interaction/toxicity:** Barbiturates decrease effects of theophylline. β-Adrenergic blockers, corticosteroids, tricyclic antidepressants, and MAOIs increase action.

SODIUM BICARBONATE (VARIOUS)

- **Uses:** correct metabolic acidosis
- **Dose:** Adults, children, and infants: (IV) dosage based on following formula if blood gases and pH measurements available: HCO_3 (mEq) = 0.3 × weight (kg) × base deficit (mEq/L). Administer half dose initially, then remaining half dose over the next 24 h. If acid-base status not available dose for older children and adults, use 1–2 mEq/kg infusion over 4–8 h; subsequent doses should be based on acid-base status.

- Site of clearance: lungs
- t$^{1}/_{2}$: N/A
- Interaction/toxicity: Increase sodium retention, intracerebral bleed (neonates); urinary alkalinization increases duration of action of certain drugs.

SUCCINYLCHOLINE (ANECTINE) **BBW**

- Uses: depolarizing neuromuscular blocker
- Dose: Adults: (IV) 1–1.5 mg/kg, up to 150 mg total dose; continuous infusion 10–100 mcg/kg/min (dilute to concentration of 1–2 mg/mL in D$_5$W or NS). Children: (IV) initial 1–2 mg/kg, maintenance 0.3–0.6 mg/kg. Because of the risk of malignant hyperthermia, use of continuous infusions is not recommended in infants and children.
- Site of clearance: plasma cholinesterase enzyme
- t$^{1}/_{2}$: 1 min
- Interaction/toxicity: Elevates serum potassium, especially in burn patients and patients with spinal cord injury or progressive neuromuscular disease; trigger for MH, causes increased IOP. Can cause bradycardia, especially with repeated administration at short intervals (<5 min). Cross-sensitivity in patients allergic to other muscular relaxants.

SUFENTANIL (SUFENTA)

- Uses: analgesia
- Dose: *Anesthetic adjunct:* Adults: (IV) 1.0–2 mcg/kg, maintenance 10–25 mcg prn (in obese, use lean body weight). Children: (IV) 0.5–2 mcg/kg, maintenance infusion 1.0–3 mcg/kg/h. *Main anesthetic:* (IV) 10–15 mcg/kg.
    Premedication: (intranasal) 2 mcg/kg.
- t$^{1}/_{2}$: 158–164 min
- Site of clearance: hepatic
- Interaction/toxicity: Benzodiazepines potentiate hypotensive action; truncal muscle rigidity may be seen during induction and emergence. Bradycardia.

SUMATRIPTAN SUCCINATE (IMITREX)

- Uses: migraine and cluster headaches
- Dose: (SQ) 6 mg, second injection 60 min later, NTE 2 injections in 24 h; (nasal spray) 5–20 mg, MR after 2 h, max daily dose 40 mg; (PO) initial 25–100 mg at onset of headache, MR q2h, max daily dose 300 mg.
- Site of clearance: enzymatic

- $t^1/_2$: 2 h
- **Interaction/toxicity:** Contraindicated in patients with CAD or coronary vasospasm and uncontrolled HTN, and in patients being treated with ergotamines. Administer with caution to patients with hepatic dysfunction.

TERBUTALINE (BRETHAIRE, BRICANYL)

- **Uses:** bronchodilator; premature labor
- **Dose:** *Premature labor:* Acute: (IV) 2.5–10 mcg/min, increase gradually q10–20min. Effective max dosages from 17.5–30 mcg/min have been used with caution. Duration of infusion is at least 12 h. Maintenance: (PO) 2.5–10 mg q4–6h for as long as necessary to prolong pregnancy depending on patient tolerance.

  Bronchoconstriction: Adults and children >15 yr: (PO) 5 mg q6h tid; if side effects occur reduce dose to 2.5 mg q6h, NTE 15 mg in 24 h; (SC) 0.25 mg repeated once in 15–30 min, NTE total dose of 0.5 mg within 4 h period. Children 12–15 yr: (PO) 2.5 mg q6h tid, NTE 7.5 mg/24 h. Children <12 yr: (PO) 0.05 mg/kg tid, increased gradually, max 0.15 mg/kg tid–qid or 5 mg/24 h; (SC) 0.005–0.01 mg/kg (max dose 0.3 mg) q15–20 min for 3 doses.
- **Site of clearance:** hepatic
- $t^1/_2$: 11–26 h
- **Interaction/toxicity:** Potentiates MAOIs; halogenated anesthetics sensitize (especially halothane) myocardium to sympathomimetic effects (dysrhythmias).

TETRACAINE (PONTOCAINE)

- **Uses:** regional/topical anesthesia
- **Dose:** spinal 4–15 mg; topical 80 mg.
- **Site of clearance:** plasma cholinesterase, hepatic
- $t^1/_2$: N/A
- **Interaction/toxicity:** Beta-blockers decrease hepatic clearance; cimetidine increases serum level. Plasma concentration >8 mcg/mL may cause seizures, respiratory/cardiac depression.

THEOPHYLLINE (VARIOUS)

- **Uses:** bronchodilator
- **Dose:** Adults: (IV) loading 6 mg/kg over 20–30 min, then 0.5–1.0 mg/kg/h, NTE 25 mg/min; maintain serum levels at 10–20 mcg/mL; (PO) loading 5 mg/kg, then 4 mg/kg q6h. Children: (IV) 5 mg/kg, then 0.5–1.0 mg/kg/h; (PO) loading 5 mg/kg, then

3–4 mg q6h, max daily dose 18–24 mg/kg. Each 0.5 mg/kg administered as loading dose increases serum theophylline levels by 1.0 mcg/mL.
■ **Site of clearance:** hepatic
■ $t^1/_2$: highly variable and dependent on age, liver function, cardiac function, lung disease and smoking history.
■ **Interaction/toxicity:** Contraindicated in patients with poorly controlled dysthymias, peptic ulcer disease, or uncontrolled seizure activity. May cause dysrhythmias with halogenated anesthetics and seizures with ketamine. The following can decrease theophylline levels: barbiturates, carbamazepine, sympathomimetics, phenytoin, and loop diuretics. The following can increase theophylline levels: beta-blockers, calcium channel blockers, antibiotics, steroids, cimetidine, and CHF. Antagonizes effects of hydantoins, lithium, and nondepolarizing muscle relaxants. Parenteral preparations may contain alcohol or preservatives and should not be used in children.

THIOPENTAL (PENTOTHAL)

■ **Uses:** induction agent
■ **Dose:** *Induction anesthesia:* Adults: (IV) 3–5 mg/kg. Children 1–12 yr: (IV) 5–6 mg/kg. Infants: (IV) 5–8 mg/kg.
    Maintenance anesthesia: Adults: (IV) 25–100 mg prn. Children: (IV) 1.0 mg/kg prn.
    Increased intracranial pressure: Adults and children: (IV) 1.5–5 mg/kg, repeat prn to control intracranial pressure.
■ **Site of clearance:** hepatic
■ $t^1/_2$: 3–11.5 h, decreased in children
■ **Interaction/toxicity:** Releases histamine; may cause hypotension or respiratory depression; may trigger porphyria, allergic reaction.

TRAMADOL (ULTRAM)

■ **Uses:** analgesic
■ **Dose:** (PO) 50–100 mg tid, NTE 400 mg/day.
■ **Site of clearance:** renal
■ $t^1/_2$: 6 h
■ **Interaction/toxicity:** Carbamazepine increases tramadol metabolism. Quinidine increases plasma tramadol levels. Increased seizure risk with concomitant administration of SSRIs, tricyclic antidepressants, opioids, MAOIs, neuroleptics. Potentiate respiratory depression of anesthetics. Impaired renal function results in decreased clearance.

TRIMETHAPHAN (ARFONAD)

- **Uses:** vasodilator (ganglionic blocker)
- **Dose:** Adults: (IV) 2–4 mg/min (dilute 500 mg in 500 mL D_5W). Children: (IV) 50–150 mcg/kg/min.
- **Site of clearance:** plasma cholinesterase
- $t^1/_2$: N/A
- **Interaction/toxicity:** Histamine release. Produces mydriasis, ileus, dilation, and respiratory depression.

d-TUBOCURARINE (VARIOUS)

- **Uses:** nondepolarizing neuromuscular blocker
- **Dose:** (IV) 0.3–0.5 mg/kg.
- **Site of clearance:** renal
- $t^1/_2$: 173 min
- **Interaction/toxicity:** Potentiated by volatile anesthetics, hypokalemia, antibiotics (aminoglycosides), lithium, magnesium, local anesthetics, procainamide, quinidine, monoamine oxidase inhibitors, trimethaphan, and propranolol. Prolongation of neuromuscular blockade may occur in patients with renal and/or hepatic disease. Releases histamine.

VALDECOXIB (BEXTRA) (CURRENTLY NOT AVAILABLE IN THE US) `BBW`

- **Uses:** nonsteroidal analgesic (selective COX-2 inhibitor)
- **Dose:** (PO) 10 mg/day.
- **Site of clearance:** hepatic
- $t^1/_2$: 8–11 h
- **Interaction/toxicity:** Corticosteroids may increase risk of GI ulceration. GI bleeding (including ulceration and perforation), liver dysfunction, renal impairment, and worsening of aspirin-sensitive asthma have been reported. Aspirin potentiates GI ulceration. Avoid in patients with history of allergic response to sulfonamides. Cyclosporine, dextromethorphan, lithium levels increased. Serum concentrations/toxicity of methotrexate may be increased. Use increases the risk of cardiovascular events such as heart attack and stroke.

VANCOMYCIN (VARIOUS)

- **Uses:** antibiotic
- **Dose:** (IV) 1.0 g q12h, max daily dose 4 g.
    Pseudomembranous colitis produced by Clostridium difficile: Adults: (PO) 125 mg q6h, max daily dose 2 g. Children:

(IV) 40 mg/kg/day divided q6–8h, max daily dose 2 g. Dosing intervals should be extended in patients with renal impairment.
- **Site of clearance:** renal
- **t$^1/_2$:** adults 5–11 h, children (>3 yr) 2.2–3 h, ESRD 200–250 h.
- **Interaction/toxicity:** Reduce dose in renal dysfunction or with patients receiving nephrotoxic or ototoxic drugs. Administer as infusion over 60 min. Rapid IV infusion associated with "red man syndrome" (hypotension with vasodilation due to histamine release). Potentiates nondepolarizing neuromuscular blockers and histamine release of anesthetic drugs.

VASOPRESSIN (PITRESSIN)

- **Uses:** vasoconstrictor, neurogenic diabetes insipidus
- **Dose:** *Vasodilatory shock/septic shock:* (IV) 0.01–0.04 units/min. Doses >0.05 units/min may have more cardiovascular side effects.
  Cardiac arrest: (IV): 40 units IV push may be given via ETT one time.
  Abdominal distention: (IM) 5 units stat, 10 units q3–4h.
  Diabetes insipidus: Adults: (IM, SC) 5–10 units bid–qid prn. Children: (IM, SC) 2.5–10 units bid–qid prn. Adults and children: (IV) 0.0005 unit/kg/h continuous infusion, double dosage prn q30min to max of 0.01 unit/kg/h.
- **Site of clearance:** hepatic, renal
- **t$^1/_2$:** 10–20 min
- **Interaction/toxicity:** Coronary artery vasoconstriction, allergic reactions, HTN.

VECURONIUM (NORCURON) **BBW**

- **Uses:** nondepolarizing neuromuscular blocker
- **Dose:** *Surgery:* Adults and children >1 yr: (IV) loading 0.08–0.1 mg/kg or 0.04–0.06 mg/kg after initial dose of succinylcholine for intubation; maintenance 0.01–0.015 mg/kg 25–40 min after initial dose, then 0.01–0.015 mg/kg q12–15 min, may be administered as a continuous infusion at 0.8–2 mcg/kg/min. Infants >7 wk to 1 yr: (IV) loading 0.08–0.1 mg/kg, maintenance 0.05–0.1 mg/kg q60min prn.
  ICU: (IV) 0.05–0.1 mg/kg bolus followed by 0.8–1.7 mcg/kg/min once initial recovery from bolus observed or 0.1–0.2 mg/kg q1h.
- **Site of clearance:** hepatic, renal
- **t$^1/_2$:** 51–80 min

■ **Interaction/toxicity:** Potentiated by volatile anesthetics, hypokalemia, antibiotics (aminoglycosides), magnesium, local anesthetics, procainamide, quinidine. Conditions associated with increased volume of distribution (e.g., slower circulation time, edematous states, and old age) may be associated with delay in onset. Prolongation of neuromuscular blockade may occur in patients with renal and/or hepatic disease. Theophylline and phenytoin decrease effects. Bradycardia may occur with rapid administration in patients receiving opioids.

VERAPAMIL (CALAN, ISOPTIN)

■ **Uses:** antidysrhythmic, antihypertensive
■ **Dose:** *Dysrhythmia (SVT):* Adults: (IV) 2.5–5 mg over 2 min, second dose of 5–10 mg (~0.15 mg/kg) may be given 15–30 min after the initial dose if patient tolerates but does not respond to initial dose; max total dose 20 mg. Children <1 yr: (IV) 0.1–0.2 mg/kg over 2 min, MR q30min prn. Children 1–15 yr: 0.1–0.3 mg/kg (max 5 mg) over 2 min, MR in 15 min if adequate response not achieved, max for second dose 10 mg.

Angina: (PO) initial 80–120 mg bid (elderly or small stature 40 mg bid), range 240–480 mg/day tid–qid.

HTN: (PO) immediate release 80 mg tid, usual dose range 80–320 mg/day divided bid; sustained release 240 mg/day, usual dose range 120–360 mg/day qd or divided bid (120 mg/day in elderly or small patients). No evidence of additional benefit in doses >360 mg/day.
■ **Site of clearance:** renal
■ **t^1/$_2$:** Adults single dose 2–8 h, multiple doses up to 12 h.
■ **Interaction/toxicity:** Potentiates beta-blockers, theophylline; increases digoxin levels. Barbiturates may decrease bioavailability. Cimetidine increases bioavailability.

WARFARIN (COUMADIN)

■ **Uses:** anticoagulant
■ **Dose:** (PO) 5–10 mg. Adjust dose for prothrombin time 1.5–2.0 times control.
■ **Site of clearance:** hepatic
■ **t^1/$_2$:** 20–60 h
■ **Interaction/toxicity:** Platelet aggregation inhibitors (e.g., salicylates, dipyridamole, indomethacin), procoagulant inhibition factors (e.g., quinidine) increase risk of hemorrhage. Decreased effect with enzyme inducers (e.g., barbiturates, phenytoin).

APPENDIX H ■ HERBAL MEDICATIONS

The authors and publisher have exerted every effort to ensure that the drug selection and dosage set forth in this appendix are in accord with current recommendations and practice at the time of publication. However, in view of ongoing research, changes in government regulations, and the constant flow of information relating to drug therapy and drug reactions, the reader is urged to check the package insert for each drug for any change in indications and dosage and for added warnings and precautions. This is particularly important when the recommended agent is a new or infrequently used drug.

The editors wish to acknowledge the contribution of Stella A. Haddadin, BSc, PharmD, Yale–New Haven Hospital, Department of Pharmacy Services, in the preparation of this appendix.

ALFALFA
Uses: Diuretic, kidney, bladder and prostate conditions, hyperglycemia, asthma, arthritis, indigestion
Interaction/toxicity: Excessive use may interfere with anticoagulant therapy, potentiate drug-induced photosensitivity, and interfere with hormone therapy.

ANGELICA ROOT
Uses: Gastrointestinal spasm, loss of appetite, feeling of fullness, and flatulence
Interaction/toxicity: Can cause photodermatitis, claims to increase stomach acid, therefore, interferes with antacids, sucralfate, H2 antagonists, and proton pump inhibitors. Potentiates the effects and adverse effects of anticoagulants and antiplatelet drugs.

ANISE
Uses: Dyspepsia and as a pediatric antiflatulent and expectorant
Interaction/toxicity: Excessive doses can prolong coagulation, increasing PT/INR because of coumarin contained in anise. An interaction exists with anticoagulant therapy, MAOIs, and hormone therapy. Catecholamine activity might increase blood pressure and blood pressure readings and increase heart rate.

ARNICA FLOWER
Uses: Antiphlogistic, antiseptic, anti-inflammatory, analgesic
Interaction/toxicity: Potentiates anticoagulant and antiplatelet effect of drugs and possibly increases risk of bleeding.

ASAFOETIDA
Uses: Chronic bronchitis, asthma, pertussis, hoarseness, hysteria, flatulent colic, chronic gastric, dyspepsia, irritable colon, and convulsions
Interaction/toxicity: Might increase the risk of bleeding, and excessive doses might interfere with blood pressure control. Can irritate GI tract and is contraindicated in patients with infectious or inflammatory GI conditions.

BOGBEAN
Uses: Rheumatism, loss of appetite, dyspepsia
Interaction/toxicity: Potentiates anticoagulant and antiplatelet drugs and possibly increases risk of bleeding.

BROMELAIN
Uses: Acute postoperative and posttraumatic conditions of swelling, especially of the nasal and paranasal sinuses, osteoarthritis
Interaction/toxicity: Potentiates anticoagulant and antiplatelet drugs and possibly increases risk of bleeding. Increases plasma and urine tetracycline level.

CAYENNE
Uses: Muscle spasms, chronic pain
Interaction/toxicity: Overdose may cause hypothermia. May cause skin blisters.

CELERY
Uses: Rheumatism, gout, hysteria, nervousness, weight loss as a result of malnutrition, loss of appetite, exhaustion, sedative, mild diuretic, urinary antiseptic, digestive aid, antiflatulent, blood purification
Interaction/toxicity: Potentiates anticoagulant and antiplatelet drugs and possibly increases risk of bleeding. There is an additive effect with drugs with sedative properties and may cause increase in phototoxic response to psoralen plus ultraviolet light A (PUVA) therapy because of its psoralen content.

CHAMOMILE
Uses: Flatulence, nervous diarrhea, restlessness, insomnia, antispasmodic

Interaction/toxicity: Concomitant use with benzodiazepines might cause additive effects and side effects. Potentiates anticoagulant and antiplatelet drugs and possibly increases risk of bleeding. Is an inhibitor of the cytochrome p450 3A4 enzyme system.

CLOVE
Uses: Flatulence, nausea, and vomiting
Interaction/toxicity: Potentiates anticoagulant and antiplatelet drugs and possibly increases risk of bleeding.

DANSHEN
Uses: Circulation problems, cardiovascular diseases, chronic hepatitis, abdominal masses, insomnia because of palpitations and tight chest, acne, psoriasis, eczema, aids in wound healing
Interaction/toxicity: Potentiates anticoagulant and antiplatelet drugs and possibly increases risk of bleeding. Increases the cardiovascular effects and side effects of digoxin.

DEVIL'S CLAW
Uses: Osteoarthritis, rheumatoid arthritis, gout, myalgia, fibrositis
Interaction/toxicity: Can affect heart rate, contractility of heart, and blood pressure. Might decrease blood glucose levels and have additive effects with medications used for diabetes. May cause an increase in gastric acid secretions.

DONG QUAI
Uses: Gynecologic ailments, menopausal symptoms
Interaction/toxicity: Potentiates anticoagulant and antiplatelet drugs and possibly increases risk of bleeding.

ECHINACEA
Uses: Common colds, urinary tract infections
Interaction/toxicity: May cause hepatotoxicity especially with other concomitant hepatotoxins. Antagonizes steroids and immunosuppressants. May possess immunosuppressive activity after long-term use.

EPHEDRA
Uses: Diet aid, bacteriostatic, antitussive
Interaction/toxicity: May cause arrhythmias with inhalation anesthetics and cardiac glycosides. Life-threatening reaction with MAOIs. May cause depletion of catecholamines and lead to perioperative hemodynamic instability. Can cause death.

FENUGREEK
Uses: Lower blood sugar in diabetics

Interaction/toxicity: Potentiates anticoagulant and antiplatelet drugs and possibly increases risk of bleeding. Inhibits corticosteroid drug activity, interferes with hormone therapy, can alter blood glucose control, and potentiate effect of MAOIs.

FEVERFEW
Uses: Migraine prophylaxis, antipyretic
Interaction/toxicity: Inhibit platelet activity. Potentiates anticoagulants. Abrupt withdrawal may cause rebound headaches. Uterine stimulant. Associated with serotonin syndrome.

GARLIC (PERTAINS TO SUPPLEMENT PRODUCT)
Uses: Lower lipids, antihypertensive, antiplatelet, antioxidant, antithrombolytic
Interaction/toxicity: Potentiates anticoagulants, especially in the presence of drugs that inhibit platelet function. Potentiates vasodilator drugs and antihypertensives. May decrease blood glucose levels as a result of increased serum insulin levels.

GINGER (PERTAINS TO SUPPLEMENT PRODUCT)
Uses: Antinauseant, antispasmodic
Interaction/toxicity: Inhibits thromboxane synthetase. Potentiates anticoagulants. May alter effects of calcium channel blockers

GINKGO
Uses: Circulatory stimulant, inhibit platelets
Interaction/toxicity: Potentiates anticoagulants, especially in the presence of aspirin, NSAIDs, heparin, and warfarin.

GINSENG
Uses: Antioxidant
Interaction/toxicity: Antagonize anticoagulants. Avoid use of sympathetic stimulants, which may result in tachycardia or hypertension. Possesses hypoglycemic effect. Potentiates digoxin and MAOIs.

GOLDENSEAL
Uses: Diuretic, anti-inflammatory, hemostatic
Interaction/toxicity: May worsen edema and hypertension. Oxytocic possesses activity.

GREEN TEA
Uses: Improves cognitive performance, lowers cholesterol and triglycerides, aids in the prevention of breast, bladder, esophageal, and pancreatic cancers. Decreased risk of Parkinson's disease, gingivitis, obesity

Interaction/toxicity: Concomitant use might inhibit effect of adenosine and antagonize effect of warfarin. Because of the caffeine content, there is an increase in cardiac inotropic effects of beta-adrenergic agonist drugs, an increase in the effects and toxicity of clozapine, and an increased risk of agitation, tremors, and insomnia in combination with ephedrine. It might precipitate hypertensive crisis with MAOIs as well. Might reduce sedative effects of benzodiazepines.

HORSE CHESTNUT
Uses: Varicose veins and relieving pain, tiredness, tension , swelling in legs, itching, and edema
Interaction/toxicity: Potentiates anticoagulant and antiplatelet drugs and possibly increases risk of bleeding, hypoglycemic effects, might interfere with binding of protein binding drugs.

KAVA-KAVA
Uses: Anxiolytic, analgesic
Interaction/toxicity: Potentiates barbiturates, opioids, and benzodiazepines.

LICORICE
Uses: Heal gastric and duodenal ulcers
Interaction/toxicity: May cause hypertension, hypokalemia, and edema.

LOVAGE ROOT
Uses: Used for inflammation of the lower urinary tract and prevention of kidney gravel; in "irrigation therapy," it is used as a mild diuretic
Interaction/toxicity: Might increase sodium retention and interfere with diuretic therapy.

MEADOWSWEET
Uses: Supportive therapy for colds
Interaction/toxicity: Can potentiate narcotic effects. Contains a salicylate constituent.

ONIONS
Uses: Loss of appetite, preventing atherosclerosis, dyspepsia, fever, colds, cough, tendency toward infection, and inflammation of the mouth and pharynx
Interaction/toxicity: May enhance antidiabetic drug effects and alter blood sugar control. Might enhance antiplatelet drug activity and increase bleeding risk.

PAPAIN
Uses: Inflammation and swelling in patient with pharyngitis
Interaction/toxicity: Concomitant use with anticoagulant and antiplatelet drugs may increase risk of bleeding.

PARSLEY
Uses: Breath freshener, for urinary tract infections, and kidney or bladder stones
Interaction/toxicity: Might interfere with oral anticoagulant therapy because of the Vitamin K contained in parsley. May interfere with diuretic therapy by enhancing sodium retention. Might potentiate MAOI drug therapy.

PASSION FLOWER
Uses: Generalized anxiety disorder
Interaction/toxicity: Concomitant use with barbiturates can increase drug-induced sleep time; can potentiate the effects of sedatives and tranquilizers, including sedative effects of antihistamines.

QUASSIA
Uses: Anorexia, indigestion, fever, mouthwash, as an anthelmintic for thread worms, nematodes, and ascaris
Interaction/toxicity: Stimulates gastric acid and might oppose effect of antacids and H2 antagonists. Excessive doses might have additive effects with anticoagulant therapy with Coumadin. Concomitant use of potassium-depleting diuretics or stimulant laxative abuse might increase risk of cardiac glycoside toxicity as a result of potassium loss.

RED CLOVER
Uses: Hot flashes
Interaction/toxicity: Can increase the anticoagulant effects and bleeding risk because of its coumarin content. May interfere with hormone replacement therapy or oral contraceptives, and may interfere with tamoxifen because of its potential estrogenic effects. Can inhibit cytochrome P450 (cyp450) 3A4.

SAW PALMETTO
Uses: Benign prostatic hypertrophy, antiandrogenic
Interaction/toxicity: Potentiates birth control pills and estrogens. May cause hypertension.

ST. JOHN'S WORT
Uses: Depression, anxiety
Interaction/toxicity: Possible interaction/toxicity with MAOIs and meperidine. May prolong anesthetic effects. Potentiates digoxin.

May decrease effects of warfarin, steroids, and possibly benzodi-azepines and calcium channel blockers.

SWEET CLOVER
Uses: Chronic venous insufficiency, including leg pain and heaviness, night-time leg cramps, itching and swelling, for supportive treatment of thrombophlebitis, lymphatic congestion, postthrombotic syndromes, and hemorrhoids
Interaction/toxicity: Use with hepatotoxic drugs might increase risk of hepatotoxicity. Concomitant use with anticoagulant and antiplatelet drugs may increase risk of bleeding.

TUMERIC
Uses: Dyspepsia, jaundice, hepatitis, flatulence, abdominal bloating
Interaction/toxicity: Concomitant use with anticoagulant and antiplatelet drugs may increase risk of bleeding.

VALERIAN
Uses: Sedative, anxiolytic
Interaction/toxicity: Potentiates barbiturates and anesthetics. May blunt symptoms of benzodiazepine withdrawal.

VITAMIN E
Uses: Vitamin E deficiency, heart disease
Interaction/toxicity: Concomitant use with anticoagulant and antiplatelet drugs may increase risk of bleeding. Might prevent tolerance to nitrates

WILLOW BARK
Uses: Lower back pain, fever, rheumatic ailments, headache
Interaction/toxicity: Enough salicylate is present in willow bark to cause drug interactions common to salicylates or aspirin. Can impair effectiveness of beta-adrenergic blockers, probenecid, and sulfinpyrazone. Can increase effects, side effects, or toxicity of alcohol, anticoagulants, carbonic anhydrase inhibitors, heparin, methotrexate, NSAIDs, sulfonylureas, and valproic acid.

The authors thank the authors and publishers listed below for permission to reprint the following materials:

Figure 6-1: From Pancrazio JJ, Lynch C: Snails, spiders and sterospecificity—Is there a role for calcium channels in anesthetic mechanisms? Anesthesiology 81:1, 1994.

Figures 11-1 and 11-2: From Wood AJJ: Drug disposition and pharmacokinetics. In Wood M, Wood AJJ (eds): Drugs and Anesthesia: Pharmacology for Anesthesiologists. Baltimore, Williams & Wilkins, 1990.

Figure 11-4: From Stanski DR, Watkins WD: Drug Disposition in Anesthesia. New York, Grune & Stratton, 1982.

Figure 13-2: From Van Hemelrijck White PF: Use of intravenous sedative agents. In Rogers MC *et al* (eds): Principles and Practice of Anesthesiology. St. Louis, CV Mosby, 1992.

Figure 13-3: From White PF, Vascones LO, Mathes SA *et al*: Comparison of midazolam and diazepam for sedation during plastic surgery. J Plast Reconstr Surg 81:703, 1988.

Figure 13-4: From White PF: Clinical uses of intravenous anesthetic and analgesic infusions. Anesth Analg 68:161, 1989.

Figure 13-5: From Glass PSA, Shafer SL, Jacobs JR, Reves JG: Intravenous drug delivery systems. In Miller's Anesthesia, 4th ed, p 391. New York, Churchill Livingston, 1994.

Figure 14-1: From Shafer SL, Varvel JR: Pharmacokinetics, pharmacodynamics, and rational opioid selection. Anesthesiology 74:53, 1991.

Figure 14-2: From Egan TD, Lemmens HJM, Fiset P *et al*: The pharmacokinetics of the new short acting opioid remifentanil (G187084B) in health adult male volunteers. Anesthesiology 79:881, 1993.

Figure 15-12: Adapted from Goff MJ, Arain SR, Ficke DJ *et al*: Absence of bronchodilation during desflurane anesthesia: A comparison to sevoflurane and thiopental. Anesthesiology 93:404, 2000.

Figure 15-13: Adapted from Pagel PS, Fu JL, Damask MC *et al*: Desflurane and isoflurane produce similar alterations in systemic and pulmonary hemodynamics and arterial oxygenation in patients undergoing one-lung ventilation during thoracotomy. Anesth Analg 87:800, 1998.

Figure 15-15: Adapted from Kharasch ED, Hoffman GM, Thorning D *et al*: Role of the renal cysteine conjugate β-lyase pathway

1118

in inhaled compound A nephrotoxicity in rats. Anesthesiology 88: 1624, 1998.

Figure 16.2: From Taylor P: Are neuromuscular blocking agents more efficacious in pairs? Anesthesiology 63:1, 1985.

Figures 25-4 and 25-5: From Mulroy MF: Regional Anesthesia: An Illustrated Procedural Guide. Boston, Little Brown, 1989.

Figure 25-7: From Bonica J, Kennedy W, Ward R, Toals A: A comparison of the effects of high subarachnoid and epidural anesthesia. Acta Anaesthesiol Scand 23:429, 1966.

Figure 28-3: From West JB, Dolley CT, Naimark A: Distribution of blood flow in isolated lung: Relation to vascular and alveolar pressures. J Appl Physiol 19:713, 1964.

Figure 29-1: From Neustein SM, Cohen E: Preoperative evaluation of thoracic surgical patients. In Cohen E (ed): The Practice of Thoracic Anesthesia. Philadelphia, JB Lippincott, 1995.

Figure 40-1: From Horlocker TT, Cucchiari RF, Ebersold MJ: Vertebral column and spinal cord injury. In Cuchiari RF, Michenfelder JD (eds): Clinical Neuroanesthesia. New York, Churchill Livingstone, 1990.

Figure 42-1: From Hon EH: An Introduction to Fetal Heart Rate Monitoring. New Haven, Connecticut, Harty Press, 1969.

Figure 46-1: From Medidy HW: Criteria for selection of ambulatory surgical patients and guidelines for anesthetic management: A retrospective study of 1553 cases. Anesth Analg 61:921, 1982.

Figure 47-3: From Jacobs JR, Reves JG, Marty JWD, et al: Aging increases pharmacodynamic sensitivity to the hypnotic effects of midazolam. Anesth Analog 80:143, 1995.

Figure 48-2: From Rooke GA, Schwid HA, Shapira Y: The effect of graded hemorrhage and intravascular volume replacement on systolic pressure variation in humans during mechanical and spontaneous ventilation. Anesth Analg 80:925, 1995.

Figure 48-3: From Capan LM, Gottlieb G. Rosenberg A: General principles of anesthesia for major acute trauma. In Capan LM, Miller SM, Turndorf H (eds): Trauma: Anesthesia and Intensive Care, p 259. Philadelphia, JB Lippincott, 1991.

Figure 49-2: From Levy JH: Identification and Treatment of Anaphylaxis: Mechanisms of Action and Strategies for Treatment Under General Anesthesia. Chicago, Smith Laboratories.

Page numbers followed by t and f indicate tables and figures, respectively.

A

Abdominal aortic aneurysms, 562
Abdominal injury, 794–795
Abdominal insufflation
  respiration, 640t
ABO
  Rhesus typing, 105
Abruptio placentae, 704
Absorption
  in drug interactions, 820
ACE inhibitors. *See* Angiotensin-converting
  enzyme (ACE) inhibitors
Acetaminophen (Paracetamol-APAP),
  1037–1038
  for children, 738–740
  pharmacokinetics of, 886t
  pharmacology of, 884
  for postoperative pain in children,
  900t
  for thyroid storm, 681t
Acetazolamide, 1038
  anesthetic ramifications of, 576
Acetic acids
  pharmacokinetics of, 885t
Acetylcholine (ACh), 141
  metabolism of, 142f
  synthesis of, 142f
ACh. *See* Acetylcholine (ACh)
Acid-base balance, 75f
Acid-base equilibrium, 74
  with trauma, 806
Acid-base interpretation
  practical approach to, 80–81
  sequential approach to, 81t
Acidosis. *See also* Metabolic acidosis
  rapid correction of, 709
  respiratory, 78–79
    anesthetic implications of, 79–80
  causes of, 80t
ACL. *See* Anterior cruciate ligament
  (ACL)
ACLS. *See* Advanced cardiac life support
  (ACLS)
Acquired immunodeficiency syndrome
  (AIDS), 705–706
  chronic pain in, 915
Acromegaly, 692–693, 693t
ACT. *See* Activated clotting time (ACT)
Action potentials, 506, 507f
Actiq. *See* Fentanyl Oralet (Actiq)
Activated clotting time (ACT), 112
Activated protein C
  for septic shock, 930
Active transport, 120
Acupressure
  for postoperative nausea and vomiting,
  765t
Acute cocaine intoxication, 823
Acute fatty liver of pregnancy, 654
Acute hemolytic transfusion reactions
  (AHTR), 98
Acute ischemic stroke, 924
Acute liver failure, 863
Acute lung injury (ALI), 931–932

Acute postoperative pain
  adjuvant analgesia for, 890
  analgesia methods for, 891–899
  management of, 881–902
  postoperative analgesia service, 899–901
Acute pulmonary edema, hypotension, and
  shock
  algorithm for, 1013f–1014f
Acute quadriplegic myopathy, 941
Acute renal failure, 601–602, 601f, 601t,
  932
  osmolality in, 933t
  urinalysis in, 933t
  urine chemistry in, 933t
Acute respiratory distress syndrome
  (ARDS), 931–932
Acute respiratory failure, 930–932
  critical care medicine, 930–932
Adalat. *See* Nifedipine (Procardia, Adalat)
Addison's disease. *See* Adrenal insufficiency
  (Addison's disease)
Adductor pollicis, 249
A delta fibers, 881
Adenocard. *See* Adenosine (Adenocard)
Adenoidectomy, 583–585
Adenosine (Adenocard), 1035
Adenosine triphosphate (ATP), 143, 158
Adjustable gastric banding, 624
Adjuvant analgesia
  for acute postoperative pain, 890
Adjuvant drugs
  for chronic pain, 911–912
Adrenal cortex, 683–686
Adrenalectomy, 685t
Adrenal function
  in critical illness, 934
Adrenal insufficiency (Addison's disease),
  683
Adrenal medulla, 686–687
Adrenergic agonists, 151–157
  action sites, 152t
  doses of, 152t
  hemodynamics, 151, 153t
Adrenergic antagonists-sympatholytics,
  159–161
Adrenergic receptors, 144–148
  classification of, 146t
  numbers or sensitivity, 148–149
Adult emergency cardiopulmonary
  resuscitation
  algorithm for, 946f
Advanced cardiac life support (ACLS), 944,
  952–953
  defibrillation, 952
  defibrillators, 952–953
  pharmacologic therapy, 954t
  transthoracic impedance, 953, 953t
AEG. *See* Atrial electrogram (AEG)
Aging. *See also* Elderly
  anesthesiologists, 30–31
  concepts of, 741
  diseases, 751t
  inhalation anesthesia, 750f
  injection anesthesia, 750f

Aging (*cont.*)
  and organ function, 741–744
  population
    effect on critical care, 919
    respiratory function changes, 467,
      467t
Agitation
  in ICU patients, 935
AHA. *See* American Heart Association
    (AHA)
AHF. *See* Factor VIII (Antihemophiliac
    factor, AHF)
AHTR. *See* Acute hemolytic transfusion
    reactions (AHTR)
AICD. *See* Automatic implantable
    cardioverter-defibrillator (AICD)
AIDS. *See* Acquired immunodeficiency
    syndrome (AIDS)
Air embolism
  venous
    diagnosis of, 455t
    treatment of, 455t
Air-trapping, 931
Airway, 465. *See also* Difficult airway
  anatomy, 341–343
  anesthesia, 420–421
  artificial
    epiglottitis, 590t
  classification systems, 274t
  compromise with trauma, 803
  control, 4
  emergencies
    pediatric otolaryngologic surgery,
      588–590
  evaluation of, 583
  functional divisions of, 465t
  with laser surgery, 590
  management, 341–356
    anesthesia induction, 344
    awake with difficult airway, 353–354
    with BLS, 946
    in children, 737–738
    with difficult airway, 351–356
    minimally invasive procedures for,
      641
    patient history and physical exam,
      342–343
    preoxygenation, 343–344
    with supraglottic airways, 344–345
    tracheal intubation, 346–351
  obesity, 621, 625
  with otolaryngologic surgery, 586–588
  preoperative evaluation of, 273–274
  reflexes
    fentanyl, 196
    protective in gastrointestinal disorders,
      630–631
  resistance
    desflurane, 227f
    sevoflurane, 227f
  securing in otolaryngologic surgery, 593
  surgery, 586–588
  trauma evaluation and intervention,
    782–784, 783f
  traumatized upper in otolaryngologic
    surgery, 595
  upper in otolaryngologic surgery, 592
Albumin, 81
  serum, 648
Albuterol, 1039

Alcohol, 914t
Alcohol abuse
  postoperative morbidity, 646f
Aldomet. *See* Methyldopa (Aldomet,
    Methyldopate)
Alfalfa, 1107
Alfenta. *See* Alfentanil (Alfenta)
Alfentanil (Alfenta), 194, 198–199, 207f,
    1039
  dosage for in elective surgery, 210t
  evoked potentials, 447t
  recovery curves, 206f
ALI. *See* Acute lung injury (ALI)
Alkaline phosphatase (AP), 648
Allergic drug reactions, 815–816, 816t.
    See also Anaphylaxis
  agents implicated in, 817–818
  evaluation of, 817
  immunologic mechanisms of, 816
  tests for, 817t
Allergic reactions, 24, 808–818
  immunologic principles, 808
  intraoperative, 811–815
Allergies
  latex, 25, 818
  perioperative management of, 815–817
  testing for, 817
Alpha 1 acid glycoprotein
  drugs binding to, 128t
Alpha agonists
  adverse effects of, 151
Alpha antagonists, 159
Alpha blockers
  effects during anesthesia, 823t
Alpha 2 blockers
  with preoperative vascular surgery, 554t
Alpha error. *See* Type I (alpha) error
Alpha particles, 963t
Alpha receptors
  in cardiovascular system, 144–148
Alteplase (rt-PA)
  for acute ischemic stroke, 924
Alternating currents, 61
Alveolar-arterial oxygen gradient, 973
Alveolar-capillary membrane, 465
Alveolar dead space, 473
Alveolar oxygen tension, 973
Alzheimer's disease, 306–307
Ambulatory ECG
  preoperative evaluation, 279
Ambulatory laparoscopic cholecystectomy,
    643
Ambulatory surgery, 755–766
  anesthesia effect on recovery time, 756f
  anesthetic premedication, 759–761
  fluid and food restriction for, 759
  general anesthesia, 763–764
  intraoperative anesthetic management,
    761–764, 761t
  nausea and vomiting, 765, 765t
  pain, 765
  patient anxiety, 757–758
  patient discharge, 765–766
  postanesthesia care, 764–766
  preoperative evaluation, 757–759
  preoperative sedation for, 759t
  in preterm infants, 757
  regional techniques, 762–763, 762t
  unlikely candidates for, 756t
  URI in children, 758, 758t

Americaine. *See* Benzocaine (Americaine, Hurricaine)
American Heart Association (AHA) resuscitation protocols, 1003–1023
American Society for Testing and Materials (ASTM)
  manufactured workstations standards, 329t
American Society of Anesthesiologists (ASA), 8
  safety guidelines, 843
  standards, 828, 1024–1029
  web site, 8
Ames bacterial assay, 23
Ames test, 229
Amidate. *See* Etomidate (Amidate)
Aminocaproic acid, 1039
Aminophylline, 1040
Amiodarone (Cordarone), 1039–1040
  for ACLS, 954t
  for CPR, 955
Amitriptyline, 1040–1041
Amobarbital, 1041
Amoxicillin, 1041
Ampicillin, 1041–1042
Ampofol
  physiochemical properties, 175
Amrinone, 158
  for congenital heart defects, 541t
Analgesia. *See also* Anesthesia
  adjuvant
    for acute postoperative pain, 890
  central neuraxial, 891–895
  definition of, 832t
  delivery routes for, 891t
  order sheet, 899t
  patient-controlled, 891, 892t
  postoperative
    epidural, 893t
    latency and duration of, 896t
    patient-controlled, 899t
  service
    for acute postoperative pain, 899–901
    postoperative, 899–901
Analysis of variance (ANOVA), 18
Anaphylaxis. *See also* Allergic reactions
  chemical mediators of, 813t
  during general anesthesia, 812t
  during regional anesthesia, 812t
Anectine. *See* Succinylcholine (Anectine)
Anemia, 307–310, 307t, 934
  conditions decreasing tolerance for, 102t
  hemolytic, 308
  iron deficiency, 308
  isovolemic
    vs. acute blood loss, 101–103
  nutritional deficiency, 308
  with preterm infants, 757
Anesthesia. *See also* Analgesia
  cellular and molecular mechanisms of, 40–743
  complication of, 39t
  definition of, 40
  education about, 6–7
  before ether, 1
  face mask, 344
  history of, 1–7
  lipid theories of, 45
  machines, 4, 328
  measurements, 40–41

organizations, 6–7
pharmacogenoics, 54–57
protein theories of, 46
provided at alternate sites, 828–842
  care, 829–833
  dental surgery, 841–842
  equipment, 828–829
  gastroenterology, 838–839
  patient factors, 831t
  patient transport, 842
  radiation therapy, 833–836
  radiology, 831t, 833–836
  three-step approach to, 829t
  related deaths, 38t
  ventilators, 338
  workstations
    checking, 329t
    pneumatics, 328–331
    variations, 339–340
Anesthesia Patient Safety Foundation (APSF), 843
Anesthesia preoperative evaluation clinic (APEC), 14
Anesthesiologists
  aging, 30–31
  mortality among, 31
  role in bioterrorism, 966
Anesthesiology practice
  administrative components of, 8–9
Anesthetic, 849
  agents
    genetic variability, 56
    molecular targets *vs.* intact organism, 46–48
  circuits, 333–337
  gases
    hazards of, 22–23
  monitoring
    ASA standards for, 1022–1023
  target sites
    chemical nature of, 44–45
Aneurysms
  aortic, 561–562
  intracranial, 457–458
  thoracic, 563
Angelica root, 1110
Angiography
  cardiac, 503–504
  coronary, 281
Angiomax. *See* Bivalrudin (Angiomax)
Angiotensin-converting enzyme (ACE) inhibitors
  effects during anesthesia, 823t
  preoperative, 547t
  preoperative vascular surgery, 555t
Angiotensin II
  liver, 647
Anise, 1107
Ankle blockade, 435
  landmarks for, 436f
Ankle surgery, 669, 670t
ANOVA. *See* Analysis of variance (ANOVA)
Anoxic brain injury, 924
ANS. *See* Autonomic nervous system (ANS)
Antacids
  dose, 287t
Antepartum hemorrhage, 704
Anterior cruciate ligament (ACL)
  repair, 669

Anterior ischemic optic neuropathy
  with ophthalmic surgery, 581–582
Anthranilic acids
  pharmacokinetics of, 886t
Anthrax, 965
Antibody screen, 105
Anticholinergic drugs, 150–151, 290–291,
    292t
  for neonates, 716
Anticholinesterase, 150
  doses of, 253t
  pharmacokinetics of, 252t
  pharmacology of, 251
Anticoagulation
  with interventional neuroradiology, 834
Anticonvulsants, 305t
  for chronic pain, 912–913
  side effects of, 912t
Antidepressants
  side effects of, 912t
Antiemetics, 5, 290, 291t
Antigens, 808
Antihemophiliac factor. *See* Factor VIII
    (Antihemophiliac factor, AHF)
Antihypertensive drugs
  effects during anesthesia, 824t
Antilirium. *See* Physostigmine (Antilirium)
Antiplatelets
  neuraxial anesthesia, 548t
Antiproliferative drugs, 859
Antithrombin III (Thrombate III), 1042
Antitrust, 12
Anxiety
  with ambulatory surgery, 757–758
Anxiolysis
  definition of, 832t, 1028
Aorta
  anatomy of, 501
Aortic aneurysms
  abdominal, 562
  endovascular surgery, 564–565, 564t
Aortic cross-clamping and unclamping
  hemodynamic changes during, 562t
Aortic insufficiency, 523–524
Aortic-mesenteric revascularization,
    563
Aortic occlusion, 562–563
Aortic pressure
  coronary flow, 509f
Aortic reconstruction, 563
  monitoring and anesthetic choices,
    565–566
Aortic regurgitation, 524f
Aortic reperfusion, 562–563
Aortic stenosis, 281, 522–523, 523f
Aortic surgery
  elective, 566–567
  emergency, 567–568
Aortorenal revascularization, 564
AP. *See* Alkaline phosphatase (AP)
APEC. *See* Anesthesia preoperative
    evaluation clinic (APEC)
Apgar score
  calculation of, 709t
Apresoline. *See* Hydralazine (Apresoline)
Aprotinin (Trasylol), 526–527, 1039
APSF. *See* Anesthesia Patient Safety
    Foundation (APSF)
AquaMephyton. *See* Phytonadione
    (AquaMephyton, Konakion)

Aquavan
  physiochemical properties of, 175
Aqueous humor, 574
Arachnoid mater, 393
Aramine. *See* Metaraminol bitartrate
    (Aramine)
Ardeparin (Normiflo), 1042–1043
ARDS. *See* Acute respiratory distress
    syndrome (ARDS)
Arduan. *See* Pipecuronium (Arduan)
Arfonad. *See* Trimethaphan (Arfonad)
Argatroban, 1043
Arm
  dermatome of, 423f
  upper, 666–667
Arnica Flower, 1111
Arterial baroreceptors, 149–150
Arterial blood pressure
  indirect measurement of, 371–372
  invasive measurement of, 372–373
Arterial blood pressure monitoring
  cannulation site, 375t
Arterial cannulation, 373–374
Arterial hemoglobin saturation with
    oxygen, 370f
Arterial oxygenation
  assessment of, 475
Arterial oxygen content, 973
Arterial pressure waveform, 925
Arterial pulses, 513–514
Arterial-to-alveolar oxygen ratio,
    973
Arterial-venous oxygen content difference,
    973
Arteriovenous malformations (AVM),
    459–460
Arthroplasty
  total hip
    deep venous thrombosis with, 673
  total knee, 669
Arthroscopy
  knee, 669
  temporomandibular joint, 592
Artificial airway
  epiglottitis, 590t
ASA. *See* American Society of
    Anesthesiologists (ASA)
Asafoetida, 1111
Ashman beats
  EKG of, 977
Aspirin
  pharmacokinetics of, 885t
  preoperative, 546t
Asthma, 282
  in children, 729
ASTM. *See* American Society for Testing
    and Materials (ASTM)
Asystole
  algorithm for, 1007f
Atenolol (Tenormin), 1043–1044
  effects during anesthesia, 823t
Atherosclerosis, 543, 543t, 544–545
Ativan. *See* Lorazepam (Ativan)
Atorvastatin
  preoperative vascular surgery, 554t
ATP. *See* Adenosine triphosphate (ATP)
Atracurium (Tracrium), 242–243, 1044
  for children, 734t
  clearance, 244t
  comparative pharmacology of, 242t

dosing for obesity, 623t
pharmacokinetics of, 241t
Atrial electrogram (AEG)
    EKG of, 999
Atrial fibrillation
    EKG of, 977
Atrial flutter
    EKG of, 977
Atrial pacing
    EKG of, 998
Atrial systole, 504
Atrioventricular block, first degree
    EKG of, 979
Atrioventricular block, second degree
    Mobitz type II
        EKG of, 981
    Wenckebach
        EKG of, 980
Atrioventricular block, third degree
    complete heart block
        EKG of, 982
Atrioventricular dissociation
    EKG of, 983
Atrium
    anatomy of
        left, 500
        right, 499
Atropine, 1044–1045
    adjustments for elderly, 753t
    for CPR, 956
    dose of, 287t
    for nerve agent poisoning, 967
    oculocardiac reflex, 575
Automated oscillometry, 372
    mechanical errors, 372t
Automatic implantable
        cardioverter-defibrillator (AICD),
        70, 837
Autonomic hyperreflexia, 661t
Autonomic innervation, 141
Autonomic nervous system (ANS)
    clinical pharmacology of, 150–158
    efferent
        schematic diagram of, 140f
    elderly, 748–749
    functional anatomy of, 137–140
    hemodynamics, 151
    homeostasis, 139f
    hyperreflexia, 137
    inhalation anesthesia, 223
    neurotransmission, 141–143
    physiology and pharmacology of,
        137–166
    reflexes, 149–150
AVM. See Arteriovenous malformations
        (AVM)
Awake airway management
    difficult airway, 353–354
Axillary technique
    for peripheral nerve blockade, 424–426,
        425f
Azathioprine
    side effects of, 859

B
Backache
    with epidural and spinal anesthesia, 412
Baclofen
    for cancer pain, 914
Bain circuit, 334, 335f

Barbiturates
    for carotid endarterectomy, 558
    for elderly, 174, 753t
    physiochemical properties, 174–175
Baroreceptors
    arterial, 149–150
    venous, 150
Baroresponse, 716
Basic life support (BLS), 944, 946–951
    airway management, 946
    circulation, 948–949
    foreign body airway obstruction, 947
    ventilation, 947–948
Bayesian analysis
    perioperative laboratory testing, 283
B-cell lymphocytes. See Bursa-derived
        lymphocytes (B-cell lymphocytes)
Benadryl. See Diphenhydramine (Benadryl)
Benzocaine (Americaine, Hurricaine), 1042
    clinical profile of, 267t
Benzodiazepines, 288
    adjustments for elderly, 753t
    for ambulatory surgery, 760
    with chronic renal failure, 604
    dosages of, 775t
    for monitored anesthesia care, 773–775
    physiochemical properties, 177–178
    for TBI, 921
Beta-2 agonists
    anesthetic drug interaction, 705
    side effects, 705t
Beta antagonists, 159
    pharmacokinetics of, 160t
    side effects, 159
Beta blockers
    effects during anesthesia, 823t
    preoperative, 547t
    preoperative vascular surgery, 554t
Beta error. See Type II (beta) error
Beta particles, 963t
Beta-1 selectivity, 161
Bextra. See Valdecoxib (Bextra)
B fibers, 881
Bicarbonate, 74
    effects on arterial pH and serum
        bicarbonate, 76t
    retention or elimination, 75f
Bier block, 426
Billing, 12
Binding proteins, 126
Bioavailability, 121
Biochemical monitoring, 708
Biologic agents
    used for warfare, 964t
Biologic disasters, 964–966
Biologic terrorism, 964–965
Biophysical monitoring, 706–707
Bioterrorism
    anesthesiologists role in, 966
Bipolar ESU, 70
Bisoprolol (Zebeta), 1042
Bivalrudin (Angiomax), 1043
Bladder
    innervation of, 596
Blankets
    cooling
        for thyroid storm, 681t
Bleeding time, 111
Bleomycin pulmonary toxicity, 618t
Blinding, 16

Blister agents, 968
Blockade. *See also* Intercostal nerve
    blockade; Peripheral nerve blockade
    ankle, 435
        landmarks for, 436f
    celiac plexus, 433
        complications of, 434t
        landmarks for, 434f
    central neuraxis, 257–258
    cervical plexus, 420, 421t
    hypogastric plexus, 433–434
    ilioinguinal, 431
    nondepolarizing neuromuscular
        characteristics of, 239t
    penile, 431
    stellate ganglion, 431–433
        complications, 433t
        landmarks for, 432f
    sympathetic, 431–434
    sympathetic nervous system (SNS)
        following stellate ganglion block, 432t
Blood agents
    in bioterrorism, 967–968
Blood conservation techniques, 104t
Blood flow
    distribution of, 472, 473f
Blood pressure, 514
    arterial
        indirect measurement of, 371–372
        invasive measurement of, 372–373
    factors controlling, 515f
    systemic monitoring during anesthesia,
        4–5
    systolic, 802f
Blood pressure monitoring, 370–375
    arterial
        cannulation site, 375t
    noninvasive automatic cycled cuff-based,
        373t
Blood product administration
    infectious risks associated with, 98, 99t
    risks of, 98–101
Blood products
    collection and preparation of for
        transfusion, 104–107
Blood typing
    Rhesus
        ABO, 105
Blood volume
    conditions associated with deficits in, 85t
BLS. *See* Basic life support (BLS)
Blunt cardiac injury, 794
Board certification, 9
Body composition
    age-related changes in, 747f
Body fluid compartments, 81–82
Body temperature monitoring
    ASA standards for, 1027
Bogbean, 1111
Bonica, John J., 3
Botulism, 966
Bovie, William T., 68
Bovie pencil, 68
Brachial plexus block
    anatomic approach to, 422t
Brachial plexus injuries
    with dorsal decubitus positions,
        358–360, 360t
Bradycardia
    algorithm for, 1008f

Brain
    dead donors
        anesthetic management of, 855–856
    death
        determination of, 856t
    injury
        anoxic, 924
    metabolism, 438
    neurophysiology, 438–441
        drug effects, 442t
    pathways, 438
    protection, 443–444
    tissue oxygenation, 920
        neurosurgery anesthesia, 448
    trauma
        neurophysiology, 441
    tumors
        neurophysiology, 441
Brain, A.I.J., 4
Breast, 849
Breath holding, 470
Breathing
    chemical control of, 470
Brethaire. *See* Terbutaline (Brethaire,
        Bricanyl)
Bretylium (Bretylol), 1046
Bretylol. *See* Bretylium (Bretylol)
Brevibloc. *See* Esmolol (Brevibloc)
Brevital. *See* Methohexital (Brevital)
Bricanyl. *See* Terbutaline (Brethaire,
        Bricanyl)
Bromelain, 1111
Bronchopleural fistula and empyema,
        494–495, 494t
Bronchoscopy, 492, 587–588
Bubonic plague, 965
Bullae, 495
Bumetanide
    effects during anesthesia, 823t
Bundle-branch block-left (LBBB)
    EKG of, 984
Bundle-branch block-right (RBBB)
    EKG of, 985
Bupivacaine (Marcaine, Sensorcaine),
        1046–1047
    cardiovascular toxicity of, 265
    for children, 739
    clinical profile of, 266t
    dose and duration of, 406t
    epidural, 893t
        with epinephrine, 260t
    for neonates, 719
    peak plasma concentrations of, 262t
    physiochemical properties of, 259t
    toxicity of, 268t
    uses for surgical epidural anesthesia, 407t
Buprenex. *See* Buprenorphine (Buprenex)
Buprenorphine (Buprenex), 203,
        1047–1048
    with PCA, 892t
Burns, 795–797
    airway complications with, 795–796
    anesthesia, 805
    carbon monoxide toxicity, 796
    cyanide toxicity, 796
    fluid replacement for, 796–797
    intensive care, 796
    ventilation with, 796
Bursa-derived lymphocytes (B-cell
        lymphocytes), 808

Butorphanol (Stadol), 202, 1048
  pharmacokinetics of, 888t

C
CAD. *See* Coronary artery disease (CAD)
Cadaveric lung donors
  ideal, 857t
Caffeine
  in preterm infants, 757
Calan. *See* Verapamil (Calan, Isoptin)
Calcineurin inhibitors, 858–859
Calcium, 93–94
  for CPR, 956–957
Calcium channel blockers
  effects during anesthesia, 823t
  for ischemia, 521–522
  preoperative, 547t
  preoperative vascular surgery, 555t
Calcium chloride, 1048–1049
Calcium entry blockers, 161–163, 163
  comparative effects of, 162t
Calcium gluconate, 1049
Cancer pain, 913–915
Capacitance, 61
Capnogram, 365, 366f, 368t
Capnography, 366
Capnometry, 365–366
Capoten. *See* Captopril (Capoten)
Capsaicin, 1046
Captopril (Capoten), 1049
  effects during anesthesia, 823t
Carbamazepine, 305t, 1050
Carbocaine. *See* Mepivacaine (Carbocaine)
Carbon dioxide, 74
  absorbers, 231f
  effects on
    arterial pH and serum bicarbonate, 76t
  elimination, 75f
  end-tidal, 366, 367t
  retention, 75f
  transport of, 472–475
  ventilatory response curves, 471f
  ventilatory response to, 471t
Carbon monoxide
  poisoning
    in PACU, 876
  toxicity
    symptoms of, 796t
Carbon monoxide diffusing capacity
    (DLCO), 477
Carcinoid heart disease, 635
Carcinoid patient
  perioperative management of, 635–636
Carcinoid syndrome, 635
Carcinoid tumors, 634–636
Cardene IV. *See* Nicardipine (Cardene IV)
Cardiac. *See also* Heart
  angiography, 503–504
  catheterization, 503, 836–837
    normal data, 504t
  conduction system, 501
  cycle, 504–506, 505f
  ejection fraction
    assessment of, 281
  electrophysiology, 506–507
  injuries
    anesthesia, 804–805
    blunt, 794
  massage
    for neonatal depression, 709

  nerves, 502–503
  physiology of, 508
  output, 510
    distribution of, 513t
    noninvasive techniques, 383
  physiology, 504–515
  pump mechanism, 949
  receptors, 502–503
  surgery, 518–542
    cardiopulmonary bypass, 526–528
    coronary artery disease, 518–521
    incision to bypass, 530–532
    induction and intubation, 530
    intraoperative management, 530–539
    opioids for, 529–530
    postcardiopulmonary bypass, 536–537
    postoperative considerations, 537–539
    postoperative exploration, 537t
    preincision period, 530
    preinduction period, 530
    preoperative evaluation, 528–530,
      528t
    renal dysfunction with, 608
    valvular heart disease, 522–526
  tamponade
    after cardiac surgery, 537, 538t
  work, 511
Cardiac index (CI), 972
Cardiac magnetic resonance imaging
    (CMRI), 503
Cardiogenic shock, 151, 926–927
Cardiopulmonary bypass, 526–528, 527f,
    527t, 540
  cardiovascular dysfunction following,
    535t
  checklist for, 531t–532t
  discontinuation, 533
  intraoperative management, 532–533
  monitors, 529t
  renal dysfunction with, 608
  rewarming, 533
  ventricular dysfunction after, 534t
Cardiopulmonary function status
  tests determining, 486f
Cardiopulmonary resuscitation (CPR),
    943–958
  adult
    algorithm for, 946f
    blood flow distribution during, 949
  circulation assessment during, 951
  emergency
    adult, 946f
  gas transport during, 949
  history of, 944t
  pharmacologic therapy, 953–957, 954t
  successful, 951t
Cardiopulmonary system
  transition of, 711–712
Cardiovascular anatomy, 499–503
Cardiovascular diagnostic procedures,
    503–504
Cardiovascular system
  beta receptors in, 148
Cardioversion, 837–838
Cardizem. *See* Diltiazem (Cardizem)
Carotid endarterectomy, 553–561
  anesthetic and monitoring choices,
    559t
  barbiturates, 558
  monitoring, 557–560

Carotid endarterectomy (*cont.*)
  postoperative management, 560–561, 560t
  preoperative evaluation and preparation, 557
Case control studies, 17
Case discussion, 11
Catapres. *See* Clonidine (Catapres)
Catecholamines, 143
  for CPR, 954–955
  inactivation of, 143
  synthesis of, 144t
Caudal anesthesia
  with ambulatory surgery, 762–763
Caudal block
  for children, 739
Caudal epidural block
  for neonates, 718–719
Causalgia, 908–909
Cayenne, 1111
Cefazolin, 1050–1051
Cefotan. *See* Cefotetan (Cefotan)
Cefotaxime (Claforan), 1051
Cefotetan (Cefotan), 1051–1052
Celebrex. *See* Celecoxib (Celebrex)
Celecoxib (Celebrex), 1052
  pharmacokinetics of, 886t
Celery, 1111
Celiac plexus blockade, 433
  complications of, 434t
  landmarks for, 434f
Cellular electrophysiology, 506
Central anticholinergic syndrome, 150–151
Central autonomic nervous system organization, 137
Central chemoreceptors, 469–470
Central location, 18
Central nervous system, 41–42
  depressants
    drug interactions between, 825t
  diseases, 302–307
  elderly, 747–748
  respiratory centers, 468f
Central neuraxial analgesia, 891–895
Central neuraxis blockade, 257–258
Central venous catheters
  fiberoptic, 925
  neonatal placement of, 725
Central venous monitoring, 375–378
Central venous pressure cannulation sites, 376f
Central venous pressure catheter placement techniques
  complications, 381t
Central venous pressure waveforms, 380f
  diagnostic value of, 380t
Cerebral blood flow, 439–440
  perfusion pressure, 439f
Cerebral cortex, 42
Cerebral oxygenation/metabolism monitors
  neurosurgery anesthesia, 448
Cerebral preconditioning, 443
Cerebral vasomotor center, 502
Cerebral vasospasms
  after subarachnoid hemorrhage, 923
Cerebrospinal fluid, 440
Cerebrospinal malformations, 457–460
Cervical plexus blockade, 420, 421t
Cesarean section
  anesthesia for, 699–700

C fibers, 881
Chamomile, 1111–1112
Chemical agents, 966t
Chemical warfare, 966–968
Chemoreceptors
  central, 469–470
Chernobyl, 962
Chest compressions
  closed, 950, 950t
    circulation during, 948–949
Chest injury, 793–794
Chest wall injury, 793–794
Chest x-rays, 285
Children, 727–740. *See also* Neonates
  acetaminophen for, 738–740, 900t
  acute pain management in, 901–902
  airway management in, 737–738
  ambulatory surgery in
    midazolam for, 761
  anatomical and physiological distinction from adults, 727t–728t
  anesthetic agents, 730–732
  antiemetics for, 735
  asthma in, 729
  atracurium for, 734t
  breathing circuits in, 738
  bupivacaine for, 739
  caudal block for, 739
  cisatracurium for, 734t
  coexisting health conditions, 727–730
  dexamethasone for, 735
  droperidol for, 735
  endotracheal tubes for, 737
  epidural anesthesia for, 740
  fluid and blood product management, 735–737, 737t
  ibuprofen for, 739
  inhalation anesthesia for, 730–731, 731
  intravenous agents for, 732–735
  ketamine for, 732
  ketorolac for, 739
  laboratory evaluation, 730
  laryngeal mask airway for, 737–738
  with liver transplantation, 863
  lung transplantation in, 866
  mask induction pharmacology of for, 730
  maximum local anesthetic doses of in, 901t
  minimal alveolar concentration, 731
  mivacurium for, 734t
  monitoring of, 738
  muscle relaxants for, 733
  nondepolarizing muscle relaxants for, 733, 734t
  obstructive sleep apnea in, 727–729
  office-based anesthesia for, 851t
  ondansetron for, 735
  opioids for, 733
  outpatient surgery, 850
  pain management in, 738–740
  pancuronium for, 734t
  in postanesthesia care unit, 739t
  postoperative pain in
    codeine for, 900t
    fentanyl for, 900t
    ibuprofen for, 900t
    meperidine for, 900t
    naproxen for, 900t
  postoperative pain medications, 900t

preoperative evaluation of, 727–730, 729t
preoperative fasting, 730
preoperative sedatives, 730, 731t
propofol for, 732
radiation therapy for, 836t
regional anesthesia for, 739–740
renal transplantation in, 860
reversal agents for, 735
rocuronium for, 734t, 735
sedative-hypnotics for, 732–733
sevoflurane for, 731
spinal anesthesia for, 739
succinylcholine for, 731t, 733
URI in, 727
ambulatory surgery, 758, 758t
vecuronium for, 734t
Chirocaine. *See* Levobupivacaine (Chirocaine)
Chloral hydrate, 1052
Chloramphenicol, 1052–1053
Chlordiazepoxide (Librium), 1053
Chloroform
and obstetrics, 2
4-chloro-m-cresol, 319
Chloroprocaine (Nesacaine), 1053
clinical profile of, 267t
dose and duration, 406t
with epidural and spinal anesthesia, 414
with epinephrine, 260t
physiochemical properties, 259t
toxicity of, 268t
uses for surgical epidural anesthesia, 407t
Chlorpromazine (Thorazine), 1053–1054
Cholecystectomy
ambulatory laparoscopic, 643
Cholestatic jaundice
renal dysfunction with, 609
Cholinergic drugs, 150–151
Cholinergic receptors, 143
Cholinesterase, 325t
disorders, 323–326
enzyme, 324t
mivacurium disposition, 326
Chronic hypercapnia, 79
Chronic immune suppression
multisystem complications of, 859t
Chronic pain
in AIDS, 915
management, 903–917
cancer pain, 913–915
HIV/AIDS, 915
interventional techniques for, 916t
psychological interventions for, 915–917, 916t
pharmacologic treatment of, 911–913
psychological factors associated with, 915t
syndromes, 903–910
Chronic renal failure, 602, 602t
CI. *See* Cardiac index (CI)
Cigarette smoking
effect on pulmonary function, 480–481, 480t
Ciliary body
anatomy of, 572
Cimetidine (Tagamet), 1054
dose of, 287t
CIPNM. *See* Critical illness polyneuropathy and myopathy (CIPNM)

Cipro. *See* Ciprofloxacin (Cipro)
Ciprofloxacin (Cipro), 1054–1055
Circadian disruption, 27
Circle breathing systems, 334, 336f, 336t
Circulation monitoring
ASA standards for, 1027
Circulatory failure, 926–927
clinical management of, 927–928
Circumcision, 719
Cirrhosis
decreasing drug clearance, 123
uncommon causes of, 654t
Cisatracurium, 243
for children, 734t
clearance, 244t
comparative pharmacology of, 242t
dosing for obesity, 623t
pharmacokinetics of, 241t
Cisatracurium besylate (Nimbex), 1055
Citanest. *See* Prilocaine (Citanest)
Claforan. *See* Cefotaxime (Claforan)
Claims, 12
Clarke, William E., 1
Clindamycin, 1055
Clinical electrophysiology, 506–507
Clinical pharmacology, 120–136
Clinical privileges, 8
Clonazepam, 305t, 1055–1056
Clonidine, 293
clinical uses of, 157
preoperative vascular surgery, 554t
side effects of, 157
Clonidine (Catapres), 1056
Clopidogrel
preoperative, 546t
Closed chest compressions, 950, 950t
circulation during, 948–949
Clove, 1112
Clover, Joseph, 4
Clover bag, 4
CME. *See* Continuing medical education (CME)
CMRI. *See* Cardiac magnetic resonance imaging (CMRI)
Coagulation
abnormalities
with trauma, 805–806
amplification of, 107
characteristics of, 109t
factor V, 53
laboratory evaluation of, 111–112
with liver transplantation, 862
mechanism of, 107–108
profiles, 116, 116t
propagation of, 107
regulation and control of, 110t
studies, 284
tests
interpretation of, 114t
with trauma, 803
Cobra pharyngeal laryngeal airway, 346
Cocaine, 706t, 1056–1057
acute intoxication, 827
clinical profile of, 267t
introduction as topical anesthetic, 3
maternal use during pregnancy, 719
Codeine, 1057
genetic variability in response to, 57
pharmacokinetics of, 888t
for postoperative pain in children, 900t

Coexisting diseases. *See* Rare and coexisting
    diseases
Cognitive dysfunction
    postoperative
        of elderly, 753–754
Cohort studies, 17
Collagen vascular diseases, 310–314, 311t
    medication adverse effects, 313t
Collecting, 12
Colloids, 83–85
    vs. crystalloid intravenous fluids, 84t, 85
Colton, Gardner Quincy, 1
Combined spinal-epidural anesthesia,
    401–402
Compartment syndrome, 795
Compatibility testing, 105
    blood selection in absence of, 106t
Compazine. *See* Prochlorperazine
    (Compazine)
Complement, 810–811
Complete blood count, 283
Complete heart block
    EKG of, 982
Complex disease
    genetic analysis, 50–51
Complex regional pain syndrome (CRPS),
    907–910
Complex regional pain syndrome (CRPS) I,
    907–908, 908t
Complex regional pain syndrome (CRPS) II,
    908–909
Computed tomography (CT), 834–835
Computerized electroencephalogram
    processing
    neurosurgery anesthesia, 444–446
Conductive flooring, 71
Confusion
    in ICU patients, 935
Congenital diaphragmatic hernia, 720–721,
    721t
Congenital heart defects
    cardiopulmonary bypass, 540
    classification of, 538t
    continuous intravenous infusion, 541t
    postoperative ventilation, 540
    tracheal extubation, 540, 542t
Congenital heart disease, 539–542
    induction anesthesia, 540
    maintenance anesthesia, 540, 541t
    premedication, 540
    preoperative evaluation of, 539t
Congenital nonhemolytic jaundice, 656
Congestive heart failure
    decreasing drug clearance, 123
Conjunctiva
    anatomy of, 572
Conscious sedation
    definition of, 832t
Continuing medical education (CME), 9
Continuous brachial plexus anesthesia
    orthopedic surgery, 668
Continuous epidural anesthesia, 3,
    400–401
Continuous epidural infusion regimens,
    895t
Continuous epidural technique
    safety of, 897t
Continuous quality improvement (CQI),
    35–36
Continuous spinal anesthesia, 398

Contracture test
    halothane-caffeine, 319
Contrast agents
    intravenous
        for alternate site anesthesia, 833
Control groups, 16
Convection, 472
Convenience sampling, 16
Converting enzyme inhibitors, 163
Cooling blankets
    for thyroid storm, 681t
Coomb's test
    indirect, 105
Cordarone. *See* Amiodarone (Cordarone)
Corlopam. *See* Fenoldopam (Corlopam)
Cormack and Lehane laryngeal view
    scoring system, 350f–353f
Cornea
    anatomy of, 572
Corneal abrasion
    with ophthalmic surgery, 580
Corning, Leonard, 3
Coronary angiography, 281
Coronary arteries
    alpha-receptors in, 144
    circulation distribution, 502t
Coronary arteriography, 504
Coronary artery disease (CAD), 518–521
    genetics, 53
    and valvular heart disease, 522
Coronary autoregulation, 508–509
Coronary blood flow, 518–519, 519t
Coronary circulation, 501, 501f
Coronary circulation physiology, 508
Corticosteroids, 6, 282, 859
    comparative pharmacology of, 684t
    for septic shock, 930
    for supratentorial intracranial tumors,
        451
Cost, 14–15
    of drugs, 15
    of PACU, 871t
Coumadin. *See* Warfarin (Coumadin)
CPR. *See* Cardiopulmonary resuscitation
    (CPR)
CQI. *See* Continuous quality improvement
    (CQI)
Cranial nerve monitoring
    neurosurgery anesthesia, 446
Craniosacral (parasympathetic) nervous
    system
    schematic distribution of, 138f
Credentialing, 8
Cricoid cartilage, 342
Cricothyroid membrane, 341
Cricothyrotomy, 355
Crigler-Najjar syndrome, 656
Crile, George W., 4
Critical care medicine, 918–942
    acquired neuromuscular disorders in,
        941–942
    acute renal failure, 932
    acute respiratory failure, 930–932
    anemia and transfusion therapy in, 934
    cardiovascular and hemodynamic aspects
        of, 924–930
        monitoring, 924–925
    endocrine aspects of, 932–934
    nutrition in, 935
    sedation, 935–936

Critical illness polyneuropathy and myopathy (CIPNM), 941
Crossmatch, 105
Cross sectional studies, 17
CRPS. *See* Complex regional pain syndrome (CRPS)
CRPS I. *See* Complex regional pain syndrome (CRPS) I
CRPS II. *See* Complex regional pain syndrome (CRPS) II
Cryoprecipitate
  collection and preparation of, 107
  indications for administration of, 104t
  transfusion thresholds, 103
Crystalloid, 83–85
Crystalloid intravenous fluids *vs.* colloids, 84
CT. *See* Computed tomography (CT)
Curare, 6
Curbelo, Martinez, 3
Cushing, Harvey, 4
Cushing's syndrome, 683, 685t
Cyclopentolate
  anesthetic ramifications of, 575
Cystectomy
  radical, 618
Cystourethroscopy, 609
Cytochromes P450, 126–127, 127t
Cytokines, 810, 810t

D
Dalmane. *See* Flurazepam (Dalmane)
Dalteparin (Fragmin), 1057–1058
Damages, 32
Danaparoid (Organan), 1058
Danshen, 1112
Dantrium. *See* Dantrolene (Dantrium)
Dantrolene (Dantrium), 1058–1059
Data collection, 37
Data structure, 18
Datex-Ohmeda Aladin Cassette Vaporizer, 333
Datex-Ohmeda S/5 ADU, 339
Datex-Ohmeda Tec 6 vaporizer, 332
DDAVP. *See* Desmopressin acetate (DDAVP, Stimate)
D-dimer, 113
Dead space, 366
  alveolar, 473
Deaths, 39
  anesthesia-related, 37
Decadron. *See* Dexamethasone (Hexadrol, Decadron)
Deep peroneal nerve block, 437
Deep sedation
  definition of, 832t, 1028–1029
Deep venous thrombosis
  regional anesthesia, 674t
  with total hip arthroplasty, 673
Defibrillation
  in ACLS, 952
Defibrillators
  in ACLS, 952–953
Delayed ischemic neurological deficits (DIND), 923
Delivery room
  newborn resuscitation in, 708–709
Delta-tubocurarine, 1107
Demerol. *See* Meperidine (Demerol)
Dental surgery, 841–842

Dentistry, 850
Depolarizing blocking drugs, 237–241
Depolarizing muscle relaxants
  for myasthenia gravis, 497–498
Depression
  neonatal, 708t
Dermatome, 393, 394f
  of arm, 423f
Dermatomyositis, 313–314
Descriptive statistics, 18
Desflurane
  airway resistance, 227f
  for ambulatory surgery, 764
  autonomic nervous system, 223
  brain neurophysiology, 442t
  carbon dioxide absorbers, 230
  with cardiac surgery, 521
  chemical structure of, 209f
  clinical overview of, 216
  coronary steal, 223
  creation of, 3
  evoked potentials, 447t
  for neonates, 716
  shunt fraction, 228f
  stress hormone response, 224f
Desipramine, 1059
Desmopressin acetate (DDAVP, Stimate), 527, 1059
Devil's claw, 1112
Dexamethasone (Hexadrol, Decadron), 1060
  for children, 735
Dexmedetomidine (Precedex), 158, 293, 1060
  with chronic renal failure, 604
  dosages of, 775t
  for ICU patients, 936
  for monitored anesthesia care, 776–777
Dextromethorphan
  genetic variability in response to, 57
Dextrose, 82
Diabetes, 282
Diabetes insipidus, 692–693
Diabetes mellitus, 687–692
  classification of, 688t
  emergencies, 690–691
  glycemic goals, 690
  intraoperative management, 691t
  preoperative evaluation of, 689t
  treatment of, 689t, 690t
Diabetic ketoacidosis, 690–692, 691t, 692t
Diaphragmatic injury, 794
Diaschisis, 443
Diazepam (Valium), 288, 1060
  for ambulatory surgery, 759t
  chemical structure of, 169f
  dosages of, 287t, 775t
  evoked potentials, 447t
  physicochemical properties of, 177, 178
Diazoxide, 166
Dibenzyline. *See* Phenoxybenzamine (Dibenzyline)
Diclofenac, 1061
  pharmacokinetics of, 886t
Difficult airway, 351–356
  algorithm for, 351–353, 354f, 1034f
  awake management of, 353–354
  cause of, 352
  fiberoptic bronchoscope, 354–355
  management of, 343t

Difunisal
  pharmacokinetics of, 885t
Digitalis effect
  EKG of, 986
Digoxin (Lanoxin), 158–159, 1061
  for thyroid storm, 681t
Dilantin. *See* Phenytoin (Dilantin)
Dilaudid. *See* Hydromorphone (Dilaudid)
Diltiazem (Cardizem), 163, 1061–1062
  effects during anesthesia, 823t
  genetic variability in response to, 57
  for ischemia, 521
DIND. *See* Delayed ischemic neurological
  deficits (DIND)
Diphenhydramine (Benadryl), 1062
  dose of, 287t
Diprivan. *See* Propofol (Diprivan)
Dipyridamole, 1062
Direct airway injury, 785t
Direct currents, 61
Direct thrombin inhibitors, 119
Disaster preparedness, 960–962
  government role, 961–962
Disasters
  biologic, 964–966
  resulting in mass casualties, 961t
Disease
  genetic basis of, 49–50
Disk herniation
  pain distribution associated with, 905t
Diuretics
  effects during anesthesia, 823t
  preoperative, 547t
DLCO. *See* Carbon monoxide diffusing
  capacity (DLCO)
Dobutamine (Dobutrex), 156, 1062
  for congenital heart defects, 541t
  for shock, 929
Dobutamine echocardiography
  preoperative evaluation, 279
Dobutrex. *See* Dobutamine (Dobutrex)
Dolophine. *See* Methadone (Dolophine)
Dong quai, 1112
Donor proteins
  reactions to, 100
Donors
  anesthetic management of, 855–858
    kidney, 857
    liver, 857–858
    lung
      cadaveric, 857t
Dopamine (Intropin), 143, 156–157,
  1062–1063
  clinical uses of, 157
  combination therapy, 157
  for congenital heart defects, 541t
  preoperative evaluation of, 279
  for shock, 929
  side effects of, 157
Dopram. *See* Doxapram (Dopram)
Dorsal decubitus positions, 357–360, 358t
  physiology, 357
Double lumen endobronchial tube, 4, 488
  malposition of, 491f
  verifying position, 489t, 490f, 490t
Double-lung transplantation, 865–866
Doxacurium (Nuromax), 245, 1063
  clearance, 244t
  comparative pharmacology of, 242t
  pharmacokinetics of, 241t

Doxapram (Dopram), 1063
Draeger Medical Narkomed 6000 series,
  339
Droperidol (Inapsine), 6, 1063–1064
  for children, 735
  for postoperative nausea and vomiting,
    765t
Drotrecogin alfa (Xigris), 1064
Drugs
  absorption, 121
  administration routes, 121t
  agonists, 134t
  allergy
    immunologic mechanisms of, 816
    tests for, 817t
  binding to plasma proteins, 128–130
  binding to proteins, 129t
  biotransformation reactions, 126–127,
    128t
  compartmental pharmacokinetic models,
    130–131
  concentration-response relationships, 133
  cost of, 15
  distribution, 121–122
    volumes of, 130
  dose-receptor interactions, 133
  dose-response curve
    slope, 132
  dose-response curves, 132–133
    and drug interactions, 819
  efficacy of, 132
  elimination, 123–125
  half times, 129
  hepatic blood flow, 124f
  hepatic drug clearance, 123–125
  induced sedation
    for TBI, 921
  infusions
    pharmacokinetic principles of, 136
  interactions, 135t, 819–827
    drug-drug interactions, 819
    pharmaceutical interactions, 819
    pharmacodynamic, 821t, 822–823
    pharmacodynamic interactions
      affecting hemodynamics, 824–827
    pharmacokinetics of, 820–821
  metabolism, 126–128
  molecular properties of, 120–121
  pharmacokinetic principles of, 129–130
  placental transfer of, 122
  potency of, 132
  rate constants, 129
  receptor interactions, 134t
  redistribution of, 122
  renal clearance of, 125–126, 126t
  rise to steady-state concentration, 136
  transfer across membranes, 120–121
  variability of, 133
Duchenne's muscular dystrophy, 295–297
Duragesic. *See* Fentanyl (Duragesic,
  Sublimaze)
Dura mater, 392–393
Duranest. *See* Etidocaine (Duranest)

E
Ear surgery, 586
ECC. *See* Emergency cardiac care (ECC)
ECG. *See* Echocardiography (ECG)
Echinacea, 1112
  toxicity of, 825t

Echocardiography (ECG), 926. *See also*
    Transesophageal echocardiography
    (TEE)
  ambulatory
    preoperative evaluation, 279
  dobutamine
    preoperative evaluation, 279
  stress
    preoperative evaluation, 279
Echothiophate
  anesthetic ramifications of, 575
Eclampsia, 702–703
ECT. *See* Electroconvulsive therapy (ECT)
Edecrin. *See* Ethacrynic acid (Edecrin)
Edrophonium (Tensilon), 1064
  adjustments for elderly, 753t
  for neonates, 717
  pharmacokinetics of, 252t
Efferent autonomic nervous system
  schematic diagram of, 140f
EKG. *See* Electrocardiograph (EKG)
Elbow
  peripheral nerve blockade, 427, 427t
  surgery, 667
Elderly, 741–754. *See also* Aging
  analgesic and anesthetic requirement,
    749–751
  anesthetic adjustments in, 753t
  autonomic nervous system, 748–749
  body composition, 746–747
  cardiopulmonary function in, 744–745
  central nervous system, 747–748
  common drugs for, 752t
  hepatorenal and immune function,
    745–746
  metabolism, 746–747
  perioperative management and outcome,
    751–752
  peripheral nervous system, 748
  pharmacokinetics of, 746–747
  postoperative cognitive dysfunction,
    753–754
Elective aortic surgery, 566–567
Elective lower extremity revascularization,
    569–570, 570t
Elective oral tracheal intubation
  first use of, 4
Electrical and fire safety, 61–73
Electrical power
  grounded, 63
  ungrounded, 63
Electrical shock hazards, 62–68
Electricity
  principles of, 61
Electrocardiogram-cardiac cycle, 977
Electrocardiogram (EKG), 977–985
  atlas, 975–999
  exercise
    preoperative evaluation, 279
  lead placement for, 975
  preoperative evaluation of, 279
  three-lead systems, 976
Electroconvulsive therapy (ECT), 70,
    838–841, 840t
Electroencephalogram (EEG), 385–386
  neurosurgery anesthesia, 444, 444t,
    445t
  computerized processing, 444–446
Electrolyte disturbances, 986
  with trauma, 806

Electrolytes, 87–97, 283
  composition of fluid losses, 83
  physiologic role of, 88t
Electrolyte therapy
  in neonates, 714
Electromagnetic interference (EMI), 71
Electrophysiology
  cardiac, 506–507
  cellular, 506
  clinical, 506–507
  procedures for, 837
Electrosurgery, 68–69
Electrosurgical unit (ESU), 68
  bipolar, 70
  return plate, 69f, 70t
  unipolar, 70
Emergency aortic surgery, 567–568
Emergency cardiac care (ECC)
  algorithm for, 1004f
Emergency cardiopulmonary resuscitation
  adult
    algorithm for, 946f
Emergency preparedness
  JCAHO, 959–960
EMI. *See* Electromagnetic interference
    (EMI)
EMLA. *See* Lidocaine/prilocaine (EMLA)
Emotional considerations, 29–30
Empyema
  bronchopleural, 494–495
Enalapril
  effects during anesthesia, 823t
Endobronchial tube
  double lumen, 4, 488
  malposition of, 491f
    verifying position, 489t, 490f, 490t
  placement, 489f
Endocardial/epicardial flow ratio, 509
Endocrine system, 677–693
  adrenal medulla, 686–687
  diabetes mellitus, 687–692
  parathyroid glands, 682–683
  pituitary gland, 692–693
  thyroid gland, 677–682
Endogenous opioids, 186
Endoscopic retrograde
    cholangiopancreatography (ERCP),
    651, 838–839
Endoscopy
  gastrointestinal, 849–850
Endotracheal tubes, 591f
  for children, 737
  as fire hazards, 72, 73
Endourologic procedures, 609t
  anesthesia for, 609–610
Endovascular surgery
  aortic aneurysms, 564–565, 564t
End-stage liver disease
  multisystem complications of, 861t
End-tidal carbon dioxide, 366, 367t
Enflurane
  brain neurophysiology, 442t
  chemical structure of, 209f
  clinical overview of, 215
  creation of, 2–3
  evoked potentials, 447t
Enoxaparin (Lovenox), 1061–1062
Environmental hazards, 71
Ephedra, 1112
  toxicity of, 825t

•

Ephedrine, 1065
    clinical uses of, 155
    side effects of, 155
Epidemiologic studies, 22
Epidermolysis bullosa, 314
Epidural analgesia
    postoperative, 893t
        order sheet, 898t
Epidural anesthesia, 390, 398–399,
        405–407, 894t
    adjustments for elderly, 753t
    with ambulatory surgery, 762–763
    anatomy, 390–394
    cardiovascular physiology, 409–411,
        410–411, 410t
    for children, 740
    complications of, 412–416
    continuous, 3, 400–401
    duration, 408t
    endocrine-metabolic physiology, 412
    gastrointestinal physiology, 412
    for labor and vaginal delivery, 697–698
    pharmacology of, 402–407
    physiology, 407–412
    respiratory physiology, 411
    risk of, 415t
    selection of, 416t
    technique, 394–396
Epidural fat, 392
Epidural opioids
    latency and duration of, 896t
Epidural space
    anatomy of, 391–392
Epidural steroid injections
    for lumbosacral radiculopathy, 904
    for sciatica, 906t
Epidural test dose, 401
Epiglottitis, 588
    artificial airway, 590t
Epilepsy, 303–304
Epinephrine, 143, 1063
    for ACLS, 954t
    for allergic reactions, 814
    chloroprocaine with, 260t
    clinical uses of, 154–155
    for congenital heart defects, 541t
    for CPR, 954–955
    for intraocular surgery, 579
    metabolism of, 145f
    for shock, 929
    side effects of, 154
    stress hormone response, 224f
    test-dose algorithm for inadequate, 897f
Epinephrine, racemic (Vaponefrin,
        Micronefrin), 1066
ERCP. *See* Endoscopic retrograde
        cholangiopancreatography (ERCP)
Ergonovine (ergotrate), 1066
Ergotrate. *See* Ergonovine (ergotrate)
ERV. *See* Expiratory reserve volume (ERV)
Erythromycin, 1066–1067
Esmolol (Brevibloc), 161, 1067
    for thyroid storm, 681t
Esophageal pressure, 466
Esophageal tracheal combitube, 355–356
Esophagus, 629–630
ESU. *See* Electrosurgical unit (ESU)
Ethacrynic acid (Edecrin), 1067
Ether
    anesthesia before, 1

Ether inhalers
    creation on, 4
Ethosuximide, 305t
Etidocaine (Duranest), 1067–1068
    physiochemical properties of, 259t
    toxicity of, 268t
    uses for surgical epidural anesthesia, 407t
Etodolac
    pharmacokinetics of, 885t
Etomidate (Amidate), 1068
    adjustments for elderly, 753t
    brain neurophysiology, 442t
    chemical structure of, 169f
    with chronic renal failure, 604
    evoked potentials, 447t
    physiochemical properties, 179–180
Etomidate-induced myoclonus, 575
Evoked potential monitoring, 387
    neurosurgery anesthesia, 446
    sensory pathways, 388t
Evoked potentials, 447t
Exclusive service contracts, 13
Exercise electrocardiogram (EKG)
    preoperative evaluation, 279
Expanded interstitial fluid
    mobilization of, 83
Experimental design, 16–21
Expiratory reserve volume (ERV), 974
Expired gas monitoring, 365–368
External jugular vein catheter placement
    anatomic approach for, 378f
Extracellular fluid volume
    conditions associated with deficits in, 85t
    regulation of, 82
Extracorporeal shock wave lithotripsy
        (SWL), 613–615
Extremity injury, 795

F
Facial nerve function monitoring, 387
Factor IX concentrate, 1068–1069
Factor VII a recombinant (Novoseven),
        1068
Factor VIII (Antihemophiliac factor, AHF),
        1068
Familial dysautonomia. *See* Riley-Day sun
        (familial dysautonomia)
Familial periodic paralysis, 298–299, 298t
Familial unconjugated hyperbilirubinemia,
        656
Famotidine (Pepcid), 1069
    dose of, 287t
Fat
    embolus syndrome, 672–673, 673t
    epidural, 392
FDP. *See* Fibrin degradation products (FDP)
Felbamate, 305t
Fenamates
    pharmacokinetics of, 886t
Fenoldopam (Corlopam), 1069
Fenoprofen
    pharmacokinetics of, 885t
Fentanyl (Duragesic, Sublimaze), 5,
        194–197, 207f, 289, 1069–1070,
        1070
    airway reflexes, 196
    for ambulatory surgery, 759t
    brain neurophysiology, 442t
    for cardiac surgery, 529
    cardiovascular effects, 196

CNS effects, 195
    for congenital heart disease, 540
    disposition kinetics, 196
    dosage of, 196–197, 210t, 287t, 623t,
        775t
    effect on volatile anesthesia MAC, 195
    endocrine effects, 196
    evoked potentials, 447t
    gastrointestinal effects, 196
    for labor and vaginal delivery, 696
    latency and duration of, 896t
    for neonates, 717
    with PCA, 892t
    for postoperative pain in children, 900t
    recovery curves, 206f
    respiratory depression, 195
    smooth muscle, 196
    transdermal
        for cancer pain, 914
Fentanyl Oralet (Actiq), 1067
Fenugreek, 1112–1113
Fetus
    biophysical monitoring of, 706t
    circulation, 696t, 711
    exposure to anesthetic drugs, 694–695
    heart rate, 707f
    monitoring, 706–708
    pulse oximetry, 707–708
Fever
    postoperative, 443–444
Feverfew, 1113
Fiberoptic central venous catheters, 925
Fibrin degradation products (FDP), 109,
    113
Fibrinogen level, 113
Fibrinolysis, 108–109
    laboratory evaluation of, 113
Fire
    extinguishing, 73
    safety, 61–73, 72–73
    triad, 72t
        interruption of, 73
Fistula
    bronchopleural, 494–495
Flail chest
    mechanical ventilation in, 787t
Flaxedil. *See* Gallamine (Flaxedil)
Flecainide
    genetic variability in response to, 57
Flow-volume loops, 477
Fluid management
    physiology of, 81–82
Fluid replacement therapy, 82–83
    for burns, 796–797
    for hypotension, 927–928
    in neonates, 714
Fluid status
    assessment and monitoring of, 85–87
    intraoperative clinical assessment of,
        86–87
Flumazenil (Mazicon), 1070
    chemical structure of, 169f
    for monitored anesthesia care, 774f, 774t
    physiochemical properties, 178
Fluoride-induced nephrotoxicity, 232
Flurazepam (Dalmane), 1068
Folic acid deficiency, 308
Foot surgery, 669, 670t
Foreign body airway
    BLS, 947

Foreign body aspiration, 589–590
4-chloro-m-cresol, 319
Fragmin. *See* Dalteparin (Fragmin)
FRC. *See* Functional residual capacity
    (FRC)
Fresh frozen plasma (FFP)
    collection and preparation of, 106
    indications for administration of,
        103t
    transfusion thresholds, 103
Full disclosure, 12
Functional hemodynamic monitoring
    for critical care medicine, 925–926
Functional reserve
    age-related decrease in, 743f
Functional residual capacity (FRC), 974
    operative site, 481t
Fungal infections
    in ICU, 938
Furosemide (Lasix), 1068
    effects during anesthesia, 823t

G
GABA. *See* Gamma-aminobutyric acid
    (GABA)
Gabapentin (Neurontin), 305t, 1068
Gallamine (Flaxedil), 1071–1072
Gamma-aminobutyric acid (GABA)
    activated ion channels, 43–44
    postsynaptic receptor sites, 170f
Gamma-rays, 963t
Garlic, 1110
    toxicity of, 825t
Gas
    analysis, 369t
    bulk flow of, 472
    diffusion, 472
    monitoring
        inspiratory and expired, 365–368
Gastric banding
    adjustable, 624
Gastric electrical stimulation, 625
Gastric fluid
    pH and volume, 289–290, 291t
Gastroenterology, 838–839, 838t
Gastroesophageal reflux
    LMA, 345
Gastrointestinal disorders, 629–636
    anesthetic management of, 636
    carcinoid tumors, 634–636
    esophagus, 629–630
    intestines, 632–634
    perioperative aspiration risk, 631–632,
        631t
    protective airway reflexes, 630–631
    stomach, 630
Gastrointestinal endoscopy, 849–850
Gastrointestinal hemorrhage
    in ICU, 938–939
General anesthesia
    for ambulatory surgery, 763–764
    anaphylaxis management during, 812t,
        815t
    for cesarean section, 700–701, 701t
    definition of, 832t, 1029
General damages, 32
Genetic
    variability
        for prolonged postoperative
            mechanical ventilation, 54

Genetics, 50
    analysis
        of complex disease, 50–51
    association studies, 51
    of coronary artery disease, 53
    disease, 49–50
    ethical considerations, 59
    inhalation anesthesia, 229–230
    malignant hyperthermia, 56
    polymorphisms, 58t
    susceptibility to adverse perioperative
        outcomes
        cardiovascular, 53
        neurologic, 53–54
        renal, 54
    targeted drug development, 59
    variation
        of anesthetic agents, 56
        human, 49–50
        perioperative event-free survival, 53
        in response to codeine, 57
Genitourinary system, 850
    anatomy and innervation of, 596
Genomics, 52–53
    and critical care, 57–59
Genotype, 50f
Gentamicin, 1072
Geriatrics. *See also* Aging; Elderly
    concepts of, 741
Gilbert's syndrome, 656
Ginger, 1113
    toxicity of, 825t
Ginkgo, 1113
    toxicity of, 825t
Ginseng, 1113
Glasgow Coma Scale, 460, 460t
Glaucoma, 574
Glomerular filtration, 597–598
    rate
        autoregulation of, 598–599, 599f
Gloves
    latex
        reactions to, 26t
Glucagon. *See* Glucagon (Glucagon)
Glucagon (Glucagon), 1072
    liver, 647
Glucocorticoid excess, 683, 685t
Glucose
    in critical illness, 932
Glutamate, 438
Glutamate activated ion channels, 43
Glycogen storage disease, 327
Glycoprotein alpha-1 acid
    drugs binding to, 128t
Glycoprotein IIb/IIIa platelet receptor, 53
Glycopyrrolate (Robinul), 1072–1073
    dose of, 287t
Goldenseal, 1113
    toxicity of, 826t
Goldman risk index, 275
Graft-*versus*-host disease (GVHD), 100
Granisetron (Kytril), 1073
Green tea, 1113–1114
Griffith, Harrold, 6
Ground fault circuit interrupter, 66–67
Ground plate, 68
Ground wires
    equipment with, 64f
    equipment without, 62f
Gudel, Arthur, 4

Guillain-Barre syndrome, 301–302
GVHD. *See* Graft-*versus*-host disease
        (GVHD)
GW280430A, 245
Gynecology, 850

H
Haldol. *See* Haloperidol (Haldol)
Hall, Richard, 3
Haloperidol (Haldol), 1073
Halothane
    blood pressure, 221f
    brain neurophysiology, 442t
    caffeine contracture test, 319
    carbon dioxide absorbers, 230
    cardiac index, 222f
    chemical structure of, 209f
    clinical overview of, 215
    creation of, 2
    evoked potentials, 447t
    hemodynamics, 220
    hepatic blood flow, 229f
    hepatitis, 232–234
    history of, 205
    metabolism, 233f
Halsted, William, 3
Hand surgery, 667–668
HCV. *See* Hepatitis C virus (HCV)
Head and neck surgery, 584t
Head injury, 460–463, 791t
    anesthesia, 804
    early management of, 788–792
    emergency treatment, 461t
    preanesthetic management, 462t
    systemic sequelae, 463t
Health care
    safety standards for, 919
Health Insurance Portability and
        Accountability (HIPAA), 13–14
Hearing loss
    with epidural and spinal anesthesia, 413
Heart. *See also* Cardiac
    anatomy of, 499–500, 500f
    autonomic innervation, 141
    neonatal, 714–716
    rate
        of fetal, 707f
    transplantation, 866–867
        with nontransplant surgery and
            anesthetic management, 868–869
Heart disease. *See also* Valvular heart
        disease
    carcinoid, 635
    with labor, 704
HELPP syndrome, 654
Hemodynamic control, 6
Hemodynamic formulas, 972
Hemodynamic monitoring
    functional
        for critical care medicine, 925–926
    with trauma, 797
Hemodynamic values, 510t
Hemoglobin concentration, 283
Hemoglobinopathies, 308–310
Hemolytic anemia, 308
Hemorrhage
    antepartum, 704
    gastrointestinal
        in ICU, 938–939
Hemorrhagic fever, 966

Hemorrhagic shock
advanced trauma life support
classification of, 789t
Hemostasis, 107–119
acquired disorders of, 117–119, 118t
diagnosis, 117t
disorders of, 116–119
hereditary disorders of, 116, 117t
laboratory evaluation of, 110–116
tests interpretation, 113–114
Hemotherapy, 98–119
Henderson-Hasselbalch equation, 74, 74f
Heparin, 1070–1071
in cardiopulmonary bypass, 119
reversed with protamine, 536
Hepatic. See Liver
Hepatitis
halothane, 232–234
Hepatitis C virus (HCV)
with blood product administration, 98
Hepatobiliary imaging, 650–651
Hepatocellular carcinoma, 654
Herbal medications, 1110–1116
neuraxial anesthesia, 548t
toxicity of, 825t–826t
Hering-Breuer reflex, 469
Heritability, 50. See also Genetics
Hernia
congenital diaphragmatic, 720–721, 721t
Herpes zoster, 910, 910t
Hespan. See Hetastarch (Hespan)
Hetastarch (Hespan), 1074
Heterozygous, 50f
Hexadrol. See Dexamethasone (Hexadrol,
Decadron)
High-frequency jet ventilation, 494
HIPAA. See Health Insurance Portability
and Accountability (HIPAA)
Hip arthroplasty
total
deep venous thrombosis with, 673
Hip surgery, 668
Histamine
nonimmunologic release of, 814
HIV. See Human immunodeficiency virus
(HIV)
HMG COA reductase inhibitors
preoperative, 546t
Holter monitoring
preoperative evaluation, 279
Homozygous, 50f
Horner's syndrome, 432t
Horse chestnut, 1114
Hospital subsidies, 13
Host defense systems, 808
HPA axis. See Hypothalamic-pituitary
adrenal (HPA) axis
Human factors, 26
Human genetic variation, 49–50
Human Genome Project, 59
Human immunodeficiency virus (HIV),
705–706
with blood product administration, 98
chronic pain in, 915
Hurricaine. See Benzocaine (Americaine,
Hurricaine)
Hydralazine (Apresoline), 165, 1074
effects during anesthesia, 823t
Hydrocodone
pharmacokinetics of, 888t

Hydrocortisone (Solu-Cortef), 1074
for thyroid storm, 681t
Hydrogen cyanide, 968
Hydromorphone (Dilaudid), 1075
with PCA, 892t
pharmacokinetics of, 888t
Hyperbaric local anesthetic solutions
in supine position, 404f
Hyperbicarbonatemia, 75
Hyperbilirubinemia, 648, 650t
Hypercalcemia, 94–95
signs and symptoms of, 95t
Hypercapnia
chronic, 79
Hyperglycemia, 932
Hyperkalemia, 92–93
with chronic renal failure, 604t
signs and symptoms of, 93t
treatment of, 93t
Hypermagnesemia, 97
signs and symptoms of, 97t
Hypernatremia, 89–90
signs and symptoms of, 90t
treatment of, 90t
Hyperosmolar nonketotic coma, 691t
Hyperparathyroidism, 682–683
Hyperphosphatemia, 95
Hyperreflexia, 137
autonomic, 661t
Hypersensitivity
classification of, 811t
Hypertension
intracranial
emergency treatment, 461t
postoperative, 874t
Hyperthyroidism, 677–681
preparation of, 680t
Hypertonic fluid administration
clinical implications of, 85
Hypertonic solutions, 83–85
Hypertrophic cardiomyopathy, 523
Hyperventilation
supratentorial intracranial tumors, 452
for TBI, 922–923
Hypervolemia, 83
Hypervolemic/hypertensive and
hemodilution
for subarachnoid hemorrhage, 923–924
Hypnotics
for ICU patients, 936
Hypocalcemia, 93–94, 683t
signs and symptoms of, 94t
treatment of, 94t
Hypogastric plexus blockade, 433–434
Hypoglycemia, 692
Hypokalemia, 90–91
signs and symptoms of, 91t
treatment of, 92t
Hypomagnesemia, 96–97
signs and symptoms of, 96t
treatment of, 96t
Hyponatremia, 88
after subarachnoid hemorrhage, 924
signs and symptoms of, 89t
Hypoparathyroidism, 683
Hypotension
algorithm for, 1013f–1014f
with obstetric anesthesia, 702t
in PACU, 873t
postoperative, 873, 873t

Hypotension (*cont.*)
  refractory, 815
  with trauma, 805
Hypothalamic-pituitary adrenal (HPA) axis, 685
Hypothalamus, 137
Hypothermia, 443–444
  with trauma, 805
Hypothesis formulation, 17
Hypothyroidism, 681–682, 681t
Hypoventilation
  postoperative, 875t
Hypovolemia
  in hypotensive and tachycardiac patients, 790t
  laboratory evidence of, 86, 86t
  signs and symptoms of, 85t
  with trauma, 803–804

I
Ibuprofen, 1075
  for children, 739, 900t
  pharmacokinetics of, 885t
IC. *See* Inspiratory capacity (IC)
ICG. *See* Indocyanine green (ICG)
ICP. *See* Intracranial pressure (ICP)
ICU. *See* Intensive care unit (ICU)
IGS. *See* Implantable gastric stimulator (IGS)
Ileus
  postoperative, 633, 634t
Ilioinguinal blockade, 431
Imipenem and cilastin (Primaxin), 1072
Imipramine, 1075–1076
Imitrex. *See* Sumatriptan succinate (Imitrex)
Immersion lithotripsy, 613, 614t
Immune response
  cells, 810, 810t
Immune suppression
  chronic
    multisystem complications of, 859t
Immunoglobulins, 809t
Immunomodulation, 100–101
Impedance, 61
Implantable gastric stimulator (IGS), 625
Inamrinone (Inocor), 1076
Inapsine. *See* Droperidol (Inapsine)
Increased intracranial pressure
  signs, 450t
Indels, 49
Inderal. *See* Propranolol (Inderal)
Indicator dilution applications, 379–382
Indirect Coomb's test, 105
Indocyanine green (ICG), 649–650
Indomethacin, 1076
  pharmacokinetics of, 885t
Infants
  complicating anatomic factors in, 715f
  MAC, 718t
  maximum local anesthetic doses in, 901t
  postoperative apnea, 720
Infection, 27–29
  nosocomial
    in ICU, 936–938
  sources from patients, 28t
Inferential statistics, 18–19
Information resources, 8
Information technology
  preoperative evaluation, 272–294

Infraclavicular approach
  to peripheral nerve blockade, 424
Infratentorial intracranial tumors, 454–456
Inguinal hernia, 723
Inhalation anesthesia, 205–234, 213f, 219f
  absorbent interaction, 338, 338t
  age-related, 750f
  anesthetic metabolism, 232–234
  autonomic nervous system, 223
  bronchiolar smooth muscle tone, 225
  carbon dioxide, 225
    absorbers, 230–232
  carbon monoxide and heat, 231–232
  for cardiac surgery, 520–521, 529
  chemical structure of, 209f
  for children, 730–731, 731
  circulatory system, 220–223
  clinical overview of, 215–217
  delivery systems for, 328–340
  elimination of, 215f
  exhalation and recovery, 214
  genetic effects, 229–230
  hemodynamics, 220–221
  hepatic arterial blood flow, 645
  hepatic effects, 227–228
  history of, 205–206
  hypoxemia, 225
  intracranial pressure, 220
  for labor and vaginal delivery, 699
  malignant hyperthermia, 228–229
  minimum alveolar concentration, 217–219, 218t
  minute ventilation, 225f
  myocardial contractility, 223
  myocardial ischemia, 223
  for neonates, 716
  neuromuscular effects, 228–229
  neuropharmacology of, 217–220
  obstetric effects, 230
  overpressurization, 212
  perfusion effects, 213–214
  pharmacoeconomics, 234
  pharmacokinetics of, 210–214
  physical characteristics, 210t
  pulmonary system, 223–227
  pulmonary vascular resistance, 227
  respiratory rate, 225f
  second generation of, 2–3
  tidal volume, 225f
  value-based decisions, 234
  ventilation effects, 213
  ventilatory mechanics, 224
Injection anesthesia
  age-related, 750f
Injury
  functional genomics of, 59
  genetic variability in response to, 57–59
Inocor. *See* Inamrinone (Inocor)
Inomax. *See* Nitric oxide (Inomax)
Inotropes
  for shock, 928–929
INR. *See* International normalized ratio (INR)
Insertion-deletion polymorphisms, 50f
Inspiratory and expired gas monitoring, 365–368
Inspiratory capacity (IC), 974
Inspiratory reserve volume (IRV), 974
Intensive care unit (ICU)
  complications in, 936–942

Interactions. *See also* specific drugs
  pharmacokinetics of, 820–821
Intercostal nerve blockade, 428–430
  complications of, 431t
  hand and needle positions for, 430f
  landmarks, 429f
Interleukins, 810
Internal jugular vein catheter placement
  anatomic approach for, 377f
International normalized ratio (INR), 112,
  649
Internet, 8
Interpleural anesthesia, 430–431
Interscalene approach
  to brachial plexus, 423t
  to peripheral nerve blockade, 422
Interventional neuroradiology, 833–834
  for alternate site anesthesia, 833–834
  anticoagulation with, 834
  complications of, 834t
  for subarachnoid hemorrhage, 924
Intestinal obstruction, 723
Intestines, 632–634
Intra-aortic balloon pump, 534, 536t
Intracranial aneurysms, 457–458
Intracranial hypertension
  emergency treatment, 461t
Intracranial pressure (ICP), 440
  colloidal infusions implications, 84
  controlling, 451t
  crystalloid infusions implications, 84
  increased, 450t
  inhalation anesthesia, 220
  intracranial volume, 441f
  measuring, 448f
  monitoring, 385
  neurosurgery anesthesia, 446
Intraocular pressure, 574
Intraoperative blood volume replacement
  clinical indicators of, 87t
Intraoperative death
  with trauma, 806
Intrapulmonary shunt, 973
Intraspinal opioids
  for cancer pain, 914
Intrathecal opioid administration, 891
Intravascular catheter-associated bacteremia
  in ICU, 937–938
Intravenous anesthetics
  for anesthesia maintenance, 183–185,
    184f
  clinical pharmacological properties of,
    174–181
  clinical uses of, 181–185
  for congenital heart disease, 540
  context-sensitive half-time, 171
  desirable characteristics of, 168t
  efficacy of, 172
  elimination half-time, 171
  factors influencing dose requirements,
    183t
  hemodynamic effects, 173t
  hypersensitivity of, 173–174
  as induction agents, 181–183, 182t
  for neonates, 717
  neurophysiology, 443
  perfusion-limited clearance, 171
  pharmacodynamic effects of, 171–172
  pharmacokinetics of, 170t
    interpatient variability in, 171t

physiochemical properties of, 174–181
  potency, 172
  for sedation, 185
Intravenous contrast agents
  for alternate site anesthesia, 833
Intravenous infusion pumps
  desirable features of, 136t
Intravenous medications, 5–6
  pharmacokinetics of, 134–136
Intravenous sedative hypnotics
  with cardiac surgery, 521
Intropin. *See* Dopamine (Intropin)
Intubating laryngeal mask airway, 349
Invasive arterial monitoring
  complications of, 374
Ion channels, 43
Ionizing radiation, 963t
  potential sources of exposure to, 962–963
  protection from, 833
Ion trapping, 120–121
Iron deficiency anemia, 308
IRV. *See* Inspiratory reserve volume (IRV)
Ischemia
  EKG of, 987
Ischemic optic neuropathy
  with ophthalmic surgery, 580–582
Islet transplantation, 863
Isoflurane, 226f
  autonomic nervous system, 223
  brain neurophysiology, 442t
  carbon dioxide absorbers, 230
  with cardiac surgery, 521
  carotid endarterectomy, 558
  chemical structure of, 209f
  clinical overview of, 215–216
  for congenital heart disease, 540
  coronary steal, 223
  creation of, 2–3
  evoked potentials, 447t
  hepatic blood flow, 229f
  for neonates, 716
  shunt fraction, 228t
  stress hormone response, 224f
Isolated power system
  decision to install, 71–72
  safety feature of, 65f
Isolation precautions, 27–29
Isolation transformer, 64f
Isoproterenol (Isuprel), 155–156, 1077
  adjustments for elderly, 753t
  clinical uses of, 156
  for congenital heart defects, 541t
  side effects of, 156
Isoptin. *See* Verapamil (Calan, Isoptin)
Isosorbide
  effects during anesthesia, 823t
Isovolemic anemia
  vs. acute blood loss, 101–103
Isovolemic hemodilution
  compensatory mechanisms maintaining
    oxygen delivery during, 102t
Isuprel. *See* Isoproterenol (Isuprel)

J
JCAHO. *See* Joint Commission on the
  Accreditation of Healthcare
  Organizations (JCAHO)
Jehovah's Witnesses, 34–35
  transfusions, 104
Job market, 12

Johnson, Enid, 6
Johnstone, Michael, 2
Joint Commission on the Accreditation of
    Healthcare Organizations (JCAHO),
    9, 10, 12, 35
  emergency preparedness, 959–960
  patient safety goals, 36t
  preoperative evaluation, 272
  quality improvement, 36
  standards, 828–833
Joule, 61
Journal
  first anesthetic, 7
Journal articles
  reading, 21
Jugular venous bulb oximetry
  neurosurgery anesthesia, 448

K
Kanamycin (Kantrex), 1077
Kantrex. *See* Kanamycin (Kantrex)
Kava-kava, 1114
  toxicity of, 826t
Ketalar. *See* Ketamine (Ketalar)
Ketamine (Ketalar), 5, 1077
  brain neurophysiology, 442t
  chemical structure of, 169f
  for children, 732
  with dental surgery, 841
  dosages of, 775t
  evoked potentials, 447t
  for labor and vaginal delivery, 697
  for monitored anesthesia care, 776
  for neonates, 717
  for office-based anesthesia, 852
  physiochemical properties, 180–181
  with renal failure of, 602
Ketoprofen
  pharmacokinetics of, 885t
Ketorolac (Toradol), 1078
  for children, 739
  pharmacokinetics of, 885t
Kidney donors
  living
    anesthetic management of, 857
Kidneys. *See also* Renal
  alpha receptors in, 148
  anatomy and physiology of, 596–600
  anatomy of, 597f
  beta receptors in, 148
  physiology of, 597–600
Kirstein, Albert, 4
Knee arthroplasty
  total, 669
Knee arthroscopy, 669
Koller, Carl, 3
Konakion. *See* Phytonadione
    (AquaMephyton, Konakion)
Korotkoff sounds
  auscultation, 371–372
Kyphoscoliosis, 295
Kytril. *See* Granisetron (Kytril)

L
Labetalol (Normodyne, Trandate), 161,
    1078
  effects during anesthesia, 823t
Labor and delivery
  anesthesia for, 696–699
Laboratory studies, 23, 284t

Lambert-Eaton syndrome. *See* Myasthenic
    syndrome (Lambert-Eaton
    syndrome)
Lamotrigine, 305t
Landsteiner, Karl, 6
Lanoxin. *See* Digoxin (Lanoxin)
Laparoscopic surgery
  carbon dioxide surgery, 638
  cardiovascular effects, 638
  cerebral blood flow, 640
  gas exchange effects, 640
  neurohumoral response, 638
  nitrous oxide as fire hazard during, 73
  patient position, 640
  physiologic changes, 639f
  physiologic effects of, 638–640
  pneumoperitoneum mechanical effects,
    638
  renal blood flow, 640
  splanchnic blood flow, 640
  urologic surgery, 616
  VATS, 642t, 643
Large-scale gene and protein expression
    profiling, 51–52
Laryngeal mask airway (LMA), 4, 344–345
  bronchospasms, 345
  for children, 737–738
  complications of, 346t
  contraindications to, 345t
  in failed airway, 355
  Fastrach, 349
  gastroesophageal reflux, 345
  intubating, 349
  positive-pressure ventilation, 345
  proseal, 345, 346t
  remifentanil, 201
Laryngeal tube, 345
Laryngoscope blade, 347
  straight, 4
Laryngoscopy
  for tracheal intubation, 346–347
Laryngospasm
  causing difficult airway, 350
Laryngotracheobronchitis, 588–589
Larynx
  innervation of, 341
  skeleton of, 341
Laser plumes
  viruses in, 29
Lasers, 590t
  urologic surgery, 616
Lasix. *See* Furosemide (Lasix)
Lateral decubitus positions, 360–361, 360t
Latex allergy, 25, 818
Latex gloves
  reactions to, 26t
Lawen, Arthur, 6
Lawsuits. *See* Malpractice suits
LBBB. *See* Bundle-branch block-left (LBBB)
Leapfrog Group, 919
LeFort classification of fractures, 592
LeFort III fractures, 594–595
Left atrium
  anatomy of, 500
Left ventricle
  anatomy of, 500
Left ventricular stroke work index
    (LVSWI), 972
Lepirudin (Refludan), 1078–1079
LES. *See* Lower esophageal sphincter (LES)

Levetiracetam, 305t
Levobupivacaine (Chirocaine), 1079
  cardiovascular toxicity of, 265
  clinical profile of, 266t
  toxicity of, 268t
Levophed. *See* Norepinephrine (Levophed)
Librium. *See* Chlordiazepoxide (Librium)
Licorice, 1114
  toxicity of, 826t
Lidocaine (Xylocaine), 1079
  for ACLS, 954t
  clinical profile of, 266t, 267t
  for congenital heart defects, 541t
  for CPR, 955
  dose and duration of, 406t
  dose-dependent systemic effects of, 268t
  with epinephrine, 260t
  neural toxicity of, 269
  peak plasma concentrations of, 262t
  physiochemical properties of, 259t
  test-dose algorithm for inadequate, 897f
  toxicity of, 268t
  uses for surgical epidural anesthesia, 407t
Lidocaine/prilocaine (EMLA), 1079–1080
Lidocaine topical patches, 890
Ligaments
  anatomy of, 391
Ligand gated channels, 43
Limb replantation
  microvascular surgery, 671t
Line isolation monitor, 65–66, 66f
Linkage analysis, 51
Lipid *versus* protein targets, 45
Liposuction, 849
Lisinopril
  effects during anesthesia, 823t
Lithotripsy
  immersion, 613, 614t
Liver, 644–658
  anatomy of, 644–646
  biopsy, 652
  blood flow regulation, 646–647
  cholestatic disease, 656
  cirrhosis
    pathophysiology of, 652t
  drug metabolism, 822t
  extraction ratios, 124f, 125t
  failure
    acute, 863
    renal dysfunction with, 609
  function assessment, 647–653, 648t
  hematoma, 654
  humoral regulators, 647
  infarct, 654
  innervation of, 645–646
  intrahepatic circulation, 645
  laboratory evaluation, 647–650, 649t
  living donors
    anesthetic management of, 857–858
  lobes *vs.* segments, 644
  lymphatic system, 646
  postoperative dysfunction, 656
    etiology, 658t
    prevention and treatment of, 656–658
  pregnancy-related disorders, 654
  rupture, 654
  transformations in drug interactions, 821–822
  transplantation, 860–863
  vascular supply of, 644–645

Liver disease, 282
  azotemia, 653t
  classification of, 651t
  end-stage
    multisystem complications of, 861t
    perioperative management of, 657t
    preoperative approach to, 655f
Living donors
  anesthetic management of
    kidney, 857
    liver, 857–858
LMA. *See* Laryngeal mask airway (LMA)
Local anesthetics, 255–271
  adjustments for elderly, 753t
  allergic reactions to, 271
  with alpha-2 adrenergic agonists, 261
  cardiovascular toxicity of, 265–266
  clinical pharmacokinetics of, 264
  clinical profile of, 266t
  clinical use of, 264t
  with clonidine, 261
  distribution of, 263
  elimination of, 263–264
  with epinephrine, 260t, 261
  mechanism of action, 255–258
  molecular mechanisms of, 257
  neural toxicity of, 269
  with opioids, 261
  pharmacodynamics of, 258–261
  pharmacokinetics of, 261–264, 263t
  pharmacology of, 258–261
  physiochemical properties of, 259t
  spreading in epidural space, 408t
  spreading in subarachnoid space, 404t
  systemic absorption of, 263t
  systemic toxicity of
    treatment of, 268–269, 269t
  toxicity of, 264–271
  uses for surgical epidural anesthesia, 407t
Locus, 50f
Logic of proof, 17
Long, Crawford Williamson, 1
Long Island Society of Anesthetists, 7
Longitudinal studies, 17
Lopressor. *See* Metoprolol (Lopressor)
Lorazepam (Ativan), 288, 1080
  chemical structure of, 169f
  dosage of, 287t
  physiochemical properties of, 177, 178
Losartan
  effects during anesthesia, 823t
Loss of resistance technique
  locating epidural space, 399, 400f
Lovage root, 1114
Lovenox. *See* Enoxaparin (Lovenox)
Low back pain, 903
Lower esophageal sphincter (LES), 629, 631t
Lower extremities
  elective revascularization, 569–570
  orthopedic surgery, 668–669
Lower gastrointestinal obstruction, 724t
Low-molecular weight heparin
  neuraxial anesthesia, 548t
Low-output syndrome, 151
Ludwig's angina, 592
Lumbar epidural anesthesia
  for cesarean section, 700, 700t

Lumbar epidural catheter
  tests ruling out intrathecal or
    intravascular placement of, 697t
Lumbar puncture
  introduction of, 3
Lumbosacral arthropathy, 907
Lumbosacral radiculopathy, 903–904
Lungs
  capacities, 477, 477f, 974
  cysts, 495
  donors
    cadaveric, 857t
  elastic work, 466
  functional anatomy of, 464–466
  gas flow resistance, 466–467
  increased airway resistance, 467
  mechanics of, 466–467
  neonatal
    circulatory changes associated with
      initial expansion, 712t
  structures of, 464–465
  transplantation, 864–866
  transplant recipients
    anesthetic management of, 868
  volume reduction surgery, 495–496
  volumes, 477, 477f, 974
LVSWI. *See* Left ventricular stroke work
    index (LVSWI)

M
MAC. *See* Minimal alveolar concentration
    (MAC)
Macewan, William, 4
Macintosh, Robert, 4
Macintosh blade, 347, 349f
Macintosh laryngoscope, 355
Macroshock, 63
Magnesium, 95, 1080–1081
Magnetic resonance imaging (MRI),
    834–835
Malignant hyperthermia, 315–323, 316t
  classic, 315–316
  clinical presentation of, 315
  diagnosis of, 319–320
  drugs triggering, 318t
  epidemiology of, 319
  genetics of, 56
  grading of, 320t
  incidence of, 319
  inhalation anesthesia, 228–229
  inheritance of, 319
  late onset of, 317
  molecular genetic testing, 321
  protocol for, 1032–1033
  syndrome resembling, 318t
  treatment of, 321–322, 321t, 322t, 323t
Mallampati classification, 274
Malpractice, 32
  proving, 33t
Malpractice insurance, 12
Malpractice suits
  causes of, 33
  named in, 34
Managed care, 13
Mannitol (Osmitrol), 1081
  for head injury, 792
Manufactured workstations
  ASTM standards, 329t
MAO interactions. *See* Monoamine oxidase
    (MAO) interactions

MAP. *See* Mean arterial pressure (MAP)
Mapleson systems, 334, 334t
Marcaine. *See* Bupivacaine (Marcaine,
    Sensorcaine)
Marijuana
  maternal use during pregnancy, 719
Mask induction pharmacology
  for children, 730
Mass casualties
  anesthesiologists role in managing, 962
  disasters resulting in, 961t
Massive blood transfusions
  consequences of, 101t
Mastoidectomy, 586t
Maternal cocaine
  during pregnancy, 719
Maternal marijuana
  during pregnancy, 719
Maternal monitoring, 706–708
Maternal mortality
  with obstetric anesthesia, 702t
Maxillofacial surgery, 850
Maxillofacial trauma, 591–592
Mazicon. *See* Flumazenil (Mazicon)
McMechan, Francis Hoffer, 7
Meadowsweet, 1114
Mean arterial pressure (MAP), 972
Mechanical ventilation, 4
  for acute respiratory failure, 930–931
  weaning from, 479t
Meclofenamate
  pharmacokinetics of, 886t
Meconium aspiration, 713
Mediastinoscopy, 492–493, 493t
Medical staff, 9
Medical therapies
  evaluating evidence for, 919t
Medications. *See* Drugs
Meetings, 11
Mefanamic acid
  pharmacokinetics of, 886t
Membrane disordering, 45–46
Membrane expansion, 45
Membrane perturbation, 45
Membrane potentials, 438
Meninges
  anatomy, 392–393
Meningomyelocele, 724t
Meperidine (Demerol), 193–194, 289, 1078
  for labor and vaginal delivery, 696
  latency and duration of, 896t
  with PCA, 892t
  pharmacokinetics of, 888t
  for postoperative pain in children, 900t
  for thyroid storm, 681t
Mephentermine (Wyamine), 1081–1082
Mepivacaine (Carbocaine), 1082
  clinical profile of, 266t
  with epinephrine, 260t
  peak plasma concentrations, 262t
  physiochemical properties of, 259t
  toxicity of, 268t
  uses for surgical epidural anesthesia,
    407t
Meropenem (Merrem), 1082
Merrem. *See* Meropenem (Merrem)
Mesenteric traction syndrome, 633–634
Mestinon. *See* Pyridostigmine (Regonol,
    Mestinon)

Metabisulfite
  allergic reactions to, 271
Metabolic acidosis
  anesthetic implications of, 78t
  bicarbonate, 75–77
  classification of, 77t
  physiologic effects produced by, 77t
  treatment of, 78t
Metabolic alkalosis, 75t
  bicarbonate, 74
  physiochemical effects produced by, 76t
  treatment of, 77t
Metabolism
  in drug interactions, 820
Metaproterenol, 1082
Metaraminol bitartrate (Aramine), 1083
Methadone (Dolophine), 194, 1083
  latency and duration of, 896t
  with PCA, 892t
  pharmacokinetics of, 888t
Methergine. See Methylergonovine
    (Methergine)
Methohexital (Brevital), 1083
  chemical structure of, 169f
  physiochemical properties of, 174
Methoxamine (Vasoxyl), 151, 1083–1084
Methyldopa (Aldomet, Methyldopate),
    1084
Methyldopate. See Methyldopa (Aldomet,
    Methyldopate)
Methylene blue, 1084
Methylergonovine (Methergine), 1084
Methylmethacrylate, 24, 673–675
Methylparaben
  allergic reactions to, 271
Methylprednisolone (Solu-Medrol),
    1084–1085
  for lumbosacral radiculopathy, 904–907
Metoclopramide (Reglan), 1085
  dosage of, 287t
Metocurine (Metubine), 1085
Metoprolol (Lopressor), 1086
  effects during anesthesia, 823t
Metronidazole, 1086
Metubine. See Metocurine (Metubine)
Meyer-Overton rule, 44–45, 46
Microdialysis, 920
Micronefrin. See Epinephrine, racemic
    (Vaponefrin, Micronefrin)
Microsatellite polymorphisms, 50f
Microsatellites, 49
Microshock, 67–68
Midazolam (Versed), 288, 1086–1087
  for ambulatory surgery, 759t
  for ambulatory surgery in children, 761
  brain neurophysiology, 442t
  chemical structure of, 169f
  dosages of, 287t, 775t
  dose-response relationships, 172f
  evoked potentials, 447t
  as induction agents, 181–183
  for monitored anesthesia care, 773–775
  for obesity, 623t
  physiochemical properties of, 177, 178
Miller, Robert, 4
Miller blade, 347, 349f
Milrinone (Primacor), 158, 1087
Mineralocorticoid excess, 683
Minimal access intraabdominal gynecologic
    procedures, 637

Minimal access procedures
  intraoperative complications, 642t
Minimal alveolar concentration (MAC)
  in children, 731
Minimally invasive cardiac surgery, 537
Minimally invasive procedures, 637–643
  airway management, 641
  ambulatory laparoscopic
    cholecystectomy, 643
  anesthetic technique, 640–641
  laparoscopy
    nitrous oxide as fire hazard during,
      73
    physiologic effects, 638–640
  minimal access intraabdominal
    gynecologic procedures, 637
  monitoring, 641
  nitrous oxide, 641
  postoperative complications, 641–643
  surgical technique, 638
  of trachea, 355
Minimal sedation
  definition of, 832t, 1025
Minimum alveolar concentration (MAC),
    40–41
  inhalation anesthesia, 217–219, 218t
Mitochondria
  cycle of aging, 742f
Mitral regurgitation, 525, 526f
Mitral stenosis, 524–525, 525f
Mivacron. See Mivacurium (Mivacron)
Mivacurium (Mivacron), 245, 1087–1088
  for children, 734t
  clearance of, 244t
  comparative pharmacology of, 242t
  pharmacokinetics of, 241t
Mixed antagonists, 161
Mixed venous oximetry, 378
Mixed venous oxygen content, 973
Mobitz type II
  EKG of, 981
Moderate sedation
  definition of, 832t, 1025
Modified Child-Pugh score, 653t
Monitored anesthesia care, 767–781, 779t
  accumulation, 769–772, 770f
  agitation during, 769t
  distribution, 769–772, 770f
  drug administration optimization, 769
  drug interactions in, 772–773
  drugs used in, 773–777
  duration of action, 769–772, 770f
  elimination, 769–772, 770f
  nonanesthesiologist sedation and
    analgesia, 781
  PCA, 777
  preoperative assessment, 767–768
  respiratory function and sedative
    hypnotics, 777–778
  techniques of, 768
  terminology for, 767
Monitoring, 365–385
  anesthetic
    ASA standards for, 1025–1027
  biochemical, 708
  biophysical, 706–707
Monoamine oxidase (MAO) interactions,
    820–821
Monoclonal antibodies, 859
Morbidity, 39

Morphine, 189–193, 289, 1088
  analgesia, 189–193
  for cancer pain, 914
  cardiovascular effects of, 192–193
  CNS effects of, 192
  disposition kinetics of, 193
  dosage of, 193, 287t
  effect on volatile anesthetic minimum
    alveolar concentration, 192
  epidural, 893t
  latency and duration of, 896t
  for neonates, 717
  with PCA, 892t
  pharmacokinetics of, 888t
  for postoperative pain in children, 900t
  respiratory depression, 192
Morphine, controlled release (MS Contin),
  1088
Mortality, 37, 38t
  anesthesia-related, 37
  maternal
    with obstetric anesthesia, 702t
Morton, William T.G., 1–2
Motor evoked potentials, 387
  drug effects on, 447t
  neurosurgery anesthesia, 446
MRI. *See* Magnetic resonance imaging
  (MRI)
MS Contin. *See* Morphine, controlled
  release (MS Contin)
Multiple expired gas analysis, 368
Multiple sclerosis, 302–303
Multivisceral transplantation, 863–864
Muscle relaxants, 6
  allergenic potential of, 818
  autonomic effects of, 243t
  for children, 733
  with chronic renal failure, 605
  depolarizing
    for myasthenia gravis, 497–498
  drug interactions of, 248t
  histamine-releasing effects of, 243t
  supratentorial intracranial tumors, 453
Muscular dystrophy, 295–297
  Duchenne's, 295–297
Musculoskeletal disorders, 283
Mutation, 49
Myasthenia gravis, 299–301, 300t
  vs. myasthenic syndrome, 302t
Myasthenic syndrome (Lambert-Eaton
  syndrome), 301
  vs. myasthenia gravis, 302t
Myocardial infarction, 987
Myocardial ischemia
  intraoperative
    treatment of, 521–522, 522t
  monitoring for, 519t
Myocardial mechanics, 511
Myocardial metabolism, 511
Myocardial oxygen supply, 512t,
  518–519
Myocardium
  alpha receptors in, 148
  beta receptors in, 148
Myoclonus
  etomidate-induced, 575
Myofascial pain, 907–908
Myoglobinuria
  late onset of, 317
Myotonias, 297–302

Myotonic dystrophy (Steinert's disease),
  297–302
Myringotomy, 586
Myxedema
  treatment of, 682t

N
Nafcillin, 1089
Nalbuphine (Nubain), 202, 1089
Nalmefene hydrochloride (Revex), 1089
Naloxone (Narcan), 203, 1089
  for labor and vaginal delivery, 697
Naltrexone, 203
Naprosyn. *See* Naproxen (Naprosyn)
Naproxen, 1089–1090
  pharmacokinetics of, 885t
  for postoperative pain in children,
    900t
Narcan. *See* Naloxone (Narcan)
Naropin. *See* Ropivacaine (Naropin)
Narrow-complex supraventricular
  tachycardia
  algorithm for, 1010f
Nasal surgery, 590
National Fire Protection Association
  (NFPA)
  health care facilities standards, 71
National Institute for Occupational Safety
  and Health (NIOSH), 24
National Pharmaceutical Stockpile (NPS)
  CDC, 961
National Practitioner Data Bank, 8–9, 35
Natrecor. *See* Nesiritide (Natrecor)
Nausea and vomiting
  with ambulatory surgery, 765, 765t
  PACU, 878–879
  postoperative, 765t
Neck injury, 793
Neck surgery, 584t
Necrotizing enterocolitis, 723, 724t
Needle-based ophthalmic anesthesia
  complications of, 577t
Needles
  for epidural and spinal anesthesia,
    394–396, 395f
Nembutal. *See* Pentobarbital (Nembutal)
Neonates, 711–725
  anatomic and maturational factors of,
    714–716
  anesthetic drugs for, 716–717
  anesthetic management of, 717–719
  anticholinergic drugs for, 716
  arterial blood gas values, 712t
  cardiovascular maturational factors,
    714–716
  circulatory system transition, 711–713
  depression, 708t
  exposure to anesthetic drugs, 694–695
  lungs
    circulatory changes associated with
      initial expansion of, 712t
  MAC, 719t
  pulmonary maturational factors, 714
  regional anesthesia, 718–719
  renal system transition, 714
  resuscitation, 709t
  resuscitation with rapid rhythm and poor
    perfusion, 1020f
  surgical procedures in, 720–725
  tracheal intubation of, 717–718
Neoplasms, 23

Neostigmine (Prostigmin), 1090
  adjustments for elderly, 753t
  for neonates, 717
  pharmacokinetics of, 252t
Neo-Synephrine. *See* Phenylephrine
  (Neo-Synephrine)
Nephrectomy
  radical, 618
Nephron
  anatomy of, 597, 598f
Nerves
  agents, 966–967
  anatomy of, 255
  blocks
    with ambulatory surgery, 763
  fibers
    classification of, 256t
  injury
    with obstetric anesthesia, 702t
Nervous system
  electrophysiologic function, 42–43
Nesacaine. *See* Chloroprocaine (Nesacaine)
Nesiritide (Natrecor), 1090
Neural conduction
  electrophysiology of, 255–257
Neural impulses
  dynamic modulation of, 882–883
  supraspinal modulation of, 883
Neuraxial opioids
  complications of, 893t
  ventilation delayed depression, 898t
Neuroanesthesia, 442–443
Neurogenesis, 443
Neurohumoral response
  laparoscopic surgery, 638
Neuroleptic malignant syndrome,
  317–318
Neurological critical care, 919–924
Neurologic functioning monitoring,
  385–387
Neurologic injury
  with epidural and spinal anesthesia,
  414
Neurolytic blocks, 914t
  for cancer pain, 914
Neuromuscular blocking agents (NMBA),
  235–254
  altered responses to, 248t
  antagonism of, 249t, 251–254
  for cardiac surgery, 530
  cardiovascular effects of, 253–254
  clinical application of, 250
  for congenital heart disease, 540
  for ICU patients, 936
  monitoring of, 248–250
  for neonates, 716–717
  pharmacology of, 235–237
  physiology of, 235–237
  presynaptic events, 237
  reversal of, 253t
Neuromuscular junction, 236f
Neuronal excitability, 42
Neurontin. *See* Gabapentin (Neurontin)
Neuroplasticity, 882
Neuroradiology, 449, 449t
Neurosurgery anesthesia, 438–463
  monitoring, 444–448
Neurosurgical critical care, 919–924
Neutrons, 963t
Newborn. *See* Neonates

New York Society of Anesthetists, 7
NFPA. *See* National Fire Protection
  Association (NFPA)
Nicardipine (Cardene IV), 163, 1090
  effects during anesthesia, 823t
Nicotinic acetylcholine receptor, 236f
Nifedipine (Procardia, Adalat), 162–163,
  1091
  effects during anesthesia, 823t
  for ischemia, 521
Night call, 26–27
Nimbex. *See* Cisatracurium besylate
  (Nimbex)
Nimodipine (Nimotop), 163, 1091
Nimotop. *See* Nimodipine (Nimotop)
NIOSH. *See* National Institute for
  Occupational Safety and Health
  (NIOSH)
Nipride. *See* Nitroprusside (Nipride,
  Nitropress)
Nitric oxide (Inomax), 1091
Nitroglycerin (Tridil, Nitrol IV, Nitrostat
  IV), 165–166, 1091
  for congenital heart defects, 541t
  effects during anesthesia, 823t
  for ischemia, 521
  preoperative vascular surgery, 555t
Nitrol IV. *See* Nitroglycerin (Tridil, Nitrol
  IV, Nitrostat IV)
Nitropress. *See* Nitroprusside (Nipride,
  Nitropress)
Nitroprusside (Nipride, Nitropress), 165,
  1092
  side effects of, 165
Nitrostat IV. *See* Nitroglycerin (Tridil,
  Nitrol IV, Nitrostat IV)
Nitrous oxide, 214f
  for ambulatory surgery, 764
  brain neurophysiology, 442t
  for cardiac surgery, 530
  cellular effects of, 23
  chemical structure of, 209f
  clinical overview of, 217
  evoked potentials, 447t
  as fire hazard during laparoscopic
  surgery, 73
  with gastrointestinal disorders, 634
  myocardial contractility, 223
  for neonates, 716
NMBA. *See* Neuromuscular blocking
  agents (NMBA)
NMDA. *See* N-methyl-D aspartate
  (NMDA)
N-methyl-D aspartate (NMDA)
  receptors, 43
Nociception, 881
  modulation of, 882
Noise pollution, 25–26
Nonadrenergic sympathomimetic agents,
  158–159
Nondepolarizing agents
  for neonates, 716–717
Nondepolarizing muscle relaxants
  adjustments for elderly, 753t
  for children, 733, 734t
  clearance, 244t
  for congenital heart disease, 540
  for intraocular surgery, 579
  for myasthenia gravis, 497
  pharmacokinetics of, 241t

Nondepolarizing neuromuscular blockade
  characteristics of, 239t
Nondepolarizing neuromuscular blocking
  drugs, 241–247
  comparative pharmacology of, 242t
  duration of action, 241–242
  pharmacokinetics of, 241
Nonheart-beating donors
  anesthetic management of, 856–857
Nonimmunologic histamine release
  drugs capable of, 814t
Noninvasive automatic cycled cuff-based
    blood pressure monitoring, 373t
Noninvasive cardiovascular testing
  preoperative evaluation, 279
Nonneurolytic nerve blocks
  for cancer pain, 914t
Nonopioid analgesics
  pharmacokinetics of, 885t–886t
  pharmacology of, 884–885
Nonopioid intravenous anesthesia,
    167–185
  chemical structure of, 169f
  mechanism of action, 167–168
  metabolism of, 168–171
  pharmacokinetics of, 168–171
  pharmacology of, 167–168
Nonparametric tests, 19
Nonsteroidal analgesics
  for ambulatory surgery, 760–761
Nonsurgical orthopedic procedures
  anesthesia for, 671–676
Norcuron. *See* Vecuronium (Norcuron)
Norepinephrine (Levophed), 143, 154,
    1092
  for congenital heart defects, 541t
  metabolism of, 145f
  for shock, 929
  stress hormone response, 224f
Normiflo. *See* Ardeparin (Normiflo)
Normodyne. *See* Labetalol (Normodyne,
    Trandate)
Nortriptyline, 1092–1093
Nosocomial infections
  in ICU, 936–938
Novocain. *See* Procaine (Novocain)
Novoseven. *See* Factor VII a recombinant
    (Novoseven)
NPS. *See* National Pharmaceutical Stockpile
    (NPS)
Nubain. *See* Nalbuphine (Nubain)
Nuclear accidents, 962–964, 962t
Null hypothesis, 17
Nuromax. *See* Doxacurium (Nuromax)
Nurse anesthetist
  supervision by physician, 12
Nutritional deficiency anemia, 308

O
Obesity, 619–628
  airway, 621, 625
  bariatric surgery, 624–625
  cardiovascular system, 620
  endocrine system, 621
  gastrointestinal system, 621
  intraoperative considerations, 626–628
  medical therapy for, 622–624, 623t
  with office-based anesthesia, 844–845

  pathophysiology of, 619–620
  pharmacology of, 621–622
  postoperative considerations, 628
  preoperative considerations, 625, 626t
  renal system, 621
  respiratory system, 619–620
  resuscitation, 628
Obstetrics, 694–710. *See also* Pregnancy
  anesthetic complications of, 702t
  high-risk parturient management,
    702–703
Obstructive lung disease, 478–479
  pulmonary function tests, 476t
Obstructive sleep apnea (OSA)
  in children, 727–729
  with obesity, 620
  with office-based anesthesia, 844–845
Occupational health, 22–31
Occupational Safety and Health
    Administration (OSHA) standards,
    27–29
Occurrence, 12
Octreotide, 635–636
Office-based anesthesia, 843–854, 844t
  accreditation for, 847, 848t
  business and legal aspects, 854
  causes of injuries, 844t
  children guidelines, 851t
  classification of, 848t
  contingency plans, 847t
  emergencies in, 847
  equipment for, 846t
  office selection, 845–847
  $PaCO_2$, 853
  pain, 853
  patient selection for, 843–845, 845t
  PONV, 853
  procedure selection, 847–850
  regulations governing, 854
  safety of, 843
  surgeon selection, 845
  techniques, 851–853
Ohm's law, 61
OHSA standards. *See* Occupational Safety
    and Health Administration (OSHA)
    standards
Oliguria
  postoperative, 877–878
Omphalocele-gastroschisis, 721–722, 722t
Ondansetron (Zofran), 6, 1093
  for children, 735
  for postoperative nausea and vomiting,
    765t
One-compartment model, 130
Onions, 1114
Open eye injuries
  anesthesia, 804
Operating room
  anesthetic levels in, 22–23
  construction of new, 71–72
  DNR orders in, 945t
  management, 14–15
  sources of contamination, 25t
Operational resources, 8
Ophthalmic surgery, 572–582, 850
  anatomy, 572–573, 573f
  anesthesia selection, 576t
  anesthetic ramifications of ocular drugs,
    575–576
  anesthetic techniques, 576–577

intraocular pressure, 574–575, 575t
intraocular surgery, 579–580, 579t
MAC, 578t
ocular physiology, 574
oculocardiac reflex, 575
open eye-full stomach, 577–578
postoperative complications, 581t
postoperative ocular complications, 580–582
preoperative evaluation, 576
requirements for, 573f
retinal detachment surgery, 579
strabismus surgery, 578–579
Opioid(s), 5, 186–207, 288–289
adjustments for elderly, 753t
administration of, 890
adverse effects of, 890t
agonist
dosage for in elective surgery, 210t
effects of, 191t
pharmacokinetics of, 188t
physicochemical characteristics, 188t
agonist-antagonists
receptor effects, 202t
analgesics, 887
pharmacokinetics of, 888t
antagonists, 203
biotransformation of, 189
for cardiac surgery, 520, 529–530
for children, 733
for chronic pain, 911
with chronic renal failure, 605t
clinical uses of, 204, 204t
context-sensitive half time, 204–207
dosages of, 775t
endogenous, 186
epidural
latency and duration of, 896t
excretion of, 189
for ICU patients, 936
mixed agonist-antagonists, 201–203
for monitored anesthesia care, 775, 775t
for neonates, 717
partial agonists, 201–203
pharmacodynamics of, 186–189
pharmacokinetics of, 186–189
pharmacology of, 889t
plasma concentration, 190t
potencies of, 190t
receptors, 186
classification of, 187t
side effects of, 289t
Opsonization, 808, 810
Oral and maxillofacial surgery, 850
Oral hypoglycemics
preoperative, 547t
Oral medications
for cancer pain, 913t
Organ donors
anesthetic management of, 855–858
Organ failure
definition of, 928t
Organ perfusion
with trauma, 799–802
Organ transplantation, 855–869
heart, 866–867
immunosuppressive drugs, 858–859
islet, 863
kidneys, 859–860

liver, 860–863
lung, 864–866
multivisceral, 863–864
pancreas, 863
small bowel, 863–864
Organan. *See* Danaparoid (Organan)
Orlistat
for obesity, 622–624
Orthopedic surgery, 659–676, 850
antithrombotic therapy, 676
analgesia, 675t
neuraxial anesthesia, 676
lower extremities, 668–669
postoperative analgesia, 669
preoperative assessment, 659
regional *vs.* general anesthesia, 660t
spine, 659–665
thromboembolism prevention, 674t
upper extremities, 665–668
OSA. *See* Obstructive sleep apnea (OSA)
Oscillometry
automated, 372
mechanical errors, 372t
Osmitrol. *See* Mannitol (Osmitrol)
Osteoarthritis, 283
Osteogenesis imperfecta, 327
Otolaryngologic surgery, 583–595, 850
airway surgery, 586–588
anesthesia for, 590–592
awake intubation, 593–594
ear surgery, 586
extubation, 595
LeFort III fractures, 594–595
patient evaluation, 593
pediatric airway emergencies, 588–590
securing airway, 593
temporomandibular joint arthroscopy, 592
traumatized upper airway, 595
tumors, 592
upper airway infection, 592
Outcome measurement
difficulty in, 36
Outpatient anesthesia
questionnaire before, 758t
Outpatient setting
regional anesthesia in, 672
Oxacillin, 1093
Oxicams
pharmacokinetics of, 886t
Oximetry
jugular venous bulb
neurosurgery anesthesia, 448
transcranial
neurosurgery anesthesia, 448
Oxycarbazepine, 305t
Oxycodone, controlled release (Oxycontin), 1093
pharmacokinetics of, 888t
Oxycontin. *See* Oxycodone, controlled release (Oxycontin)
Oxygen
consumption, 973
delivery, 87
tension
alveolar, 973
transport of, 472–475, 973
Oxygenation
arterial
assessment of, 475

Oxygenation (*cont.*)
  brain tissue, 920
    neurosurgery anesthesia, 448
  cerebral
    neurosurgery anesthesia, 448
  monitoring, 368–370
    ASA standards for, 1026
Oxymorphone
  with PCA, 892t
  pharmacokinetics of, 888t
Oxytocin (Pitocin), 1093–1094

P
PA. *See* Partial pressure (PA)
PAC. *See* Premature atrial contraction
    (PAC); Pulmonary artery catheter
    (PAC)
Pacemakers
  EKG of, 996
  evaluation of, 997
  failure of, 997
$PaCO_2$, 74
  effects on arterial pH and serum
    bicarbonate, 76t
  retention or elimination, 75f
PACU. *See* Postanesthesia care unit (PACU)
Pain. *See also* Acute postoperative pain;
    Chronic pain
  acute *vs.* chronic, 902
  adverse physiologic sequelae of, 883t
  after cardiac surgery, 537–538
  with ambulatory surgery, 765
  cancer, 913–915
  changes accompanying, 904t
  cognitive modulation of, 883
  genetic variability in response to,
    57
  low back, 903
  myofascial, 907–908
  pathophysiology of, 883–884
Paired t test, 18
PALS. *See* Pediatric Advanced Life Support
    (PALS)
P-aminophenols
  pharmacokinetics of, 886t
Pancreas transplantation, 863
Pancuronium (Pavulon), 246, 1094
  for children, 734t
  clearance, 244t
  comparative pharmacology of, 242t
  pharmacokinetics of, 241t
Papain, 1115
Paracetamol-APAP. *See* Acetaminophen
    (Paracetamol-APAP)
Parasympathetic nervous system. *See*
    Craniosacral (parasympathetic)
    nervous system
Parasympathetic nervous system (PNS),
    137, 141–143
  neurotransmission, 141–143
Parathyroid glands, 682–683
Parkinson's disease, 304–306, 306t
Paroxysmal atrial tachycardia (PAT)
  EKG of, 988
Parsley, 1115
Partial pressure (PA), 40–41
Partial thromboplastin time (PTT), 111,
    112
Passion flower, 1115
Passive diffusion, 120

PAT. *See* Paroxysmal atrial tachycardia
    (PAT)
Patent ductus arteriosus, 712, 725
Patient anxiety
  with ambulatory surgery, 757–758
Patient-controlled analgesia (PCA), 891,
    892t
  postoperative order sheet, 899t
Patient discharge
  after ambulatory surgery, 765–766
Patient monitoring, 4–5
Patient positioning, 357–364
  dorsal decubitus positions, 357–360
  head-elevated positions, 362
  lateral decubitus positions, 360–361
  perioperative peripheral neuropathies,
    362–364, 364t
  ventral decubitus (prone) positions,
    361–362, 362t
Patient safety, 4
  JCAHO goals, 36t
Patient transport, 842
Pattern generators, 42
Pavulon. *See* Pancuronium (Pavulon)
PCA. *See* Patient-controlled analgesia (PCA)
Pediatric. *See also* Children
  airway emergencies, 588–590
    otolaryngologic surgery, 588–590
  cardiopulmonary resuscitation, 957
  orthopedic surgery, 670–671
  otolaryngologic surgery, 583–586
    adenoidectomy, 583–585
    tonsillectomy, 583–585
Pediatric Advanced Life Support (PALS)
  bradycardia
    algorithm for, 1017f
  pulseless arrest
    algorithm for, 1018
  tachycardia
    algorithm for, 1019f–1020f,
      1021f–1022f
Peer review, 37
Peer review organization (PRO), 11
Pelvic injury, 794–795
Pelvis
  fractures of, 795
Pemphigus, 314
Penetrating cardiac injury, 794
Penicillin G, 1094
Penile blockade, 431
Penile urethra
  innervation of, 596
Penis
  innervation of, 596
  ring block of, 719
Pentazocine (Talwin), 1094
  with PCA, 892t
  pharmacokinetics of, 888t
Pentobarbital (Nembutal), 1095–1096
Pentothal. *See* Thiopental (Pentothal)
Pepcid. *See* Famotidine (Pepcid)
Percutaneous renal procedures, 615–616
Percutaneous transtracheal jet ventilation,
    355, 356t
Performance improvement quality
    assurance
  events triggering chart reviews, 846t
Perfusion
  distribution of, 472
  to ventilation relationships, 474f

Peribulbar blocks
 in ophthalmic surgery, 576
Pericardial tamponade, 794, 804–805
Perioperative evaluation
 AHA/ACC guidelines, 280f
Perioperative fluid management, 83
Perioperative hypothermia, 387–388
Perioperative laboratory testing, 283–285
Perioperative medicine
 genetic polymorphisms, 58t
 genomic basis of, 49–60
Perioperative profiling, 52–53
Peripheral autonomic nervous system
 organization, 137–138
Peripheral circulation, 515–517
 autonomic innervation, 141
Peripheral circulation physiology, 513
Peripheral nerve afferent fibers, 881
Peripheral nerve blockade, 257, 417–437
 axillary technique for, 424–426
 contraindications, 419t
 discharge criteria, 419–420
 distal upper extremity, 427–428
 elbow, 427, 427t
 equipment, 418
 head and neck techniques, 420–421
 intravenous regional anesthesia, 426–427
 local anesthetic drug selection and doses
  of, 417
 lower extremity, 434–437
 monitoring, 419
 nerve localization, 417
 nerve stimulator, 417
 patient preparation, 419–420, 419t
 patient selection, 419
 premedication, 419
 trunk, 428–434
 upper extremity techniques, 422–426
 wrist, 427
Peripheral nervous system
 elderly, 748
Peripheral vascular disease, 544–545
 coexisting medical problems, 556t
 coronary artery disease with, 545–553
Peripheral vascular insufficiency
 emergency surgery for, 570–571
Peripheral vasculature
 neural supply of, 503
Peripheral vessels
 alpha receptors in, 148
 beta receptors in, 148
Peritonsillar abscess, 585
Peroneal nerve block
 deep, 437
Persistent pulmonary hypertension, 712,
  713t
PH
 defined, 74
Pharmaceutical interactions, 819
Pharmacodynamics, 55f
 principles of, 132–133
Pharmacokinetics of interactions, 820–821
Pharmacologic stress thallium imaging
 preoperative evaluation, 279
Phenacetin
 pharmacokinetics of, 886t
Phenergan. *See* Promethazine (Phenergan)
Phenobarbital, 305t, 1095–1096
Phenol, 914t
Phenotype, 51f

Phenoxybenzamine (Dibenzyline),
  1099
 effects during anesthesia, 823t
Phentolamine (Regitine), 159, 1096
 for congenital heart defects, 541t
 effects during anesthesia, 823t
Phenylacetic acids
 pharmacokinetics of, 886t
Phenylephrine (Neo-Synephrine), 151,
  1096
 anesthetic ramifications of, 575
 clinical uses of, 154
 for congenital heart defects, 541t
 for ischemia, 521
 side effects of, 154
Phenytoin (Dilantin), 305t, 1097
Pheochromocytoma, 687, 687t, 688t
Phosgene, 967
Phosphate, 95
Physical hazards, 22–23
Physiologic dead space, 473, 973
 assessment of, 473
Physiologic shunt, 474–475
 assessment of, 475
 calculation, 475
Physostigmine (Antilirium), 1097
Phytonadione (AquaMephyton, Konakion),
  1097
Pia mater, 393
Pipecuronium (Arduan), 1098
Piroxicam
 pharmacokinetics of, 886t
Pitocin. *See* Oxytocin (Pitocin)
Pitressin. *See* Vasopressin (Pitressin)
Pituitary gland, 692–693
Pituitary tumors, 456–457
Placental transfer
 of anesthetic drugs, 694–695, 695t
Plague, 965
Plasma cholinesterase
 disorders, 323–326
 enzyme, 324t
 mivacurium disposition, 326
Plasma volume, 81
Plasmin
 excess circulating, 109–110
 formation of, 108–109
Plasminogen activator inhibitor-1, 53
Platelet count, 110–111
Platelets
 collection and preparation of, 106
 indications for administration of, 103t
 transfusion thresholds, 103
Pleura, 464
Pleural injury, 794
Pneumonic plague, 965
PNS. *See* Parasympathetic nervous system
  (PNS)
Podiatry, 850
Policy and procedure manual, 11
Polyclonal antibodies, 859
Polymorphisms, 49
 categories of, 50f
 insertion-deletion, 50f
 microsatellite, 50f
Polymyositis/dermatomyositis, 313–314
Polyuria
 postoperative, 878
Pontocaine. *See* Tetracaine (Pontocaine)
Porphyrias, 326–327, 326t

Positive-pressure ventilation
LMA, 345
Postanesthesia care
admission report to, 871t–873t
with ambulatory surgery, 764–766
ASA standards for, 1031–1032
assessing value of, 870
Postanesthesia care unit (PACU)
admission to, 870–871
anesthetic levels in, 24
assessment before discharge from, 872t
coma in, 880t
complications in, 878–879, 879t
cost of, 871t
electrolyte changes in, 878t
glucose changes in, 878t
metabolic derangements in, 878t
monitoring in, 872t
nausea and vomiting in, 878–879
persistent sedation in, 880
temperature in, 879
Postanesthetic discharge scoring, 766t
Postcardiopulmonary bypass, 536–537
Postdural puncture headaches
with obstetric anesthesia, 702t
Posterior fossa surgery
postoperative concerns, 456t
Posterior ischemic optic neuropathy
with ophthalmic surgery, 582
Posterior tibial nerve block, 436
Postherpetic neuralgia, 911f
Postoperative
hypertension, 873–874
Postoperative analgesia
latency and duration of, 896t
Postoperative analgesia service, 899–901
for acute postoperative pain, 899–901
Postoperative anastomotic leakage, 633
Postoperative arterial hypoxemia, 876t
Postoperative cardiac dysrhythmias,
874–875, 874t, 875t
Postoperative cognitive dysfunction
of elderly, 753–754
Postoperative epidural analgesia, 893t
Postoperative epidural analgesia order
sheet, 898t
Postoperative fever, 443–444
Postoperative hypertension, 873–874,
874t
Postoperative hypotension, 873, 873t
Postoperative hypoventilation, 875t
Postoperative ileus, 633, 634t
Postoperative nausea and vomiting, 765t
Postoperative oliguria, 877–878
Postoperative pain management
in children
morphine for, 900t
in PACU, 871
pharmacology of, 884–890
Postoperative patient-controlled analgesia
order sheet, 899t
Postoperative polyuria, 878
Postoperative pulmonary complications,
481–482
Postoperative pulmonary function, 481–482
Postoperative recovery, 870–880
cardiovascular complications, 873–875
perioperative aspiration, 877
pulmonary dysfunction, 875–876
renal complications, 877–878

Postoperative renal failure
risk factors, 606t
Postoperative voiding, 877
Postresuscitation care, 957–958
Postsynaptic effects, 42
Postural puncture headache
with epidural and spinal anesthesia,
412–413
Potassium, 81, 90–92
maintenance requirements for, 82
Potassium channels, 43
Practice guidelines, 10
Prader-Willi syndrome, 327
Pralidoxime chloride
for nerve agent poisoning, 967
Prazosin, 159
effects during anesthesia, 823t
Preanesthesia care
ASA standards for, 1030
Precedex. *See* Dexmedetomidine (Precedex)
Prednisolone, 1098
Preeclampsia, 654, 702–703, 703t
Pregnancy
acute fatty liver of, 654
anesthesia for nonobstetric surgery, 710,
710t
maternal drug use during, 719
physiologic changes of, 694, 695t
Pregnancy testing, 285
Premature atrial contraction (PAC)
EKG of, 989
Premature ventricular contraction (PVC)
EKG of, 990
Preoperative cardiac risk stratification,
549t
Preoperative evaluation, 272–294
with cardiac disease, 274–278, 275t
cardiac testing, 279–281
with endocrine disease, 282
exercise tolerance, 278
of healthy patient, 273–274
with pulmonary disease, 275t, 281–282
Preoperative medications, 285–294, 286t
adult *vs.* pediatric, 293–295
dose, 287t
selection of, 287t
Preoperative pulmonary assessment, 477,
478t
Preoperative sedation
for ambulatory surgery, 759t
Pressure reversal, 45
Pressure-volume loops, 511, 512f
Presynaptic effects, 42
Preterm delivery, 704, 705t, 729
Preterm infants
ambulatory surgery in, 757
anemia with, 757
Prilocaine (Citanest), 1098
clinical profile of, 267t
physiochemical properties, 259t
toxicity, 268t
Primacor. *See* Milrinone (Primacor)
Primaxin. *See* Imipenem and cilastin
(Primaxin)
Primidone, 305t
PRO. *See* Peer review organization (PRO)
Procainamide (Pronestyl), 1098–1099
Procaine (Novocain), 1099
clinical profile of, 267t
introduction of, 3

physiochemical properties, 259t
toxicity, 268t
Procardia. *See* Nifedipine (Procardia, Adalat)
Prochlorperazine (Compazine), 1099
Professional liability, 32–33
Promethazine (Phenergan), 1099–1100
  dose, 287t
  for postoperative nausea and vomiting, 765t
Prone position, 663f
Pronestyl. *See* Procainamide (Pronestyl)
Propafenone
  genetic variability in response to, 57
Propionic acids
  pharmacokinetics of, 885t
Propofol (Diprivan), 5, 1100
  adjustments for elderly, 753t
  for ambulatory surgery, 761, 764
  brain neurophysiology, 442t
  chemical structure of, 169f
  for children, 732
  with chronic renal failure, 604
  dosages of, 775t
  dosing for obesity, 623t
  with ECT, 840–841
  evoked potentials, 447t
  as induction agents, 181–183
  for monitored anesthesia care, 773
  physiochemical properties, 175–176
  for postoperative nausea and vomiting, 765t
  for TBI, 921
Propoxyphene
  pharmacokinetics of, 888t
Propranolol, 161
  effects during anesthesia, 823t
  for thyroid storm, 681t
Propranolol (Inderal), 1100
Propylthiouracil
  for thyroid storm, 681t
Prospective studies, 17
Prostaglandin E1, alprostadil (Prostin VR), 1100–1101
  for congenital heart defects, 541t
Prostate
  innervation of, 596
Prostatectomy
  radical, 617
Prostigmin. *See* Neostigmine (Prostigmin)
Prostin VR. *See* Prostaglandin E1, alprostadil (Prostin VR)
Protamine, 1101
  side effects of, 537t
Protective airway reflexes, 630–631
  gastrointestinal disorders, 630–631
Proteins
  anesthetic binding to, 46
  binding, 126
    to drugs, 128–130, 129t
  expression, 52f
    profiling, 51–52
  vs. lipid targets, 45
  reactions to, 100
  for septic shock, 930
  theories
    for anesthesia, 46
Prothrombin time (PT), 111, 649
Pseudocholinesterase, 143
Pseudocholinesterase deficiency, 56

Psychological interventions
  for postoperative analgesia, 895–896
Psychoprophylaxis
  for labor and vaginal delivery, 696
PT. *See* Prothrombin time (PT)
PTT. *See* Partial thromboplastin time (PTT)
Pudendal nerve, 596
Pulmonary agents, 967
Pulmonary artery
  anatomy of, 499
Pulmonary artery catheter (PAC), 925
  accuracy, 383t
  complications, 382t
  flotation of, 381f
Pulmonary artery monitoring, 375–378, 376–377
Pulmonary aspiration
  fasting, 290t
  with obstetric anesthesia, 702t
  prevention of, 632
Pulmonary circulation, 515–516, 516t
Pulmonary embolus
  with total hip arthroplasty, 673
Pulmonary function tests, 285, 475–478
Pulmonary system
  transition of, 711–712
Pulmonary vascular resistance (PVR), 972
Pulmonary vascular systems, 466
Pulseless electrical activity
  algorithm for, 1006f
Pulse oximetry, 368–370
  accuracy, 371t
  fetal, 707–708
  introduction of, 5
Pulse waveform, 514f
Punitive damages, 32
Pupil
  anatomy of, 572
PVC. *See* Premature ventricular contraction (PVC)
PVR. *See* Pulmonary vascular resistance (PVR)
Pyloric stenosis, 724t, 725, 725t
Pyridostigmine (Regonol, Mestinon), 1101
  for nerve agent poisoning, 967
  pharmacokinetics of, 252t

Q
Quadriplegic myopathy
  acute, 941
Quality
  improvement, 12, 34–36
  measuring, 37
Quassia, 1115
Queen Victoria, 2
Quincke, Heinrich, 3
Quinidine
  genetic variability in response to, 57
Quinidine gluconate, 1101
Quinsy tonsil, 585
Q waves
  preoperative evaluation, 279

R
Racemic epinephrine, 1066
Radial artery cannulation, 374f
Radiation
  types of, 963t
Radiation exposure, 25
Radiation therapy, 836

Radical cystectomy, 618
Radical nephrectomy, 618
Radical prostatectomy, 617
Random allocation of treatment groups, 16
Random sampling, 16
Ranitidine (Zantac), 1101–1102
  dosage of, 287t
Rapacuronium, 246
Rapid-sequence induction
  tracheal intubation, 347–349
Rare and coexisting diseases, 295–304
  anemias, 307–310
  central nervous system diseases, 302–307
  collagen vascular diseases, 310–314
  muscular dystrophy, 295–297, 296t
  myotonias, 297–302
  skin disorders, 314
RBBB. *See* Bundle-branch block-right (RBBB)
Receptors, 143–149
  adrenergic, 144–148
    classification of, 146t
    numbers or sensitivity, 148–149
  cardiac, 502–503
  cholinergic, 143
  opioid, 186
    classification of, 187t
Recurrent laryngeal nerve, 341
Red blood cells
  collection and preparation of for transfusion, 104–105
  surface antigen incidence, 105t
  transfusion thresholds, 101–102
Red clover, 1115
Reflex sympathetic dystrophy, 907–908
Refludan. *See* Lepirudin (Refludan)
Refractory hypotension, 815
Regional anesthesia
  anaphylaxis management during, 812t
  for cesarean section, 699–700
  for deep venous thrombosis, 674t
  of head and neck, 420t
  introduction of, 3
  for labor and vaginal delivery, 697
  peak plasma concentrations, 262t
Regitine. *See* Phentolamine (Regitine)
Reglan. *See* Metoclopramide (Reglan)
Regonol. *See* Pyridostigmine (Regonol, Mestinon)
Remifentanil (Ultiva), 5, 199–201, 207f, 1102
  analgesia, 200
  for congenital heart disease, 540
  disposition kinetics, 200–201
  dosage of, 201, 210t, 623t, 775t
  effect on volatile anesthetic MAC, 200
  LMA, 201
  for monitored anesthesia care, 201, 776
  for office-based anesthesia, 851
Renal blood flow
  autoregulation of, 598–599
  laparoscopic surgery, 640
Renal circulation, 598
Renal disease, 282
Renal dysfunction
  and anesthesia, 600–605
Renal failure. *See also* Acute renal failure
  anesthetic agents in, 602–605
  chronic, 602, 602t

postoperative
  risk factors, 606t
Renal function tests, 607t
Renal system
  transition and maturation of, 714
Renal transplantation, 859–860
Renal transplant patient
  with nontransplant surgery
    anesthetic management of, 868
Renal vasodilator mechanisms, 600
Renin-angiotensin aldosterone system, 600
Reperfusion
  with liver transplantation, 862
Reproductive outcomes, 22–24
Reptilase time, 113
Rescue breathing, 948t
Research design
  types of, 17
Research studies
  design of, 16–17
Residents
  duty hours standards, 27
  sleep deprived, 27
Residual volume (RV), 974
Res ipsa loquitur
  proving, 33t
Respiration
  abdominal insufflation, 640t
Respiratory acidosis, 79
  anesthetic implications of, 79–80
  causes of, 80t
Respiratory alkalosis, 78
  causes of, 79t
  physiologic effects produced by, 79t
Respiratory distress syndrome, 719
Respiratory failure
  acute, 930–932
    critical care medicine, 930–932
Respiratory formulas, 973
Respiratory function, 464–482
  aging changes in, 467, 467t
Restrictive lung disease, 479–480
  pulmonary function tests, 476t
Results
  interpretation of, 21
Resuscitation
  AHA protocols for, 1003–1023
  neonatal, 709t
  obesity, 628
  for TBI, 920–921
Reticular activating system, 41
Retina
  anatomy of, 572
Retinal detachment surgery, 579
Retinopathy of prematurity, 720
Retrobulbar blocks
  in ophthalmic surgery, 576
Retrograde wire intubation, 355
Retrospective studies, 17
Reversal agents
  for ambulatory surgery, 764–765
  for children, 735
  for neonates, 717
Revex. *See* Nalmefene hydrochloride (Revex)
Rhabdomyolysis, 625
RhDsus typing
  ABO, 105
Rheumatoid arthritis, 310–311, 312t

Right atrium
anatomy of, 499
Right ventricle
anatomy of, 499
Right ventricular stroke work index
(RVSWI), 972
Riley-Day sun (familial dysautonomia), 327
Risk management, 12, 34–35
Ritodrine (Yutopar), 1102
anesthetic drug interaction, 705
Riva Rocci cuff, 5
Robershaw, Frank, 4
Robershaw tube, 488
Robinul. *See* Glycopyrrolate (Robinul)
Robustness, 19
Rocuronium, 246–247
for children, 734t, 735
clearance, 244t
comparative pharmacology of, 242t
dosing for obesity, 623t
for neonates, 716–717
pharmacokinetics of, 241t
Rofecoxib (Vioxx), 1102
pharmacokinetics of, 886t
Root cause analysis, 36
Ropivacaine (Naropin), 1103
cardiovascular toxicity of, 265
clinical profile of, 267t
with epinephrine, 260t
for neonates, 719
peak plasma concentrations, 262t
physiochemical properties of, 259t
toxicity of, 268t
uses for surgical epidural anesthesia, 407t
Rt-PA. *See* Alteplase (rt-PA)
RV. *See* Residual volume (RV)
RVSWI. *See* Right ventricular stroke work
index (RVSWI)
Ryanodine, 319

S
Sacral hiatus
anatomy of, 390
Safety
ASA guidelines for, 843
of continuous epidural technique, 897t
electrical and fire, 61–73
of office-based anesthesia, 843
patient, 4
JCAHO goals, 36t
standards for, 919
SAH. *See* Subarachnoid hemorrhage (SAH)
Salicylates
pharmacokinetics of, 885t
Sampling, 16
Saphenous nerve block, 436
Saw palmetto, 1115
Scapulocostal syndrome, 907
Scavenging, 23, 339
hazards introduced by, 340t
Sciatic nerve block, 435
landmarks for, 435f
Scleroderma, 311–313
Scoliosis surgery
anesthesia for, 662t
Scopolamine, 1103
dose of, 287t
Screening spirometry, 475
Secobarbital (Seconal), 1103
Seconal. *See* Secobarbital (Seconal)

Second messenger activated ion channels,
44
Sedation
with ambulatory surgery, 763
ASA levels of, 852t
ASA standards for, 1028–1029
conscious
definition of, 832t
critical care medicine, 935–936
deep
definition of, 832t, 1028–1029
drug-induced
for TBI, 921
Sedative-hypnotics
for children, 732–733
Seizures, 304t
neurophysiology of, 441
with obstetric anesthesia, 702t
SEMI. *See* Subendocardial myocardial
infarction (SEMI)
Sensorcaine. *See* Bupivacaine (Marcaine,
Sensorcaine)
Sensory evoked potential monitoring
neurosurgery anesthesia, 446
Sensory evoked potentials
drug effects on, 447t
Sentinel events, 36
Sepsis
definition of, 928t
Septic shock, 151, 927, 930
Serum albumin, 648
Sevoflurane
airway resistance, 227f
autonomic nervous system, 223
blood pressure, 221f
brain neurophysiology, 442t
carbon dioxide absorbers, 230
with cardiac surgery, 521
chemical structure of, 209f
for children, 731
clinical overview of, 216–217
for congenital heart disease, 540
coronary steal, 223
creation of, 3
evoked potentials, 447t
hemodynamics, 220–221
for neonates, 716
oxidative metabolism, 233f
SF6. *See* Sulfur hexafluoride (SF6)
Shattock, Samuel, 6
Shivering
meperidine for, 194
Shock
algorithm for, 1013f–1014f
clinical management of, 927–928
sources of, 62
Shock wave lithotripsy (SWL), 615t
extracorporeal, 613–615
Shoulder surgery, 666–667
Shunt, 366
effect, 475
SI. *See* Stroke index (SI)
SIADH. *See* Syndrome of inappropriate
antidiuretic hormone secretion
(SIADH)
Sibutramine
for obesity, 622
Sickle cell disease, 308–310, 309t
SIDS. *See* Sudden infant death syndrome
(SIDS)

Silent heart
    algorithm for, 1007f
Simpson, James Young, 2
Single blind study, 16
Single gene paradigm, 59
Single-lung transplantation, 865
Single nucleotide polymorphisms (SNP), 49,
    50f
Sinusitis
    in ICU, 936–937
Sinus tachycardia
    EKG of, 991
Sitting position
    complications of, 363t
Skin disorders, 314
Sleep deprivation, 16
Small bowel transplantation, 863–864
Smallpox, 965
Smoking
    drug metabolism, 128
    effect on pulmonary function, 480–481,
        480t
Smoking cessation, 282
Sniff position, 348f
Snow, John, 2, 4
SNP. *See* Single nucleotide polymorphisms
    (SNP)
SNS. *See* Sympathetic nervous system (SNS)
Sodium, 81, 87
    maintenance requirements for, 82
    tubular resorption of, 599–600
Sodium bicarbonate, 1103–1104
    for ACLS, 954t
    for CPR, 955–956
Sodium channel blockers
    for chronic pain, 913
Sodium iodide
    for thyroid storm, 681t
Sodium mustard, 968
Solu-Cortef. *See* Hydrocortisone
    (Solu-Cortef)
Solu-Medrol. *See* Methylprednisolone
    (Solu-Medrol)
Solvent detergent plasma
    collection and preparation of, 106
Somatostatin, 635
Somatotropic function
    in critical illness, 934
Special damages, 32
Spina bifida, 816
Spinal anesthesia, 3, 390–416, 894t. *See
    also* Epidural anesthesia
    adjustments for elderly, 753t
    with ambulatory surgery, 762
    cardiovascular physiology, 409–410
    for cesarean section, 700
    for children, 739
    continuous, 398
    dose and duration, 406t
    duration, 407t
    for labor and vaginal delivery, 698
    lumbosacral approach, 398
    midline approach, 397, 398f
    myotoxicity, 270
    paramedian approach, 397
    patient position for, 396–397, 396t
    pharmacology of, 402–405
    surgical procedures for, 403t
    transient neurologic symptoms after,
        269–270, 270t

Spinal cord, 41, 882
    anatomy of, 393–394
    injury, 659, 792–793
Spinal hematoma
    with epidural and spinal anesthesia,
        414–416
Spinal modulation, 882
Spine
    anatomy of, 390–391
    injury, 792–793
Spine surgery, 659–665
    blood loss, 664–665
    degenerative vertebral column disease,
        662–663
    epidural and spinal anesthesia after, 665,
        666t
    orthopedic surgery, 659–665
    postoperative care, 665
    scoliosis, 661–662
        monitoring, 663t
    spinal cord monitoring, 664
    succinylcholine-induced hyperkalemia,
        661
    temperature control, 661
    tracheal intubation, 659–660
    venous air embolus, 665
    visual loss after, 665
Spirogram, 476f
Spirometry
    screening, 475
Splanchnic blood flow, 633
    laparoscopic surgery, 640
St. John's wort, 1115–1116
    toxicity of, 826t
Stable ventricular tachycardia
    algorithm for, 1111f
Stadol. *See* Butorphanol (Stadol)
Stamina, 30
Standard of care, 9, 10, 32–33
Standards
    ASA, 828, 1024–1032
Standards of practice, 9
Starling function curve. *See* Ventricular
    (Starling) function curve
Statistical testing, 17–21
Statistics, 16–21
    descriptive, 18
    inferential, 18–19
Steinert's disease. *See* Myotonic dystrophy
    (Steinert's disease)
Stellate ganglion blockade, 431–433
    complications of, 433t
    landmarks for, 432f
Steroid(s)
    with adrenal cortex surgery, 685–686,
        686t
    epidural
        for lumbosacral radiculopathy,
            904
        for sciatica, 906t
Stimate. *See* Desmopressin acetate (DDAVP,
    Stimate)
Stomach, 630
Straight laryngoscope blade, 4
Stray capacitance, 62
Stress, 29–30
    echocardiography
        preoperative evaluation, 279
    hormone response
        desflurane, 224f

response
 to surgery, 53
 ulcers
 in ICU, 938–939
Stridor, 586–587, 587t
Stroke
 acute ischemic, 924
 suspected
 algorithm for, 1015f–1016f
Stroke index (SI), 972
Stroke volume (SV), 972
Student's t test, 18
Subarachnoid hemorrhage (SAH), 923–924
 preoperative evaluation of, 458t
 treatment of, 459t
Subarachnoid space, 393
Subclavian vein catheter placement
 anatomic approach for, 379f
Subendocardial myocardial infarction
 (SEMI), 987
Sublimaze. *See* Fentanyl (Duragesic,
 Sublimaze)
Substance abuse, 30, 706
Substance dependence, 30
Substance P, 882
Succinylcholine (Anectine), 6, 237–241,
 1104
 adductor pollicis, 238t
 adjustments for elderly, 753t
 for children, 733
 clinical uses of, 240
 for congenital heart disease, 540
 contraindications for children, 731t
 dosing for obesity, 623t
 intraocular pressure, 574
 for neonates, 716
 neuromuscular effects of, 238–239
 pharmacology of, 239
 side effects of, 240t
Succinylcholine-related apnea, 323–326
Suckling, Charles, 2
Sudden infant death syndrome (SIDS), 720
Sufenta. *See* Sufentanil (Sufenta)
Sufentanil (Sufenta), 194, 197–198, 207f,
 1104
 for cardiac surgery, 529
 dosage for, 210t, 623t
 evoked potentials, 447t
 latency and duration of, 896t
 with PCA, 892t
 recovery curves, 206f
Suicide, 31
Sulfur hexafluoride (SF6)
 anesthetic ramifications of, 576
Sulindac
 pharmacokinetics of, 885t
Sumatriptan succinate (Imitrex), 1104–1105
Superficial peroneal nerve block, 437
Superior laryngeal nerve block, 421,
 593–594
 through thyrohyoid membrane, 421f
Supplemental oxygen
 in PACU, 876
Supraclavicular approach
 to peripheral nerve blockade, 422–424
Supraglottic airways
 airway management, 344–345
Suprascapular block, 427–428
Supratentorial intracranial tumors,
 450–454

Supraventricular tachycardia
 narrow-complex
 algorithm for, 1010
Sural nerve block, 436
Surgery
 fluid shifts during, 83
Surgical fires
 risk of, 70
Surgical fluid requirements, 83
Surgical stress
 components of, 883–884
 endocrine response to, 693
Surgical stress response
 anesthesia influence on, 884
Suspected stroke
 algorithm for, 1015f–1016f
SV. *See* Stroke volume (SV)
SVR. *See* Systemic vascular resistance (SVR)
Sweet clover, 1116
SWL. *See* Shock wave lithotripsy (SWL)
Sympathetic blockade, 431–434
Sympathetic nervous system (SNS), 137
 blockade
 following stellate ganglion block, 432t
 neonatal, 714–716
 neurotransmission, 143
 schematic distribution of, 138f
Sympathetic system, 502
Synaptic function, 42
Synaptic transmission, 438
Synchronized cardioversion
 algorithm for, 1012f
Syndrome of inappropriate antidiuretic
 hormone secretion (SIADH), 88
 precipitating causes of, 89t
Systematic review, 21
Systemic lupus erythematosus, 311
Systemic toxicity
 with epidural and spinal anesthesia, 413
Systemic vascular resistance (SVR), 972
Systolic blood pressure, 802f

T
T3. *See* Triiodothyronine (T3)
T4. *See* Thyroxine (T4)
Tachycardia
 algorithm for, 1009f
 narrow-complex supraventricular
 algorithm for, 1010f
 PALS
 algorithm for, 1019f–1020f
 with rapid rhythm and poor perfusion,
 1020f–1022f
 paroxysmal atrial
 EKG of, 988
 sinus
 EKG of, 991
 stable ventricular
 algorithm for, 1011f
 ventricular
 EKG of, 994
Tagamet. *See* Cimetidine (Tagamet)
Talwin. *See* Pentazocine (Talwin)
Target-controlled infusions (TCI), 135
Target population, 16
TBI. *See* Traumatic brain injury (TBI)
TCD ultrasonography. *See* Transcranial
 Doppler (TCD) ultrasonography
T-cell lymphocytes. *See* Thymus-derived
 lymphocytes (T-cell lymphocytes)

TCI. *See* Target-controlled infusions (TCI)
TEE. *See* Transesophageal
    echocardiography (TEE)
Temperature monitoring, 387–389
Temporomandibular joint arthroscopy,
    592
Tenormin. *See* Atenolol (Tenormin)
Tensilon. *See* Edrophonium (Tensilon)
Terbutaline (Brethaire, Bricanyl),
    1105
  anesthetic drug interaction, 705
Terrorism
  biologic, 964–965
Testicular cancer
  radical surgery for, 618
Tetracaine (Pontocaine), 1105
  clinical profile of, 267t
  dose and duration, 406t
  with epinephrine, 260t
  neural toxicity of, 269
  physiochemical properties of, 259t
  toxicity of, 268t
THC. *See* Transhepatic cholangiography
    (THC)
Theophylline, 1105–1106
Thermodilution cardiac output
    determination, 379
Thiamylal
  chemical structure of, 169f
  physiochemical properties of, 174
Thiazides
  effects during anesthesia, 823t
Thiopental (Pentothal), 5, 1106
  brain neurophysiology, 442t
  chemical structure of, 169f
  dosing for obesity, 623t
  evoked potentials, 447t
  physiochemical properties of, 174
  with renal failure, 602
Thoracic aneurysm repair, 563
Thoracic aneurysms, 563
Thoracic aortic injury, 794
Thoracic aortic surgery, 564
  spinal cord protection during, 565t
Thoracic pump mechanism, 949
Thoracic surgery, 483–498
  anesthesia for diagnostic procedures,
    492–494
  anesthesia selection, 492
  complications of, 485t
  history of, 484t
  hypoxic pulmonary vasoconstriction,
    492
  intraoperative monitoring, 484–485
  invasive monitoring, 487t
  laboratory studies, 485t
  myasthenia gravis, 496–498
  one-lung ventilation, 486–487
    indications for, 487t
    management of, 490–491
    optimizing oxygenation during, 491t
    physiology of, 485–486
  physical examination, 484t
  postoperative complications of, 498t
  preoperative evaluation of, 483
  preoperative laboratory studies, 483
  preoperative preparation, 484
Thoracolumbar nervous system
  schematic distribution of, 138f
Thorazine. *See* Chlorpromazine (Thorazine)

Three-compartment model, 132, 132f
Three-ring syringe, 418f
Thrombate III. *See* Antithrombin III
    (Thrombate III)
Thrombin time (TT), 112
Thromboelastogram, 113, 803f
Thrombolysis
  for acute ischemic stroke, 924
Thrombolytics
  neuraxial anesthesia, 548t
Thromboprophylaxis
  neuraxial anesthesia, 548t
Thymectomy
  for myasthenia gravis, 496–4997
Thymus-derived lymphocytes (T-cell
    lymphocytes), 808
Thyroid gland, 677–682
  complications following surgery, 680t
  in critical illness, 934
  function, 677
  metabolism, 677
  tests, 679t
Thyroid hormone
  synthesis of, 678f
Thyroid storm, 681t
  acetaminophen for, 681t
Thyroxine (T4), 677
Tiagabine, 305t
Tidal volume (TV), 974
Timolol, 161
  anesthetic ramifications of, 576
TIPS. *See* Transjugular intrahepatic
    portosystemic shunt (TIPS)
Tissue plasminogen activator (t-PA), 109
TLC. *See* Total lung capacity (TLC)
TMI. *See* Transmural myocardial infarction
    (TMI)
TNS. *See* Transient neurologic symptoms
    (TNS)
Tobacco, 281
Tomecin
  pharmacokinetics of, 885t
Tonsillectomy, 583–585
  postoperative complications of, 585t
Topical anesthesia
  for ophthalmic surgery, 577
Topiramate, 305t
Toradol. *See* Ketorolac (Toradol)
Torsades de pointes
  EKG of, 992
Tort system, 32
Total body water, 81
Total drug clearance, 130
Total hip arthroplasty
  deep venous thrombosis with, 673
Total knee arthroplasty, 669
Total lung capacity (TLC), 974
Total quality management (TQM), 36
Total spinal anesthesia
  with epidural and spinal anesthesia, 414
Tourniquets, 672
T-PA. *See* Tissue plasminogen activator
    (t-PA)
TQM. *See* Total quality management
    (TQM)
Trace anesthesia
  effects on psychomotor skills, 24
Trachea, 464
Tracheal extubation, 349–351, 540
  weaning from, 479t

Tracheal intubation, 342
  airway management, 346–351
  development of, 4
  elective oral
    first use of, 4
Tracheal resection, 496t
Tracheoesophageal fistula, 722–723, 722t,
    723t
Tracrium. *See* Atracurium (Tracrium)
TRALI. *See* Transfusion-related acute lung
    injury (TRALI)
Tramadol (Ultram), 1106
Trandate. *See* Labetalol (Normodyne,
    Trandate)
Transcranial Doppler (TCD)
  ultrasonography, 920
  neurosurgery anesthesia, 448
Transcranial oximetry
  neurosurgery anesthesia, 448
Transdermal fentanyl
  for cancer pain, 914
Transesophageal echocardiography (TEE),
    383–385
  indications for, 384t
  intracardiac filling pressures, 384
  intraoperative, 520t
  left ventricular contractility, 384
  myocardial ischemia, 385
  with trauma, 797
Transfusion, 6, 934
  blood products for, 104–107
  immunologically mediated reactions,
    98–100
  massive
    consequences of, 101t
Transfusion-related acute lung injury
    (TRALI), 100
Transfusion-transmitted disease
  rates of, 99t
Transhepatic cholangiography (THC),
    650
Transient neurologic symptoms (TNS)
  with epidural and spinal anesthesia, 414
Transjugular intrahepatic portosystemic
    shunt (TIPS), 838, 838t
Transmural myocardial infarction (TMI),
    988
Transplantation
  double-lung, 865–866
  heart, 866–867
  heart-lung, 866
  islet, 863
  liver, 860–863
  lung, 864–866
  multivisceral, 863–864
  pancreas, 863
  renal, 859–860
  single-lung, 865
  small bowel, 863–864
Transplant patient
  with nontransplant surgery
    anesthetic management of, 867–869
Transurethral resection of bladder tumors
    (TURB), 612–613
Transurethral resection of the prostate
    (TURP), 610–612
  anesthesia for, 612
  complications of, 611–612, 613t
  future of, 612
  irrigating solutions for, 610t

Transurethral resection (TUR) syndrome,
    610–611, 611t
Trasylol. *See* Aprotinin (Trasylol)
Trauma, 782–807
  airway evaluation and intervention,
    782–784, 783f
  baseline neurologic examination of, 791t
  breathing abnormalities, 785–786
  cervical spine injury, 785
  early management of, 788–795
  early postoperative considerations, 807
  equipment and supplies for, 799t
  with full stomach, 784
  head, open eye injuries, 784–785
  hypotension with, 787t
  initial evaluation and resuscitation,
    782–788
  intraoperative complications, 805–806
  intraoperative management of, 798t
  monitoring, 797–802, 800t–801t
  operative management of, 797–806
  postoperative period, 806t
  shock, 786–788
Traumatic brain injury (TBI), 920–923
  ICU management of, 922t
  outcomes, 921t
  secondary injury prevention, 921
Tricyclic antidepressants
  for chronic pain, 911–912
Tridil. *See* Nitroglycerin (Tridil, Nitrol IV,
    Nitrostat IV)
Triiodothyronine (T3), 677, 678t
Trimethaphan (Arfonad), 1107
TT. *See* Thrombin time (TT)
Tube test, 803t
Tularemia, 965
Tumeric, 1116
Tuohy, Edward, 3
Tuohy needle, 3
TUR. *See* Transurethral resection (TUR)
    syndrome
TURB. *See* Transurethral resection of
    bladder tumors (TURB)
TURP. *See* Transurethral resection of the
    prostate (TURP)
TV. *See* Tidal volume (TV)
Two-compartment model, 130–131, 131f
Two-gas anesthesia machine, 330f
Tympanoplasty, 586t
Type I allergic reaction, 813f
Type I (alpha) error, 17
Type II (beta) error, 17
Type I immediate hypersensitivity reactions,
    812f

U
UES. *See* Upper esophageal sphincter (UES)
Ulnar neuropathy
  with dorsal decubitus positions, 358
Ultiva. *See* Remifentanil (Ultiva)
Ultram. *See* Tramadol (Ultram)
Unconscious patient
  standard approach to, 945t
Unfractionated heparin
  neuraxial anesthesia, 548t
Unipolar ESU, 70
Univent tube, 487
Universal precautions, 27–29, 29t
Unpaired t test, 18
Upper arm surgery, 666–667

Upper esophageal sphincter (UES), 629
Upper extremities
  injuries with dorsal decubitus positions,
    358–361, 360t
  orthopedic surgery, 665–668
Upper gastrointestinal endoscopy, 838
Upper gastrointestinal obstruction, 723t
Upper respiratory infection (URI)
  in children, 727, 758
Uremia, 603t
Ureteral procedures, 609
Ureters
  anatomy of, 597f
URI. *See* Upper respiratory infection (URI)
Urinary tract infection (UTI)
  in ICU, 938
Urine output
  with trauma, 797–799
Urologic surgery, 596–618
  anesthesia for, 609–616
  high-risk procedures, 606–607
  laparoscopy, 616
  lasers, 616
  nephrotoxins during perioperative
    period, 607t
  radical cancer surgery, 616–618
  renal anatomy and physiology,
    596–600
  renal function preservation, 605–606
UTI. *See* Urinary tract infection (UTI)
Uveal tract
  anatomy of, 572

V
Vaginal delivery
  anesthesia for, 696–699
Valdecoxib (Bextra), 1107
Valerian, 1116
  toxicity of, 826t
Valium. *See* Diazepam (Valium)
Valproate, 305t
Valsalva maneuver
  blood pressure and heart rate response
    to, 149f
Valsartan
  effects during anesthesia, 823t
Value based anesthesia practice, 13
Valvular heart disease, 522–526
  aortic insufficiency, 523–524
  aortic stenosis, 522–523
  hypertrophic cardiomyopathy, 523
  mitral regurgitation, 525
  mitral stenosis, 524–525
Vancomycin, 1107–1108
VAP. *See* Ventilator-assisted pneumonia
  (VAP)
Vaponefrin. *See* Epinephrine, racemic
  (Vaponefrin, Micronefrin)
Variability, 18
Variable bypass vaporizers, 332–333, 332t
  hazards associated with, 333t
Vascular disease, 543–545
  atherosclerosis, 543, 543t, 544–545
  peripheral vascular disease, 544–545,
    545
    coronary artery disease with, 545–553
Vascular nerves, 502–503
Vascular surgery, 543–571
  aortic reconstruction, 561–568
  cardiac function testing, 551t

carotid endarterectomy, 553–561
  cerebral perfusion, 556t
  history, 549t
  increased perioperative cardiovascular
    risk, 550t
  lower extremity revascularization,
    568–571
  myocardial ischemia perioperative
    monitoring, 552t
  perioperative cardiac risk reduction
    strategies, 552–553
  perioperative myocardial ischemia,
    551–552
  pharmacologic prophylaxis, 554t–555t
  physical examination, 549t
  preoperative coronary revascularization,
    551
  renal dysfunction with, 608
Vasodilators, 163–166
  action sites, 164t
  doses of, 164t
  effects during anesthesia, 823t
Vasopressin (Pitressin), 158, 1108
  for congenital heart defects, 541t
  for CPR, 955
  for shock, 929–930
Vasopressors
  for CPR, 954–955
  for shock, 928–929
Vasoxyl. *See* Methoxamine (Vasoxyl)
VATS. *See* Video-assisted thoracoscopic
  surgery (VATS)
VC. *See* Vital capacity (VC)
Vecuronium (Norcuron), 247, 1108–1109
  for children, 734t
  clearance, 244t
  comparative pharmacology of, 242t
  dosing for obesity, 623t
  pharmacokinetics of, 241t
Venous air embolism
  diagnosis of, 455t
  treatment of, 455t
Venous baroreceptors, 150
Venous return, 517
Venous system physiology, 516–517
Venous thromboembolism (VTE)
  in ICU, 939–941
  risk factors for, 940t
Ventilation
  control of, 467–471
  distribution of, 472
  monitoring
    ASA standards for, 1026–1027
  muscles of, 464
  neonates *vs.* adults, 715t
  to perfusion relationships, 474f
  reflex control of, 468–469
Ventilator-assisted pneumonia (VAP)
  in ICU, 937
Ventilators
  hazards associated with, 340t
Ventilatory pattern, 468
Ventricle
  anatomy of
    left, 500
    right, 499
Ventricular assist device, 534
Ventricular fibrillation
  algorithm for, 1005f
  EKG of, 993

Ventricular (Starling) function curve, 511
Ventricular pacing
  EKG of, 998
Ventricular pulseless VT
  algorithm for, 1005f
Ventricular tachycardia
  EKG of, 994
Verapamil (Calan, Isoptin), 162, 1109
  effects during anesthesia, 823t
  for ischemia, 521
Versed. *See* Midazolam (Versed)
Vertebrae
  anatomy of, 390–391
Vertebral column
  anatomy of, 391f
Vertebral interspaces
  landmarks for, 392t
Vesicants, 968
Video-assisted thoracoscopic surgery
  (VATS), 493–494, 642t, 643
Video-Macintosh laryngoscope, 355
Vioxx. *See* Rofecoxib (Vioxx)
Vital capacity (VC), 974
Vitamin B12, 308
Vitamin E, 1116
  toxicity of, 826t
Vocal cord, 341
Voiding
  postoperative, 877
Volatile anesthetics
  adjustments for elderly, 753t
  cardioprotection from, 223
  clinical utility, 234
  neurophysiology, 442–443
  physiochemical properties of, 210t
Voltage dependent calcium channels, 43
Voltage dependent ion channels, 43
Vomiting
  with ambulatory surgery, 765, 765t
  PACU, 878–879
  postoperative, 765t
VTE. *See* Venous thromboembolism (VTE)

W
Wake-up test, 664
Warfare
  biologic agents used for, 964t
Warfarin (Coumadin), 1109
  neuraxial anesthesia, 548t
Washington, George, 6
Water
  composition of fluid losses, 83
  maintenance requirements for, 82, 82t
  tubular resorption of, 599–600
Watts, 61
Wells, Horace, 1
Wenckebach
  EKG of, 980
White cell-related transfusion reactions, 100
Willow bark, 1116
Wolff-Parkinson-White syndrome (WPW), 162
  EKG of, 995
Works hours, 26–27
WPW. *See* Wolff-Parkinson-White
  syndrome (WPW)
Wrist
  terminal nerves at, 428f
Wrist surgery, 667–668
Wyamine. *See* Mephentermine (Wyamine)

X
Xenon
  clinical overview of, 217
Xigris. *See* Drotrecogin alfa (Xigris)
X-rays, 963t
Xylocaine. *See* Lidocaine (Xylocaine)

Y
Yutopar. *See* Ritodrine (Yutopar)

Z
Zantac. *See* Ranitidine (Zantac)
Zebeta. *See* Bisoprolol (Zebeta)
Zofran. *See* Ondansetron (Zofran)
Zonisamide, 305t